Family Interaction and Psychopathology

Theories, Methods, and Findings

APPLIED CLINICAL PSYCHOLOGY

Series Editors:
Alan S. Bellack, *Medical College of Pennsylvania at EPPI, Philadelphia, Pennsylvania,*
and Michel Hersen, *University of Pittsburgh, Pittsburgh, Pennsylvania*

Current Volumes in this Series

CHILDHOOD AGGRESSION AND VIOLENCE
Sources of Influence, Prevention, and Control
Edited by David H. Crowell, Ian M. Evans, and Clifford R. O'Donnell

FAMILY INTERACTION AND PSYCHOPATHOLOGY
Theories, Methods, and Findings
Edited by Theodore Jacob

HANDBOOK OF ASSESSMENT IN CHILDHOOD PSYCHOPATHOLOGY
Applied Issues in Differential Diagnosis and Treatment Evaluation
Edited by Cynthia L. Frame and Johnny L. Matson

HANDBOOK OF BEHAVIORAL GROUP THERAPY
Edited by Dennis Upper and Steven M. Ross

A PRIMER OF HUMAN BEHAVIORAL PHARMACOLOGY
Alan Poling

THE PRIVATE PRACTICE OF BEHAVIOR THERAPY
Sheldon J. Kaplan

RESEARCH METHODS IN APPLIED BEHAVIOR ANALYSIS
Issues and Advances
Edited by Alan Poling and R. Wayne Fuqua

SEVERE BEHAVIOR DISORDERS IN THE MENTALLY RETARDED
Nondrug Approaches to Treatment
Edited by Rowland P. Barrett

SUBSTANCE ABUSE AND PSYCHOPATHOLOGY
Edited by Arthur I. Alterman

TREATING ADDICTIVE BEHAVIORS
Processes of Change
Edited by William R. Miller and Nick Heather

A Continuation Order Plan is available for this series. A continuation order will bring delivery of each new volume immediately upon publication. Volumes are billed only upon actual shipment. For further information please contact the publisher.

Family Interaction and Psychopathology

Theories, Methods, and Findings

Edited by
Theodore Jacob
University of Arizona
Tucson, Arizona

Plenum Press • New York and London

Library of Congress Cataloging in Publication Data

Family interaction and psychopathology.

  (Applied clinical psychology)
  Includes bibliographies and index.
  1. Mentally ill—Family relationships. 2. Family—Mental health. 3. Psychology,
Pathological. I. Jacob, Theodore. II. Series. [DNLM: 1. Family. 2. Interpersonal
Relations. 3. Mental Disorders. 4. Psychopathology—methods. WM 100 F1985]
RC455.4.F3F38 1987   616.89   87-2570
ISBN 0-306-42357-X

© 1987 Plenum Press, New York
A Division of Plenum Publishing Corporation
233 Spring Street, New York, N.Y. 10013

Printed in the United States of America

To my family

Contributors

Angela Arrington, Department of Psychology, University of California at Los Angeles, Los Angeles, California

Andrew Christensen, Department of Psychology, University of California at Los Angeles, Los Angeles, California

James C. Coyne, Department of Family Practice, University of Michigan, School of Medicine, Ann Arbor, Michigan

Jean E. Dumas, University of Western Ontario, London, Ontario, Canada

Michael J. Goldstein, Department of Psychology, University of California at Los Angeles, Los Angeles, California

Ian H. Gotlib, Department of Psychology, University of Western Ontario, London, Ontario, Canada

John M. Gottman, Department of Psychology, University of Washington, Seattle, Washington

Theodore Jacob, Division of Family Studies, University of Arizona, Tucson, Arizona

Neil S. Jacobson, Department of Psychology, University of Washington, Seattle, Washington

Jana Kahn, Mental Research Institute, Palo Alto, California

David Klein, Department of Sociology, University of Notre Dame, Notre Dame, Indiana

Gloria Krahn, Crippled Children's Division, Oregon Health Sciences University, Portland, Oregon

Gayla Margolin, Department of Psychology, University of Southern California, Los Angeles, California

Howard J. Markman, Department of Psychology, University of Denver, Denver, Colorado

Barclay Martin, Department of Psychology, University of North Carolina, Chapel Hill, North Carolina

Clifford I. Notarius, Department of Psychology, Catholic University of America, Washington, DC

Michael F. Pogue-Geile, Department of Psychology and Department of Psychiatry, University of Pittsburgh, Pittsburgh, Pennsylvania

David Reiss, Department of Psychiatry and Behavioral Sciences, Center for Family Research, George Washington University Medical Center, Washington, DC

Elizabeth A. Robinson, Department of Psychology, University of Washington, Seattle, Washington

Richard J. Rose, Department of Psychology and Department of Medical Genetics, Indiana University, Bloomington, Indiana

Ruth Ann Seilhamer, Department of Psychology, University of Pittsburgh, Pittsburgh, Pennsylvania

Harvey A. Skinner, Addiction Research Foundation, 33 Russell Street, Toronto, Ontario, Canada

Peter Steinglass, Center for Family Research, Department of Psychiatry and Behavioral Sciences, George Washington University, School of Medicine, Washington, DC

Paul D. Steinhauer, Department of Psychiatry, Hospital for Sick Children, 555 University Avenue, Toronto, Ontario, Canada

Angus M. Strachan, Department of Psychology, University of California at Los Angeles, Los Angeles, California

Daniel L. Tennenbaum, Department of Psychiatry, University of Pittsburgh, Pittsburgh, Pennsylvania

Robert G. Whaler, Child Behavior Institute, University of Tennessee, Knoxville, Tennessee

Preface

Throughout the past 30 years, there have been significant developments in theory and research relating family variables to various psychopathologies. The potential importance of such efforts is obviously great, given the implications that reliable and valid findings would hold for treatment and preventive interventions across a variety of settings and populations. The purpose of this volume is to present a critical evaluation of this field of inquiry through a detailed assessment of the theoretical perspectives, the methodological issues, and the substantive findings that have characterized family studies of psychopathology during the past several decades. The book is divided into four parts, each containing contributions from leading researchers and theorists in the field.

The first part, "Background," presents a review of the major streams of influence that have shaped the development and the present character of the field.

The second part, "Conceptual Foundations," contains presentations of general models and orientations relevant to family studies of psychopathology. In most cases, a particular theoretical perspective provides the primary underpinning of the approach, the exception to this format being the family model of David Reiss based on the concept of the *family paradigm*. The major objective of this part is to present a broad yet detailed set of chapters that address the conceptual status of the field. It is hoped that this material will provide a rich background against which subsequent discussions of specific theories, methods, and findings can be more fully appreciated.

The third part, "Methodological Issues and Strategies," surveys the critical issues that have characterized family studies of psychopathology since the mid-1960s. Each contributor to this section discusses a key methodological topic (or set of related issues) that is of particular importance to the quality of data the researcher obtains in his or her attempt to probe family-interaction–psychopathology associations. The topics of these six chapters are: (a) design and research strategies; (b) reliability and validity issues in the use of observation data; (c) coding systems in marital and family research; (d) self-report procedures in family assessment; (e) sequential analysis of family data; and (f) participant observation procedures in family assessment.

The final part, "Family Research on Specific Psychopathologies," contains a set of contributions that summarize the current state of knowledge regarding the family's role in four types of disordered behavior: (a) schizophrenia; (b) child-hood disturbance; (c) alcoholism; and (d) depression. Because it was not reasonable to expect contributors to this section to have expertise in both psychosocial and genetics literatures, a final chapter reviews the evidence for hereditary influences in major and minor psychopathologies.

Currently, no single publication exists that presents a comprehensive, up-to-date contribution to this field. Rather, material relevant to family studies of psychopathology is scattered across various disciplines and research provinces, and there is too little awareness and appreciation of the broader field of inquiry within which separate investigations and theory developments are housed. Given the breadth and depth of coverage to which this book aspires, it should become a major resource in evaluating the complex and increasingly voluminous literature on family studies of psychopathology. It is hoped that the critical appraisals and insights of the contributors to this volume will sharpen our view of the field and will significantly enhance the quality of subsequent efforts in this domain of study.

Contents

xi

Chapter 5

DEVELOPMENTAL PERSPECTIVES ON FAMILY THEORY AND
PSYCHOPATHOLOGY   163

Barclay Martin

Chapter 6

PARADIGM AND PATHOGENESIS: A FAMILY-CENTERED
APPROACH TO PROBLEMS OF ETIOLOGY AND TREATMENT OF
PSYCHIATRIC DISORDERS   203

David Reiss and David Klein

PART III   METHODOLOGICAL ISSUES AND STRATEGIES

Chapter 7

RESEARCH ISSUES AND STRATEGIES   259

Andrew Christensen and Angela Arrington

Chapter 8

FACTORS INFLUENCING THE RELIABILITY AND VALIDITY OF
OBSERVATION DATA   297

Theodore Jacob, Daniel L. Tennenbaum, and Gloria Krahn

Chapter 9

CODING MARITAL AND FAMILY INTERACTION: CURRENT
STATUS   329

Howard J. Markman and Clifford I. Notarius

Chapter 12

THE SEQUENTIAL ANALYSIS OF FAMILY INTERACTION   453

John M. Gottman

PART IV FAMILY RESEARCH ON SPECIFIC PSYCHOPATHOLOGIES

Chapter 13

THE FAMILY AND SCHIZOPHRENIA   481

Michael J. Goldstein and Angus M. Strachan

Chapter 14

DEPRESSION   509

James C. Coyne, Jana Kahn, and Ian H. Gotlib

Chapter 15

ALCOHOLISM AND FAMILY INTERACTION   535

Theodore Jacob and Ruth Ann Seilhamer

Chapter 16

FAMILY FACTORS IN CHILDHOOD PSYCHOLOGY: TOWARD A COERCION–NEGLECT MODEL

Chapter 17

PSYCHOPATHOLOGY: A BEHAVIOR GENETIC PERSPECTIVE

PART I

BACKGROUND

CHAPTER 1

Family Interaction and Psychopathology

Historical Overview

THEODORE JACOB

INTRODUCTION

Throughout the past century, clinical researchers have been increasingly drawn to explorations of the family's role in the etiology, course, treatment, and prevention of psychopathological disorders. In attempts to unravel and elucidate relationships involving family life and disordered behavior, various theoretical perspectives and research strategies have been exploited, each of which has been directed toward a somewhat different level, aspect, or concomitant of the family matrix. For the most part, however, investigators have emphasized either the characteristics of individual family members or the family group as a totality. Although interest in relational parameters has been strongly implied throughout much of this literature, programmatic studies of interaction *per se* have been undertaken only since the mid-1950s.

Early clinical case studies, for example, often alluded to and implicated the family's role in disordered behavior (Fromm-Reichman, 1948; Lewis, 1937), as did a large number of subsequent empirical studies aimed at detailing the personality characteristics of disturbed family members and their significant others (Jacob, Favorini, Meisel, & Anderson, 1978). Similarly, investigations of psychiatrically disturbed parents have been directed toward documenting and explicating the degree and nature of impact that parental psychopathology exerts on the psychosocial and psychiatric status of children during early childhood and adolescence; the most recent representative of this interest has involved "high-risk" samples studied within prospective research designs (Garmezy, 1974a,b). A third area of interest, the study of family genetics, as conducted since the mid-1930s,

---

THEODORE JACOB • Division of Family Studies, 210 Family and Consumer Resources Building, University of Arizona, Tucson, AZ 85721.

has also focused on individual outcomes—in this case, the degree to which psychiatric disorders have a hereditary foundation and the search for biological markers associated with the major psychiatric disorders (Fieve, Rosenthal, & Brill, 1975; Gershon, Matthysse, Breakfield, & Ciaranello, 1981; Gottesman & Shields, 1982).

In addition to these interests in the status and functioning of individual family members, other family researchers have focused on group-level characteristics of the family, which, in turn, have been related to the health—illness status of individual members. Psychiatric epidemiologists, for example, have investigated the impact of differing family structures on the psychosocial development of young children, suggesting that a considerable proportion of the outcome variance can be accounted for by differences in family composition (Kellam & Ensminger, 1980; Kellam, Ensminger, & Turner, 1977). Still others have emphasized the impact of such molar variables as social class and ethnicity on patterns of socialization and the fostering of social deviance and psychopathology (Cooper & Gath, 1977; Langner, Gersten, Eisenberg, Green, & Herson, 1986; Mintz & Schwartz, 1964).

Although each of these foci has contributed significantly to our understanding of family factors and psychopathology, none has given primary emphasis, theoretically or methodologically, to family interaction *per se* and to those family patterns and processes that are related to the development and perpetuation of disordered behavior. As will be detailed subsequently, this emphasis on interaction has gained distinction only within relatively recent times, notwithstanding references to and nonscientific analyses of relationship variables that can be traced back to the turn of the century. In retrospect, it now seems clear that the family interaction model was most importantly influenced and shaped by the contributions of several disciplines, including theoretical and methodological efforts of family sociologists and social psychologists during the second quarter of this century; the "paradigm-forging" work of systems and communications researchers and the development of family theories of and treatments for schizophrenia; the rigorous and elegant work of child development and developmental psychologists aimed at elucidating the process and outcome of childhood socialization; and the conceptual, data-analytic, and treatment contributions arising from behavioral psychology in general and social learning theory in particular.

As suggested, research on family interaction represents only one aspect of the broader field of inquiry referred to as *family studies of psychopathology*. Many levels of family influence must certainly be integrated within a multidimensional model before we can hope to appreciate the family's role in psychopathology. Nevertheless, it is still of vital importance to develop a more precise understanding of each source or level of influence. Consolidation and integration must surely be pursued; yet without detailed knowledge of the different sources of influence, the complex models that we aspire to develop may be less compelling and illuminating than anticipated. It is for precisely this reason that we seek to present and evaluate—in one volume—the theoretical, methodological, and substantive status of the field of inquiry that we have come to call *family interaction and psychopathology*.

The theoretical and methodological perspective we refer to as *family interaction* embodies two major commitments: (a) to identifying family patterns and processes that are precursors, concomitants, and consequences of disordered behavior, and (b) to the integration of this knowledge into the broader family studies literature concerned with the independent and interdependent effects of genetic, sociocultural, and personality factors on the development and perpetuation of psychopathology.

In this chapter, I provide a brief historical overview of the major intellectual influences that have shaped the present character of family research in general, and of research on family interaction and psychopathology in particular. The structure for this review—involving discussion of contributions from family sociology, systems and communications theory, child and developmental psychology, and social learning theory—evolved nearly 15 years ago when I first developed a graduate seminar in "Family Theory, Research, and Therapy." Survey of the field at that time revealed little in the way of a unified theory relating family process to disordered behavior. Instead, there appeared to be a loosely constructed model of family interaction that had achieved considerable recognition and acceptance among small groups of researchers and clinicians—a model that had clearly been influenced by larger conceptual perspectives primarily identified with the disciplines of sociology, psychology, and communication theory. Although there have certainly been significant developments in conceptualization and methodology since that time, formal theories have remained elusive, and the larger, overarching "theoretical perspectives" have continued to guide much of the work in this area of inquiry. In light of this reality, the following review describes and highlights the major contributions that each of these perspectives has made to the development and the present character of family studies of psychopathology.

Before presenting this overview, two points should be made. First, Part II of this volume includes detailed and critical evaluations of these four major perspectives, each written by a family scholar who presents a relatively comprehensive discussion of a particular model's contributions to family studies of psychopathology (see the chapters by Martin, by Robinson and Jacobson, by Steinglass, and by Steinhauer). In addition, Reiss's important work on family paradigms—which builds on several conceptual bases in an attempt to develop a more truly family-level framework—is presented with great care and scope in the last chapter of this section (see the chapter by Reiss and Klein). Obviously, the reader will find a wealth of detailed and critical analyses in each of these chapters that will give substance to the mere scaffolding that is attempted in this introductory presentation. On the other hand, the present overview—because it is an overview—can perhaps reveal the peaks and valleys of this considerable territory in a way that is not possible when there is such concentrated focus on only one conceptual model.

Second, although each of these perspectives has been given a separate description, implying that the contributions of each tradition have been made independently of knowledge development in other areas, this is certainly not the case. In many instances, cross-fertilization between domains has been clear, and concepts originating in one field have been translated into models and language systems associated with another area of inquiry. In other cases, a larger social or intellectual zeitgeist can be seen to have provided a common background and motivation for similar theoretical developments occurring in seemingly distinct disciplines. The format we have selected, then, is an aid to expository clarity and not necessarily a reflection of actual independence among the various sources of influence.

FAMILY SOCIOLOGY

Sociology and anthropology were the first formal disciplines to give serious attention to the study of family behavior—a commitment that became evident only during the 1920s. Before that time, discussion and analysis of families and family behavior had been found primarily within the domains of philosophy, literature, journalism, theater, and social history. The involvement of psychiatry and psychology in the study of family behavior has occurred only in quite recent times, notwithstanding the general contributions of major personality theorists such as Freud, Lewin, and Erickson (Handel, 1965).

In his classic volume on family and marital studies, Christensen (1964a) divided the history of the field into four major stages: *preresearch,* which dates back to before 1850; *social Darwinism,* which spans the period from 1850 to 1900; *emerging science,* evident from 1900 to 1950; and *systematic theory building,* which began around 1950 and continues into the present time. Briefly, the preresearch period was a time when family phenomena were largely within the province of novelists, philosophers, and social historians, who drew primarily on family lore, speculation, and individual insights.

The second stage, social Darwinism, was a period of "grand theory" in which major attention was directed at the social evolution of marriage and family forms in a broad historical and institutional perspective. Answers to central questions—including the origins and primitive forms of family life—were sought in historical documents, folklore, and myths. These efforts were guided by the underlying assumption that the contemporary family could be understood in terms of a long evolutionary process and was not in need of direct study.

During the early years of the twentieth century, however, rapidly unfolding social changes called attention to problems of the contemporary family, particularly those of poverty and readily visible suffering. For many who sought change in these social conditions, it became critical to document the actual conditions of life in the cities of both Europe and America—concerns that stimulated a variety of studies on poverty and the economic conditions of the family. Soon thereafter, other problems, just as disturbing as poverty, became apparent: increasing divorce and separation, decreasing birth rates, women's suffrage, and the "individuation" of the family and its members, the latter stimulating considerable discussion regarding the continued existence of the family as a group. As noted by Bell and Vogel (1960),

> as individuation proceeded it was recognized that more than satisfactory economic conditions were necessary for families to be stable and for family members to be

adjusted. Comfortably situated families had problems of personal and sexual adjustments and they were turning to expert sources outside the family for consultation and help. (p. 4)

Similarly, Burr, Hill, Nye, and Reiss (1979) noted that "problems of interpersonal relations in the family pressed for public attention [problems that were salient enough so] that the American Sociological Society meeting (of 1908) was devoted entirely to them" (p. 4). As a result of this motivation to understand and change problem aspects of family life, the field was moved to study more molecular and definable family variables and to make increasing use of empirically based procedures, including the survey method and the analysis of quantitative data (Christensen, 1964b).

For many, the field of family studies was formally launched with the publication of Ernest Burgess's seminal paper, "The Family as a Unit of Interaction Personalities" (1926). As noted by Handel (1965), this position paper—published more than 60 years ago—anticipated many concepts and perspectives that are now critical ones in the current literature on family theory and research. Four examples can be noted. First, Burgess conceived of the family as a group of interacting personalities that "has its existence in the interaction of its members" (p. 5). Within this framework, Burgess emphasized the process versus the content of interaction and the family group as the unit of study—emphases that can be seen as important forerunners of later views of the family from the systems and small-group perspectives.

Second, Burgess was clear in noting that this interaction principle applied not only to communication within families but to relationships between the family and the larger social environment within which the family operates. In reviewing work attempting to relate family types to areas of the city, for example, Burgess concluded that "the pattern of family life develops under certain life conditions and thrives in conformity with the folkways and mores of the local community" (p. 4). From this analysis, there would appear to be strong encouragement for examining the social and physical environment as a major influence on family life—a perspective that is certainly compatible with the current emphasis on ecological and cultural influences on individual and family development (Moos & Moos, 1983).

Third, Burgess raised central research problems for family investigation when he encouraged efforts (a) to conceptualize the family as a unit of study; (b) to study the personalities of several members and the interrelationships among them; and (c) to analyze family life in terms of family patterns and roles. In many ways, family research is still struggling with some of these basic issues, namely, how to conceptualize the family group and what to assess.

Finally, Burgess's early writings can even be read as a forerunner of current family theories of psychopathology and of family therapy as a treatment intervention. In speaking of a case study involving a disturbed child, for example, Burgess (1926) noted that "any program of treating this case would lie not in assessing the proportional share of blame on the father, mother, or child, but understanding their attitudes in light of each one's conception of his role in the family" (p. 9).

During the 30-year period from 1920 to 1950, the discipline of sociology certainly made the most significant contributions to the general field of family studies. Of particular importance, this time period witnessed the development of major theoretical frameworks within which family behavior was conceptualized and studied, including the institutional, structural-functional, symbolic-interactional, situational, and family-developmental approaches (Christensen, 1964a; Hill & Hansen, 1960). Furthermore, various programmatic research efforts were initiated during this time, many of which became cornerstones of family theory and practice during the years ahead. Of particular importance, studies of marital satisfaction and stability, initiated by Burgess and Cottrell (1939) during the 1930s, spawned dozens of investigations, not only of marital relationships but of parent–child relationships as well. Finally, the development of new laboratory methodologies as well as the refinement of various report procedures became evident during these years, allowing for the more reliable and complex assessment of key family variables.

Contributing to all of these directions was the work of Talcott Parsons and Robert Bales (Bales, 1950; Parsons & Bales, 1955). Although this brief introduction does not allow for an extensive discussion of their efforts, their major contributions must at least be acknowledged. First, Parson's structural-functional model of group process, emphasizing the importance of role behavior and task performance, was extremely influential in subsequently developed models of direct relevance to conceptualizing and treating disordered behavior within the family context (Steinhauer, 1987; Tharp, 1965). Second, Parson's primary dimensions of group functioning, instrumental and socioemotional role functions, still represent major dimensions of family interaction thought to be relevant to an understanding of the emergence and/or the perpetuation of psychopathology within the family. Third, the collaboration between Parsons and Bales resulted in the development of interaction process analysis (IPA), an observational coding system for analyzing group process in *ad hoc* problem-solving groups. Both the methodology (i.e., direct observations of ongoing interaction) and the key variables assessed (instrumental and socioemotional communications) provided the basis for numerous coding systems that were developed over the next 20 years, aimed at assessing the problem-solving and naturalistic interactions of disturbed individuals and their families.

From 1950 to the present time, small-group theory and research on families have grown rapidly. In a review of one segment of this literature, Klein and Hill (1979) identified four major activity centers: (a) studies of the family as the context in which social and interpersonal problems develop (including psychiatric disorders); (b) developments in theory and research concerned with the family's response to crises; (c) attempts to conceptualize and measure change in family relationships over the family life cycle; and (d) studies of the problem-solving, decision-making characteristics of family groups. Many of these efforts have been of direct relevance to family studies of psychopathology and have contributed significantly to the conceptual foundations on which clinical theories of child and family disturbance have been based. Furthermore, various family-assessment procedures in current use owe a large intellectual debt to the theoretical and methodological contributions of family sociology and to the social psychology of small-group behavior, for example, the revealed-difference technique (Strodtbeck, 1951), the card sort task (Reiss, 1981), and the various observational coding systems that were strongly influenced by Bales's studies with interaction process analysis. (For further discussion of these issues see Burns, 1973; Steinhauer, 1987; Walters, 1982.) It is our contention that the concepts, methods, and theories that have been developing within family sociology have made and continue to make significant contributions to an understanding of the family's role in psychopathology.

SYSTEMS AND COMMUNICATIONS THEORY

In addition to the theories and methods that have arisen within family sociology, several other forces have fostered and shaped the present character of family research on psychopathology. The most significant of these influences was the emergence of the "family theories" of schizophrenia during the 1950s— in particular, the work of Bowen; of Jackson, Bateson, Haley, and Weakland; of Lidz; and of Wynne (for reviews of these frameworks, see Mishler & Waxler, 1965). Common to all of these efforts was the primary emphasis on family communications and their distortions as the cause of psychopathology, that is, the etiological role of family interaction in the genesis of severe psychiatric disorder and its emergence during adolescence. Distorted role structures and communications were certainly highlighted by all of these clinical theories, although the major theoretical and conceptual underpinnings of the various positions were quite different. In the case of Lidz's writings (Lidz, Cornelison, Fleck, & Terry, 1957) on marital schism and skew, the intellectual debt to Parsons's theory of role structure and differentiation was clearly acknowledged, as was the link to traditional psychodynamic formulations of children's psychosexual development. Wynne's notions of "transactional thought disorder and pseudomutuality," on the other hand, were embedded in a conceptual framework characterized by a mix of psychodynamic, existential, and role theories (Wynne, Ryckoff, Day, & Hersch, 1958).

Notwithstanding the significant contributions of Lidz, Wynne, and Bowen, the most provocative perspective on the family's role in the development and perpetuation of schizophrenia was to come from the collaborations of an anthropologist, several "radical" psychiatrists, and a budding young communications specialist with a background in the dramatic arts. The theoretical centerpiece of this effort was the development of the double-bind hypothesis, whose historical roots can be traced most directly to the cybernetics revolution of the 1940s.

As described by Gottman (1979), the efforts of Norbert Wiener, an MIT mathematician who conducted early studies on computer technologies and antiaircraft artillery, provided critical foundations for the design of servomechanisms involving error-activated feedback mechanisms. The translation of concepts from control engineering to the realm of communication, however, was most fully accomplished by Wiener's student, Claude Shannon, whose "classic 1949 paper became the landmark paper in the mathematical definition of the amount of information transmitted in a communication channel" (p. 15). A key concept that came to characterize this area of study, first used by Wiener himself, was *cybernetics*—a term that describes the process of self-regulation by which the present and future states of a system are determined. By the late 1940s, a series of conferences on the topic of cybernetics and feedback was established through the Macy Foundation and involved participants from various social, biological, and physical sciences. Among the participants in these conferences was Gregory Bateson. Profoundly influenced by these meetings, Bateson soon began work with Jurgen Ruesch at the Langley Porter Clinic and, throughout the next decade, collaborated with a group of "maverick psychiatrists" interested in new approaches to the study of schizophrenia. Supported by a grant from the Rockefeller Foundation, Bateson, with Donald Jackson, Jay Haley, and John Weakland, attempted to understand the nature of schizophrenia as a disorder of communication that developed and was maintained within the family system. The result of this collaboration, of course, was the publication, of the seminal paper on the double-bind hypothesis, which, in effect, presented a clinical-theoretical model emphasizing the multilevel nature of human communication and the contention that seemingly aberrant behavior can result from attempts to resolve and respond to communications conveying contradictory meanings.

The communication theory of the Palo Alto group, as well as the cybernetics literature that provided one of its critical underpinnings, can be "nested" within an even broader intellectual zeitgeist that had been evolving during the previous 30 years: general systems theory (GST). In tracing the history and key features of this evolution, Steinglass (1978) provided the following account:

> In 1928, Ludwig von Bertalanffy introduced the first of a series of concepts that, taken together, were intended to develop an "organismic" approach to biological problems. In 1945 these concepts were collectively given the title General Systems Theory (von Bertalanffy, 1968). Historically, these concepts were developed in response to major dilemmas that had been arising in the biological sciences, dilemmas which von Bertalanffy felt were related primarily to limitations imposed on scientific explanation by existing theoretical approaches to science. The core of the problem as he saw it was the exclusive reliance on what has been called the reductionistic/mechanistic tradition in science. In essence, the reductionistic/mechanistic approach explains events by developing a linear series of stepwise cause and effect equations, each of which is intended to unearth a fundamental precedent event assumed to be causally explanative of the final behavior under study. In psychology, the stimulus–response model is perhaps the clearest example of this approach: an attempt to explain behavior as a series of two-step events, one being the cause or stimulus, the other being the behavior or response. Von Bertalanffy attempted to reverse this prevailing trend in science by urging that attention be paid not only to reductionistic principles, but also to those more general principles that might be used to explain biological processes that lead to increasing complexity of organization for the organism. (pp. 300–301)

The Society for General Systems Research, founded in the mid-1950s, sought to further the development of theoretical systems applicable to more than one of the traditional departments of knowledge. Consistent with this objective, inspection of the various systems principles associated with GST indicates that they have been derived from a number of formal disciplines as well as from specific, interdisciplinary research domains such as cybernetics, information theory, and decision theory. Many systems concepts appear to be particularly relevant to the study of family systems, be they disordered or not. Most important, the distinction between open and closed systems reminds us that families (as open systems) maintain their constancy through a continuous exchange and flow of information; that is, the identity and functioning of an open system depends on communication within the system and between the system and the external environment. From this deceptively simple concept can be derived a series of characteristics, operating principles, and developmental processes that characterize any open system, including the family: *constancy* is achieved through continuous communication within the family and between the family and the external environment; *adaptiveness and change* can occur in response to fluctuating internal and external stimulation; *order and organization* not only are possible but are expected to occur over time; *subsystems, boundaries, and their permeability* serve to differentiate the family system and to define the nature of relationships within the family and between the family and the external environment; *equifinality* informs us that the same final state can be reached from different initial conditions and, as a result, directs attention away from one-cause—one-effect models and toward different developmental pathways; and *positive and negative feedback processes* enable the investigator to approach questions of how change occurs and how sameness remains.

In brief, the systems and communications perspective offered a new model within which to view disordered behavior—a model that first and foremost emphasized the primacy of the interactional context in attempts to understand any behavior, be it deviant or normative. The "strong" variant of this model suggested that it is not even meaningful to discuss psychopathology from an individual perspective because behavior is inextricably intertwined with an interpersonal context and has meaning only when viewed within this context. If this position is accepted, one would conclude that the smallest appropriate unit of analysis is not an individual's behavior but an interactional sequence involving a pattern of exchange that occurs between individuals; in a word, the unit of importance is the system of members in mutual and interdependent relationships with one another, not individual behavior in isolation from this context.

Since the mid-1950s, this framework has had a significant impact on both clinical developments and research efforts concerned with linking family interaction and psychopathology (Steinglass, 1978, 1987). Regarding the former, beginning interests in and curiosity about family treatment approaches in psychiatry grew into a major treatment modality and, for some, an intellectual and personal "movement." Various schools of family therapy were spawned during the 1960s and 1970s, each associated with a group of dedicated adherents and with clinicians of great charisma and influence. Second, the general model was of importance in stimulating a considerable amount of empirical research on family interaction and psychopathology from 1960 to 1980, although most of these efforts were not initiated by the original theorists or clinicians themselves but arose within the larger clinical research community (Jacob, 1975). Third, the systems model not only has been accepted as a primary rationale for intervention and prevention efforts focused on the family but has been incorporated into other theories of family dysfunction and clinical models of treatment (Vincent, 1980). Finally, this perspective, more than any of the others, underscores the complexity of relationships that can exist between family influences and psychopathology; the continuing incorporation of systems principles into small-group, developmental, and behavioral approaches to family disturbance clearly attests to its compelling nature.

CHILD AND DEVELOPMENTAL PSYCHOLOGY

A third stream of influence that has provided a critical cornerstone of family studies of psychopathology involves the contributions from child and developmental psychology. As noted by Achenbach (1982), the study of childhood and its disorders achieved formal status only during the present century. Various intellectual and social forces contributed to this evolution, the most important including the development of intelligence tests for schoolchildren; the growth of the child study movement stimulated by the pioneering efforts of G. Stanley Hall and Lightner Witner; the formulation and dissemination of psychoanalysis; and the growth of child guidance clinics and the child guidance movement. Throughout the second quarter of the century, psychoanalysis, in pure or revised form, dominated conceptualizations and treatments of childhood disorders in which therapy was "aimed at assisting the child in modifying basic underlying personality structure" (Ollendick & Hersen, 1983, p. 9). Athough early parent–child relationships were assumed to be important contributors to development gone awry, it was the work of researchers in developmental psychology and learning theory, rather than of the child clinicians, that would eventually give elaboration and full meaning to the role of these parent–child relationships.

From the seminal writings of Symonds (1939) to the elaborated, circumplex models of Becker (1964), Schaefer (1959), and Seigelman (1965), a great deal of theoretical and empirical effort has been directed toward explicating parental behaviors related to children's cognitive and social-emotional development. Since the mid-1940s, these efforts have identified, replicated, and elaborated three primary dimensions of parental behavior—affect, control, and consistency—which have been linked to a wide range of child outcomes related to personality, social-interpersonal, and cognitive variables (Rollins & Thomas, 1979).

In reviewing this period of research, Hartup (1977) characterized the emergent parent–child conceptualizations as "social mold theories" in which influences were assumed to be unidirectional: the parent acted and the child responded. Several other areas of investigation, however, which soon gained greater recognition, began to characterize the child as an "active" organism that contributed significantly to the nature and course of the evolving parent–child relationship. Piaget's descriptions (1970), of organismically based schemas and White's competency-based view (1959) of motivation sensitized researchers to the child's "choosing, action-producing" nature (Rollins & Thomas, 1979), whereas studies of child temperament invigorated theoretical and empirical interests in biologically rooted child variables and their impact on patterns of parent–child relationships (Thomas & Chess, 1977). The linking of parental behaviors to variations in child temperament was impressively forged by Bell in his classic 1968 paper, "A Reinterpretation of the Direction of Effects in Studies of Socialization." From there, it was clear that the next generation of models would be truly interactional in that a process of mutual influence would compete with simpler, unidirectional conceptualizations of parent–child relationships (Maccoby & Martin, 1983; Parke, 1984).

The contributions of child development and developmental psychology to family studies of psychopathology are obviously critical, alerting us to age- and stage-related changes in behavior. The "constancy of change" is ensured by the inevitable developmental changes that occur in the psychosocial, cognitive, and social characteristics of both children and parents and in the patterns of relationships that link members to one another over time. From the various literatures that have contributed to the developmental model, we are told that the child's behavior—and our evaluation of its "deviance"—must be evaluated within a temporal context. Without this context—ideally based on both theory and normative data—it is extremely difficult to anticipate whether the behavior is likely to change, over what period of time, to what degree, and in what direction. When speaking of behaviors that have clinical or psychiatric significance, such knowledge can be of critical importance to issues of course, outcome, and treatment alternatives.

Furthermore, knowledge of developmental parameters can be of great value in evaluating family theories of child psychopathology. One example will suffice. In a recent review of the literature on inconsistent communication and family disturbance, Jacob and Lessin (1982) found only mixed support for the contention that incongruities in verbal and nonverbal communications are reliably associated with childhood disorders. In considering this issue in greater detail, it was suggested that the child's level of cognitive and linguistic development was a potentially key variable that had been given only scant attention in this literature. In essence, verbal content is much more influential in message interpretations by younger children than are voice tone and nonverbal cues. Only as children approach preadolescence do the paralinguistic and facial cues take on marked importance in the decoding of incongruent messages. The major implication of such data is that the perception of a message as incongruent is importantly related to the child's developmental stage, and that incongruent messages will be disturbing—that is, have an impact—only if the child is old enough to recognize and appreciate the channel discrepancy.

The developmental tradition has also contributed importantly to the assessment of child psychopathology within the family, underscoring the need to measure the key parenting dimensions of acceptance, control, and consistency (Jacob & Tennenbaum, 1986). Child and developmental psychology have also made notable contributions to the development of the observational procedures used in both laboratory (Hughes & Haynes, 1978) and naturalistic settings, as

well as to various report procedures concerning children's perception of parents
(e.g., Margolies & Weintraub, 1977). Finally, theory and research within the
developmental tradition have been integrated into other models and thus have
resulted in more compelling theories and methodologies than existed before.

In the same way that the field of cybernetics can be nested within a broader
conceptual framework (i.e., GST), issues of individual development can, and in
the present context should, be seen as one component of a family development
model. The original impetus for this perspective comes from family sociology, in
which the family life cycle and changing role relationships were the key to
understanding temporal aspects of family life. As a major conceptual perspective
within family sociology (Hill & Mattessich, 1979), the family developmental approach was never a pure strain; instead, it drew its character and strength from
the application and integration of concepts from other areas of inquiry: stages of
the family life cycle from rural sociology; "career" as a series of role sequences
from the sociology of professions; the concepts of position, role, and norm from
symbolic interactionism; and developmental needs and tasks from child psychology. As described by Hill (1964):

> The family developmental approach views the family as a small group system, intri-
> cately organized internally into paired positions of husband-father, wife-mother, son-
> brother, and daughter-sister. Norms prescribing the appropriate role behavior for each
> of these positions specify how reciprocal relations are to be maintained, as well as how
> role behavior may change with changing ages of the occupants of these positions. The
> group has a predictable natural history, designated by stages, beginning with the simple
> husband–wife pair and becoming more complex as members are added. The number
> of interpersonal relations are [sic] highest with the birth of last child, stabilizing for a
> brief period, to become less complex with the progressive launching of adult children
> in jobs and marriage as the group contracts in size once again to the dyadic interactions
> of husband–wife pair. As age composition changes, so do the age role expectations for
> occupants of the positions in the family, and so does the quality of interaction among
> family members.
>   There can be identified several stages of the family life cycle—each with unique
> conflicts, interaction patterns and solidarity. Each stage may be seen in three dimen-
> sions of increasing complexity: (1) changing developmental tasks and role expectations
> of children as they age, (2) changing developmental tasks and role expectations of
> parents, and (3) the developmental tasks of the family as family which emerge from
> cultural imperatives placed upon the family at each stage of growth. (pp. 188–189)

Although the family developmental model has not been systematically exploited by psychopathology researchers, there are numerous empirical studies
(scattered as they may be) that support the value of this perspective in understanding relationships between changes in family-life-cycle characteristics and
disordered behavior. In some cases, these findings are directly relevant to psychopathological outcomes, whereas in other instances, the links between family
development and disordered behavior are implied and in need of more explicit
study. Several examples can be noted: family developmental crises are significantly related to the onset of symptomatic behavior (Hadley, Jacob, Milliones,
Caplan, & Spitz, 1974); changes in family power structure not only occur across
the preadolescent–adolescent time period but are importantly influenced by
variations in social class (Jacob, 1974); newly married couples become in-

creasingly differentiated as they negotiate the early stages of marriage and parenthood (Raush, Marshall, & Featherman, 1970); birth order and spacing—which are correlated with differences in family stage and the quality of marital, parent–child, and sibling interaction—are related to children's psychosocial and psychiatric status (see the chapter by Martin); and marital satisfaction exhibits a curvilinear relationship with family development and, by implication, is related to the quality and quantity of family interaction (Anderson, Russell, & Schumm, 1983; Rollins & Galligan, 1978).

Notwithstanding these supportive findings, Martin (see Chapter 5) reminds us that single variables—be they individual or family parameters—are unlikely to be robust or to demonstrate generalizable relationships with the development of psychopathology. The complexity of our task *requires* the incorporation of other individual and system variables into our inquiry, most importantly, the genetic-biological and interaction histories of family members. The temporal unfolding and interaction of these various sources of influences must eventually be the researcher's major concern if she or he is to provide significant progress in our understanding of the family's contribution to the development of psychopathology.

SOCIAL LEARNING THEORY

A final influence on family studies of psychopathology has been behavioral psychology in general and social learning theory (SLT) in particular. SLT is certainly not independent of the other influences, nor is it a homogeneous, tightly defined set of concepts drawn from and evaluated within a single discipline. This approach is characterized by certain features, however, that give it a strong identity in the literature.

The roots of this tradition can be traced back to the early years of the current century—a period of time that witnessed the emergence of the first scientific studies of learning processes. Most important, the work of two Russian physiologists, Pavlov and Bekhterev, resulted in the formalization of two major learning paradigms that would become the dominant perspectives in experimental psychology during the next 50 years: classical (respondent) and operant (instrumental) conditioning. At about the same time, and independent of Bekhterev's work, an American psychologist, Edward Thorndike (1898), reported similar findings involving the impact of rewards on subsequent behavior—a relationship that was simply yet elegantly referred to as the *law of effect*. With the publication of "Psychology as the Behaviorist Views It," John Watson (1913) brought the learning position into full relief, arguing that observable behavior and how it is learned—without resort to introspection and issues of consciousness—should be the only legitimate concern of psychology.

During the second quarter of the century, the full impact of these seminal works was to be realized in the elegant and highly influential theories of Hull, Spence, and Skinner, along with several competing models stressing cognitive variables (e.g., Hilgard & Bowers, 1966; Tolman, 1932). It was not until the late

1950s and early 1960s, however, that principles derived from the classical and operant conditioning models were applied to the analysis and treatment of major clinical disorders, in particular, Wolpe's reciprocal inhibition (1958) in the treatment of anxiety-based disorders and application of operant conditioning techniques to the treatment of a wide range of human maladaptations (Ayllon & Azrin, 1968; Hersen, Kazdin, & Bellack, 1983).

By that time, the "pure" strains of learning theory—the Hull–Spence and the Skinnerian paradigms—were being challenged by rapid developments in cognitive theory and research, as well as the competing paradigm proposed by Albert Bandura. Briefly, Bandura sought to broaden earlier learning models through greater emphasis on the social aspects of learning and the mutual, interactive effects of behavior, person, and environment (Bandura, 1977; Bandura & Walters, 1963). The focus on the interplay among these several sources of influence emphasized the importance of cognitive variables, in particular, the contention that learning through observing complex behaviors and then modeling such patterns is the source by which the most important learning of the social world takes place. Consistent with this emphasis, Bandura's theoretical framework became known as *social learning theory*.

During the next two decades, SLT was revised, elaborated, and integrated with other frameworks and models within the social sciences. Although still referred to as SLT, the approach is now a diverse and rich one, containing several subapproaches that vary in the relative emphasis given to key concepts and methodologies. As noted by Vincent (1980), "Social learning theory is not a unified, original statement of propositions; instead, the theory is an assemblage of several models" (p. 3). The most prominent components in the framework are operant learning and social exchange theory, plus a more recent integration with concepts from general systems theory and attribution theory. Notwithstanding this diversity, the general model can be characterized by several distinguishing features, the most important of which are (a) a focus on behavioral systems and on the reciprocal, bidirectional interactions among members; (b) a continuing emphasis on variations in behavior as a function of changes in the environment, notwithstanding the necessity for the continued incorporation of cognitive variables into the model; (c) a preference for the naturalistic study of families; (d) a commitment to clinical application and development; and (e) an overriding investment in the study and treatment of disordered behavior via scientific, methodologically rigorous procedures.

The contributions that SLT has made to the study of psychopathology within the family context have been significant. Conceptually, the sustained efforts of various family researchers have resulted in further delineation and elaboration of two key constructs in developing models of family interaction and psychopathology: coercion and reciprocity. Given the dynamic interplay between conceptualization, empirical assessment, and model revision that characterizes the SLT model, these key concepts have been refined significantly since the mid-1960s. As noted earlier, the model is now characterized by greater appreciation of the cognitive, individual, and extrafamilial influence that impact on the more molecular and momentary patterns of behavioral interaction.

Another major contribution made by the behavioral approach has involved the development and validation of a number of observational coding systems for use in both laboratory and naturalistic settings—procedures that have allowed for the rigorous and rich description of interaction relevant to theory development and treatment evaluation in the area of child psychopathology and marital dysfunction (see Chapter 9 by Markman and Notarius). In addition, various statistical methods for analyzing complex patterns of interaction have been offered by researchers in this area, the most notable involving the application of sequential and time-series analyses aimed at clarifying the contingent and temporal nature of complex patterns of family interaction (Gottman, 1979, 1982; see Chapter 12 by Gottman).

A final contribution made by behavioral family researchers has involved the development and evaluation of family-based treatment programs for child, marital, and family disturbance (Jacobson & Margolin, 1979; Patterson, 1982). The early parent-training, child-management models of Patterson, Wahler, and Bernal—although modified and elaborated significantly since the mid-1970s—still represent major clinical strategies in the treatment of childhood conduct disorders. Similarly, behavioral marital therapy approaches have been subjected to a tremendous amount of evaluation and revision since the mid-1970s, incorporating concepts from cognitive theory and techniques from other schools of family therapy in search of maximally effective interventions for marital discord (Hahlweg & Jacobson, 1984). Given the commitment to both scientific rigor and clinical relevance, it is anticipated that the behavioral approach will continue to offer significant theoretical insights and clinical intervention relevant to the family context of psychopathology.

SUMMARY

The field of inquiry that we refer to as *family interaction and psychopathology* has been and continues to be influenced by four major perspectives: sociological, developmental, systems and communications, and behavioral. Each of these influences has provided critical theoretical, methodological, and clinical foundations on which the family interaction model is currently based. From the sociological tradition, we have come to conceptualize the family as a small group, characterized by structural arrangements based on variations in age and sex composition; processes reflecting the exchange of instrumental and social-emotional information; and norms and values that convey expectations regarding the behavior among family members, as well as relationships between the family and the nonfamily institutions in the larger community. In addition, the sociological tradition has directed our attention toward laboratory assessments of family process, emphasizing the problem-solving nature of family groups and the importance of observing and systematically coding patterns of intrafamily communications.

From the developmental perspective, the family and its members are seen to undergo age- and stage-related changes in individual, dyadic, and system functioning. Key dimensions of parenting behavior have been identified by developmental investigators, together with report and laboratory assessment procedures aimed at measuring these dimensions.

Since the mid-1970s, interactional parameters have become increasingly emphasized in attempts to more accurately account for the relationship between family and child functioning over time. The systems and communications perspective represents the broadest framework within which to view the family. Deriving its substance and support from diverse disciplines and interest areas, systems theory has provided a major scaffolding and rationale on which many family efforts have been based since the mid-1950s. Most often linked with processes and outcomes of interpersonal communication, the systems perspective has offered an alternative and powerful prism through which constancy and change can be viewed. The increasing incorporation and integration of systems concepts into sociological, developmental, and behavioral models of family process during the past several decades attests to the compelling nature of this framework.

Finally, social learning theory has exerted a most significant impact on the study of family interaction and psychopathology. The early efforts of Patterson, Wahler, and Weiss attempted to exploit laboratory-based learning paradigms in the interests of describing and modifying problem parent–child and marital interactions. In turn, these pioneering efforts stimulated the development of a whole generation of behavioral and cognitive-behavioral scientists, who have contributed so importantly to theoretical, methodological, and treatment advances in the field as we view it today. As with the other perspectives, the concepts and principles associated with the SLT perspective have become increasingly integrated with those of other models.

Future studies of family interaction and psychopathology will no doubt continue to be influenced by these major frameworks, building on progress made within each domain as well as contributions that emerge from the interrelating of several models and their associated concepts. Given the complexity of issues involved in conceptualizing and studying family influences, it is unlikely that any one framework alone is sufficiently comprehensive to account for substantial and clinically meaningful portions of variance associated with psychopathological processes and outcomes. The integration of concepts from various models has occurred and will continue to occur—a process of cross-fertilization that will hopefully produce more robust and valid theories of family influence than are possible through exclusive reliance on one set of relatively narrow constructs and methods.

Beyond the continued exploitation and integration of these major frameworks, future studies of family process and disordered behavior must become integrated with at least two additional perspectives: psychiatric epidemiology and family genetics. From the former, we have learned that much clinical research—based on relatively small and questionably representative samples—may be only modestly generalizable to the larger community of families and psychiatric disorders. Given these threats to external validity (Campbell & Stanley, 1963), future studies should certainly consider a multilevel approach to sampling and assessment. That is, large community samples would be drawn and carefully described along structural, social, cultural, or psychiatric dimensions that are suspected to impact on patterns of family interaction. Smaller samples— selected to represent variations along one or more of these dimensions—would then be subjected to in-depth analyses of characteristic family processes and their concurrent or predictive relationship with dysfunctional behavior patterns. Given such a strategy, the investigator would derive a greater appreciation of how structural and social-environmental dimensions impact on family life, as well as of the extent to which these dimensions enhance or limit our more molecular-level findings of the relationships between interaction and psychopathology. Finally, studies of family interaction process must become increasingly integrated with and related to family genetic analyses. Thus far, such efforts have been seen only in family studies of schizophrenia in which longitudinal, prospective designs have been applied to "high-risk" samples in attempts to more carefully assess the independent and joint impact of family environmental and family genetic influences (Goldstein & Strachan, 1987). Many significant contributions have been made through these efforts since the mid-1960s; in turn, they should encourage similar efforts in studies of other forms of psychopathology and interpersonal dysfunction.

REFERENCES

Achenbach, T. M. (1982). *Developmental psychopathology.* New York: Wiley.

Anderson, S. A., Russell, C. S., & Schumm, W. R. (1983). Perceived marital quality and family life cycle categories: A further analysis. *Journal of Marriage and the Family, 45,* 127–140.

Ayllon, T., & Azrin, N. (1968). *The token economy: A motivational system for therapy.* New York: Prentice-Hall.

Bales, R. F. (1950). *Interaction process analysis.* Cambridge, MA: Addison-Wesley.

Bandura, A. (1977). *Social learning theory.* Englewood Cliffs, NJ: Prentice-Hall.

Bandura, A., & Walters, R. H. (1963). *Social learning and personality development.* New York: Holt.

Bateson, C., Jackson, D. D., Haley, J., & Weakland, J. (1956). Toward a theory of schizophrenia. *Behavioral Science, 1,* 251–264.

Becker, W. C. (1964). Consequences of different kinds of parental discipline. In M. L. Hoffman & L. Hoffman (Eds.), *Review of child development research* (Vol. 1). Chicago: University of Chicago Press.

Bell, N. W., & Vogel, E. F. (Eds.). (1960). *A modern introduction to the family.* Glencoe, IL: Free Press.

Bell, R. Q. (1968). A reinterpretation of the direction of effects in studies of socialization. *Psychological Review, 75,* 81–95.

Burgess, E. W. (1926). The family as a unit of interacting personalities. *Family, 7,* 3–9.

Burgess, E. W., & Cottrell, L. S. (1939). *Predicting success or failure in marriage.* New York: Prentice-Hall.

Burns, T. (1973). A structural theory of social exchange. *Acta Sociologica, 16,* 188–208.

Burr, W. R., Hill, R., Nye, F. I., & Reiss, I. L. (1979). *Contemporary theories about the family: Research-based theories.* New York: Free Press.

Campbell, D. T., & Stanley, J. C. (1963). *Experimental and quasi-experimental designs for research.* Chicago: Rand McNally.

Christensen, H. T. (1964a). Development of the family field of study. In H. T. Christensen (Ed.), *Handbook of marriage and the family.* Chicago: Rand McNally.

Christensen, H. T. (Ed.). (1964b). *Handbook of marriage and the family.* Chicago: Rand McNally.

Cooper, B., & Gath, D. (1977). Psychiatric illness, maladjustment and juvenile delinquency: An ecological study in a London borough. *Psychological Medicine, 7*, 465–474.

Fieve, R. R., Rosenthal, D., & Brill, H. (Eds.). (1975). *Genetic research in psychiatry.* Baltimore: Johns Hopkins University Press.

Fromm-Reichman, F. (1948). Notes on the development of treatment of schizophrenics by psychoanalytic psychotherapy. *Psychiatry, 11*, 263–273.

Garmezy, N. (1974a). Children at risk for the antecedents of schizophrenia: 1. Conceptual models and research methods. *Schizophrenia Bulletin, 8*, 14–90.

Garmezy, N. (1974b). Children at risk: The search for the antecedents of schizophrenia: 2. Ongoing research programs, issues, and intervention. *Schizophrenia Bulletin, 9*, 55–125.

Gershon, E. S., Matthysse, S., Breakfield, X. A., & Ciaraenllo, R. D. (Eds.). (1981). *Genetic research strategies in psychobiology and psychiatry.* Pacific Grove, CA: Boxwood Press.

Goldstein, M. J., & Strachan, A. (1987). The family and schizophrenia. In T. Jacob (Ed.), *Family interaction and psychopathology: Theory, methods and findings.* New York: Plenum Press.

Gottesman, I. I., & Shields, J. (1982). *Schizophrenia: The epigenetic puzzle.* London: Cambridge University Press.

Gottman, J. M. (1979). *Marital interaction: Experimental investigations.* New York: Academic Press.

Gottman, J. M. (1982). *Time-series analysis: A comprehensive introduction for social scientists.* New York: Cambridge University Press.

Hadley, T., Jacob, T., Milliones, J., Caplan, J., & Spitz, D. (1974). The relationship between family developmental crisis and the appearance of symptoms in a family member. *Family Process, 13*, 207–214.

Hahlweg, K., & Jacobson, N. W. (1984). *Marital interaction: Analysis and modification.* New York: Guilford Press.

Handel, G. (1965). Psychological study of whole families. *Psychological Bulletin, 63*, 19–41.

Hartup, W. W. (1977). Perspectives on child and family interaction: Past, present, and future. In R. M. Lerner & G. B. Spanier (Eds.), *Child influences on marital and family interaction.* New York: Academic Press.

Hersen, M., Kazdin, A. E., & Bellack, A. S. (Eds.). (1983). *The clinical psychology handbook.* New York: Pergamon Press.

Hilgard, E. R., & Bowers, G. H. (1966). *Theories of learning.* New York: Appleton-Century.

Hill, R. (1964). Methodological issues in family development research. *Family Process, 3*, 186–206.

Hill, R., & Hansen, D. (1960). The identification of conceptual frameworks utilized in family study. *Marriage and Family Living, 22*, 299–311.

Hill, R., & Mattessich, P. (1979). Family development theory and life span development. In P. B. Baltes & O. G. Brim (Eds.), *Life span development and behavior* (Vol. 2). New York: Academic Press.

Hughes, H. M., & Haynes, S. N. (1978). Structured laboratory observation in the behavioral assessment of parent–child interactions: A methodological critique. *Behavior Therapy, 9*, 428–447.

Jacob, T. (1974). Patterns of family conflict and dominance as a function of child age and social class. *Developmental Psychology, 10(101)*, 1–12.

Jacob, T. (1975). Family interaction in disturbed and normal families: A methodological and substantive review. *Psychological Bulletin, 82*, 33–65.

Jacob, T., & Lessin, S. (1982). Inconsistent communication in family interaction. *Clinical Psychology Reviews, 2*, 295–309.

Jacob, T., & Tennenbaum, D. (1986). Family methods in the assessment of child and adolescent psychopathology. In M. Rutter, H. Tuma, & I. Lann (Eds.), *Assessment and diagnosis of child and adolescent psychopathology.* New York: Guilford Press.

Jacob, T., Favorini, A., Meisel, S., & Anderson, C. (1978). The spouse, children and family interactions of the alcoholic: Substantive findings and methodological issues. *Journal of Studies on Alcohol, 39*, 1231–1251.

Jacobson, N. S., & Margolin, G. (1979). *Marital therapy: Strategies based on a social learning and behavior exchange principles.* New York: Brunner/Mazel.

Kellam, S. G., & Ensminger, M. E. (1980). Theory and method in child psychiatric epidemiology. In F. Earls (Eds.), *Studies of children.* New York: Prodist (Neal Watson Academic Publications).

Kellam, S. G., Ensminger, M. E., & Turner, R. J. (1977). Family structure and the mental health of children: Concurrent and longitudinal community-wide studies. *Archives of General Psychiatry, 34,* 1012–1022.

Klein, D. M., & Hill, R. (1979). Determinants of family problem-solving effectiveness. In W. R. Burr, R. Hill, R. I. Nye, & I. L. Reiss (Eds.), *Contemporary theories about the family* (Vol. 1). New York: Free Press.

Langner, T. S., Gersten, J. C., Eisenberg, J. G., Green, E. L., & Herson, J. H. (1986). *Children under stress: Family and social factors in the behavior of urban children and adolescents.* New York: Columbia University Press.

Lewis, M. (1937). Alcoholism and family casework. *Family, 18,* 39–44.

Lidz, T., Cornelison, A., Fleck, S., & Terry, D. (1957). The intrafamilial environment of schizophrenic patients: II. Marital schism and marital skew. *American Journal of Psychiatry, 114,* 241–248.

Maccoby, E. E., & Marin, J. A. (1983). Socialization in the context of the family: Parent–child interaction. In P. Mussen (Ed.), *Handbook of child psychology* (Vol. 4). New York: Wiley.

Margolies, P. J., & Weintraub, S. (1977). The revised 56-item CRPBI as a research instrument: Reliability and factor structure. *Journal of Clinical Psychology, 33,* 472–476.

Mintz, N. L., & Schwartz, D. T. (1964). Urban ecology and psychosis: Community factors in the incidence of schizophrenia and manic-depression among Italians in Greater Boston. *International Journal of Social Psychiatry, 10,* 101–118.

Mishler, E., & Waxler, N. (1965). Family interaction patterns and schizophrenia: A review of current theories. *Merrill-Palmer Quarterly, 11,* 269–315.

Moos, R. H., & Moos, B. S. (1983). Adaptation and the quality of life in work and family settings. *Journal of Community Psychology, 11,* 158–170.

Ollendick, T. H., & Hersen, M. (1983). A historical overview of child psychopathology. In T. H. Ollendick & M. Hersen (Eds.), *Handbook of child psychopathology.* New York: Plenum Press.

Parke, R. (Ed.). (1984). *Review of child development research: Vol. 7. The Family.* Chicago: University of Chicago Press.

Parsons, T., & Bales, R. (1955). *Family socialization and interaction process.* Glencoe, IL: Free Press.

Patterson, G. R. (1982). *A social learning approach: Vol. 3. Coercive family process.* Eugene, OR: Castalia.

Piaget, J. (1970). Piaget's theory. In P. E. Mussen (Ed.), *Carmichael's manual of child psychology* (3rd ed. Vol. 1). New York: Wiley.

Raush, H. L., Marshall, K. A., & Featherman, J. M. (1970). Relations at three early stages of marriage as reflected by the use of personal pronouns. *Family Process, 9,* 69–82.

Reiss, D. (1981). *The family's construction of reality.* Cambridge: Harvard University Press.

Rollins, B., & Galligan, R. (1978). The developing child and marital satisfaction of parents. In R. M. Lerner & G. B. Spanier (Eds.), *Child influences and marital and family interaction.* New York: Academic Press.

Rollins, B. C., & Thomas, D. L. (1979). Parental support, power, and control techniques in the socialization of children. In W. R. Burr, R. Hill, F. I. Nye, & I. L. Reiss (Eds.), *Contemporary theories about the family: Research based theories* (Vol. 1). New York: Free Press.

Schaefer, E. S. (1959). The circumplex model for maternal behavior. *Journal of Abnormal and Social Psychology, 59,* 226–235.

Seigelman, M. (1965). Evaluation of Bronfenbrenner's questionnaire for children concerning parental behavior. *Child Development, 36,* 164–174.

Shannon, C. E. (1949). The mathematical theory of communication. In C. E. Shannon & W. Weaver (Eds.), *The mathematical theory of communication.* Urbana, IL: University of Illinois Press.

Steinglass, P. (1978). The conceptualization of marriage from a systems theory perspective. In T. Paolino & B. McCrady (Eds.), *Marriage and marital therapy: Psychoanalytic, behavioral and systems theory perspectives.* New York: Brunner/Mazel.

Steinglass, P. (1987). A systems view of family interaction and psychopathology. In T. Jacob (Ed.), *Family interaction and psychopathology: Theory, methods and findings.* New York: Plenum Press.

Steinhauer, P. D. (1987). The family as a small group: The process model of family functioning. In T. Jacob (Ed.), *Family interaction and psychopathology: Theories, methods and findings.* New York: Plenum Press.

Strodtbeck, F. L. (1951). Husband–wife interaction over revealed differences. *American Sociological Review, 16,* 468–473.

Symonds, P. (1939). *The psychology of parent–child relationships*. New York: Appleton-Century-Crofts.

Tharp, R. (1965). Marriage roles, child development and family treatment. *American Journal of Orthopsychiatry, 35,* 531–538.

Thomas, A., & Chess, S. (1977). *Temperament and development*. New York: Brunner/Mazel.

Thorndike, E. L. (1898). Animal intelligence: An experimental study of the associative processes in animals. *Psychological Review Monograph Supplement, 2:8 (4)*.

Tolman, E. C. (1932). *Purposive behavior in animals and men*. New York: Appleton-Century-Crofts.

Vincent, J. (1980). The empirical-clinical study of families: Social learning theory as a point of departure. In J. Vincent (Ed.), *Advances in family intervention, assessment and theory* (Vol. 1). Greenwich, CT: JAI Press.

von Bertalanffy, L. (1968). *General systems theory*. New York: George Braziller.

Walters, L. H. (1982, November). Are families different from other groups? *Journal of Marriage and the Family, 44,* 841–850.

Watson, J. B. (1913). Psychology as the behaviorist views it. *Psychological Review, 20,* 158–177.

White, R. W. (1959). Motivation reconsidered: The concept of competence. *Psychological Review, 66,* 297–333.

Wolpe, J. (1958). *Psychotherapy by reciprocal inhibition*. Stanford, CA: Stanford University Press.

Wynne, L. C., Ryckoff, I., Day, J., & Hirsch, S. (1958). Pseudomutuality in the family relations of schizophrenics. *Psychiatry, 21,* 205–220.

PART II

CONCEPTUAL
FOUNDATIONS

CHAPTER 2

A Systems View of Family Interaction and Psychopathology

Peter Steinglass

INTRODUCTION

In this book, we have taken on a challenging task: to examine key links between family organizational and behavioral variables and the major types of psychopathology. Whenever one approaches a subject of such inherent complexity, it is critically important that it be done within the perspective of a clearly articulated theoretical orientation. Otherwise, it is all too easy to become lost in a flood of subjectively powerful data, a victim of empirical speculations.

Imagine for example, that one is a therapist interviewing a family for the first time. In a typical interview, the therapist finds himself or herself rapidly engulfed in an overwhelming stew of facts, communicational acts, compositional and demographic data, emotions, conflicting histories, and so on. Family members first will not talk, then all talk simultaneously. Incidents are alluded to, family secrets are kept at a tantalizing distance, coalitions and alliances between family members wax and wane as the session proceeds, and there may be little agreement about even the chief complaint that brought the family to the therapist in the first place. How does one survive in such a clinical situation? Only by having a theoretical model inside one's head that serves to guide and structure the therapy session as it proceeds. Questions asked, answers attended to or ignored, even decisions made about whom to include in the session—all respond to the guidelines provided by such a model.

The researcher faces a similar dilemma. Who should be included in the

PETER STEINGLASS • Center for Family Research, Department of Psychiatry and Behavioral Sciences, George Washington University, School of Medicine, Washington, DC 20037.

study? Where should the family be observed? In its home; in a laboratory setting; in a treatment environment? What aspects of behavior should be measured? Or is behavior of any interest at all? Should subjects' attributions on projective test results be emphasized less than, equally with, or more than directly observed behavior? Clearly, here as well, it is the theoretical model that guides not only the interpretations of findings, but also the selection of research settings and designs in the first place.

Hence, we start the book with a section on theory. In this first of a series of chapters devoted to descriptions of the more influential models of family functioning, we take on the mandate of discussing the model that has had perhaps the greatest impact on thinking and practice in the family field: family systems theory.

The family systems model is one that has tended to generate strong feelings pro and con. On the one hand, its supporters have hailed it as a revolutionary approach to our understanding of clinical problems and therapeutic interventions. A bevy of laudatory and grandiloquent terms have been used to underscore this view. Systems thinking has been called a new "scientific paradigm" (Gray, Duhl, & Rizzo, 1969), a new "world view" (Ritterman, 1977), and a new "epistemology" (Dell, 1982).

On the other hand, its detractors have argued that systems theory is not a theory at all, but merely a descriptive language for underscoring relationships that are commonsensical and hence not particularly useful (from a scientific perspective). In particular, these critics decry an absence of rigor not only in the definition of terms, but also in the pinpointing of exclusionary criteria defined by the model. It is a model, they say, that is incapable of scientific examination. That is, it cannot generate testable hypotheses because it is incapable of defining the circumstances under which rejection of hypotheses would be warranted. And last, they say that, because it is by-and-large useless as a framework for predicting consequent results given certain antecedent circumstances, it fails to pass one of the most important tests of a first-rate scientific theory.

It is frankly beyond the scope of this chapter to attempt to resolve this controversy. In fact, it could be argued that it is a controversy beyond adequate resolution. If, as many systems theorists claim, the central contribution of systems theory is its introduction of a fundamentally different approach to our understanding of cause and effect, then the controversy becomes a largely irrelevant one. That is, a critique of systems theory should focus not primarily on how well it stacks up against customary scientific standards but on an explication of what the unique aspects of this approach actually are, and on why it is or is not a useful clinical model.

Suffice it to say the systems view of family interaction and psychopathology, in that it is as much a way of thinking as it is a set of theoretical postulates, has generated not one but a number of systems models of families. Many of the more popular family-therapy approaches, for example, make liberal reference to their roots in systems theory. Structural family therapy (Minuchin, 1974; Minuchin & Fishman, 1981), the various strategic family-therapy models (Haley, 1976; Madanes, 1981; Selvini-Palazzoli, Cecchin, Prata, & Boscolo, 1978), and the Bowen model (1976) have all been advertized as family systems models. Clearly, however, their various interpretations of systems principles have led to quite different models of therapy, with the differences including not only styles of therapeutic intervention but also the content of the therapy session (the clinical data they choose to focus on), decisions about who should be included in the treatment process (membership criteria), and the perceived role of the therapist.

Further, these models have quite different views of what constitutes family psychopathology. In one instance, pathology might be defined primarily in terms of alliances and coalitions, the relative permeability of systemic boundaries, and the nature of hierarchical distributions of power within the system (Aponte & Van Deusen, 1981). In another instance, the primary emphasis might be on communication (information exchange), with relative clarity, redundancy, and directness of communication channels being used as the criteria for judgments regarding the health or the dysfunctional quality of the family system (Watzlawick, Beavin, & Jackson, 1967).

Yet, despite these differences, a closer examination reveals that the differences result more from the degree of emphasis that each model places on one or another of a series of *core constructs* associated with general systems theory than from fundamental disagreements about theory. What they all share is the conceptualization of the family as an operational system and the embracing of a set of notions that we will subsume under the term *systems perspective*. These commonly embraced notions are themselves so profoundly important an influence as to make the differences between the various family systems models of far less import than the contrast between systems approaches and more traditional models, such as the psychodynamic or behavioral ones.

Because this chapter deals primarily with theory rather than clinical technique, our emphasis will be on an explication of the above-mentioned systems perspective and on a discussion of the core constructs of family systems theory. Discussing these constructs, all of which are derived from a focus on the family as a *living system*, will therefore be the major emphasis of this chapter.

THE SYSTEMS PERSPECTIVE

In his 1979 essay, "Medical Lessons from History," Lewis Thomas made the following assertion:

> For every disease there is a single key mechanisms that dominates all others. If one can find it, and then think one's way around it, one can control the disorder. This generalization is harder to prove, and arguable—it is more like a strong hunch than a scientific assertion—but I believe that the record thus far tends to support it. The most complicated, multi-cell, multi-tissue, and multi-organ diseases I know of are tertiary syphilis, tuberculosis, and pernicious anemia. In each, there are at least five major organs and tissues involved, and each appears to be affected by a variety of environmental influences. Before they came under scientific appraisal, each was thought to be what we now call a multi-factorial disease—far too complex to allow for a single causative mechanism and yet, when all the necessary facts were in, it was clear that by

simply switching off one thing—the spirochete, the tubercle bacillus or a single vitamin
deficiency—the whole array of disordered and seemingly unrelated pathological mechanisms could be switched off, at once. (p. 140)

What Lewis Thomas was stating here, in eloquent fashion, is the *reductionistic-mechanistic approach* to causation, an approach that has dominated nine-
teenth- and twentieth-century scientific thinking. This approach attempts to
explain events by the development of a linear series of stepwise cause-and-effect
equations, each of which is intended to identify a fundamental precedent event
assumed to be causally explanatory of the final behavior under study. The
assumption underlying the approach is what might be called the belief in ultimate causality. In the Lewis Thomas version, the "cause" of tertiary syphilis is
the spirochete organism; of pernicious anemia, the specific vitamin deficiency.

Clearly, the examples that Thomas supplied are compelling evidence not
only of the validity of the reductionistic-mechanistic approach, but also of its
value in directing us toward specific interventions that can powerfully influence
(cure) the diseases in question. Yet infectious diseases and deficiency syndromes
are not the only examples that Thomas feels can be solved by a scientific exploration directed by a reductionistic philosophy. He went on to say, "I believe that a
prospect something like this is the likelihood for the future of medicine. . . . I
think that schizophrenia will turn out to be a neurochemical disorder with some
central, *single* chemical event gone wrong" (p. 141).

That is, the seeming complexity of psychopathological conditions like
schizophrenia is illusory, just as the seeming complexity of tertiary syphilis is
illusory. Behind the complex and intricately connected series of psychological,
behavioral, cognitive, and interpersonal difficulties associated with schizophrenia lies a simple and beautifully straightforward causative agent—a single
neurochemical reaction gone awry. It is this neurochemical "deficit," speculated
Thomas, that will prove to be responsible for the initiation of a series of consequent dysfunctional reactions that, as they multiply, produce the complex
clinical picture associated with schizophrenia. Eliminate the neurochemical malfunction, and you will have before you a normally functioning individual. Identify the neurochemical defect, and you have discovered the "cause" of schizophrenia. Rectify or eliminate the defect, and you have discovered the "cure" as
well.

Juxtaposed with the traditional reductionistic approach represented by the
Thomas view is a second approach—usually called an *interactionalist* or *contextual
approach*—which has taken a very different stance with regard to the issue of
causality. Instead of seeing pathology as the result of a linear chain of cause-and-
effect reactions, this second approach views pathology in terms of malfunctional
interactions between factors or components within a system. The actual emergence of "pathology," according to this view, results from a *combination* of interacting elements that, when they interact in certain ways, *destabilize* a previously
smoothly functioning system.

In medicine, for example, this second view is well represented in George
Engel's influential essay, "The Need for a New Medical Model: A Challenge for
Biomedicine" (1977). In this essay, Engel explored the relative utility of the

traditional model of disease, which limits itself to somatic parameters, as contrasted with a "new model that attempts to incorporate psychosocial parameters as well" (p. 130). Thus, argued Engel, a medical model capable not only of understanding the determinants of a disease, but also of providing direction regarding rational treatments and patterns of health care, "must also take into account the patient, the social context in which he lives, and the complimentary system devised by society to deal with the disruptive effects of illness, that is, the physician role and the health care system" (p. 132).

In like fashion, epidemiologists like Cassel (1975) have, in their writings, taken on an area that has been one of the triumphs of the reductionistic-mechanistic scientific approach: the etiology of infectious disease. In keeping with the approach advocated by Engel, Cassel has argued that an appreciation of the factors leading to the onset of a disease (that is, the emergence of a pathological condition) requires a sophisticated understanding of the complex interactions that exist between infectious agent, host, and host environment. Thus, although in the classical laboratory experiment the "etiology" of a particular infectious disease was clearly shown to have been "caused" by a specific infectious agent, when one returned to the real-life situation it became quite apparent that the presence of the infectious agent *alone* did not invariably produce the disease condition. Instead, the emergence of pathology appeared to be influenced by a highly complex set of factors, many of which were related to the host environment. Thus, an understanding of pathology in the *in vivo* situation required a sophisticated appreciation of host–agent interaction.

Hence, argue interactionalists like Cassel, the crucial question becomes one of identifying the factors leading to a "breakdown" in the customary systemic regulatory processes. In the absence of agent-produced toxins, the unique pattern that the breakdown takes would not occur, and the specific infectious disease—say, pneumonia or syphilis—would not occur. But an appreciation of why bodily defenses were in some situations adequate and in others inadequate becomes as crucial an issue as the identification of the infectious agent itself. The "vulnerability" model of schizophrenia espoused by Zubin (1977) is an example of this approach applied to a psychopathological condition, and it illustrates how sharply the interactionalist perspective contrasts with the reductionist view of schizophrenia held by Lewis Thomas.

General Systems Theory

This debate, reflected in the juxtapositioning of the views of Lewis Thomas and of George Engel, is neither a new one nor one limited to the field of biomedicine. It has been enjoined in no small part because of the growing influence of concepts subsumed under the term *general systems theory*, a set of concepts that were specifically developed because of dissatisfaction with traditional reductionist-mechanistic approaches. As early as 1928, when Ludwig von Bertalanffy, the "father" of general systems theory, first introduced a series of concepts intended to provide the basis for an "organismic" approach to biology, he was doing so because of his belief that certain fundamentally important questions in biological science required a new and different approach. In particular, it was his feeling that an understanding of phenomena like growth and development could be substantially improved if attention were paid to those biological processes that lead to the increasing complexity of organization (of biological organisms).

Forty years later, von Bertalanffy (1968), still impressed by the currency of the inherent conflicts between reductionist and interactionalist approaches, provided the following historical view:

> In the biological, behavioral and sociological fields, there exist predominant problems which were neglected in classical science, or rather which did not enter into its considerations. If we look at a living organism, we observe an amazing order, organization, maintenance in continuous change, regulation and apparent etiology. Similarly, in human behavior goal-seeking and purposiveness cannot be overlooked, even if we accept a strictly behaviorist standpoint. However, concepts like organization, directiveness, etiology, etc., just do not appear in the classic system of science. As a matter of fact, in the so-called mechanistic world view based on classical physics, they were considered elusory or metaphysical. This means, to the biologist for example, that just the specific problems of living nature appeared to lie beyond the legitimate field of science. (p. 2)

The solution offered by von Bertalanffy is the *organismic* viewpoint, simply stated as follows: "In one brief sentence it means that organisms are organized things and, as biologists, we have to find out about it" (p. 2).

Almost 60 years after von Bertalanffy introduced the first of his systems concepts, general systems theory has found wide applicability in fields as diverse as community planning, computer science, systems engineering, operations research, human engineering, and, of course, family systems theory and family therapy. However, despite these successes, general systems theory still seems to many an unapproachable, foreign, and unfathomable set of concepts, best left to "think-tank" theoreticians or researchers well versed in multivariate statistics and computer simulation techniques. Given a choice, most of us would still prefer to see the world as structured along the lines proposed by classical reductionistic-mechanistic science. That is, we are preferentially drawn toward linear cause-and-effect models, impressed by their seeming clarity and elegance, and willing to put into action the "solutions" suggested by such equations.

This pull to the linear causal model seems particularly strong when we are dealing with pathological situations. Take the case of psychopathological behavior—our interest in this book. The emergence of hallucinations or of debilitating phobias, for example, is invariably viewed as evidence of a functional breakdown. Something has gone wrong, and reparative action (treatment) is therefore in order. As clinicians, we are under the gun; we are under pressure to appear sure-footed and to delineate a straightforward, confident treatment plan. Methods of problem analysis that yield clear-cut statements about the source and sight of pathology also tend to generate clear-cut instructions about how to rectify the deficit. Hence, they are powerfully attractive to us as conceptual models for exploring pathology and its treatment.

The systems theorists, however, tell us that such an approach to clinical problems is an illusory one. It is not that it is incorrect. After all, it is surely the case that syphilis will not occur in the absence of the specific infectious agent that initiates a functional destabilization of the human organism. Further, it is also the case that the use of medication specifically targeted at this infectious agent will arrest the pathological process. But it is not necessarily the case that this is the best solution to the pathological situation. Insofar as advocates of the reductionist approach reach the conclusion that the infectious agent is the "cause" of the disease process, the only logical treatment is one directed explicitly at this agent.

But if one says, instead, that dysfunctional or pathological situations are those in which breakdown of customary regulatory processes is undermining optimal organization of the organism's internal environment, then any action that helps the organism restore the integrity of its internal environment is an excellent "treatment" for the pathological condition. Removal of a noxious agent—be it a bacterial pathogen, an environmental toxin, a destabilizing drug like heroin or alcohol, or a sociopathic family member—is surely one possible solution. But an equally acceptable and, in some cases, more effective strategy is the bolstering of systemic regulatory processes—whether those be immunological defense mechanisms, support of cardiovascular stability, a societal policy that reduces the presence of noxious substances in the external environment, or bolstering of family communication networks to improve information processing within the family.

Thus, juxtaposed with the traditional explanatory approach to scientific questions is a new approach that focuses on interactions between elements in a system. Further, the particular focus of this new approach is on those patterns of interaction that serve to make possible and to sustain complexity and constancy of systemic organization and function. And this systemic approach is being urged on us, as clinicians, for two main reasons: first, because in many instances an adequate appreciation of pathology is best achieved within the context of a knowledge of the systemic properties of the organism under study; and second, because efficacious "treatment" of pathology is best planned if one keeps in mind the effect of various interventions on the organism as a system. Thus, a reductionist approach to pathology that, in the process of inquiry, leaves the original organism in unrecognizable shape can often lead the clinician astray. And correction of pathology in one part of the system may well overtly correct the presenting complaint, but only at the expense of a fundamental distortion of the organism's natural architecture and functional integrity.

In systems terms, the above two factors are encompassed in the deceptively simple axiomatic phrase, "The whole is greater than the sum of its parts." This statement, if taken at face value, means that no complex system can be fully understood if one adopts a strategy of breaking it down into its component and subcomponent parts. Instead, it has a uniqueness, an additional element, that is a product of the intricate structural and functional integration of these parts into a unified whole. So neither pathology nor treatment should be explored in the absence of a sophisticated understanding of this uniqueness.

So now we come to the issue of the family. But it has been preceded by the above long introduction because the clinician must understand, first and foremost, why one would advocate a family-focused approach to psychopathology in the first place. Why work with a system of such inherent complexity (the family) when a far less complex one (the individual) is readily available? Why take on a system that hasn't even been satisfactorily defined? (We are still struggling to come up with uniform criteria for determining family membership, for example, particularly as nontraditional families increase in number and variety.)

Individuals have obvious biological and physical integrity. They are clearly bounded in space. They have a relatively clear-cut inception (birth), life cycle, and demise. Although they are open systems, interacting with their environments, they carry out recognizable actions, have their own thoughts, have clearly defined anatomies, and so on. The inception and demise of a family, on the other hand, is an artificially and externally imposed punctuation of an ongoing, relatively continuous process. The family life cycle, a concept we will discuss at length later in the chapter, is in many ways an equally artificial concept. Family boundaries are more metaphorical than real. Family-level thought processes—be they myths, patterns of communication, family affective levels, or family paradigms—simply can't be grabbed hold of with the same sense of conviction as individual-level thought processes.

Clinical work with families can be equally puzzling and frustrating. The clinician takes on the task of meeting with a group of individuals who have an already established and shared history, an established set of rules and values, private codes for communication, and so on, all of them initially unknown to the therapist, and very different from—and for many clinicians, far more taxing than—the experience of interviewing and assessing an individual who has come alone to a strange environment (the clinician's office) to ask for help.

In the end, researchers and clinicians work with families because they believe that these naturally occurring behavioral systems simply cannot be ignored. Families clearly fit the most popular working definition of a system—a set of units with relationships among them—even if, at times, it is hard to identify all the units that should be included within a particular family. Defining the family as a system not only implies that the family is comprised of a set of units or elements (individuals) standing in some consistent relationship to one another, but further, that the behavior of the family system is best understood as a *product* of its organizational characteristics. Another way to say this is that individuals within the system are not entirely free to behave according to their individually determined drives, motivations, personality attributes, and so on; rather, they are constrained and shaped in their behavior by the nature of the relationships that they have with the other elements of the family system.

Here, then, is the same set of issues that we have been discussing up to this point, this time applied to the family. Instead of assuming that behavior is the product of a linear causal chain of factors and events (e.g., that depression is caused by an imbalance of CNS neurotransmittors, or that dissatisfaction in marriage is caused by an inability to resolve conflicting feelings toward parental love objects), behavior is seen as the product of the various interactive relationships and organizational characteristics of the family as a whole (e.g., problem hyperactivity in a child is seen as the product of a poor "goodness of fit" between the child's temperamental characteristics and the temperamental characteristics of the family as a system, or marital dysfunction is seen as a product of malfunctioning communication channels within the family system).

Note that this different way of defining pathology is applicable to an understanding of both individual and family-level pathological behavior. In the first instance, we talk about individual-level pathology as being influenced and shaped by the family context within which the individual lives. In the second instance, we talk about systemic properties of the family as contributing to dysfunctional outcomes. To be entirely consistent, of course, we should also talk about the nature of the fit between the family and its external environment. To be sure, this "ecological" approach to family pathology has had its strong proponents (Barker, 1968; Speck & Attneave, 1974). But the majority of clinicians have limited themselves to the two above areas, namely, the influence of the family environment on individual behavior and the conceptualization of pathology as family-system malfunctioning.

Both these approaches, of course, insofar as they introduce a systemic approach to the definition of pathology, have required us to discuss more fully the organizational characteristics of the family as a system. Paramount in these efforts has been the focus on organizational *patterns*—hence the focus on interactional behavior, structural patterning, and the balance or the stability of the system as a whole. The types of coalitions existing within the families, the way in which the families are organized into subsystems (e.g., parental subsystem and marital subsystem), and the nature of the family's internal and external boundaries have also received a great deal of attention as useful ways of describing systemic characteristics of the family.

But it is important to note as well that whether the primary focus is on the family as a family or on the family as the environmental context for the individual, treatment approaches in both instances suggest that efforts directed at changing the nature of families' organizational properties will be efficacious in diminishing pathological behavior. In the first instance, the attraction of family therapy as a clinical intervention is obvious. But even in the second instance, the premise that individual behavior is significantly determined and shaped by the organizational characteristics of the family in which the individual lives is also the single most compelling reason for family therapy as an intervention technique. For if this premise is true, then presumably individual behavior can also be effectively changed by altering the organizational and functional characteristics of the family system.

Thus, even if pathology is defined in individual terms (as it has been and for the most part probably will continue to be in those diagnostic systems in widespread clinical use), it is nevertheless plausible that a more efficacious way of altering pathological behavior is to address the systemic environment in which the behavior is occurring—hence the development of family therapy approaches for the treatment of behavioral disorders, addictions, individual developmental crises, sexual dysfunction, psychomotor abnormalities, management of chronic illness, and the like—all individually based disorders.

But in this chapter, we will be focusing primarily on the family as a system in its own right. It is with this goal in mind that we move on to a discussion of the core constructs of living systems as applied to the family.

THE CORE CONCEPTS OF FAMILY SYSTEMS THEORY

Although family systems theory comes in many shapes and forms, all versions owe primary allegiance to general systems concepts as applied to living systems. In their book *General Systems Theory and Psychiatry* (1969), Gray, Duhl, and Rizzo described this general systems perspective as follows. Systems theory is

> a logical-mathematical field which deals with the new scientific doctrines of wholeness, dynamic interaction, and organization. It is a new approach to the unity-of-science problem which sees organization rather than reduction as the unifying principal, and which therefore searches for general structural isomorphisms in systems. (p. 7)

The most widely accepted definition of a system is that it is a series of elements arranged in some consistent and enduring relationship with each other (Miller, 1965). The key to the definition is therefore the notion of consistency of relationships. The arrangement of elements is not random, but patterned— hence the focus on the way these elements are organized and on a description not only of the relationships themselves but of the organization of the whole. Thus, the key notions introduced in systems theory are *wholeness, organization,* and *relationships.* These notions, in turn, are being championed instead of the reductionist, cause-and-effect, and mechanistic-functional views.

Living systems (such as families) are unique in two additional respects. The first is that they are *open* systems. That is, their boundary characteristics allow for selective and patterned input of energy from the surrounding environment. The availability of an external supply of energy, in turn, permits growth to occur; that is, living systems tend to become increasingly complex over time. The second unique characteristic of living systems is their ability to reproduce themselves.

The application of general systems concepts to living systems, therefore, places particular emphasis on the above two characteristics. Family systems theory, one such application, has as its primary goals the following tasks: (a) a description of the unique organizational characteristics of families; (b) an identification of the dynamic qualities of family functioning and family structures that help families regulate (pattern) the constancy of their internal and external relationships; and (c) a description of family growth and development with particular emphasis on the factors that make *patterned* growth possible.

With these tasks in mind, we can say that family systems theory can be seen to comprise three core concepts, all of them distillations of basic tenets of "pure" systems theory as applied to living systems:

The first of these concepts is *organization.* Family systems theory borrows from general systems theory a series of descriptive and often metaphorical constructs in an effort to succinctly and constructively draw attention to the important organizational characteristics of families as systems.

The second core concept is *morphostasis*. This term refers to a fundamentally important characteristic of all living systems, namely, that living systems function as *steady states*. That is, despite their dynamism, families are able to maintain a remarkable consistency of their organizational characteristics over time. In an effort to appreciate better the functional characteristics of living systems that allow them to maintain this constancy, systems theorists have hypothesized the existence of a series of control or regulatory mechanisms. Thus, a discussion of this second core concept will lead us to an examination of the regulatory mechanisms characteristic of family systems.

The third core concept is *morphogenesis*. Here, the focus is not so much on mechanisms of control and on constancy of relationships over time as on systemic growth and development. Once again largely descriptive, this core concept addresses both the characteristic ways in which family systems change over time (the family life cycle) and the energy sources that fuel this increase in organizational complexity.

Another way of looking at these three core concepts is to appreciate that family systems are the product of the constant dynamic interplay of morphogenetic (growth) forces and morphostatic (control) forces. This dynamic interplay, structured, in turn, by the organizational characteristics of the system, produces both the patterned internal relationships *and* the patterned changes over time that differentiate a living system from a random and functionally unrelated set of phenomena.

In large part, the differences that have emerged in the various versions of family systems theory that have been advanced over the years are the products either of an emphasis placed on one core concept to the detriment of others, or of a selective embracing of one or two of the many constructs that have been advanced as descriptive metaphors for the core concept of organization. We will be illustrating some of these differences at a later point in the chapter. But suffice it to say at this point that whatever its individual coloration, all versions of family systems theory are built around the three core concepts of living systems noted above.

The Concept of Organization

The core concept of organization is the most fundamental one in systems theory. In effect, it is virtually synonymous with the concept of a system. After all, if our definition of a system is that it is a set of elements in a consistent relationship or interactional stance to each other, this definition clearly implies that any system is composed of elements that are *organized* because and by the nature of their relationships. Because living systems are dynamic in their characteristics, the consistency of the organizational relationships between elements is clearly relevant. But this relativity is highly skewed in the direction of patterning and predictability.

When describing family systems, the convention is to think of the systemic elements as the individuals within the family. Functional family systems, therefore, must have relative membership constancy. Although it is possible to build a case that family membership may include persons who are not functionally involved in the daily life of the family—for example, family heroes or rogues who play mythic roles in family discussions explicating behavioral rules or values—most family therapists have identified the functional family system as those individuals whose constancy of contact and relationships produce predictable patterns of functional behavior, behavior that, in turn, can be relied on for systems maintenance.

On the other hand, it is possible to say that the elements in the family system are behaviors rather than individuals. Within such a conceptualization, organizational constancy describes the relationships that exist between types of behaviors. The individuals carrying out these behaviors are of secondary importance within such a model. A descriptive model centered on the concept of functional role—one of the popular sociological views of family—would be an example here (Parsons & Bales, 1955; Pitts, 1964). Although in traditional families role distribution may be such that the same individuals carry out a particular role time after time, nontraditional family forms incorporate flexibility of role behavior.

In some ways, this "behavioral" model is more consistent with a pure systems approach than is the "membership" approach. Behavioral analyses, for example, have led to suggestions that balanced family systems must include certain mixtures of growth-inducing and systems-maintaining behaviors. Within such an analysis, the behavior of any individual within the family is, to a significant degree, *constrained* and *dictated* by the behavior of other members of the system. "Radical" behavior on one member's part establishes a context that is likely to induce "conservative" behaviors elsewhere within the family system. The overall *combination* of behaviors, however, remains within some relatively consistent range characteristic of that particular family system. It is an analysis of this type that has led to the suggestion that aberrant (pathological) behavior on the part of an individual within the family is not so much the product of a diathesis within that individual as it is the product of the overall combination of behaviors within the system—hence the suggestion, for example, that acting out behavior on the part of an adolescent is the product of or is made possible because of system-level incongruities or regulatory mechanism failures, rather than the product of a personality or conduct disorder in the individual herself or himself.

Thus, the concept of organization, although a basic one for all systemic models of the family, nevertheless leaves ample room for a wide diversity of descriptive models to have emerged. Nevertheless, if one reviews these various models, it becomes apparent that all models rely heavily on three principles in describing the organizational characteristics of families. These principles are that of the "wholeness" of a family system; the functional significance of "boundaries" in defining the family's organizational characteristics; and the importance of "hierarchical" structures as organizational patterns.

Wholeness. This principle refers to the system axiom that the whole is greater than the additive sum of its separate parts. As has already been mentioned, although deceptively simple as a statement and by now quite familiar because of its repetition in theoretical writings about the family, it remains perhaps the most radical statement in family systems theory. It proposes, in effect, that no family can be adequately understood or totally explained once it has been subdivided into its component parts. Whether by *parts* a clinician is referring to the individuals in the family or to the functional components of the system, the statement still applies. Furthermore, this principle implies that no single element or subgroup of elements within the family can be thought of as acting independently. Instead, the family must be thought of as an organized entity in which "the state of each unit is constrained by, conditioned by, or dependent on the state of other units" (Miller, 1965, p. 68).

The implications of this principle for our understanding of family psychopathology lie mainly in the area of causality. According to this principle, descriptive terms such as *flexibility* and *rigidity, reactivity,* and *affective warmth* and *coolness* are terms that can be appropriately applied to the family group as a system. Further, one must not assume that a dimension of the family (e.g., its characteristic affective level) can be understood as the simple combination of the characteristic affects displayed by the various family members. The holistic systems approach has also forced on us the use of a *descriptive* language, rather than a causative language, in attempting to understand family behavior. For example, pathology in a family system might be defined in terms of the relative coherence or lack of coherence of the various elements of the system as they attempt to establish a unified whole (Dell, 1982). "Goodness-of-fit" models, therefore, become attractive; linear causal models are, of course rejected.

Nevertheless, it has thus far proved to be an insurmountable challenge to develop an adequate descriptive language for the principle of wholeness that can be used as the basis of a theory of family pathology. Suffice it to say for now that the most important consequence of the application of the principle of wholeness to family systems is the recognition that a language describing family *personality* is a legitimate venture. Hence, efforts to describe phenomena such as family cognitive styles, family share constructs (paradigms), family temperament, and family sense of coherence are all legitimized.

Boundaries. If systems are elements relating in a consistent fashion, then they are also elements bounded by the nature of the relationships between them. This bounding process can be thought of as taking place either in a spatial context or in a time context, but for both these contexts, the clarity of the boundary that emerges is directly proportional to the clarity of the pattern determined by relationships.

The notion that families can be thought of as bounded in space and time is an extremely popular one. Most versions of family systems theory place great emphasis not only on family boundaries, but also on the metaphor of boundary permeability (the ease or difficulty that outside persons or elements experience in moving into or out of the family system). In some models, most notably the structural model, the characteristics of family boundaries are perhaps the single most important determinant of relative functionality or dysfunctionality of the family system.

Nevertheless, it is important to remember that the concept of boundaries as applied to the family system is largely a metaphorical one. When the relationship of elements in space is so highly patterned that a physical boundary can be easily identified, the system identified can be physically perceived (seen, felt). A single ·cell, or an animal, is an example. The concept of a family system obviously has no such clear-cut boundaries, but notions of organization demand that they be described. Most diagrammatic illustrations of family structure invariably include these metaphorical boundaries, with solid or dotted lines used to represent the relative permeability of the boundaries being described.

It is relatively easy in looking at these diagrams to conjure up physical images of family boundaries and to supply anecdotal material in support of these images. One can imagine, for example, that a family boundary could be likened to the physical boundaries that families set up in their homes. The family that lives with constantly locked doors, electronic alarm systems, and high bushes seems quite different in character from one in which the door always seems to be open and the movement of neighborhood children in and out of the family's home occurs without a second thought. It must be kept in mind, of course, that such pictures are merely surface phenomena reflective of a presumed underlying structure that cannot be directly assessed, as would be the case if one were assessing membrane permeability in a living cell.

Most systems models emphasizing boundary permeability as a central concept suggest that semipermeable boundaries are the most functional. It is important to the health of the family system, according to these models, that the family have easy access to its external environment, but that movement in and out of the family not be so fluid as to cause a blurring of the family's organizational characteristics. As one example, Skynner (1976), in introducing the concept of boundary in his family systems model, described its critical importance as follows:

> Failure of the boundary to restrict exchange across it leads to a loss of difference between the living thing and its surroundings, of its separate identity; instead there develops an identity of inside and outside, one meaning of death. Too impermeable a boundary, preventing any exchange, brings another form of death, the fixed and stained tissue we see beneath the microscope. (p. 5)

Family systems models pay as much attention to the nature of internal family boundaries as they do to the boundaries between the family and its external environment. These internal boundaries serve to differentiate between the various subsystems within the family. Although the terms *coalition* and *alignment* have also been used to describe the internal organizational structure of the family, the point is that, internally, the holistic family system is, in turn, divided into a series of subsystems (e.g., parental subsystem, spouse subsystem, and sexual subsystem) (Aponte & Van Deusen, 1981; Haley, 1976). Once again, the relative permeability of these internal boundaries (often described as their relative flexibility or rigidity) is used to describe the functional constraints under which the family must operate, constraints that, in turn, define the functional adaptability of the family in the face of stressor situations (Minuchin, Rosman, & Baker, 1978).

Hierarchies. The third principle related to organization of the family system is that of hierarchical organization. The notion here is that the family's internal organizational characteristics are such that its various subsystems can be thought of as arranged in hierarchical fashion, the specifics of the hierarchy, in turn, determining the functional properties of the different subsystems. Once again, the emphasis is on a conceptualization of the family as organized along ordered and highly structured lines, with clearly identifiable differential lines of complexity that relate in logical fashion one to another.

This principle also alerts us to the importance of placing the family within an external environment that is itself hierarchically structured. Thus, community systems, religious systems, extended-family systems, national allegiances, and so on all have relevance to the intricate network of interrelationships that both provide resources to the family and operate as constraints within which the family must function in carrying out its various tasks.

The Concept of Morphostasis

The second core concept of family systems theory refers to the fact that families behave in patterned and predictable fashions because, as systems, they operate according to morphostatic (regulatory) principles. That is, families tend to establish a sense of balance or stability and to resist any change from this predetermined level of stability. A number of metaphorical terms have been used to describe this phenomenon. The two most frequently used metaphors are *homeostasis* and *cybernetic regulation.* Both these terms describe the capacity of living systems to maintain the *constancy* of their environments in the face of external change. The popularity of these metaphors reflects the fact that morphostasis, despite its name, is meant to be a dynamic concept in that it centers on a description of how families maintain organizational and functional integrity in the face of potential internal and external disruptions.

It is a basic assumption of clinicians and researchers working with families that family behavior is patterned. Yet, when one stops to think about it, the degree of regularity and stability of behavior evident in most families is a truly remarkable phenomenon. After all, the family is constantly being subjected to a potentially overwhelming series of challenges. It is challenged from outside by economic forces, political decisions, and the demands of larger organizations in which it holds membership. It is also challenged from within: its individual members have their own agendas, psychological needs, and physical requisites.

Aware of the existence of this multiplicity of internal and external stresses, the family systems theorist is impressed by the ability of the family to maintain and control these challenges. Despite living in a constantly changing environment, and despite sudden and unpredictable encounters, the family maintains a sense of balance, coherence, and regularity. It is not surprising, therefore, that systems theorists have hypothesized the existence of powerful "built-in" mechanisms, the purpose of which is to regulate family life by providing the rules and organizational structure that govern sequential behavioral processes.

Because the family behaves *as if* it is governed by underlying regulatory principles, theorists have also inferred the existence of specific *regulatory mechanisms* that bring this all about—hence the attraction not only to metaphors such as homeostasis, but the proposal, as well, of specific mechanisms that serve to regulate family life (the term *homeostatic mechanisms* is frequently applied, for example, to specific sequences of behaviors observed in clinical settings).

To summarize, systems theorists point to organizational and functional constancy as one of the core features of living systems. Family systems theorists have described a comparable phenomenon existing in families, namely, that families evidence a remarkable degree of organizational and behavioral constancy (predictability) despite the numerous challenges to stability that they experience. A corollary assumption is that this constancy is maintained because the family has available to it a set of regulatory mechanisms that are called into play whenever potential disruptions arise. However, these mechanisms remain largely metaphorical in that no successful strategies for systematically measuring them have thus far been suggested.

In the rest of this section, we will detail two of the descriptive metaphors that have been proposed as descriptors of regulatory (control) principles in families.

Family Homeostasis. Family homeostasis is a term first introduced by Don Jackson (1957, 1965b), one of the pioneers of family systems theory. It is a notion borrowed from the physiological concept of homeostasis (Cannon, 1939), but one that also relies heavily on concepts of cybernetic regulation as described by Norbert Wiener (1961).

Briefly put, the physiological-cybernetic argument is as follows: The functions that keep a biological organism "alive" all operate most efficiently when the organism's internal environment is maintained within certain optimal ranges. For the human being, these internal environmental factors are temperature, rates of oxygenation, barometric pressure, electrolyte balance, and so on. But the external environment does not restrict itself to these optimal limits. Hence, mechanisms exist that ensure a consistent internal environment despite a potentially hostile external environment (hostile in the sense that it is too hot or too cold, or too wet or too dry, and so on).

In the human organism, environmental constancy is maintained by neuronal and hormonal mechanisms, which Cannon called collectively "homeostatic mechanisms." The key elements in this process are a series of peripheral "servomechanisms" that act as sensory devices appraising the current state of the environment and feeding this information to a central processing unit, the brain. Output (action) takes the form of an integrated series of responses that are constantly being adjusted or modified as revised information about the environment is fed back to the central processing unit by the peripheral sensors.

Thus, the essential features of this model of regulation are threefold: (a) the need to maintain the internal environment within its limited range because optimal functioning is achieved within that range; (b) the existence of sensory devices to continually monitor important environmental parameters; and (c) the presence of coordinated input–output mechanisms arranged in a series of reverberating circular loops (feedback loops).

Jackson's application of the concept of homeostasis to family systems closely followed the physiological version. Thus, emphasis was placed on the need to maintain internal stability and to resist any change from that predetermined level of stability, presumably because optimal family functioning occurs within the range established by the organizational and behavioral balances that the family has established. Further, Jackson proposed that a series of mechanisms whose primary purpose is the maintenance of an acceptable behavioral balance within the family can be identified. Clinical observations of sequential patterns of behavior within the family in the face of disruptive events were hypothesized to represent the family equivalent of positive and negative feedback loops as postulated in the physiological model.

Also implied in Jackson's version of family homeostasis are a set of devices or mechanisms within the family, devices that "go off" when stability is threatened and set in motion the behavioral mechanisms that restore the family to its prior organizational and functional balance. Clinical examples of these processes at work often suggest that one member of the family serves as a family thermostat or servomechanism (a term borrowed from cybernetics) and, through exaggerated or symptomatic behavior, initiates a sequence of interactional behaviors that are the surface manifestations of underlying regulatory mechanisms at work. For example, a clinician may hypothesize that the promiscuous behavior of an adolescent family member is a reaction to a growing estrangement in the marital subsystem (perhaps stimulated by disruptive forces coming from involvement in external work or social networks), an estrangement that threatens the fundamental balance and stability of the family (Haley, 1980). The consequence of the adolescent's behavior, the reengagement of the parents, restores the prior organizational balance of the family and is thus seen as a type of homeostatic mechanism at work. As another example, alcoholic behavior has, in some instances, been seen as serving the purpose of maintaining the relative impermeability of some alcoholic families vis-à-vis a potentially intrusive external environment (Steinglass, Davis, & Berenson, 1977).

Family homeostasis, were it to closely follow the example of its physiological-cybernetic cousin, would be viewed as a largely positive and necessary component of family life that serves the purpose of keeping the family on an even keel. The mechanisms that families mobilize to deal with environmental challenges are as important to the ongoing viability of the family system as, for example, temperature regulation is to the viability of the biological organism. However, it has become common parlance in clinical settings to apply the term *homeostasis* instead to situations in which therapeutic change is being *resisted* by the family.

Increasingly, this tendency to equate homeostasis with resistance has given the term a pejorative quality. This trend is an unfortunate one. We must be impressed with the intricate and delicate series of mechanisms that families bring to bear on what might otherwise be an impossibly complex and varied external and internal environment. Instead of being constantly buffeted by the vagaries of environmental demands, the mechanisms being referred to allow the family to establish constancy, to define structure, and to carry out predictable, patterned, purposeful, and, at times, even adaptive sets of behaviors. However, it is also true that these mechanisms can, in certain instances, become overbearing and rigid. In such circumstances, the status quo becomes an end in itself, in much the same fashion as bureaucracies lose sight of their original purpose and become organized around the perpetuation of the existing structure. In such circumstances, regulatory principles come to have a tyrannizing effect on the family mandating that behavior will restrict itself to certain narrow, predetermined levels. Environmental changes, instead of being assessed for their potential in offering the family interesting new life options, are seen instead only as challenges to the family's integrity. But it would be a mistake to confuse this dysfunctional extreme with the more normative situation in which family homeostasis plays a crucial *supportive* role in family life.

But what about those situations in which homeostatic mechanisms seem to have gone awry? The physiological model suggests three ways in which homeostatic mechanisms may malfunction. The first would be a failure of peripheral sensors. The sensors may, for one reason or another, simply be exhausted and unable to function properly. Or the change that is occurring in the environment is one that the sensing mechanisms are simply not in a position to ascertain. For example, biological organisms have no built-in sensors to monitor environmental levels of radiation.

Second, response patterns may be ineffective or inappropriate, perhaps because of a failure of the central processing unit to correctly interpret incoming data and to activate an appropriate response, or because of a failure of the response system itself. For example, heart disease or peripheral vessel disease makes it impossible to adequately control blood pressure no matter what signals are being set out.

And third, "failure" may occur as a result of servomechanisms that have an inappropriately "set" optimal range (that is, homeostatic mechanisms that have been set to maintain an optimal range that is either inappropriately wide or inappropriately narrow).

If we move back to families once again, we can envision failures in homeostasis arising from the same three sources. Some families simply cannot sense when their internal environment has moved an unacceptable distance from its optimal range. Other families are perfectly capable of sensing that something is wrong, but they mobilize either inappropriate or ineffective behavioral programs in response to this information. And finally, some families have established inappropriately narrow or inappropriately wide environmental limits for the activation of corrective homeostatic mechanisms. When the systems theorist talks about a family as having a dysfunctional "rigidity" of regulatory mechanisms, he or she is most likely referring to a tendency in the family to set its internal thermostats at an inappropriately narrow range. Homeostatic response mechanisms are too easily activated in such a family. The slightest change in the environment calls for reactions that, in dictatorial fashion, maintain overall stability and predictability within the family's internal environment.

Homeostasis has been the most popular metaphor yet suggested for how morphostatic principles operate in families. Recently, however, it has come under criticism as a possibly flawed concept. In particular, the concern has been that homeostasis is increasingly viewed as a causative agent rather than as a construct describing an underlying systemic property of the family. In the most influential of the published critiques of the concept of homeostasis, Dell (1982) argued that homeostasis is inappropriately defined when it is thought of as a functional and concrete entity rather than as a property of the family. As he expressed it, it is an error to talk of family behavior as occurring *because* of homeostasis, as if the behavior had been *caused* by the family's prevailing interest in maintaining the status quo. In like fashion, he was highly critical of the use of the term *homeostatic mechanism* as applied to specific behavior exhibited by the family (especially symptoms), for example, the contention that the *purpose* of a behavior like the abusive use of a drug or the expression of delusional thinking is to return the family to its homeostatic level.

Dell suggested instead that the concept of *homeostasis* really applies to a fundamental property of coherence—"a congruent interdependence in functioning whereby all the aspects of the system fit together" (p. 31)—which is characteristic of all systems. Furthermore, systemic coherence is not a static phenomenon but an evolving (changing) one: every time the system "behaves," it impacts (in recursive fashion) on all parts of the system. As Dell pointed out, the concept of *coherence* also implies that the notion of resistance is an outmoded and incorrect one. That is, it is incorrect to say that a family resists change; instead, says Dell, "it only behaves in accordance with its own organized coherence" (p. 28).

For many family clinicians, the arguments put forward by Dell, based as they are on notions of epistemology, seem overly formidable and unapproachable. Yet, at the core of his argument, Dell was alerting us to the dangers of applying too literally a set of descriptive metaphors and treating them as if they were concrete entities. At the same time, however, it is unlikely that family clinicians will agree to abandon this construct in the near future. As noted by Hoffman (1981):

> Dell replaces homeostasis with a new concept, that of coherence. Coherence has to do with how pieces of a system fit together in a balance internal to itself and external to its environment. Homeostasis has a more rubbery, punchy feel to it than coherence, which is why I hate to give it up (and won't) but coherence is purer in the epistemological sense. (p. 348)

Family Temperament. Family homeostasis is a construct that addresses the structures and behaviors used by the family to deal with potentially destabilizing forces in its environment. The emphasis is on the maintenance of an internally constant environment. Although it is acknowledged that families differ in their predilections for types of regulatory mechanisms, "optimal" behavioral ranges, and relative rigidity or flexibility of feedback mechanisms, these differences manifest themselves primarily in the interaction between the family and its environment. Less attention is paid in these constructs to the actual character of this internal environment that the family is seeking to maintain.

As any observant clinician is aware, families vary dramatically in the character and flavor of their internal environments. The degree of orderliness brought to the structuring of their daily routines, the predilection for physical and verbal contact, and the use of space at home are only three of the many ways in which these differences between families manifest themselves. The construct of *family temperament* (Steinglass, 1981) has been proposed as a useful metaphor for an underlying regulatory principle in families that may account for these dramatic differences in how families structure their internal environments.

Temperament is a psychological construct, a term originally applied to a set of enduring behavioral response styles and activity patterns in individuals that have their origins in early life (Thomas & Chess, 1977; Thomas, Chess, & Birth, 1968). As they manifest themselves in the behavior of newborns, temperamental dimensions have been described as ninefold: activity level, rhythmicity, approach–withdrawal behavior, adaptability, threshold of responsiveness, intensity of reaction, quality of mood, distractibility, and attention span and persistence. Thomas and Chess characterized these dimensions as reflecting the "how" rather than the "what" of behavior, for example, the difference between crying (a content or "what" judgment) and persistant crying (a temperament or "how" judgment). Findings from Thomas and Chess's New York Longitudinal Study suggest that early temperamental characteristics persist well into childhood (1984). There is also keen interest in demonstrating temperamental continuities into adolescent and early adult developmental stages (Lerner, Palermo, Spiro, & Nesselroade, 1982).

In developmental psychology, the concept of *temperament* has proved particularly helpful in interpreting "interactive data" and the changes in behavior that occur when individuals are placed in different environmental contexts (Goldsmith & Campos, 1981; Thomas & Chess, 1984). Why is it, for example, that the same child exhibits different patterns of behavior when placed in a closed versus an open classroom environment? The interactionalist argument is that the child's temperamental characteristics potentially "fit" with the environmental characteristic of one classroom but "clash" with another—hence the development of the "goodness-of-fit" hypothesis as an explanation for certain developmental phenomenon.

In our own work focusing on in-home observations of family behavior, we have used an on-line coding system—the Home Observation Assessment Method (HOAM) (Steinglass, 1979)—to delineate the underlying dimensions of family temperament in a study of alcoholic families. Each family was observed on nine separate occasions over a 6-month time block (Steinglass, 1981), with the aim of providing systematic recordings of seven different aspects of the subject's behavior: (a) the subject's physical location in the home; (b) the identity of other people in the room with the subject; (c) the physical distance between the subject and others in the home when they were talking to each other; (d) basic interaction rates, both physical and verbal; (e) the content of selected verbal exchanges that involved decision making; (f) the affective level of the selected verbal exchanges coded; and (g) the outcome of the verbal exchanges coded.

After the HOAM data were collected, they were factor-analyzed to disclose what, if any, underlying dimensions of family temperament were reflected in family home behavior. The most interpretable solution yielded five factors:

1. *Intrafamily engagement*—a measure of the extent to which the family members were in physical and verbal contact with each other.
2. *Distance regulation*—a measure of the family's use of space in the home,

including family members' proclivity for interacting with each other when in the same location, their rate of movement around the house, and the proportion of time they spent alone.

3. *Extrafamily engagement*—a measure of the extent to which nonfamily members were present during the coding sessions.

4. *Structural variability*—a measure of the family's variability of interactional behavior and physical movement from one coding session to another.

5. *Content variability*—a measure of the extent to which decision-making behavior and variability of affect associated with verbal interaction were characteristic of the family.

Analyses of the stability of the HOAM dimensions over the 6 months of observation indicated that they were highly stable; that is, not only was there consistency in activity levels if one compared the first 3 months of observation with the last 3 months of observation, but even more striking, the families maintained their rank order regarding their variability measures. Thus, the families that were highly predictable during the first 3 months of observation remained so for the rest of the study, whereas those families that showed much greater variability of behavior from observation session to observation session continued to do so for the second half of the study as well. These "stability" findings have been further buttressed by 2-year follow-up data collected on a subsample of the original group of families. Once again, the findings suggested that the families' rank orders remained stable over the 2-year period.

Thus, if, as we suspect, the HOAM was tapping into behavioral manifestations of underlying family temperament, these temperamental properties were quite stable across time. This stability is important to demonstrate if one is to draw analogies between the concepts of family temperament and individual temperament.

Based on the data emerging from the above study, we are currently hypothesizing that family temperament is a product of three fundamental properties of family personality: the family's energy level, its preferred interactional distance, and its characteristic behavior range. These three temperamental properties, in turn, exercise a regulatory function for the family by, in effect, establishing a set of acceptable guidelines within which family behavior tends to occur. The family's energy level establishes guidelines about behavioral activity; the family's preferred interactional distance establishes guidelines regarding boundary permeability (of both internal and external boundaries); and the family's behavioral range establishes guidelines about the degree of variability that the family manifests in its patterns of interactional behavior.

Once these guidelines are in place, we would hypothesize that the family develops a set of recognizable behavioral traits, traits that are the observable correlates of its underlying temperamental properties. These traits, in turn, are the behavioral manifestations that clinicians focus on when they use descriptive phrases like "high-energy versus low-energy" families, "hot versus cool" families, "flexible versus rigid" families (high versus low tolerance for novelty) and so forth.

This work, obviously in its infancy, has not yet tackled the question of whether different temperamental styles could be considered more or less functional for the family. Thus far, the focus has instead been on goodness-of-fit hypotheses. For example, there is considerable interest in the question of whether different temperamental styles are more or less receptive to the presence of a chronically disturbed or chronically physically ill family member. That is, does family temperament have something to do with the relative propensity of a particular family to organize its life around a chronic illness, a clinical phenomenon increasingly discussed in the literature (Steinglass, Bennett, Wolin, & Reiss, 1987)? As has been the case in developmental psychology, many questions are amenable to the goodness-of-fit hypothesis, but strategies for demonstrating their validity have thus far lagged behind hypothesis generation in this field.

The Concept of Morphogenesis: How Families Grow

We come now to the third core concept of family systems theory: morphogenesis of family growth. We noted earlier in the chapter that general systems theory first emerged out of a crisis generated by the difficulties that traditional science had in dealing with questions related to the increasing organizational complexity of living systems over time. Another way of saying this is that traditional science couldn't deal with the problem of the growth and development of living systems. It is therefore somewhat ironic that families systems theory for many years seemed to have forgotten entirely about issues related to family development. Instead, the fascination with family regulatory processes, especially homeostasis, dominated the field. Families were increasingly viewed as relatively static entities primarily interested in maintaining the status quo. Accustomed to working with families over relatively short time periods, clinicians often conceptualized their task as being the combating or altering of the stifling effects of homeostatic mechanisms within the family. Little attention was paid either to the importance of developmental transitions in generating the clinical crises in the first place, or to the growth-inducing consequences of an alteration of family regulatory processes.

In a 1970 article, Speer raised the rhetorical question "Is homeostasis enough?" as a way of drawing attention to the imbalance noted above. In this paper, Speer spelled out some of the negative consequences of a model "in which the family is viewed as a cybernetic, error-activated, self-correcting system" (p. 261). Basically, if one takes such a view of the family, any stimulus or event that produces a change in the status quo is reacted to by the family as if it were a noxious, threatening agent, one that must be overcome in the service of systems stability. There is obviously very little room in such a conceptualization for phenomena associated with systemic growth and increasing organizational complexity. If these phenomena are to be accounted for, as they obviously must be if family systems theory is to build on general systems concepts, then greater attention must be given to the core concept of morphogenesis. As Dell (1982) pointed out in reviewing Speer's critique of family systems approaches, there is a "supreme irony of founding an approach to therapeutic change on a theory of how systems do not change" (p. 23).

In the years since Speer's article was published, increasing attention has been paid to family growth and development. This interest has generated a series of concepts about family development that can be roughly divided into two groups: those that focus on *change* and those that focus on *growth*.

When the focus is on change, concepts attempt to address questions of how and why alterations occur in the systemic organization of the family. Most often, change is conceptualized as a systemic response to an event or process that is disrupting family homeostasis, a response that, rather than returning the family to a prior status quo, leads to organizational alterations. Much has been made in these discussions of the need to differentiate responses that entail a *realignment* of existing family organizational patterns (first-order change) from those that entail a *restructuring* of the family (second-order change) (Watzlawick, Weakland, & Fisch, 1974).

Second-order change, the more dramatic situation (in that it is associated with a fundamental systemic restructuring), is more likely as well to be associated with greater organizational complexity. It is characteristically described as occurring only when destabilizing crises (problems) arise that can not be managed by the family through conventional means, thereby increasing the likelihood that a nonlogical "solution" to the problem will occur, a solution that entails the systemic restructuring described above. The probability that second-order change will occur is thought to be substantially increased when the family is placed in a paradoxical situation—hence the growing popularity of therapeutic interventions based on principles of paradox (Selvini-Palazzoli *et al.*, 1978; Weeks & L'Abate, 1982).

A second construct introduced as explanatory of family systems change is the positive or "deviation-amplifying" feedback loop (Maruyama, 1963). Although initially described as a self-destructive mechanism, the positive feedback loop is now thought to have functional possibilities as well, depending on the circumstances in which it arises (Hoffman, 1971). For example, changes in family rules necessitated by biologically determined alterations in family structure (e.g., births, deaths, and natural aging processes) are facilitated by behaviors that deviate from currently accepted family norms. These behaviors, if amplified, result in systemic changes that better accommodate the family's new reality.

So much for systems concepts of change. In contrast to the more general notion of change, *growth* is a term that should be reserved for a type of change that is *predictable*. It is a term that implies a pattern of change that occurs according to a recognizable framework. Usually, this means changes that occur in a characteristic sequential order and follow a typical time sequence. Although individual variation may be great, a normative pattern can be identified, and aberrant growth patterns can therefore be clearly spotted when they are occurring. This predictable pattern of change, as it has been conceptualized in family systems theory, is encompassed in the concept of the *family life cycle*.

Just as the more general concepts of change noted above have had a major impact on clinical practice, so, too, has the concept of the family life cycle had its impact on clinical practice (e.g., Carter & McGoldrick, 1980; Haley, 1973). Not only has interest centered on the relationship between developmental crises and the emergence of clinical symptoms, but the psychoanalytic concepts of fixation and regression have also been interpreted as metaphors applicable to developmental aberrations in families (Barnhill & Longo, 1978). It is this concept of growth that probably fits more closely with the systemic notion of morphogenesis than the more general notions of change. For after all, when general systems theorists refer to characteristic increases in the organizational complexity of living systems, they are referring to predictable rather than nonrandom changes. Biological growth or development has always been thought of as patterned. Hence, we will focus this part of our discussion on the emerging concepts of the family life cycle.

A second issue arises when one is discussing growth and development in families. Not only is it important to develop descriptive models of characteristic life cycles, but it is also necessary to look for the energy source that presumably fuels this growth process. At one level, this is a relatively simple task. In that families are living systems, one can focus on the same energy sources that are traditionally thought of as the "fuel" for growth: heat, light, essential nutrients, and so on. The sociologist's emphasis on the provision of food and shelter as a fundamental task of families could easily be interpreted as an awareness of the importance of these energy sources to family growth (Duvall, 1971). But systems theorists have been more intrigued by a very different energy source—*information*—and we will therefore discuss this issue as well in this section on family growth and development.

The Family Life Cycle. The concept of the family life cycle was first suggested by the sociologists Evelyn Duvall and Reuben Hill in the late 1940s. The Duvall–Hill model (Duvall, 1971; Hill, 1970) derived directly from an application of Erik Erickson's psychosocial developmental model (1963) to families. The Eriksonian model was built around four central constructs: epigenesis, sequential developmental staging, developmental tasks, and developmental transitions. As modified for the family, a descriptive developmental model emerged in which families were seen as moving through a series of clearly definable, sequential *developmental stages*. Further, the order of these stages was thought to be invariate (in much the same way as the invariate sequential movement through the "eight stages of man" that Erikson proposed as the fundamental psychosocial life cycle of the individual). Thus, family development is seen as occurring in a fixed order, an order that is never violated. Further, each developmental step is built on the preceding steps, in hierarchical fashion. If something goes wrong at any step along the way, the foundation for the steps to follow is eroded, and subsequent development is distorted as a consequence.

In delineating the stages themselves, Duvall and Hill used three main criteria: family membership, age composition, and husband's occupational status. Each stage was seen as comprised of a "distinctive role complex" based on these three criteria (Hill & Rodgers, 1964). Particular emphasis was placed on the comings and goings of family members, especially children. Thus, specific family life stages were identified that were associated with the births of the first and second children in the family, with the oldest child leaving home, and with the youngest child leaving home.

Having delineated the different family-life-cycle stages, Duvall and Hill

TABLE 1. Stage-Critical Family Developmental Tasks through the Family Cycle[a]

Stages of the family life cycle	Stage-critical family developmental tasks
1. Married couple	Establishing a mutually satisfying marriage Adjusting to pregnancy and the promise of parenthood Fitting into the kin network
2. Childbearing	Having, adjusting to, and encouraging the development of infants Establishing a satisfying home for both parents and infant(s)
3. Preschool age	Adapting to the critical needs and interests of preschool children in stimulating, growth-promoting ways Coping with energy depletion and lack of privacy as parents
4. School age	Fitting into the community of school-aged families in constructive ways Encouraging children's educational achievement
5. Teenage	Balancing freedom with responsibility as teenagers mature and emancipate themselves Establishing postparental interests and careers as growing parents
6. Launching center	Releasing young adults into work, military service, college, marriage, and so forth, with appropriate rituals and assistance Maintaining a supportive home base
7. Middle-aged parents	Rebuilding the marriage relationship Maintaining kin ties with older and younger generations
8. Aging family members	Coping with bereavement and living alone Closing the family home or adapting it to aging Adjusting to retirement

[a] From *Marriage and Family Development* (6th ed., p. 62) by E. M. Duvall and B. C. Miller. Copyright 1985 by Harper & Row. Reprinted by permission.

further proposed that each stage has attached to it specific *developmental tasks.* Mastery or accomplishment of these tasks becomes the primary criterion of developmental success. Partial or unsuccessful mastery of these tasks produces potential distortions or developmental arrests in the families involved. That is, if family behavior related to a particular developmental task leads to either restricted or unsuccessful resolution, then subsequent development is thought to be inhibited by the partial or incomplete solution of these antecedent tasks. As originally conceived, developmental tasks were associated with three major pressures within the family: biological requirements (food, shelter, personal health, and so on); cultural imperatives (both ethnically and societally derived); and personal aspirations and values. Table 1 lists the various developmental stages and tasks proposed by the Hill–Duvall model.

Although Duvall and Hill recognized that a life-cycle model, to be complete, also needed to account for the movement of the family from one stage to the

TABLE 2. The Carter–McGoldrick Family-Life-Cycle Model[a]

Family-life-cycle stage	Emotional process of transition: Key principles	Second-order changes in family status required to proceed developmentally
1. Between families: The unattached young adult	Accepting parent–offspring separation	a. Differentiation of self in relation to b. Development of intimate peer relationships c. Establishment of self in work
2. The joining of families through marriage: The newly married couple	Commitment to the new system	a. Formation of the marital system b. Realignment of relationships with extended families and friends to include spouse
3. The family with young children	Accepting new members into the system	a. Adjusting the marital system to make space for child(ren) b. Taking on parenting roles c. Realignment of relationships with extended family to include parenting and grandparenting roles
4. The family with adolescents	Increasing flexibility of family boundaries to include children's independence	a. Shifting of parent–child relationships to permit adolescent to move in and out of system b. Refocus on midlife marital and career issues c. Beginning shift toward concerns for older generation
5. Launching children and moving on	Accepting a multitude of exits from and entries into the family system	a. Renegotiation of marital system as a dyad b. Development of adult-to-adult relationships between grown children and their parents c. Realignment of relationships to include in-laws and grandchildren d. Dealing with disabilities and death (grandparents)
6. The family in later life	Accepting the shifting of generational roles	a. Maintaining one's own and/or the couple's functioning and interests in face of physiological decline; exploration of new familial and social role options b. Support of a more central role for middle generation c. Making room in the system for the wisdom and experience of the elderly; supporting the older generation without overfunctioning for them d. Dealing with loss of spouse, siblings, and other peers and preparation for own death; life review and integration

[a]From *The Family Life Cycle: A Framework for Family Therapy* (p. 17) by E. A. Carter and M. McGoldrick. Copyright 1980 by Gardner Press. Reprinted by permission.

next, they paid relatively little attention to the behavior and tasks characteristic of transition from stage to stage. Clinicians, on the other hand, in that they often are called on during times of developmental crisis, have focused more explicitly on the issue of *developmental transitions*. As Carter and McGoldrick (1980) put it,

> The sociological literature on the family life cycle tends to convey the idea that a developmental event (such as the birth of a child or marriage) automatically moves the family from one state to the next. Family therapists are faced with those families in which the shifts are not automatic because the emotional pattern does not promote the move to the next stage. (p. 9)

Clinicians have therefore seen in an analysis of major developmental transitions a useful model for placing in proper perspective a particular request for treatment. A representative version of a clinically oriented family-life-cycle model is the one proposed by Carter and McGoldrick. As outlined in Table 2, it adopts a modified version of the Hill–Duvall staging system but adds to this framework a set of developmental tasks that have much more the flavor of family systems theory than the structural-functional sociological approach (Parsons & Bales, 1955) represented in Table 1. Note also the prominence now given to developmental transitions, which in this particular model are seen as being initiated by a set of psychologically grounded "emotional processes that are described as central to the various transitions" (p. 16).

Although the various family-life-cycle models based on Eriksonian concepts have widespread popularity, they have also proved problematic in several important ways. Most fundamental of these are the various criteria used to define the different developmental stages (and/or developmental transitions). In that they tend to be highly descriptive and concrete, the schemata they generate are too restrictive. Many families (in some cases, perhaps even a majority of families) don't follow the developmental staging sequence described by the particular model. The applicability of the Duvall–Hill model, for example, is restricted to the two-spouse, two-generational family. The life experiences of the childless couple or of the single-parent family make little sense in terms of the Hill–Duvall model's staging sequence.

Aware of this shortcoming, developmentally oriented sociologists and clinicians have proposed a series of modified life-cycle models for the "nontraditional" family. Carter and McGoldrick, for example, described a developmental sequence applicable to single-parent families and another cycle for step families. However, even these efforts fall far short of the mark. As variations in family life continue to increase, the characteristics of life-cycle staging seem to become more and more individualized. Clearly, an approach that requires so many different versions to adequately describe the variations in family types that now exist loses a great deal of its usefulness. This is particularly true regarding the clinical usefulness of such models.

The usefulness of developmental models as research tools has also been called into question (Nock, 1979; Spanier, Lewis, & Cole, 1975). It is unclear that a classification of families by developmental stage adds substantial explanatory power to more traditional variables such as social class and ethnic groupings in studies examining variance in psychopathology, functional capacity, and the like.

Nevertheless, despite the difficulties that these developmental models have had in realizing their potential, they remain highly attractive. They have an inherent "validity" in them, and it is likely that family systems theorists and clinicians will continue to struggle with different versions of family-life-cycle models as they attempt to find models that are more aesthetically and clinically pleasing.

In large part, the difficulty with the Eriksonian model is that it is linear in its approach to development. Although there is considerable dynamism in the interaction between the various elements of the model, the individual is seen as progressing through a series of linearly arranged stages starting at birth and proceeding to death. Such an approach becomes highly suspect, however, when applied to the family. Terms like *birth* and *death* make little sense when applied to the family. If anything, family development is circular. That is, families are multigenerational systems with continuity ensured by the fact that individuals are simultaneously children in their families of origin and "founders" of their own families of procreation. Thus, the typical starting point for the family suggested by most of these models—marriage—is, in fact, a starting point of convenience, a punctuation mark that officially separates one generation from another.

Therefore, there is an obvious place for a new "generation" of life-cycle models that deal more directly with this circularity and continuity of family development. Metaphors that describe processes of *systemic maturation* will, in all likelihood, be more useful than the epigenetic, stage-focused metaphors used in current life-cycle models. That is, models will have to be developed that are more firmly based in general systems theory. Such models, which would use as cornerstones of model-building those morphogenetic properties that families *share* with other living systems, will perhaps in the end prove more clinically useful than current efforts that focus instead on detailed descriptions of family developmental tasks and transition points (tasks that have proved far too idiosyncratic to each family to be useful as the basis for a general model of family growth and development). Two examples of this changed emphasis can be found in the developmental models proposed by Steinglass and his colleagues (1987) and by Wynne (1984).

Information: The Energy Source for Growth in Family Systems. Why is information seen as the primary energy source for growth in family systems? As with the other core concepts of family systems theory, the answer is that it is one of the basic constructs of general systems theory, a construct that has been extrapolated to the family by systems-oriented family therapists.

General systems theory. in addition to acknowledging the importance of traditional energy sources (heat, light, essential nutrients, etc.), also introduces a second, more complex source of energy, the concept of *entropy* (and its corollary, *negentropy*). The concept of entropy comes from studies of thermodynamics and refers to the laws that govern the degradation of energy. As it is described in thermodynamics, this concept indicates that over time, because heat energy cannot be converted into an equivalent amount of work, there will be a gradual degradational loss of energy in any particular closed system. Miller (1965) explained it as follows: "These changes, expressed statistically, constitute passing of the system from ordered arrangement into more chaotic or random distribution. The disorder, disorganization, lack of patterning or randomness of organization of the system is known as 'entropy'" (p. 60).

That is the situation in all closed systems. But as has been repeatedly alluded to, a core feature of living systems is that they manifest exactly the opposite statistical trend over time. When von Bertalanffy and others have alluded to the ability of living systems to increase in organizational complexity over time, they were implying that living systems demonstrate counterentropic qualities. In fact, it was the need to account for this tendency toward increased patterning, increased degree of organization, and more and more complex structuring over time as evidenced by living systems that stimulated the development of systems theory in the first place.

Systems theory has handled this dilemma by introducing the concept of the open or living system, and by emphasizing the different nature of boundary permeability in living and closed systems. In living systems, because external boundaries are semipermeable, energy can be freely transported in and out of the system. Thus, a tendency toward increased patterning (organization), rather than increased randomness, can be supported by the system because it has a potential source of energy. Systems theorists have used the term *negentropy* (negative entropy) in characterizing this phenomenon of open systems. However, as with many other constructs in systems theory, *negentropy* is primarily a descriptive term. It is hardly a model of energy equivalent to, for example, caloric energy. Rather, it is a principal or rule that describes how energy and matter interact in living systems.

But because it focuses on the tendency of living systems to move in a nonrandom, rather than a random, direction over time, it focuses attention on statistical probability as an energy equivalent in living systems. The argument is as follows: In a totally random situation, the likelihood that any series of elements within a field will occur in a specified sequence or combination is no more or less than that of any other combination. That a certain combination or sequence would occur at greater-than-equal or probabilistic chance implies that the elements in the field are related according to some nonrandom rules. That such a pattern or order should exist is seen as more improbable than the reverse. Looked at from the other direction, the greater the number of improbable combinations occurring in a field, the greater the potential for patterning of elements within the field, in other words, the greater the level of organizational complexity that can be achieved.

The next step is the introduction of the concept of *information*. In that information is defined largely in probabilistic terms (that is, information is directly related to the probability of occurrence of a particular event), in systems terms, information is an entropic concept. Because in information theory it is postulated that the less probable (nonrandom) the occurrence of a particular event, the more information connected with its occurrence, information is, in essence, the equivalent of negentropy. To take it to the final step, the more the information available to a particular living system, the greater the degree of nonrandomness (organizational patterning) that it can sustain. It is in this sense that information is conceptualized as the basic energy source for growth within the system.

Although information is still a descriptive concept (just as is negentropy), it has proved a highly useful and powerful one. In particular, it has helped focus our attention on those structures within living systems that are responsible for information generation, processing, and communication. Whether dealing with human language or the genetic code incorporated in the DNA molecule, the magnitude of the multiplier effect that occurs when information is appropriately and efficiently packaged is striking.

Thus, it is hardly surprising that some family systems theorists see information as so central to the healthy functioning of the family as to focus exclusively on this concept, both as the basis of a theoretical model and as the basis of an approach to therapeutic intervention (Sluzki & Ransom, 1976; Watzlawick et al., 1967, 1974). The specific focus in the therapeutic approach is on communication, the process by which information is either changed from one state to another or moved from one point to another point in space. In this model, the family is viewed as an information-processing machine, and terminology that includes information bits, programs of behavior, and decoding failure is used to analogize the family to a cybernetic, computerlike entity. The better the quality of information within the family system, and the more clearly it is communicated from one part of the system to another (from person to person within the family), the greater the capacity of the family to grow and to function effectively and adaptively within its environment.

TWO VERSIONS OF FAMILY SYSTEMS THEORY

Clinical models such as family systems theory can be thought of as serving four major functions. First, they stimulate hypothesis generation by focusing attention on critical choice points around which interesting questions can be framed. Second, they help the clinician to prioritize the importance of different types of clinical data. That is, the model provides guidelines for separating high-quality from low-quality data. Third, clinical models provide a framework for assessing pathology, for distinguishing maladaptive from adaptive behaviors, and for establishing criteria of maladjustment. Fourth, clinical models provide a blueprint for the design of effective intervention strategies. This blueprint usually includes both concepts of how and why behavioral change occurs and suggested clinical techniques for bringing such change about.

Up to this point in the chapter, we have concerned ourselves primarily with describing the core concepts of the family systems model. We have not discussed in any detail how these concepts have been interpreted by family systems clinicians. For those familiar with the family therapy field, however, it is clear that the interpretation of family systems concepts is far from uniform. Differences are most striking in the area of clinical techniques. Family therapists such as Minuchin, Bowen, and Selvini-Palazzoli, although all embracing systems concepts, are dramatically different in their clinical approaches to families. A number of those differences are more idiosyncratic than substantive, the product more of differences in clinical settings and the types of families treated than of genuine differences regarding the interpretation of systems concepts. But other aspects reflect truly different understandings of how systems concepts should be applied to families.

I would contend that the differences apparent in the myriad versions of family systems therapies currently being advocated are, at their core, a product of how each version chooses to interpret the most fundamental of systems concepts: the concept of organization. All family systems theorists see the family as a patterned (nonrandom) entity and look for ways in which family members and family behavior may be patterned. But the sources of data differ from one approach to another. One version may look for structural aspects of the family— coalition, hierarchies, and the like—as the primary data source. Another version may look to verbal and nonverbal communication to elucidate functional versus pathological patterns of behavior. Yet another version relies on three-generational transmission patterns as its data source.

Out of these differences, then, emerge family systems concepts and clinical techniques of astounding (and for some students overwhelming) variety. But these differences can be placed in a comprehensible framework if the above principle is kept in mind. I will illustrate this approach by now summarizing the two most widely known and best established of the versions of family systems theory: the communications-based model espoused by the Palo Alto Mental Research Institute (MRI) and the structural family-therapy model of Minuchin and his colleagues.

The Palo Alto Mental Research Institute Model

We have already made reference to the MRI family systems model at several earlier points in the chapter, most notably in the discussion of concepts of regulation embraced in the metaphor of family homeostasis and in the importance given to high-quality information exchange as a necessary building block for the growth and development of complex behavioral systems. In this section, I will try to summarize the main arguments being advanced by this version of family systems theory.

This model, which was one of the first of the clinical models of family behavior based on general systems theory, began with the seminal work examining communication patterns in families containing schizophrenic members (Bateson, Jackson, Haley, & Weakland, 1956) and subsequently evolved into a comprehensive series of theoretical concepts of marriage and family interaction based on communication theory (Sluzki & Ransom, 1976; Watzlawick *et al.*, 1967). Major contributors to this MRI model have included Don Jackson, Gregory Bateson, Paul Watzlawick, James Weakland, Carlos Sluzki, and Jay Haley.

Although perhaps an oversimplification of the model, it is fair to say that its basic tenet is that family systems can best be understood via the study of the family's communicational inputs and outputs. By focusing on an analysis of such inputs and outputs, and by attempting to develop a set of equations that describe the consistent relationship between these inputs and outputs, an observer can begin to delineate a set of rules that, by inference, govern the functions of the system under study (in this case, the family). Two components of this process are particularly important: first, how human communication is analyzed and, second, how concepts of psychopathology emerge from an analysis of the characteristics of functional versus dysfunctional communication patterns.

Components of Human Communication. The MRI group reminds us that there are three components in the study of human communication: syntax, semantics, and pragmatics. The first component refers to the ways in which *information is transmitted.* Such concepts as the encoding of information; channels of communication; the patterning of speech over time; and the capacity, variability, noise, and redundancy inherent in the communicational transmitting system, are derived from information theory and are applicable here. As applied to families, the syntactical component focuses on such variables as who-to-whom speech, percentage of speaking time (dominance over the channels of communication), parsimony of speech, and ratio of information to noise evidenced by family communication patterns.

The second component, semantics, focuses on the *meaning* of the communicational act. Here, the focus is on the receiver rather than on the transmitter of information. What we are most interested in is the ability of the receiver (the family member) to understand the communication being transmitted either inside or outside the family. Such aspects as clarity of language, the existence of shared private communicational systems (e.g., code words of rich symbolic meaning or private gestures), and concordance versus confusion of communication—all become areas of interest for the communications-based family systems clinician.

But the most important components of communication is the third category described within the MRI model, what these theorists call the "pragmatic" aspect of communication. *Pragmatics* here refers to the behavioral effects of communication. For example, is a message acknowledged or disavowed? Is communication within the family manifested in a manner that serves a mutually supportive function for family members, or is it a source of behavioral conflict? For the MRI group, the terms *communication* and *behavior* are virtually synonymous. Therefore, attention to the pragmatic aspect of communication is all that one need take into consideration in order to describe and define the rules of behavior that exist within a particular family.

One last aspect is also emphasized in this model. In addition to these three aspects of communication (syntax, semantics, and pragmatics), a distinction is also made between the "report" aspect of a particular communicational act and its "command" aspect. The report aspect is the actual conveying of information. The command aspect, on the other hand, is that facet of communicational behavior that serves to define the *relationship* between the communicants themselves. That is, communication in families not only serves the function of transmitting information back and forth between the component parts of the system but also is one of the most important ways in which family members define, monitor, and reinforce the nature of their relationships to each other.

Thus, one can see, incorporated in these notions of the report and command aspects of communication, the building blocks for the MRI model's understanding of how morphogenesis and morphostasis manifest themselves in family systems. The report aspect of communication, when carried out effectively (through clarity and differentiation of communicational syntax and semantics), provides the necessary building blocks for systemic growth. The command aspect of communication, on the other hand, provides the necessary channels and potential diversity of expression necessary to exercise homeostatic regulation and control of the constancy of the family's internal environment. The radical proposal encompassed in this model is the notion that careful attention to the communicational aspects of family life is *all* that is necessary to adequately describe and analyze these systematic components of family life.

Concepts of Family Psychopathology. To carry the basic argument of the MRI model forward, and to focus on the clinical aspects of the model, it follows naturally that pathological behavior, including family psychopathology, can be described adequately and sufficiently in communicational terms. Pathological behavior is synonomous with pathological communication. Further, the features that make a particular communicational act "pathological" are features identified by an analysis of the syntactical, semantic, and/or pragmatic aspect of the communicational pattern observed, with particular emphasis placed on the interface of the report and command functions being expressed. Three aspects of the MRI approach to family communication provide a flavor of how this model deals with the definition and elucidation of family-level psychopathology:

The first aspect is the emphasis placed on sequential analyses of patterns of communication. The proposal is that no single act of communication, by itself, can be judged pathological or nonpathological. Rather, that judgment emerges from an examination of a series of communications and the nature of their stochastic or patterned qualities. These qualities may be described either along dimensions defining the degree of clarity versus confusion in the communicational sequence (determined by focusing on the syntactical and semantic aspects) or along the clarity and confusion dimensions of the pragmatic aspects of the pattern of communication. In this second instance, the discriminating variables for defining communication as pathological center on clarity not of content, but of the command aspect of communication. Regarding this command aspect, the MRI model suggests that, in a sequence of communicational acts, each message transmitted can meet one of three alternative fates at the hand of the receiver: it can be *accepted*, *rejected*, or, as a potentially more omnious option, *disqualified*. This last option is a style of communication in which a person invalidates either his or her own or the other person's communications, and it is seen as one of the major types of pathological communication in families. Self-contradictions, inconsistencies, subject switches, and systematic misunderstandings are examples that lead to such a disqualification of communication.

A second major concept related to pathological communication is the notion of paradox and paradoxical communication. A paradoxical communication is one that, simply put, moves in two opposite and internally inconstant directions at the same time. It is surely a feature of everyday life and, in moderate doses, is quite manageable. However, when communication patterns take on paradoxical features at critical times in the life of the family, trouble is just around the corner. If, for example, at times of developmental crises, or as a characteristic component of family problem solving, or as a central component of child-rearing patterns, the family resorts to paradoxical communication, then the situation, according to the MRI model, becomes rapidly pathological.

The third concept addresses symptom formation; it is an attempt to conceptualize symptomatic behavior in communicational terms. The basic idea is to treat the symptom itself as a nonverbal communicational message. Although the message may be confined to the symptomatic individual alone (an expression of personal distress, an effort at stabilization of the individual's internal environment), it is also proposed that this symptom may be expressing a communicational message for the family system as a whole. For example, depression in one spouse may express a message of marital depression. Or the timing of psychotic behavior relates to the need to provide a distress signal to a complacent family otherwise unaware of a potential threat to its integrity. This view of symptomatic behavior is, of course, a highly controversial one. Suffice it to say at this point, however, that it can be thought of as a reflection of the "purity" of the MRI family systems model as regards its contention that family psychopathology can be adequately defined in communication terms.

The Structural Family Theory Model

This second version of family systems theory has been selected both because of its widespread popularity and because of its quite different approach to the definition of family psychopathology. *Structural family theory* is the name given by Salvador Minuchin and his colleagues to a strikingly differentiated style of therapy that derives from a version of family systems theory based not only on a series of clearly defined premises, but also on equally clearly defined conceptual priorities.

The name—*structural family therapy*—derives from the juxtaposition of three major assumptions made about the nature of human behavior. The first is that all individuals operate within a social context that, among other things, defines the constraints within which individual behavior must exist. The second assumption is that this social context can be seen as having a structure. The third major assumption is that some structures are good and some structures are bad. This last assumption can be restated as a belief in the existence of structural pathology. Thus, in contrast to the MRI model, which sees pathology as based in dysfunctional communication patterns, the Minuchin model defines pathology in structural terms.

What does Minuchin mean when he talks about family structure? Clearly, he is referring to those architectural properties of families that directly impact on the quality of family interactional behavior by determining the constraints within which behaviors must operate. But how does one "see" this structure? Minuchin suggests that three dimensions are particularly relevant here: (a) the family's organizational characteristics (membership, systems versus subsystems, and boundaries); (b) the patterning of family transactions over time as a measure of the internal development of the family system; and (c) the family's response to stress. This last dimension is particularly important in that it provides the rationale for Minuchin's confrontational, stress-inducing therapeutic style, a style intended in part to "flush out" the family's nascent underlying structure, where it can then be assessed and restructured as therapeutic goals dictate.

What does Minuchin mean by each of the above three dimensions? Consider first the organizational dimension. Minuchin places heavy emphasis on what, within a systems theory, could be called the *concept of level*. That is, the naturally occurring subsystems of the family—marital dyad, parental and childhood subsystems, and the like—not only are obvious component parts of the family but are parts that must be arranged in a functional hierarchy for the family to behave adaptively. Thus Minuchin's point of departure from "pure" systems theory is his belief that, for example, the marital subsystem is not merely something that exists whenever two people decide to get married. It is, in effect, an inherent and necessary part of the family system because the marital system is defined not only in terms of membership, but also in terms of function.

What about boundaries? Once again, Minuchin has used a concept from pure systems theory. The boundaries of a particular system are "the rules defining who participates, and how" (1974, p. 53). A notion central to Minuchin's thinking is that families, in order to grow and prosper, must have clear boundaries. Clear boundaries ensure that the various subsystems of the family will be protected from interference by competing subsystems, for example, that the marital subsystem is relatively free from inappropriate demands made by in-laws or children. At the same time, boundaries must not be so rigid as to prevent interaction between the family and the outside world, or between husband or wife as individuals within their separate subsystems, such as their work systems.

Clarity of boundaries, therefore, becomes a major parameter in evaluating the family's level of functioning. Minuchin has identified three general types of boundaries—disengaged, enmeshed, and clear boundaries—which he has postulated exist on a continuum. Although he has stated that these terms refer not to a qualitative difference between functional and dysfunctional types of boundaries, but to a transactional style or preference for a certain type of interaction, his theory implies that clarity of boundaries certainly makes it easier for a family to survive and thrive.

The second structural dimension that Minuchin has highlighted is the patterning of transactions. Although this dimension is analogous in many respects to the notions of homeostasis and cybernetic control postulated by the MRI model of marriage, it is more diffuse in the database it uses. Whereas the MRI model directs our attention to specific communicational acts, Minuchin's concept of patterned transactions uses a wider database. Of particular importance is his sensitivity to the relationship between context and behavior. Transactions are not merely communicational acts between transmitters and receivers; they also include intricate interrelationships between environmental contexts and individual behavior.

For example, in describing a particular marital dyad, a structural family therapist may say that it is comprised of a forceful, decision-making husband

and a quiet, reticent wife. In describing the marriage this way, the therapist is suggesting not only that she or he has observed repetitive forceful-compliant transactions, but also that these transactions are possible because of this marriage's unique structure. That is, the implication is that the husband, the wife, and the context are three parts of a jigsaw puzzle that interlock in a characteristic fashion, and that it is this interlocking structural pattern that shapes (constrains) the behavior we see. Such an image is quite different from the sequential diagrams associated with a communicational analysis of marriage.

Further, this emphasis on the fitting together of parts and on the constraints placed on behavior by the context in which the behavior occurs effectively removes the notion of motivation from transactions. It does not deny motivation; it merely indicates that it is no longer necessary to describe behavior in motivational terms. As a consequence of this stance, statements about behavior take on a distinctively nonjudgmental flavor. It no longer becomes necessary to place blame on one family member or the other for pathological transactional patterns; instead, patterns occur because a particular fit has been established. Change the fit, and the pattern of behavior will also change.

The third dimension that defines the structure of a marriage is its response to stress. Although there are four potential sources of stress on the family (interaction between individuals and extrafamilial forces, interaction between the family and extrafamilial forces, developmental transitions, and idiosyncratic sources), an underlying family structure can be identified in the common patterns of adaptation to stress that emerge. Although one can roughly distinguish two forms of attempted adaptation—one of which leads to adjustment, the other one to increased rigidity—the emphasis is on parts that fit together in a particular organizational pattern.

Many of Minuchin's concepts have a certain vagueness that makes more precise definition difficult. Nevertheless, the emphasis on structural concepts within the model has specific consequences that should be underscored. Most prominent among these is a difficulty in dealing with process variables over extended periods of time. Although Minuchin has freely acknowledged the importance of developmental issues and concepts of adaptation, both the structural model and the style of therapy that emerges from it deal very much with the here and now. The emphasis is on *maps*, in which structural variables are repesented in a spatial dimension only; past history, although interesting, does not necessarily have a logical or consistent role in the conceptualization of normality and pathology in this model.

INTEGRATING THE VARIOUS SYSTEMS MODELS

In this chapter, we have attempted to outline the basic tenets of family systems theory. We have identified three core constructs as central to an understanding of family systems theory: the concept of organization (especially how the notions of wholeness, systemic boundaries, and hierarchies apply to families); the concept of morphostasis (how families regulate their internal environments); and the concept of morphogenesis (notions of how families grow and change in complexity over time). We also attempted to provide a flavor of how the family systems theorist approaches the definition of psychopathology. In particular, we noted that pathology can be thought of not only as the product of a dysfunctional organizational pattern within the family (unstable hierarchies, boundary failure, etc.), but also as the product of an imbalance in the dynamic relationship between regulatory and growth principles within the family. This imbalance can be in the direction of either overregulation (leading to the stagnation and rigidification of functional processes) or uncontrolled growth (leading to the loss of functional coherence and integrated behaviors).

We then went on to describe two clinical models based on family systems theory: the MRI communications model and the Minuchin structural family-therapy model. These models turn out, at first glance, to be very different in their emphases, in their approach to the definitions of psychopathology, and in the types of clinical interventions they recommend. How can the same theory—family systems theory—be interpreted in such different ways? The answer lies in how the two models look for patterns within the family. The emphasis of each model on pattern recognition as the most fundamental activity to be carried out in defining the limits, the organizational characteristics, and the functional properties of the family is what makes it a systems-oriented model. But each model offers a very different set of guidelines for carrying out this pattern-recognition exercise.

As we pointed out in our discussion of the models, the MRI model looks for patterns in the *temporal* sequencing of communicational behaviors. The Minuchin model, on the other hand, looks for patterns in the *spatial* arrangements of the organizational and behavioral components of the family. In conventional terms, we call temporal patterning *process*, and we call spatial patterning *structure*.

Most family systems theorists readily acknowledge the importance of both process and structure as fundamental types of patterns in behavioral systems. The tendency, however, is to be drawn toward one or the other type of pattern as a core model around which different systems approaches are built. In fact, the relative emphasis placed on each of the three core systems concepts—organization, control, and energy—can be thought of as being determined largely by whether someone thinks structurally or sequentially in his or her approach to family systems. For example, the concept of organizational boundaries and the metaphor of boundary permeability are both structural concepts. People who use these concepts tend to have in their heads images of families represented as structural maps, with primary attention paid to the spatial distances between different family members, to the pattern of coalitions and alliances within the family, and to the rules that govern the relationships between the various subelements and organizational levels of the family system. At its extreme, this approach relies on elaborate analyses of what are, in essence, still photographs of families.

For the process-oriented family-systems theorist, on the other hand, a still photograph supplies the wrong information. What is needed instead is a motion picture. If one's goal is to look for sequential patterning, a concept like boundary permeability seems to be off the mark. The sequencing of behavioral events within the family, on the other hand, can provide a rich source of data. The image here is of a never-ending flow of events, some highly repetitive and redundant, some changing over time, but all reflecting the underlying nature of interconnectedness that makes up the behavioral system.

Another way of saying this is that the structuralist sees the system in terms of the rules and the organizational clustering of the various actors in the play, whereas the process-oriented theorist sees the system in terms of the sequential pattern of behaviors that the actors engage in. Thus, the structuralist is most interested in how the actors are placed on the stage as data for describing the central characteristics of the system under observation, whereas the process-oriented theorist is drawn instead to what the various actors are saying and how they are going about saying it.

The tendency to see systems in structural versus process terms also influences one's approach to the concept of morphogenesis. For those who see systems as primarily patterned in time, the most interesting part of morphogenesis is the notion that energy is equivalent to information—hence the emphasis on information theory, on cybernetic theory, and on game theory. The interest is in how information is packaged, transmitted, and conserved. Discontinuity and transformation (systemic growth) occur, according to this view, in association with the occurrences within the system of highly improbable events. These events are growth-inducing primarily because they introduce into the system a large quantity of new information. Further, this whole approach to information defines it in terms of the sequential probabilities of events occurring one after another. Thus, it is, at its very core, a definition of information that is virtually synonymous with the concept of patterning across time.

Structuralists, on the other hand, pay far less attention to the energy source that makes complex systems possible. Although they surely would acknowledge that high-quality information is a "food" necessary to systemic growth, their greater interest is in the growth process itself. If forced to do so, they might point to the concept of negentropy as the energy source behind morphogenesis. But as we have already pointed out, *negentropy* is primarily a descriptive term alerting us to a general principle about living system, namely, that they tend to increase in complexity over time and to behave in an increasingly nonrandom fashion.

For the structuralist, the more interesting question is *how* the pattern of growth actually plays itself out. That is, the interest is in the structuring of the developmental life cycle. Another way of putting it is that process-oriented theorists find themselves fascinated with the phenomena of discontinuous change (what the MRI group has called *second-order change*), whereas the structurally oriented theorists are interested in the constraints that systemic organization seems to place on this discontinuous change and that, in a larger context, lead to a different kind of patterning that we call the *family life cycle*.

Thus, one can see that the predilection for emphasizing one versus another systems principle and for using different dimensions as guidelines for pattern recognition leads to the development of clinical models that not only vary dramatically in flavor but also support very different styles of therapy. Had we undertaken a more comprehensive review of family systems-oriented models, the range of clinical options would have proved even more wide-ranging.

Because these models are so descriptive in nature, it is extremely difficult for us to pit them against each other to ascertain their relative merits regarding traditional measures of validity. Nor do they serve us well in generating testable hypotheses about family behavior. Thus, we will probably continue to have to live with diversity rather than homogeneity in this field.

Yet, at the same time, for those who see the world—and families, in particular—in interactionist terms (be they the "still" pictures of the structuralist or the "motion" pictures of the process-oriented theorist), the systems approach will continue to have appeal far beyond that of traditional cause-and-effect hypothesizing.

REFERENCES

Aponte, H. J., & Van Deusen, J. M. (1981). Structural family therapy. In A. S. Gurman & D. P. Kniskern (Eds.), *Handbook of family therapy.* New York: Brunner/Mazel.

Barker, R. G. (1968). *Ecological psychology.* Stanford, CA: Stanford University Press.

Barnhill, L. R., & Longo, D. (1978). Fixation and regression in the family life cycle. *Family Process, 17,* 469–478.

Bateson, G., Jackson, D. D., Haley, J., & Weakland, J. H. (1956). Toward a theory of schizophrenia. *Behavioral Science, 1,* 251–264.

Bowen, M. (1976). Theory in the practice of psychotherapy. In P. J. Guerin (Ed.), *Family therapy: Theory and practice.* New York: Gardner Press.

Cannon, W. D. (1939). *The wisdom of the body.* New York: Norton.

Carter, E. A., & McGoldrick, M. (1980). *The family life cycle: A framework for family therapy.* New York: Gardner Press.

Cassel, J. (1975). The contribution of the social environment to host resistance. *American Journal of Epidemiology, 104,* 107–123.

Dell, P. F. (1982). Beyond homeostasis: Toward a concept of coherence. *Family Process, 21,* 21–41.

Duvall, E. M. (1971). *Family development.* New York: Lippincott.

Duvall, E. M., & Miller, B. C. (1985). *Marriage and family development* (6th ed.). New York: Harper & Row.

Engel, G. L. (1977). The need for a new medical model: A challenge for biomedicine. *Science, 196,* 129–135.

Erikson, E. H. (1963). *Childhood and society* (2nd ed.). New York: Norton.

Goldsmith, H. H., & Campos, J. (1981). Toward a theory of infant temperament. In R. M. Emde & R. Harmon (Eds.), *Attachment and affiliative systems: Neurobiological and psychobiological aspects.* New York: Plenum Press.

Gray, W., Duhl, F. J., & Rizzo, N. D. (1969). *General systems theory and psychiatry.* Boston: Little, Brown.

Haley, J. (1973). *Uncommon therapy: The psychiatric techniques of Milton H. Erickson, M.D.* New York: Norton.

Haley, J. (1976). *Problem-solving therapy: New strategies for effective family therapy.* San Francisco: Jossey-Bass.

Haley, J. (1980). *Leaving home: The therapy of disturbed young people.* New York: McGraw-Hill.

Hill, R. (1970). *Family development in three generations.* Cambridge, MA: Schenkman.

Hill, R., & Rodgers, R. H. (1964). The developmental approach. In H. T. Christensen (Ed.), *Handbook of marriage and the family.* Chicago: Rand McNally.

Hoffman, L. (1971). Deviation-amplifying processes in natural groups. In J. Haley (Ed.), *Changing families.* New York: Grune & Stratton.

Hoffman, L. (1980). The family life cycle and discontinuous change. In E. A. Carter & M. McGoldrick (Eds.), *The family life cycle: A framework for family therapy*. New York: Gardner Press.

Hoffman, L. (1981). *Foundations of family therapy*. New York: Basic Books.

Jackson, D. D. (1957). The question of family homeostasis. *Psychiatric Quarterly Supplement, 31*, 79–90.

Jackson, D. D. (1965a). Family rules: The marital quid pro quo. *Archives of General Psychiatry, 1*, 589–594.

Jackson, D. D. (1965b). The study of the family. *Family Process, 4*, 1–20.

Lerner, R. M., Palermo, M., Spiro, A., III, & Nesselroade, J. R. (1982). Assessing the dimensions of temperamental individuality across the life span: The dimensions of temperament survey (DOTS). *Child Development, 53*, 149–159.

Madanes, C. (1981). *Strategic family therapy*. San Francisco: Jossey-Bass.

Maruyama, M. (1963). The second cybernetics: Deviation-amplifying mutual causal processes. *American Scientist, 51*, 164–179.

Miller, J. G. (1965). Living systems: Basic concepts. *Behavioral Sciences, 10*, 193–237.

Minuchin, S. (1974). *Families and family therapy*. Cambridge: Harvard University Press.

Minuchin, S., & Fishman, H. C. (1981). *Family therapy techniques*. Cambridge: Harvard University Press.

Minuchin, S., Rosman, B., Baker, L. (1978). *Psychosomatic families*. Cambridge: Harvard University Press.

Morris, C. W. (1938). Foundations on the theory of signs. In O. Neurath, R. Carnap, & C. O. Morris (Eds.), *International encyclopedia of united science* (Vol. 1). Chicago: University of Chicago Press.

Nock, S. L. (1979). The family life cycle: Empirical or conceptual tool? *Journal of Marriage and the Family, 41*, 15–26.

Parsons, T., & Bales, R. F. (1955). *Family, socialization and interaction process*. Glencoe, IL: Free Press.

Pitts, J. L. (1964). The structural-functional approach. In H. T. Christensen (Ed.), *Handbook of marriage and the family*. Chicago: Rand McNally.

Ritterman, M. K. (1977). Paradigmatic classification of family therapy theories. *Family Process, 16*, 29–48.

Selvini-Palazzoli, M., Cecchin, G., Prata, G., & Boscolo, L. (1978). *Paradox and counterparadox*. New York: Jason Aronson.

Skynner, A. C. R. (1976). *Systems of family and marital psychotherapy*. New York: Brunner/Mazel.

Sluzki, C. E., & Ransom, D. C. (Eds.). (1976). *Double bind: The foundation of the communicational approach to the family*. New York: Grune & Stratton.

Spanier, G. B., Lewis, R. A., & Cole, C. L. (1975). Marital adjustment over the family life cycle: The issue of curvilinearity. *Journal of Marriage and the Family, 37*, 263–275.

Speck, R., & Attneave, C. (1974). *Family networks*. New York: Vintage Books.

Speer, D. C. (1970). Family systems: Morphostasis and morphogenesis or "Is homeostasis enough?" *Family Process, 9*, 259–278.

Steinglass, P. (1979). The Home Observation Assessment Method (HOAM): Real time naturalistic observations of families in their home. *Family Process, 18*, 337–354.

Steinglass, P. (1981). The alcoholic family at home: Patterns of interaction in wet, dry, and transitional phases of alcoholism. *Archives of General Psychiatry, 38*, 578–584.

Steinglass, P., Davis, D. I., & Berenson, D. (1977). Observations of conjointly hospitalized "alcoholic couples" during sobriety and intoxication: Implications for theory and therapy. *Family Process, 16*, 1–16.

Steinglass, P., Bennett, L. A., Wolin, S. J., & Reiss, D. (1987). *The alcoholic family*. New York: Basic Books.

Thomas, A., & Chess, S. (1977). *Temperament and development*. New York: Brunner/Mazel.

Thomas, A., & Chess, S. (1984). Genesis and evolution of behavioral disorders: From infancy to early adult life. *American Journal of Psychiatry, 141*, 1–9.

Thomas, A., Chess, S., & Birth, H. G. (1968). *Temperament and behavior disorders in children*. New York: New York University Press.

Thomas, L. (1979). Medical lessons from history. In L. Thomas (Ed.), *The medusa and the snail*. New York: Viking Press.

von Bertalanffy, L. (1968). *General systems theory*. New York: George Braziller.

Watzlawick, P., Beavin, J. H., & Jackson, D. D. (1967). *Pragmatics of human communication*. New York: W. W. Norton.

Watzlawick, P., Weakland, J., & Fisch, R. (1974). *Change: Principles of problem formation and problem resolution*. New York: W. W. Norton.

Weeks, G. R., & L'Abate, L. (1982). *Paradoxical psychotherapy: Theory and practice with individuals, couples, and families*. New York: Bruner/Mazel.

Wiener, N. (1961). *Cybernetics, or control and communication in the animal and the machine*. Cambridge, MA: MIT Press.

Wynne, L. C. (1984). The epigenesis of relational systems: A model for undertaking family development. *Family Process, 23*, 297–318.

Zubin, J., & Spring, B. (1977). Vulnerability: A new view of schizophrenia. *Journal of Abnormal Psychology, 2*, 103–226.

CHAPTER 3

The Family as a Small Group
The Process Model of Family Functioning

PAUL D. STEINHAUER

INTRODUCTION

Two separate and largely unrelated streams of literature can emerge whenever several professional disciplines, each acting in isolation from the other, study a common clinical phenomenon from their own perspective and then proceed to communicate with their own colleagues via their own journals. Such was the case in the study of juvenile delinquency, where a self-report literature described a high incidence of mild and occasional antisocial behaviors. This contrasts markedly with studies of adjudicated delinquents, whose antisocial activities are more serious and more frequent and continue over a long period of time (Williams & Gold, 1972).

This same phenomenon has occurred in the study of family functioning. Practicing family therapists, on the one hand, and social psychologists and sociologists studying families as social groups, on the other, have studied families from different vantage points and with separate goals (Broderick & Pulliam-Krager, 1979; Tallman, 1970). The family therapists have applied general systems theory to explain family pathology and to develop theories of family pathology and approaches to family treatment (von Bertalanffy, 1968, 1969). The social psychologists and sociologists, however, have devised theories about family structure and functioning, seeking to determine how much and in what ways the principles that govern the behavior of *ad hoc* groups also apply to families. This approach has led to interest in the similarities and differences between family and artificially composed groups, and to an exploration of how innate structural

PAUL D. STEINHAUER • Department of Psychiatry, Hospital for Sick Children, 555 University Avenue, Toronto, Ontario, Canada M5G 1X8. Support for the development of the process model of family functioning and the Family Assessment Measure (FAM) was provided by research grants from the Hospital for Sick Children Foundation and Physicians' Services Foundation.

differences related to each type of group affect its functioning in similar situations. Because the family therapists and small-group researchers have worked largely in isolation and have published separately, the two streams of research and the respective literatures have developed relatively independently, with minimial cross-fertilization (Framo, 1965).

This chapter summarizes and compares some major areas of interest of and conclusions arrived at by both these groups. First, it puts in historical perspective the contributions of those relatively few clinicians who began to treat families by applying the techniques and theories of group therapy. After presenting the characteristics of small groups noted in families by clinicians, the chapter reviews the social-psychological literature comparing the properties of families and nonrelated groups. This section of the chapter ends by listing prerequisites for a comprehensive theory of family functioning as seen from a research perspective.

Next, the chapter presents the process model of family functioning (Steinhauer, Santa-Barbara, & Skinner, 1984). This model summarizes and integrates a broad range of clinical and research findings generated by family therapists. The process model was specifically designed to assist in the integration of family systems theory with the major psychological theories of psychopathogenesis; psychopathology and psychotherapy, including psychoanalysis; attachment theory; social learning theory; various developmental theories; crisis theory; and cognitive behavior therapy. Originating within the clinical stream, the process model is based primarily on clinical observations, and is rooted in the family therapy literature. Finally, the process model is compared to other clinical models of family functioning, and its compatibility with the major theories generated by small-group researchers who studied families is examined.

DEVELOPMENT OF FAMILY THERAPY: HISTORICAL PERSPECTIVE

Few of the pioneers in family therapy began treating families as a natural extension of work with groups. Instead, with the notable exceptions discussed below, the original family therapists came to treat families by two main routes. Some, like Ackerman, Framo, Epstein, and Minuchin, were psychoanalysts and ego psychologists who felt hampered by the traditional analytic constraints against family contacts that would complicate and contaminate transference. Aware of the importance of family interaction in perpetuating psychopathology, they chose to increase their effectiveness by seeing patients together with their families. Others, including Lidz, Bowen, Jackson, and their colleagues, were drawn to family therapy by observing the interaction of hospitalized schizophrenics with their families. This observation led to studies of communication and relationship patterns in families with a psychotic member and, eventually, to applying general systems theory to families. This latter group, the systems and communications therapists, observed exclusively highly pathological families and worked primarily from a model of family pathology, rather than from a comprehensive model of normal family functioning. Because pathological behavior is more striking than normal behavior, it is dangerous to conclude that behaviors observed in pathological families are, necessarily, pathological. Tharp stressed the importance of having a model of normal functioning, against which pathological phenomena would stand out in sharp relief (Tharp, 1965). The initial overselling of the double-bind hypothesis of schizophrenia illustrates what can happen if this warning is ignored (Berger, 1965; Grunebaum & Chasin, 1980; Watzlawick, 1963).

The systems therapists, therefore, developed theories not of family functioning, but of family pathogenesis and therapy. Twenty years after the first isolated reports of working with families had reached the literature (Bowlby, 1949; Mittelman, 1948), the Group for the Advancement of Psychiatry (GAP) reported that most family therapists still conceptualized psychopathology using individual (i.e., psychological) theories but tried to resolve the psychopathology with the techniques of group therapy (GAP, 1970). Bowen (1971) also noted the widespread use of family therapy techniques by individually oriented therapists who were empirically treating families largely intuitively with minimal reference to discordant partial theories and principles. Some early analytically oriented family therapists and sociologists did construct theories of normal family functioning. Those who did (e.g., Ackerman, 1958; Bell & Vogel, 1960; Epstein, Rakoff, & Sigal, 1962) recognized the importance of and incorporated social role theory (Parsons & Bales, 1955). Meanwhile, the family systems therapists and their heirs, the structural and strategic family therapists, extended and refined their application of systems theory to families but did not develop a comprehensive model of family functioning and paid little attention to characteristics of families also typical of small groups.

Family Group Therapy

John Bowlby is generally known not as a family therapist, but for his work on attachment theory. In 1949, in what was then a poorly circulated journal, he described the family as a structured group not dissimilar in nature and dynamics from other structured groups. In this remarkable article, presented 10 years before Ackerman published *The Psychodynamics of Family Life* (1958), Bowlby proposed family group therapy as the natural extension of the analytic group psychotherapy then being pioneered by Foulkes, and he introduced the following concepts: the family as a system in homeostatic equilibrium at the intrapsychic, interpersonal, and social levels; individual symptoms resulting from family system pathology; scapegoating; and triangulation. In the same article, Bowlby defined the goal of "family group therapy" as mobilizing the family by promoting conditions that encourage the constructive forces within it in order to allow the group to heal itself. An extended case example demonstrated the use of family sessions to sensitize alienated family members to each other's suffering and desire for change. Bowlby suggested that family therapists remain equidistant and neutral, despite family members' predictable attempts to seduce them into alliances against other members. Bowlby saw family interviewing as a still experimental technique useful chiefly in support of diagnosis, while recommending that the material so generated be worked through in individual therapy.

John Elderton Bell (1961) described family group therapy as an application of small group theory to the natural group of the family. Stressing the need to distinguish theories of family functioning from those of family therapy, Bell emphasized the obvious differences between families and artificially constituted treatment groups. He listed several parameters of normal family structure and functioning, which he attributed to attempts to accommodate the sometimes incompatible demands of a group of individuals living together as a result of biological ties. Bell defined as healthy and efficient families that provide mutual satisfaction, and he supported, when he could, the continued cohesion and effective functioning of the family group. According to Bell, symptoms result when individuals regress to more primitive communications in trying to break through family rigidity that interferes with the transmission and reception of free verbal and symbolic communication. Although not fully integrating the concept of social roles within his theory, Bell clearly recognized that, unless the source of acute symptoms is resolved, family pressure is apt to perpetuate symptomatic behavior. Symptoms then become a part of routine family life, persisting even after their communication value is long since gone. Bell's form of treatment stressed interviewing subgroups of one, two, or three members in the presence of the family. The therapist would then form subgroups with each family member, disrupt unsatisfactory patterns of communication and relationship, and demonstrate new possibilities of action and more adaptive responses. Bell's emphasis on demonstration, the achievement of understanding, and the role of the therapist in the working-through process led others to question whether his obvious awareness of systems theory and the therapeutic potential of the family group was given sufficient scope within his therapeutic method.

Bowen (1971) considered family group therapy the treatment of choice for inexperienced family therapists because it utilizes their knowledge of individual psychodynamics and group process to achieve such concrete short-term goals as improving family communication or mobilizing and assisting the work of mourning. Bowen warned of the potentially disruptive effects of uncontrolled feeling outbursts. Except for such brief and relatively limited interventions, however, Bowen considered family group therapy less effective than forms of family therapy that confront more directly the triangulation and the inadequate differentiation that he, like most family therapists, regard as being at the root of severe family pathology.

It was A. C. R. Skynner who did the most to develop family group therapy. Skynner (1981) described his method as an open-systems group-analytic family therapy. According to Skynner the family is one subsystem within a network of larger and smaller systems, an interface between the inner and outer worlds, between the individual and the group. He works equally comfortably with all three levels of the family system: the intrapsychic, interface, and interpersonal subsystems. Skynner dismisses as territorial dogmatic claims, often rationalized as a conflict of scientific principles, that have, in the past, made psychology and psychiatry appear less like a unified nation than a confederation of alienated and squabbling independent states. To Skynner, current sensory experience is determined as much by learned expectations and unconscious attitudes as by external stimuli. He considers simplistic an exclusive focus on either the intrapsychic or the interpersonal subsystems to the exclusion of the other. Rather, the therapist's job is to bridge dissociations and reestablish communication between disconnected and disowned fragments of the total family system (Skynner, 1969).

Skynner works from a sophisticated model of normal family functioning, using his expertise in psychoanalytic group psychotherapy to mobilize group processes and to catalyze change. He differs from the structural and strategic family therapists in his concept of the role of the therapist. In order to help families recognize and take responsibility for improving their functioning, he takes a position within the newly formed group consisting of family members and himself, and he uses it to lead the family toward change. In contrast, strategic and structural therapists join the family system only to gain the leverage needed to direct or manipulate the family back into health, with or without its knowledge.

Characteristics of the Family as a Small Group as Seen by Family Therapists

There is no inherent theoretical conflict between family systems theory and small-group theory. They are complementary. Each sees the family as a social system sharing some but not all of the characteristics of other task-oriented small groups. Most practicing family therapists are unfamiliar with the small-group literature on family structure and functioning. Nevertheless, several generations of clinical experience have led clinicians to a virtual consensus about the validity and usefulness of the following concepts.

The family is a small group that functions as a problem-solving unit. To solve problems, roles are defined and allocated. If this allocation is successful, role behaviors are performed automatically and effectively, and the family is spared the tensions generated by ongoing role conflict. Because roles are always reciprocal, families develop characteristic controlling mechanisms and leaders. These are needed both to regulate ongoing functioning and to accommodate to change. Members who feel appropriately included in decision making and who are prepared to accept leadership on the basis of competence feel an integral part of their family unit, thus ensuring family cohesion and continuity (Hoffman, 1965; Leavitt, 1951; Tannenbaum, 1967). Adequate communication is needed to regulate reciprocal roles, and cultural values and expectations, along with the power of the family group, exert a potent though often unrecognized pressure toward desired role behaviors. Tension and pathology result from a breakdown of role complementarity, which can lead to the transmission of role pathology from parents to children. This transmission, under certain specified circumstances, can be internalized, contributing to the development of child psychopathology. All this occurs within the context of a family system that is more-or-less self-perpetuating and therefore resistant to change (Bales & Slater, 1955; Bell, 1962; Parsons & Bales, 1955; Spiegel, 1957; Tallman, 1970; Tharp, 1965).

Similarities and Differences between Family Therapy and Treatment of Nonrelated Groups as Seen by Family Therapists

Although families share many characteristics with unrelated treatment groups, major variations in group structure contribute to differences between group and family treatment. Although some authors see no similarity between group and family therapies (Chasin & Grunebaum, 1980), most find marked similarities but equally notable differences, related to the distinctive characteristics of each type of group.

Unlike unrelated treatment groups, families enter therapy with a shared past, a shared present, and a shared future (Bowen, 1971; Steinhauer, 1964). These give them a preexisting structure and equilibrium, consisting of well-defined roles, rules, alliances, and myths. The fact that members remain together before and after treatment sessions and that, unlike members of unrelated treatment groups, they share a common destiny gives family therapy an intensity greater than that usually encountered in group therapy. The "voltage" of family therapy is further intensified because the feelings and interaction stimulated during each treatment hour spill over after each session into the family car and the home. This intensification of family process magnifies the effectiveness of family therapy (Bowen, 1971; Napier & Whitaker, 1978; Steinhauer, 1964). What Handlin and Parloff (1962) termed family therapy's "frontal assault on pathology and defences" may, for some families, increase resistance to change and the risk of serious acting-out or decompensation between treatment sessions. Although the complications described by Handlin and Parloff can occur, they generally result from inappropriate selection or ineffective technique and are not an inevitable by-product of family treatment (Bowen, 1971; Steinhauer, 1968). Indeed, most authors regard as a major advantage family therapy's ability to bring about the rapid development of improved understanding, empathy, and problem solving.

In both family and group therapies, therapists must confront both individual and group resistances. In each of them, an individually oriented therapist can regress under pressure by relating to individuals and forming multiple groups of two, largely oblivious of the effects of this patient-centered subsystem and the total group on each other (Haley, 1976; Steinhauer, 1964).

Perhaps the greatest difference between family and group therapies lies in their goals. Group therapists bring a group of unrelated strangers close enough to identify sufficiently with each other to achieve the group's tasks. Family therapists help family members to differentiate themselves from each other (Bowen, 1971; Minuchin, 1974). Group therapy uses group process to change individuals, whereas the goal of family therapy is to change the family system (Beels & Ferber, 1969; Bloch, 1973; Bowen, 1975; Minuchin, 1974; Steinhauer, 1964).

Unlike group therapy, which all members are regularly expected to attend, family therapists work with whatever combinations of family members they need to restructure the family system. Thus, one could practice family therapy by seeing an individual if, for some reason, that seemed the most effective way of bringing about a desired change (Bowen, 1975; Haley, 1978).

Another difference stems from the composition of each type of group. Unrelated treatment groups have members of roughly the same age and level of development who, ideally, have no power over each other, at least between treatment sessions. In family therapy, however, there are inevitable differences in the ages, levels of maturation, and power of the family members. Handlin and Parloff (1962) see these differences as an inherent disadvantage of family therapy. Family therapists, however, although well aware of these differences and recognizing the importance of not allowing dominant members to use therapy to impose their will on others, rarely find status differences a major obstacle. More commonly, family therapists observe and deal directly and effectively with pathological aspects of intrafamilial control as they occur (Bell, 1962; Skynner, 1969).

Transference is dealt with differently in the treatment of families and of nonrelated groups. In analytically oriented group psychotherapy, the analysis of individual and group projections onto the therapist is a major focus of the treatment. The role and analysis of transference are less prominent in family therapy, partly because, with other family members present, real interactions between members occur directly. These interactions decrease, though they by no means eliminate, the use of the therapist as a transference figure. Transference and countertransference still play a part in family therapy, and transference projections onto the therapist may play an important but rarely a dominant role in family treatment. Family therapists' greater activity and self-revelation encourage realistic perceptions and transactions between themselves and families, thus undermining the therapists' usefulness as transference figures. The therapist can deal directly with either the interactional or the transference (i.e., projective identification) components of family interactions as they occur. When dominant, transference to the therapist is noted and may be interpreted, but rather than forcing communication into a transference-dominated mold, the therapist maintains a here-and-now emphasis, with all forms of communication occurring during therapy being considered equally valid and relevant (Skynner, 1976).

Countertransference is by no means avoided in family therapy. The intensity of pathological family interaction and the pressures on the therapist to ally with one subsystem or generation against another can exert particularly potent pressures on the residual conflicts of the therapist. As long as these remain unrecognized, they can lead to selectively skewed perceptions, inappropriate processing of observations, self-serving alliances, and other forms of prolonged acting-out, which, in the family therapy literature, are referred to more often as the therapist's becoming trapped within the family system than as countertransference (Whitaker, Felder, & Warkentin, 1965).

REVIEW OF RESEARCH ON FAMILIES AS SMALL GROUPS

In 1979, Klein and Hill identified four main streams of small-group research on families. The first studied the family as the context in which such large-scale social problems as separation and divorce, illegitimacy, and physical and mental illness develop. Some studies in this group attempted to distinguish between family disorganization and family deviance (e.g., Sprey, 1966), and others tried to pinpoint what makes some families problem-prone (e.g., Beck & Jones, 1974; Brim, Fairchild, & Borgatta, 1961; Geismer & LaSorte, 1964).

A second group of studies consisted of still incomplete attempts to develop a systematic and comprehensive theory of familial responses to crisis (Farber, 1964; Hansen & Hill, 1964; Hill, 1949; McCubbin & Boss, 1980).

The third group studied how families and their individual members are affected by ongoing development. Each stage may be problematic, as it involves role confusion, transitions, and revision of preexisting role reciprocities. The developmental stream is represented by the work of Rapoport (1963), Hill, and Rodgers (1964), Duvall (1971), and Aldous (1974, 1978).

The most active stream of family research has consisted of studies of small-group problem-solving, organizational structure, and decision-making (Aldous, 1971; Bales & Strodbeck, 1951; Hill, 1970; Maier, 1967, 1970; Reiss & Oliveri, 1980; Straus, 1968; Tallman, 1970, 1971, 1972; Weiss & Margolis, 1976). These studies have included attempts to define to what extent, under what conditions, and with what modifications theories and research techniques derived from studying small *ad hoc* groups can, with validity, be applied to families. Most of these attempts were partial theories dealing with only one or two aspects of family functioning. However, despite several excellent reviews such as those of Hoffman (1965), Maier (1967), Kelley and Thibaut (1969), Klein and Hill (1979), and Holman and Burr (1980), the process of systematically integrating these theories into one comprehensive theory has just begun.

The applicability of theories derived from small-group research to families has been questioned (Burns, 1973; Haley, 1964; Murrell & Stachowiak, 1965, 1967; Walters, Miller, Rollins, Thomas, & Galligan, 1982). A number of attempts to replicate small-group research within families have proved unsuccessful (Leik, 1963; O'Rourke, 1963; Strodbeck, 1954, among others). Other studies, however, such as Kenkel's work supporting the theory of role formation in families (Kenkel, 1959a,b, 1961a,b) and that of Scott (1962) on coalition formation, have been replicated. Reviewing the discrepancies between the two series of studies, Framo (1965) attributed failures to the inability of the research design to penetrate the family's need to present an image of solidarity well enough to allow an undistorted view of its operative group processes.

But families differ fundamentally not only from other groups but also from each other. Even ideas of what constitutes a family have changed dramatically over the past two decades (Masnick & Bane, 1980). Walsh (1982, p. 7) estimated that fewer than one in four American families currently fits the classic description of the intact nuclear family of two parents and one or more children, with the father as sole breadwinner and the mother as homemaker. Therefore, theories of problem solving in *ad hoc* groups would be more useful if there were models of family functioning that applied equally well to traditional nuclear families and to their major variants, for example, single-parent families, reconstituted families, families with two working parents, families further on in the life cycle, and ethnic families. This application should be possible with models that focus on universal aspects of family functioning and common processes, rather than on specific (descriptive) content. The family variants listed above illustrate the enormous variety that exists both among and within families. The resulting differences are likely to mediate and to affect the predictability of particular families' responses to theories of small-group functioning.

COMPARISON OF PROBLEM SOLVING IN *AD HOC* AND FAMILY GROUPS

Four major sets of factors have been used to explain differences in problem solving between families and *ad hoc* groups. The first includes differences in the composition of the two types of groups. The second considers the family's unique experience of sharing a common past and a common feature. The third examines whether families and *ad hoc* groups face the same types of problems. The fourth reflects the influence of individual members on family problem-solving. Let us review the literature on each of these to see the effects of the differences between families and *ad hoc* groups on problem solving.

Differences in Composition between Family and *Ad Hoc* Groups

Family and *ad hoc* groups have very different motives for forming a group, and these affect both the nature of the group and its subsequent functioning. Unlike members of *ad hoc* groups, who are randomly selected or only broadly matched, parents choose each other on the basis of common, though often unrecognized, needs (Walters, 1982). Family members, therefore, should have more in common than the randomly selected members of *ad hoc* groups (Graziano & Musser, 1982; Tesser, 1978; Tesser & Reardon, 1981).

Unlike *ad hoc* groups, the family—at least, the nuclear family—is a kinship group whose children are biologically related to each other and to both parents. If one includes one-parent and reconstituted families, the children are still biologically related to at least one parent and, usually, to one or more siblings. The significance of the biological bond is twofold: First, it predisposes people to familylike groupings (e.g., Leibowitz, 1978). Daly and Wilson (1978) stated, "Parents maintain a benevolent interest in the welfare of their offspring for life. . . . We particularly surpass our primate kin . . . in the degree to which males are integrated into those long-term familial bonds" (p. 328). This conclusion suggests a biological inclination toward commitment to family cohesion, at least by fathers, which "may so affect family processes as to produce a quality in family groups that is not duplicated in other groups" (Walters, 1982, p. 847).

The possible effects of this enhanced commitment to sustaining family attachments will be returned to in discussing the effects of pressures toward cohesion on family problem-solving.

Second, at least some family members have greater biological similarity (i.e., siblings to siblings; children to one or both parents) than do members of *ad hoc* groups. This is likely to have some effect on temperament, as the genetic transmission of basic temperament (Thomas & Chess, 1977) has been generally accepted, even though the influence of postnatal (see Sarett, 1975) and sociocultural factors (see Sameroff & Kelly, as cited in Thomas & Chess, 1977) has not been ruled out. But although the greater biological similarity of families can hardly be contested, its effect on family functioning and motivation has not, as yet, been demonstrated.

Unlike *ad hoc* groups, whose age distribution is relatively similar, families, by definition, include members of at least two generations. Their composition is significant, because age is a major determinant of the distribution of power and leadership in families, but not in *ad hoc* groups (Aldous, 1971; Walters, 1982). Both their wider age spread, which guarantees different interests and priorities, and family members' tendencies to be less kind and more negative to each other than to strangers (Birchler, Weiss, & Vincent, 1975; Halverson & Waldrop, 1970; Ryder, 1968; Winter, Ferreira, & Bowers, 1973) favor more open (and especially more personality-oriented) conflict in families than in *ad hoc* groups. Also, conflict has been both positively and negatively correlated with increased family size (Klein & Hill, 1979; Turner, 1970). Turner (1970) and Aldous (1971) associated conflict with less risk taking and, therefore, less creative input into problem solving. Klein and Hill (1979), however, saw family size as having mixed effect on problem solving. Larger families stimulate more verbal and nonverbal communication and encourage centralization of power. These trends are opposed, however, by decreased support and legitimization of power, which counteract any increase in problem-solving effectiveness.

The greater age discrepancy in families also ensures a wider variety of attention spans, social skills, and problem-solving competencies, as well as unequal access to basic data. Attention span generally varies with age and is further compromised at times of uncertainty and tension. Because the attention span of a group is that of the member whose attention span is least, families, on this basis alone, are predisposed to favor rapid, "good-enough," as opposed to high-quality, solutions (Klein & Hill, 1979; Weick, 1971).

The presence in families of members at various stages in their life cycle guarantees a heterogeneity of interests and goals, making it harder for families to agree on the nature of a problem or, even, on whether one exists (Klein & Hill, 1979). Often, one family member or coalition tries, with variable support from others, to impose its definition of a problem on weaker members who are uninterested or oppositional. Difficulties in achieving consensus about the nature of a problem are made worse by the "confounding effect" of ongoing development (Weick, 1971). This confounding effect introduces legitimate confusion about whether many problem behaviors are merely temporary responses to developmental change, which, if ignored, will resolve spontaneously (Aldous,

1974; Duvall, 1971; Hill & Rodgers, 1964; Rapoport, 1963), or whether they require active solution (Klein & Hill, 1979; Rae-Grant, Carr, & Berman, 1983; Weick, 1971).

Walters demonstrated that role assignments are more stereotyped in *ad hoc* groups, with instrumental roles assumed by men and affective ones by women (Leik, 1963; Parsons & Bales, 1955; Strodbeck & Mann, 1956), although this pattern may be less apparent now, at least in some populations, because of the social redefinition of sex roles by the sexual revolution. Leik (1963) showed that sex in *ad hoc* groups and age in families were most important in providing status and in determining the assignment and acceptance of instrumental or affective roles. In families, however, especially when studied in their own homes, both affective and instrumental roles were taken by either parent (O'Rourke, 1963). The sex of a child was found to be more influential than sex-specific role expectations in influencing adult behavior toward that child (Bronfenbrenner, 1961).

Effects of Sharing a Common History and Future

Even more important are those differences that result from families' sharing a common history and a common future. Historical continuity has other effects on both family and group problem-solving (Aldous, 1971; Broderick & Pulliam-Krager, 1979; Klein & Hill, 1979; Reiss, 1971; Tallman, 1970, by implication; Turner, 1970; Walters, 1982; Weick, 1971). Weick (1971) suggested using an elaborate "generational metaphor" originated by Jacobs and Campbell (1961) to replicate the flow of family generations while studying long-term *ad hoc* groups. Walters (1982), however, used the work of Weiss (1975) and Rosenblatt (1977) to argue convincingly that the combination of attachment and commitment to family maintenance, though variable from family to family, is at least difficult and probably impossible to duplicate in *ad hoc* groups.

Walters also quoted Waxler and Mishler (1978), suggesting that, if Shapiro (1975) and Greenberg (1978) were correct in concluding that the prospect of future interaction affects *ad hoc* groups, "it will also affect interaction in families, since a basic characteristic of families is the prospect of future interaction" (Walters, 1982, p. 848). Klein and Hill (1979) acknowledged differences between problem-solving in families and in *ad hoc* groups but claimed that Weick failed to prove that the laws of problem solving in *ad hoc* groups do not apply to families. Although conceding that Weiss had demonstrated that family problem-solving is "a messy business . . . relatively unstructured and full of distractions and road-blocks" (Klein & Hill, 1979, p. 512), Klein and Hill underplayed the effects of a shared history and future. They argued that the discontinuity in size, gender, composition, competencies, and role relationships both within and outside the family is such that the only relatively stable elements may be the family's orderly progression through the life cycle (Klein & Hill, 1979, p. 533). They further contended that differences in "biologically ascribed and socially achieved traits such as age, gender and cognitive, interpersonal and motor skills" may affect family problem-solving more than the ever-present "integrated micro-cultural base" consisting of "shared role expectations, values, goals, family feeling, definitions of a situation and criteria for evaluating the effectiveness of problem-solving efforts" (p. 533). This view contrasts with the same authors' earlier statements acknowledging that "any group effort, no matter how novel the situation, occurs within the context of a pre-existing role structure" and that "the best predictor of how a group usually organizes to solve a problem may be its past role structure" (p. 497).

Even long-term *ad hoc* groups develop relatively stable and identifiable structural properties (Klein and Hill's integrated microcultural base), which exist already before they begin to problem-solve (Aldous, 1971; Reiss, 1971; Tallman, 1970; Weick, 1971). These stable structural properties are considered the basis of established groups' inherent resistance, at least initially, to new ideas and to the ideas of new members (Aldous, 1971; Reiss, 1971; Weick, 1971). These are important components of what the family therapy literature terms *homeostasis*. In long-term *ad hoc* groups, it is only after initial attempts at problem solving using the usual methods fail that the established structure's inherent resistance to modifying its structural patterns is overcome. This process allows roles and rules to be adjusted, permitting a new, more innovative attack on a problem (Klein & Hill, 1979). This adjustment must be even more pronounced in families, where years of living together and the prospect of a shared future have reinforced members' stake in the existing structure.

The extent to which families can accommodate new input has led to much scholarly debate. The structure and norms of some families encourage free discussion, tolerate and support broad involvement, and remain open to the new ideas and differences of opinion required for creative problem-solving and successful adaptation (Tallman, 1970; Turner, 1970; Wallach, Kagan, & Bean, 1964). In other families, a preoccupation with family cohesion leads to the avoidance of conflict at the expense of failing to find the best solution. The preoccupation with cohesion in such families suppresses participation and, especially, the expression of differences, including issue-related conflict. As a result, creativity and innovation are largely excluded (Aldous, 1971; Reiss, 1971; Rosenblatt, 1977; Straus, 1968; Weick, 1971).

Openness to new input and a willingness to tolerate disagreement are important prerequisites for adapting to changing developmental and environmental demands. Several authors have regarded the tension between the family's pressure toward cohesion and its openness to fresh input as the two irreducible axes around which a typology of clinical families can be organized (Broderick & Pulliam-Krager, 1979; Kantor & Lehr, 1975; Olson, Sprenkel, & Russell, 1979; Reiss, 1971; Straus, 1968).

A number of authors have considered the influence of family problem-solving on members' development. Children rewarded for participation in problem solving show more confidence in their ability to tackle new situations, higher self-esteem, and greater willingness to participate in future problem-solving (Tallman, 1972; Tallman & Miller, 1971; also alluded to by Reiss, 1971; Steinhauer *et al.*, 1984; Weick, 1971). Moore and Anderson (1971), Weick (1971), and Aldous (1971) have agreed that problem solving can be inherently gratifying and ego-enhancing, especially in an atmosphere of inclusion, playfulness, and en-

couragement (see also Hoffman, 1965; Leavitt, 1951; Tannenbaum, 1967). Tallman (1972, Tallman & Miller, 1974) suggested that parents resemble the grandparents in their ways of influencing their children, though Weinrich (1982)
noted that children's responses to parental modeling may be either positive or
negative (Weinrich, 1982).

Problem solving in both families and *ad hoc* groups is affected by socioeconomic status (Cohen, 1974; Haley, 1967; Straus, 1968; Strodbeck, 1951, 1958;
Weick, 1971). Most research in this area has studied whether lower-class patterns
of communication and control inhibit communication, and, thereby, creativity,
problem solving, and effectiveness, as Straus (1968) suggested. Tallman (1970)
and Turner (1970) have agreed that patterns of family communication and
leadership are class-related, but they have denied that lower-class problem-solving is necessarily inferior. Tallman argued that it is deviation from class norms
(e.g., failure of blue-collar males to dominate decision making, or of white-collar
males to share decision making from a position of strength) that is most likely to
undermine effective problem-solving (Tallman & Miller, 1974).

Tallman (1972) emphasized that many lower-class families, feeling abused
and powerless within a society that they see as depriving and excluding, tend to
be rigid and authoritarian. These tendencies inhibit participation, increase role
conflict, and threaten family cohesion. They also discourage the risk taking and
creativity needed for successful adaptation and for finding new or different
solutions. In addition, the fathers of families poorly integrated into society and
least able to protect themselves from unwanted social interventions are less likely
to be respected and to have their leadership legitimitized by other family members (Aldous, 1966; Blood & Wolfe, 1960; Tallman, 1972).

Finally, lower-class families struggling to meet basic instrumental demands
have less time, energy, or confidence to search for optimal solutions (Aldous,
1971; Millbraith, 1965; Tallman, 1972; Thibaut & Kelley, 1959). All these factors appear to undermine problem solving in disadvantaged families more than
class-related patterns of communication and leadership.

Are the Types of Problems Faced by *Ad Hoc* and Family Groups the Same?

It is in families, not *ad hoc* groups, that major social problems are experienced. But unlike those problems faced by *ad hoc* groups, family problems are so
embedded in the ongoing confusion of daily life that they are often not recognized as problems until after an initial attempt to resolve them has failed (Weick,
1971). This lack of recognition, the competition of other claims for limited time
and energy, and the fact that most family problems are solved when family
energy levels are low (i.e., before and after work and school) often cause families
to deny problems as long as they can, or to solve them as quickly as possible
(Weick, 1971). These factors make problem solving in families less thorough and
systematic than in *ad hoc* groups. The unfinished business and the dissatisfaction
remaining from earlier and unsatisfactory partial solutions feed back into the
system and add to residual levels of tension that "hitchhike" on some instrumen-

tal issue. This issue is then used as an excuse to vent the accumulated frustration, disappointment, and resentment, a process that Weick (1971) termed "problem-solving as expressive behavior."

Contributions of Individual Member Characteristics to Family Problem-Solving

The small-group problem-solving literature pays little attention to the influence of individual member characteristics, although conceding that some members may disagree about whether a problem exists or about its nature. Some may refuse to participate in finding solutions, or to implement those proposed by family leaders. Even if all participate in family problem-solving, especially in families with children of various ages, members differ in the amount and complexity of the information they can handle at a given time, in their ability to pay attention, to tolerate ambiguity and frustration, to consider alternatives, to persevere despite initial frustration, to recognize and focus on the important issues, and to think in abstract terms. Some may be intent on sabotaging the efforts of others to identify and eliminate behaviors or situations in whose continuance they have a stake. Weick (1971) and Aldous (1971) recognized the importance of problem-solving motivation and willingness to cooperate to the achievement of communal goals. Aldous (1971) and Tallman and Miller (1974) noted the effect of members' self-esteem and of individual and family status on problem solving. However, it was Weick (1971) and, more explicitly, Klein and Hill (1979) who constructed propositions that combine individual and collective units of analysis, and who suggested that attempts to explain family problem-solving that ignore the effect of individual differences on group functioning are, invariably, severely compromised. Weick, quoting Lazarus (1966) on the effects of psychological stress ("ambiguity permits maximum latitude for idiosyncratic interpretations . . . based on the individual's psychological structure," p. 118), recognized that internalized psychological influences as well as interactional ones affect perception, interpretation, and behavior. It remained for Klein and Hill (1979) to begin to integrate the many partial theories into a single comprehensive one that recognizes the importance of ongoing feedback (i.e., circular as opposed to linear causality), and that takes into account the circular effects of the group structure and the character and response style of the individuals on each other.

THE APPLICATION OF SMALL-GROUP THEORIES TO THE UNDERSTANDING OF FAMILIES

If the modifying influence of the above factors within a particular family are taken into account, one can then apply the same theories that govern problem solving in *ad hoc* groups to families. Klein and Hill's step toward a theory open enough to admit many different perspectives is an important one. Their inclusion of individual-member (i.e., psychological) characteristics as a major variable converts much of what they termed "the nonrationalistic element" in the approaches of Weick (1971) and to a lesser extent, Aldous (1971, 1974) into one that is potentially understandable given the systemic interplay between the family and its members. For example, they contrasted the different views of Aldous (1971) and Weick (1971) with those of Turner (1970) and Tallman (1970, 1972) in terms of whether stress on achieving consensus and cohesion facilitates or undermines family problem-solving. An apparent disagreement can be resolved by recognizing that what each pair of authors was discussing holds true for a different type of family. A rigid, authoritarian demand for consensus in the name of cohesion concentrates leadership on the basis of power rather than competence, discourages individual risk-taking and participation in problem solving, and undermines the creativity and innovation needed to allow for change. On the other hand, a more moderate concern about family cohesion, especially when combined with a generous distribution of support and affection, can encourage broad participation, shared leadership on the basis of competence, creativity, and flexibility, without sacrificing either individual autonomy or family ties. Clearly, any unqualified discussion of the effects of pressures for cohesion and consensus will be more confusing than enlightening unless both the degree of pressure toward conformity and the quality of family leadership or control (i.e., supportive and encouraging or intimidating and excluding) are specified and considered.

Now that we have come this far, the relative advantage of families (and *ad hoc* groups) in solving different kinds of problems is clarified. Because they are already organized, families have an advantage in solving problems similar to problems successfully resolved in the past (Aldous, 1971). However, their preexisting structure, especially when potentiated by resistance to new forms of input, puts families at a disadvantage in solving problems that need different or innovative solutions requiring broad participation, risk taking, and creativity (Reiss, 1971; Straus, 1968). Family problems require a variety of solutions and problem-solving methods at different times. For some of these, a repetition of familiar patterns of problem solving will be most effective, whereas for others, openness to new solutions and willingness to reorganize may be crucial.

Consider, also, how the effects of the family's leadership style correlate with its affective relationships. Do authoritarian families, for example, eventually pay for the short-term efficiency and conflict suppression they use to suppress whatever is interpreted as a threat to their continuity? Will these patterns, if continuous, increasingly undermine developmental flexibility, decrease responsiveness to change, and alienate members who feel excluded from what they consider their fair share of the distribution of family power, concern, support, and affection? How will family rigidity affect open and direct communication, effective role performance, and so on? Surely, in applying to families, general theories derived from *ad hoc* groups, one must recognize that families, depending on their established roles, rules, communication patterns, and other behavioral norms, will respond differently to any attempt to shift their structure and equilibrium.

In summary, then, general theories of group functioning can be applied to families, but only by first considering the filtering or potentiating effects of the particular family's composition, common history, structure, and different motivations can that family's response to a given situation be predicted. It is therefore encouraging to see newer attempts to continue the difficult task of studying the workings of group processes within families such as those of Jacob and his colleagues (Hadley & Jacob, 1976; Jacob, Kornblith, Anderson, & Hartz, 1978; Zuckerman & Jacob, 1979).

TOWARD A COMPREHENSIVE THEORY OF FAMILY FUNCTIONING

Attempts to formulate even limited aspects of family functioning that ignore the potentiating or opposing influences of other interfacing aspects of individual, family, and social functioning can be of only limited utility to clinicians who view both families and individuals from a systems perspective. Models are needed that combine and integrate the major parameters of universal family functioning with other social and intrapsychic influences, to serve as a basis for assessment procedures, therapeutic interventions, and continuing research, especially into the efficacy of various forms of intervention. The problem with multivariant models—and the process model that follows is one of these—is that they are multiplicative. As a result, although clinically useful, they are difficult to prove because the number of variables is large and because validation of the component-partial theories does not validate the model as a whole. Some have tried to circumvent these difficulties by reducing the number of essential variables even beyond what the author of this chapter considers the smallest possible number of "prime factors" that cannot be reduced further without sacrificing the model's ability to capture the richness and diversity of structure and functioning in both clinical and nonclinical families. In simplifying models in order to make them more easily researchable, there is a danger of ignoring or condensing unrelated variables, thus achieving economy at the expense of sharpness and/or validity. Should this occur, the resultant models become simplistic rather than merely simplified.

In their "theory of family problem-solving effectiveness," Klein and Hill (1979, pp. 541–542) listed a number of theoretical perspectives that they considered prerequisites of any comprehensive theory of family functioning. With a minor change indicated in brackets below, we list these as they were presented by Klein and Hill, adding the last two which we consider equally important:

1. *Systems theory,* with an emphasis on the interdependence among actors and actions, selective boundary maintenance, inputs and outputs, feedback and adaptation or structural modification.
2. *Microfunctionalism,* with an emphasis on purposive behavior geared toward its consequences and with its efficient causes rooted in structural variables, and allowing for equilibrium maintenance as well as an instrumental-expressive distinction.
3. *Cybernetic theory,* with an emphasis on information processing at both the level of individuals and that of groups.

4. *Phenomenology* and especially *symbolic interactionalism,* with an emphasis on the intersubjective [and intrasubjective] construction of meaning, and on cognition and perception.
5. *Developmentalism,* with an emphasis on changes in member characteristics, group composition, and role relations over time.
6. *Conflict theory,* with an emphasis on the productive consequences of conflict and change, and on group integration as problematic.
7. *Behaviorism,* with an emphasis on overt interaction and learning.
8. [*Psychodynamic theory,* meaning a systematic use of one or more psychological theories to provide an integrated and internally consistent explanation of the intrapsychic variables (dynamics) that affect and result from the ongoing interaction between individual members (subsystems) and the family equilibrium.]
9. [Due consideration of the *interaction at the interface* between individual subsystems (i.e., members), the interpersonal system of the family, and relevant supersystems with which the family and its members are in ongoing interaction.]

The additions of Numbers 8 and 9 suggest that an acceptable model should be open to integration with other models that explain factors governing any contained or contiguous subsystems interacting with the family system. This integration would allow systemic formulation of an individual's psychological status to include an integration of the effects of those relevant biological, familial, social, and psychological factors that predispose, precipitate, and/or perpetuate that person's current status. In the same way, a comprehensive model of the family would allow for the interacting effects of all universal parameters of family functioning and would provide entry points through which one could feed in the impact of extrafamilial influences and of individual members through their interpersonal behavior, attitudes, idiosyncratic roles, or meanings to each other. Especially since the mid-1970s, several models have been proposed that combine and integrate at least some of the available partial theories of family functioning:

1. Kantor and Lehr (1975) used patterns of information processing and strategies for maintaining distances between family members to subdivide families into three major types: closed, open, and random. Closed families stress integration and tight cohesion to ward off potential threats. Open families are more easily and adaptively responsive to developmental or environmental demands for change. Random families are much less organized, favoring greater distance and extreme autonomy at the cost of less stability and less structural cohesion. This classification resembles earlier ones of Straus (1968) and Reiss (1971), although unlike Reiss, Kantor and Lehr see both well-functioning and poorly functioning families within each major category.

2. Broderick and Pulliam-Krager (1979) manipulated distance and boundary maintenance to produce what could be seen as a forced marriage between the consensual experience theory of Reiss (1971) and an attempted rehabilitation of the double-bind hypothesis of schizophrenia (Bateson, Jackson, Haley, & Weakland, 1956). Their model exceeds the latter because, by incorporating the

work of Hess and Handel (1959) and Kantor and Lehr (1975), it looks beyond the symptom (i.e., disordered communication) to the underlying disturbance in the establishment and maintenance of boundaries that both predispose to and perpetuate the dysfunctional communication. Acknowledging its resemblance to the work of Reiss, this model has the advantage of bridging the family-therapy and the small-group literature on families. It does not, however, recognize or include the effect on families of individual-member characteristics; both biological and psychological vulnerabilities and influences are ignored. Also, although using many concepts of systems theory, the model itself employs linear rather than circular causality. Possibly its major contribution is that it moves from an additive to a multiplicative model and, at the same time, recognizes the difficulties for research that such a model presents.

3. Fleck (1980) proposed a model applicable both to clinical and to non-clinical families. It stresses the continuous dynamic interaction among five major parameters of family functioning: leadership, boundaries, affectivity, communication, and task–goal performance. A change in functioning within one of these parameters (e.g., communication) will influence the other dimensions of ongoing family life. From this model, Fleck developed a grid that can be used to locate specified aspects of family functioning along an interactional-historical continuum.

4. Olson et al. (1979) developed the "circumplex model of family functioning," which derives a family typology by locating families on a grid whose coordinates are what these authors considered the two prime dimensions of family functioning: cohesion (ranging from disengagement to enmeshment) and adaptability (too little of which leads to rigidity, whereas too much leads to disorganization). With reference to these coordinates, Olson et al. proposed a typology of 16 types of families, based on the family's perception of its place along these two prime parameters of family functioning. Those closest to the intersection of the two axes (i.e., those avoiding extremes on either dimension and therefore being most balanced) function more successfully than those closer to the periphery of the grid, in which one or both cardinal dimensions are off-balance. A self-report instrument measuring family functioning called *FACES* (Family Adaptability and Cohesion Evaluation Scales) has been derived from the circumplex model. It measures members' perception of their family's functioning along these axes, but the usefulness of the test, like that of the model, is limited by the small number of variables on which it is based.

5. Developed by Epstein, Bishop, and Levin (1978), the McMaster model of family functioning further develops the earlier family categories schema (Epstein et al., 1962), the common ancestor of both the McMaster and the process models. Focusing on the aspects of family functioning seen as central to emotional and physical health or pathology, this model equates health with normality. A highly pragmatic systems model, the McMaster model integrates many useful ideas from the authors' more than 25 years of clinical, teaching, and research experience.

The model defines and lists the major characteristics of six prime dimensions of family functioning: problem solving, communication, roles, affective responsiveness, effective involvement, and behavior control. Healthy and pathological variants of each of these are described, and this description helps to set up treatment goals within each parameter. Arguing that more than two prime dimensions are needed to capture the variety and richness of family functioning, the McMaster model, although developed primarily by and for clinicians, includes and integrates more concepts derived from small-group research (e.g., the staging of problem solving and the critical dimensions of communication and role performance) than those discussed above. Although generally using circular causality, the McMaster model formulates individual symptoms as the result of family pathology, failing to consider the reciprocal effects on the family of individual biology and psychopathology. Social influences considered in the family categories schema are downplayed in the McMaster model.

6. Widely used clinically because it is clear, simple, easy to teach, and practical, the structural model is derived from family (i.e., pathology-based) therapy rather than from a comprehensive theory of family functioning. For that reason, it will not be discussed here. However, the structural model and structural family therapy are well described in Minuchin and Fishman (1981) and in Aponte and van Deusen (1981).

THE PROCESS MODEL OF FAMILY FUNCTIONING

Introduction

Bowen's calls for an integration of individual and family systems theories (1971, 1975) have been echoed by an increasing number of individual and family therapists, among them Marmor (1975), Havens (1973), Skynner (1976), Framo (1981), Slipp (1980), Goodrich (1980), Kantor (1980), and Malone (1979). Skynner, in particular, has deplored the frequent overgeneralization of principles established within a clinical sphere that are then extrapolated to create an all-inclusive system. Several authors have pointed to the divisive effect of the in-fighting between various schools and their territorial claims and have called for a unifying conceptual framework to provide a rationale for a selective but pluralistic approach to conceptualizing and treating human behavior. Yet, despite years of valuable clinical experience and research into individual psychopathology, family functioning, and the influence of the family on the mental health of its members, there is still no standardized procedure for diagnosing family mental health or pathology (Cromwell, Olsen, & Fournier, 1965; Klein & Hill, 1979). There is a need for a comprehensive model of family functioning that integrates the complementary clinical insights and empirical data pertaining to various levels in the hierarchy of the family system (Framo, 1981; Gurman & Kniskern, 1978; Liddle & Halpin, 1978).

All but a few of the existing models of family functioning, developed by clinicians largely in isolation from each other, have failed to incorporate the generally accepted theories of individual psychopathology (Flomenhaft, 1980). Despite several attempts (Bowen, 1978; Pearce & Friedman, 1980), the interface between the family system pathology and pathology within the individual (i.e., member) subsystems has generally been ignored. Thus, individual and family approaches to formulation and treatment have developed separately, and often antagonistically.

Current literature reviews indicate a growing agreement on the essential dimensions of family functioning (Fisher, 1976). The family categories schema (Epstein *et al.*, 1962), later developed into the McMaster model (Epstein *et al.*, 1978), has provided the starting point for the process model of family functioning. Although respecting its predecessor's pioneering provision of an organizing structure, Steinhauer *et al.* (1984) felt a need for a more process-oriented and dynamic model that met the following criteria: Such a model should clearly distinguish between theories of family functioning and approaches to family treatment. It should be equally capable of describing successful and unsuccessful patterns of family structure and functioning. It should be able to serve as a framework to summarize and integrate the broad range of clinical and research findings available to date. It should provide a dynamic and process-oriented conceptual model to guide clinical assessment, ongoing treatment, and continuing research on families by defining universal dimensions of family functioning and describing interrelationships among them. It should encourage clinicians to integrate family-systems, psychoanalytic, attachment, social-learning, and crisis theories of development and psychopathology. Because no single model can, at this stage, account for the full richness of individual and family psychopathology, it should be compatible with other models of family and individual psychopathology and should begin the attempt to define the interfaces between them. Finally, such a model should generate new and researchable hypotheses about the structure and processes of family functioning. As real families are neither entirely healthy nor entirely pathological, it should describe families that function well in some areas but poorly in others and differentiate those coping well from those that cope poorly.

The process model of family functioning is one attempt to meet the above criteria. It differs from its predecessor, the family categories schema, primarily in three ways: By emphasizing the circular interaction among the major dimensions of family functioning and by its stress on the ongoing and interrelated development of individual and family, it describes not just family structure but ongoing family process. One can contrast the process model with other widely used models of family functioning (e.g., Minuchin's structural model and Epstein *et al.*'s McMaster model). The latter imply that structural relationships have an identity and a permanence of their own. The process model, however, emphasizes understanding each parameter as a separate entity and also stresses the effects of ongoing interaction at the interfaces between contiguous parameters and subsystems: parameter to parameter, intrapsychic to interpersonal (intrafamilial), interpersonal to social, and intrapsychic to social (Kantor & Lehr, 1975; Steinhauer & Tisdall, 1984; Steinhauer *et al.*, 1984). Second, the process model systematically attempts to integrate family systems theory with major theories of individual psychopathology. It does so by concentrating on the interface between individual subsystems and the family system. Examples include the discussion of how individual psychopathology affects communication and vice versa (see section headed "Communication," following); enmeshment as a phenomenon resulting from the interaction of both intrapsychic and interpersonal pathology (see "Affective Involvement"); the development and significance of the achievement of personal responsibility (see "Control"); and the origin, contribution, and influence of parental values, attitudes, and behavior on the family's values and norms (see "Values and Norms"). Third, the model builds in ways to include the influence of the greater social system of which the family is a part (see "Values and Norms"). The process model is rooted primarily in the family-therapy (as opposed to the small-group) literature, except for the contributions of Parsons and Bales (1955) and of Hill (1965). It is summarized here, and its compatibility with other models is discussed. For a more complete description of the model and its clinical applications, see Steinhauer *et al.* (1984), Steinhauer (1984), and Steinhauer and Tisdall (1984).

A hand-scored, self-report test based on the model, the Family Assessment Measure (FAM), has been developed. Already extensively used as a research tool, it is undergoing further evaluation for its ability to discriminate areas of family strength and weakness (Skinner, Steinhauer, & Santa-Barbara, 1983).

The Process Model of Family Functioning: An Overview

Like all small groups, the family and its members share common goals or objectives without which a group would not exist (Skynner, 1969; Tallman, 1970). The family's goals are to provide for the biological, psychological, and social development and maintenance of family members, thus ensuring the survival of both the family and the species (Ackerman, 1958; Murdock, 1960; Parsons & Bales, 1955). The achievement of these goals requires the execution of certain tasks. These vary over the course of the family life cycle but involve the same basic skills and processes (Brody, 1974; Glick, 1955; Scherz, 1971).

Figure 1 provides an overview of the basic model, indicating the major dimensions and their interrelationships. The superordinate goal of family functioning is the accomplishment of a variety of tasks (task accomplishment). Although some of these are culturally defined, others are unique to a particular family and are determined by that family's values and norms. These values and norms are a product of the internalized (psychological) derivatives of the parents' experience within their own families of origin; the shared history and experiences of the nuclear family; and the effects of cultural and subcultural influences. To accomplish these tasks, family members must successfully perform a variety of roles (role performance). Effective role performance demands the communication of information essential both to task accomplishment and to ongoing role definition, including the communication of feelings (affective expression), which, by its nature, can impede or facilitate task accomplishment and role performance. Members' emotional involvements with each other (affective involvement) and their ways of influencing one another (control) may either help or hinder task accomplishment.

Looking at Figure 1, one notes that values and norms are placed outside the

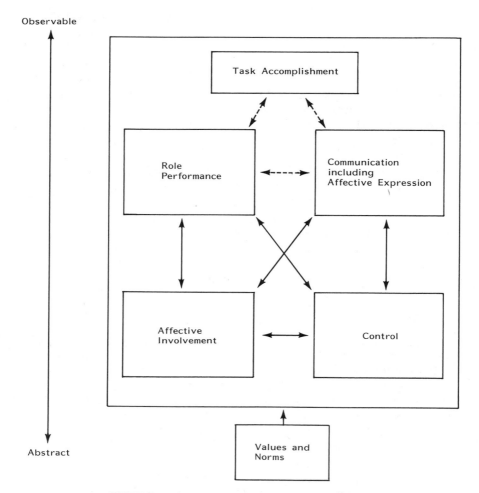

FIGURE 1. The process model of family functioning.

rectangular boundary enclosing the other major parameters of family functioning. This placement emphasizes the degree to which the other parameters are constantly being influenced by the family's values and norms. Those functions joined in the diagram by dotted arrows are more directly related to task accomplishment than those joined by solid arrows. The latter affect task accomplishment more indirectly through their influence on role performance and communication. The arrow to the left of the diagram indicates the degree of abstraction or observability of each of the major parameters in the model. One can directly observe whether or not—and by means of what steps—family tasks are accomplished. It is almost as easy to observe (though requiring more of a value judgment) whether certain defined types of communication and role performance are occurring. However, one must make more of a value judgment (rather than a direct observation) in assessing affective involvement, mechanisms of control and, still more, values and norms. These often require drawing conclusions from a mass of often contradictory data, both verbal and nonverbal. The practical significance of the "observability↔abstract" dimension is not yet clear beyond the obvious relationship between greater observability and the increased likelihood of obtaining observer agreement on a particular parameter.

This brief and greatly simplified description introduces the basic dimensions of the process model: task accomplishment, role performance, communication (including affective expression), affective involvement, values and norms, and control. The contents and processes of each of these dimensions—all of them subject to the values and norms of the particular family and the society of which the family is one subsystem—and the ways in which these parameters are interrelated are now described.

Task Accomplishment. Families achieve their biological, psychological, and social goals through successful task accomplishment. Some of these goals include ensuring the health, safety, comfort, and continuing development of all family members; providing reasonable security and autonomy for all; adapting usual patterns of functioning to meet environmental and developmental demands for change; supplying the cohesion needed to hold the family together; transmitting to the family the values of the culture; and serving as a mediator between the individual and society. With successful task accomplishment, the family functions effectively and with reasonable comfort within society. The achievement of these goals is the superordinate function of family life. The component processes involved in task accomplishment are illustrated in Figure 2.

Successful task accomplishment requires a common definition of major family tasks because, for example, if parents are upset by what they term children's misbehavior and the children resent what they define as parental overcontrol, continuing conflict rather than problem solving will occur. Successful task accomplishment is most likely if there is agreement on basic family goals and acceptance of the authority of family leaders, who encourage the expression and examination of alternative ways in which relevant family members can participate in finding generally acceptable solutions to new or different problems

ESSENTIAL PROCESSES

- Identifying the Tasks
- Exploring Alternative Approaches   } lead to TASK ACCOMPLISHMENT
- Taking Action
- Evaluating and Adjusting

CONTENTS

- Basic Tasks   - provision of necessities
- Development Tasks   - occur throughout the family life cycle
- Crisis Tasks   - task demands exceed family resources
                          (at least temporarily)

FIGURE 2. The components of task accomplishment.

(Leavitt, 1951; Tallman, 1970). Thus, one needs to understand who defines family tasks, how differences in definition and approaches to task accomplishment are reconciled, who takes responsibility for assigning tasks and following through to ensure their completion, and whether a mechanism exists for monitoring and evaluating task accomplishment and for renegotiating when necessary to devise a more successful approach.

The above discussion describes the process by which family tasks are accomplished. Specific tasks to be accomplished include ones (e.g., child rearing) that are culturally determined, so that one must understand the influences of the particular society or subculture on the family (Minuchin, 1975; Pavenstedt, 1967; Pearce, 1980; Rutter, 1976), the family's acceptance or rejection of these influences, and whatever idiosyncratic tasks and priorities the family sets for itself. Normal idiosyncracies or expressions of individual psychopathology also influence a family's definition of its essential tasks (Jackson, 1973; Johnson, 1967; Lidz, Fleck, Cornelison, & Terry, 1958; Winnicott, 1965), as does the unique nature of that family's system (Wertheim, 1973).

In day-to-day life, family problem-solving is abbreviated and much simplified, and many problems are dealt with by individuals or dyads without involving the family as a whole. Nevertheless, when problem solving becomes difficult, the above critical variables can help locate at which point(s) the problem-solving process is defective, as well as where to focus attempts at remediation.

Generally speaking, three types of tasks must be accomplished in all families:

Basic tasks are related to day-to-day survival, such as the provision of food, shelter, and health care.

Developmental tasks provide for the continuing development of all family members (Lidz, 1979; Sheehy, 1977). These tasks evolve constantly over the course of the family's life cycle and as individual members' developmental needs change (Lidz, 1970; Solnit, 1978). Thus, the type of nurturing essential for an infant would be pathogenic if imposed on an older child or an adult, although it may become necessary again as a result of illness, accident, or old age. A practical index of the successful accomplishment of developmental tasks is a family's ability to adapt its responses to the changing developmental needs of its members. Successful accomplishment of developmental tasks at one stage facilitates but does not guarantee successful development at a later stage (Barnhill & Longo, 1978; Carter & McGoldrick, 1980; Steinhauer, 1980). Unsuccessful accomplishment of developmental tasks at one stage may or may not be compensated for by catching up, or by reaching the same level by alternate developmental routes at a later date (Keniston, 1974).

Crisis tasks include the family's way of dealing with those periodic crises that occur when the number and intensity of the combined stresses confronting the family at one time temporarily exceed the skills and resources (psychological, familial, and social) available to deal with them (Hill, 1965; Steinhauer & Dickman, 1983). In a crisis, a family's capacity for successful task accomplishment is undermined, as the basic skills on which problem solving and tension relieving depend (i.e., individual cognitive capacity, integrated role behavior, and successful communication) are overwhelmed (Caplan, 1978). Families persevere in familiar patterns of task accomplishment, regardless of their appropriatness to the crisis at hand. They vary greatly in their ability to adapt problem-solving methods to meet the demands of potential crises. Their capacity to adjust communication patterns and role behavior to deal with mounting stress determines a particular family's vulnerability and ability to respond to crises (Anthony, 1978; Steinhauer, Levine, & DaCosta, 1971). A family's capacity to adapt to stress and to defuse potential crises is a strong indicator of family resilience or coping capacity (Anthony & Koupernik, 1973; Lewis, Bearer, Bassett, & Phillips, 1976).

Although it is obvious that a family's success in problem solving depends on successful communication and role performance, both of these are affected by the nature of that family's affective involvement (e.g., the degree of autonomy acceptable and the presence or absence of feelings of acceptance and support); control (e.g., the capacity for adaption when required and the constructiveness or destructiveness in the way leadership is assumed and exerted); and values and norms (e.g., the degree of freedom allowed individuals to choose how much and in which ways they will participate and consonance of family norms with those of the general society and/or the particular subgroups with which the family or its members are identified). At the same time, the nature of a family's experience in problem solving has feedback effects that will, in a circular manner, either reinforce or modify prevailing patterns of role performance, communication, affective involvement, and control.

Role Performance. Roles consist of prescribed and repetitive behaviors involving a set of reciprocal activities with other family members. Taken together, they either facilitate or interfere with successful task accomplishment. Successful role integration—achieved when all essential roles have been allocated, agreed to, and enacted—involves three distinct processes. These and their interrelationships are represented in Figure 3.

Effective role performance results in successful *role integration*. When this is achieved, all necessary tasks will be accomplished (i.e., role allocation is *comprehensive*), and roles are allocated with little overlap and inefficiency (i.e., allocations of the reciprocal and independent roles are *complementary*) (Jackson, 1957; Tharp, 1963). When roles are integrated, family members know what is expected of them and what they, in turn, can expect of others. Spiegel (1957) pointed to the association between role conflict and the contamination of (interpersonal) role behaviors by the psychopathology of individuals. Tharp (1965) demonstrated how role conflict originating in the marital dyad can spread throughout the family, leading to inappropriate role expectations and/or performance by one or more children. Although these expectations do not necessarily produce psychopathology in children, Tharp hypothesized that it is the degree and duration of the pressure on the child to assume inappropriate roles—without due consideration for that child's constitutional and psychological vulnerability—that determine whether, over time, internalized psychopathology will result from what was once interpersonal (role) pathology. Role

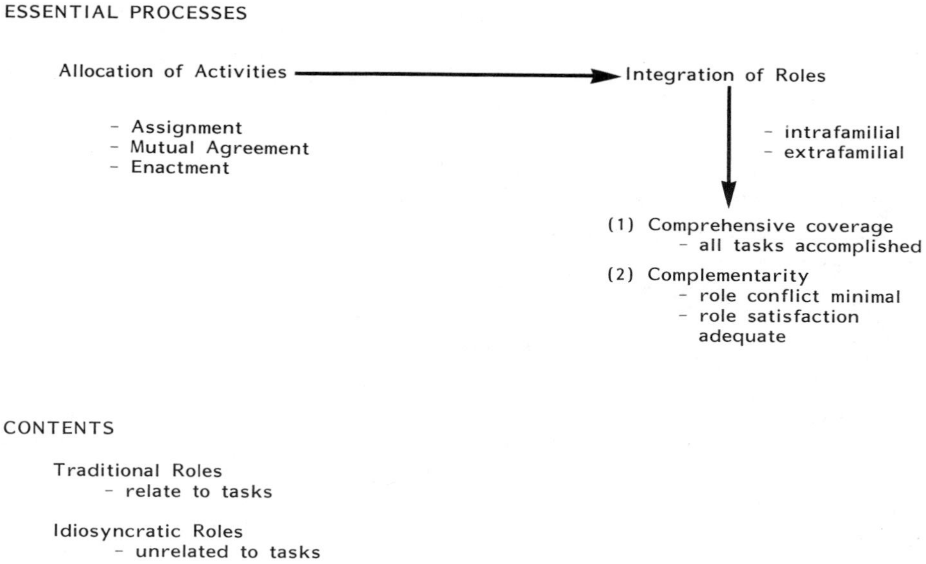

ESSENTIAL PROCESSES

Allocation of Activities ──────────────────────────▶ Integration of Roles

      – Assignment   – intrafamilial
      – Mutual Agreement   – extrafamilial
      – Enactment

                                          (1) Comprehensive coverage
                                              – all tasks accomplished
                                          (2) Complementarity
                                              – role conflict minimal
                                              – role satisfaction
                                                  adequate

CONTENTS

      Traditional Roles
          – relate to tasks

      Idiosyncratic Roles
          – unrelated to tasks

FIGURE 3. The components of role performance.

integration minimizes role conflict, increasing spontaneity and role satisfaction for all. The more members assume responsibility for enacting their assigned roles, the less pressure and conflict they and the family will exert on each other related to role behaviors.

Changing task demands require a constant monitoring and a periodic readjustment of role performance, depending on the environmental situation and the family's stage in its life cycle (Berman & Lief, 1975; Levinger, 1965). These changes necessitate continuing role realignments because changes in one member's role require reciprocal changes in the roles of others (Spiegel, 1957; Tharp, 1965). As they grow older and are increasingly involved in the world outside the family, members are assigned and assume new extrafamilial roles, which then compete with intrafamilial roles for members' energies and attention. Thus, a young boy becomes more than just a brother to his siblings and a son to his parents; he assumes the additional roles of student, member of a class, member of a hockey team, one of the boys, and so on. Excessive or conflicting role demands require resolution to prevent mounting role tension and to protect role complementarity (Spiegel & Kluckhohn, 1968).

In terms of content, roles may be classified as either traditional or idiosyncratic. *Traditional roles* contribute to the accomplishment of essential family tasks, but the definition of a traditional role (e.g., husband or wife) may vary enormously depending on the values and norms of the society and those subcultures of which the individual or the family is a part. Values and norms absorbed by modeling or identification within the parents' families of origin are transmitted across generational lines, and the internalized psychopathology of individual family members may strongly influence how a particular family defines traditional roles (Bower, 1960; Spiegel, 1957). There is no "correct" or "best" definition of a traditional role. What matters is that the family arrive at role definitions that work for it, while allowing enough flexibility to respect members' individual needs and to allow flexible adaptation, when needed, to accommodate to change.

Idiosyncratic roles do not contribute directly to task accomplishment and often express individual and family pathology. In general, idiosyncratic roles are maladaptive, draining energy away from essential family tasks, usually at a price to the individual and the family. Some families, for example, allocate one member to the role of family scapegoat, sacrificing his or her adjustment so that the family as a unit can exist in relative comfort (Ackerman, 1961; Vogel & Bell, 1960; Watzlawick, Beavin, Skiorski, & Mecia, 1970). Some scapegoats serve to bind the family together by constantly meeting the needs of others at the expense of their own. Others discharge through their behavior the hostile, antisocial, or sexual feelings disowned or repressed by others (Epstein, 1963; Johnston, 1967). Remaining trapped permanently in a scapegoat role reflects both individiaul psychopathology and pathology within the family system.

Role performance affects the accomplishment of basic, developmental, and crisis tasks. The rules regarding what kinds of communication are considered acceptable in a given family depend on role definition and on how reciprocal role behavior is orchestrated by the family's control mechanisms. At the same time, the nature of the members' affective involvement with each other, the level of their personal development, and the way in which they communicate with and control each other help to define role performance.

Communication. It is through communication that the information required for effective role performance and task accomplishment is exchanged (Alexander, 1973; Epstein *et al.*, 1962). The goal of communication—the achievement of mutual understanding—occurs if the messages sent are clear, direct, and sufficient, and if the receivers are psychologically available and open to receiving them with minimal distortion. The components of communication are outlined in Figure 4.

In content, a communication can be *affective* (i.e., expressive of feeling); *instrumental* (i.e., related to the ongoing tasks of everyday life); or *neutral* (i.e., neither instrumental nor affective) (Epstein *et al.*, 1962). At the same time, any communication ranges between *clear* and *masked* (i.e., vague, disguised, or ambiguous). Spiegel (1957) compared the function of masking at the interpersonal level of the family system to repression within the intrapsychic subsystem. The more masked the message, the more likely it is to reflect and arouse confusion, anxiety, and subsequent distortion in the receiver. The *directness* or *indirectness* of any message depends on whether it is sent to the appropriate receiver (Epstein & Bishop, 1981). Indirect communications are frequently disruptive because anyone who receives information clearly intended for someone else is thereby trapped between sender and receiver (Spiegel, 1957). Meanwhile, the intended receiver is in a bind: the content of the message invites a response, but the indirect transmission negates the invitation.

Latent content (including metacommunication, and expressed by choice of

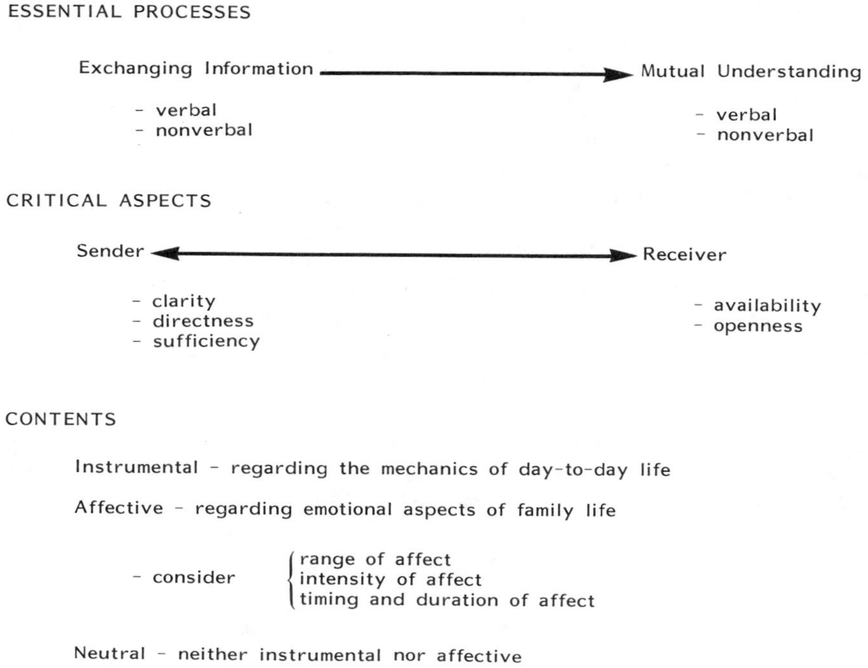

ESSENTIAL PROCESSES

Exchanging Information ⎯⎯⎯⎯⎯⎯⎯⎯⎯⎯⎯▶ Mutual Understanding

      – verbal   – verbal
      – nonverbal   – nonverbal

CRITICAL ASPECTS

Sender ◀⎯⎯⎯⎯⎯⎯⎯⎯⎯⎯⎯⎯⎯⎯⎯⎯⎯▶ Receiver

      – clarity   – availability
      – directness   – openness
      – sufficiency

CONTENTS

Instrumental – regarding the mechanics of day-to-day life

Affective – regarding emotional aspects of family life

                     ⎧ range of affect
      – consider   ⎨ intensity of affect
                     ⎩ timing and duration of affect

Neutral – neither instrumental nor affective

FIGURE 4. The components of communication.

words, tone of voice, facial expression, absence of eye contact, or body language) conveys much about the affective state of the sender and the quality of the relationship between sender and receiver. It also helps to define the cognitive and emotional responses of the receiver. When incongruity exists between manifest and latent levels of communication, the result is a paradoxical communication that invites confusion and anxiety in the receiver. But accurate perception is an active process requiring a capacity for empathy, a capacity to be attentive, and an ability to distinguish present from past and to retain and integrate messages with relevant aspects of past experience (Beavers, 1977; Skynner, 1976). Any of these component processes may be significantly distorted by the psychopathology of the receiver. Sender psychopathology can also interfere with directness and clarify or, by distorting the intensity of affect expressed or increasing the number of paradoxical messages sent, can decrease the likelihood of full and undistorted perception. For effective role allocation and task accomplishment, all necessary information must be clearly transmitted (verbally or nonverbally) and received, with minimal distortion by the appropriate receivers.

    Ambiguous communications contain either insufficient information or several unrelated but not incompatible messages leading to confusion and, frequently, anxiety. *Paradoxical* communications, however, include at least two incompatible messages, so that no matter how the receivers respond to one, they are inevitably in conflict with the other. This dilemma is greatest in the double bind (Bateson *et al.,* 1956; Watzlawick, Beavin, & Jackson, 1967), in which a relatively powerless receiver receives paradoxical communications from a family member too powerful to alienate, antagonize, or avoid. Any response to either of the incompatible messages is attacked, and family rules and/or personal psychopathology make impossible either clarification of the incompatible meanings or escape from the situation (Sluzki & Vernon, 1972; Watzlawick, 1963; Wynne, 1958).

The more disturbed the family, the greater the disruption in affective communication (Epstein, 1963). Unexpressed resentments tend to accumulate and then spill over unpredictably, contaminating first instrumental and eventually even neutral communication. In such families, any instrumental communication may be responded to as an attempt to dominate or control, which must be resisted if one is to preserve one's autonomy. Such families experience multiple power struggles because the accumulated resentments that are not recognized and/or expressed directly are displaced into the control parameter. When this displacement happens, the giving of orders or the refusal of obedience becomes (or is misinterpreted as) an indirect, masked expression of anger. Inevitably, role performance and task accomplishment suffer because the lack of effective communication blocks successful problem-solving, thus guaranteeing a perpetuation of tensions. At the same time, role conflict, the nature of affective involvement, control mechanisms, and family norms influence the nature and effectiveness of a family's communication.

Affective Involvement. The term *affective involvement* refers to the degree and quality of members' interest in and concern for one another. Optimally, the family meets all members' emotional needs, thus providing the cohesion, security, and sense of being valued that contribute to the development of trust, self-esteem, and independence. At the same time, such a family values and protects each others' right to independent thought and behavior. The development and maintenance of autonomy and security, among the most important of all developmental tasks, are intimately related to the family's affective involvement, the components of which are presented in Figure 5.

The *degree* of affective involvement is the intensity of family relationships and the members' involvement in each others' lives. The *quality* of that involvement determines whether the relationships are nurturant and supportive or destructive and self-serving (Epstein & Bishop, 1981). Unlike other models that imply that optimal affective involvement lies midway on the continuum between extreme cohesiveness and extreme disengagement (Olson *et al.*, 1979), the process model holds that the quality and degree of involvement taken together determine whether a given family will provide security and autonomy for all or, rather, will exploit and benefit only those who hold power and influence within it. The degree and quality of involvement vary independently, and together, they define a typology of affective involvements.

In the *uninvolved* family, both the degree and the quality of involvement are low. Such families resemble strangers in a boardinghouse. Their members are frequently alienated and unfulfilled. Such families also encourage premature emotional separation, often resulting in a pseudoindependence that markedly impairs the capacity to tolerate true intimacy. Uninvolved families also contrib-

ESSENTIAL PROCESSES

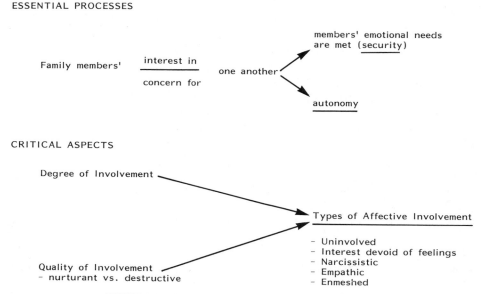

FIGURE 5. The components of affective involvement.

ute to ongoing insecurity and low self-esteem, thus blocking the development of true autonomy.

Families whose intensity and quality of involvement are only slightly greater than those of the uninvolved family may be described as showing *interest devoid of feelings*. In such families, interpersonal involvement arises more from a sense of duty, a need to control, or a basic intrusiveness than from sincere concern or empathy. Families at the higher end of this group may impart a vague sense of belonging, but the lack of true empathy usually leads to lasting frustration, insecurity, and worries about one's identity, acceptability, and self-worth.

Some families show a still higher intensity of affective involvement but withdraw their acceptance as soon as any member fails to satisfy the others' needs. Examples include parents who pressure their children to perform beyond their capacity, or who exploit and pressure them to fulfill the parents' own unachieved aspirations so that they can live vicariously through the children. Such children are faced with a Hobson's choice: to do without independence to retain parental approval, or to pursue autonomy at the expense of foregoing needed acceptance and security. Such parental *narcissistic* involvements are destructive in quality and usually excessive in degree.

Other families are high in acceptance and affection while remaining supportive of others' autonomy. Able to subordinate their own needs to those of others, members of these families share a genuine concern for each other that is truly *empathic*. In such families, members usually feel supported and cared for and experience the security and trust necessary for adequate self-esteem and true autonomy. Because such families are not threatened by autonomy, there is no need to suppress differences, and direct, clear communication and minimal role conflict allow orderly, predictable, and successful task accomplishment. Empathic families balance the autonomous needs of their members with the cohesion necessary for effective functioning as a unit.

One cannot ignore the quality dimension and directly equate degree of involvement with desirability. An even more intense but destructive involvement occurs when two or more members are *enmeshed* (Minuchin, 1974). The concept of enmeshment overlaps or is identical to those of symbiotic relationships (Mahler, Pine, & Bergman, 1975; Solnit, 1978); pseudomutuality (Wynne *et al.*, 1958); undifferentiated family ego mass (Boszormenyi-Nagy, 1965; Bowen, 1965); disruption of boundaries (Bowen, 1965; Lidz *et al.*, 1958); coherence (Bell, 1962); and the too richly cross-joined system (Ashby, 1981). Those enmeshed are trapped in a stifling and intense relationship that, although temporarily decreasing anxiety or meeting some defensive need for all involved, does so by blocking the continuing maturation of any. Enmeshments are always reciprocal (Giovacchini, 1976; Mahler *et al.*, 1975; Taylor, 1975). The adults involved have never individuated enough to establish clear and stable boundaries between themselves and those with whom they are symbiotically involved (Hoffman, 1975; Kantor & Lehr, 1975; Karpel, 1976; Slipp, 1980). Enmeshments are incompatible with the development of autonomy and usually involve tolerance, collusion, and reinforcement by other family members. Those involved are overly sensitive and react with panic or rage to any attempt by the other partner at withdrawal (Hoffman, 1976). Because of deficient ego boundaries, the enmeshment is perceived as necessary and appropriate (i.e., egosyntonic). Enmeshments are difficult to shift by confrontation, and attempts to do so threaten the family and evoke determined resistance. So crucial is the establishment of an appropriate distance within an enmeshed parent–child subsystem that many basic concepts of structural family therapy, first outlined by Minuchin (1974), are at the core of most attempts to treat families. The techniques used to counter enmeshments vary considerably, constituting one of the major differences between the various clinical approaches to family treatment (Steinhauer, 1985).

Enmeshment, therefore, indicates the existence of serious pathology at the interface between the intrapsychic and the family systems (Dell, 1982):

1. In the intrapsychic subsystem, failure of the future parents during development to achieve complete and stable ego boundaries results in a lasting inability to differentiate self from nonself. The incomplete boundaries invite excessive reliance on primitive defenses (i.e., projection, introjection, fusion, and splitting), which can occur only in the absence of sufficient boundaries (Freud, 1938, 1946; Klein, 1946). This reliance interferes with orderly communication, leading to widespread misunderstanding and constant acting-out in family relationships (Kantor & Lehr, 1975).

2. Enmeshed individuals are apt, especially under stress, to use excessively the pathological ego defenses listed above. These promote a defensive merging with other(s), thus perpetuating an enmeshed subsystem, that is, a relatively permanent fusion of individuals within which each confuses his or her thoughts, feelings, and needs with those of the partner (Boszormenyi-Nagy, 1965; Bowen,

1965). Enmeshed relationships are extremely vulnerable to circular acting-out, as all who are involved behaviorally express impulses and affects from the partner across the excessively permeable common boundary (Johnston, 1967). Any attempt by one partner to escape from an enmeshment evokes panic and entrapping behavior in the other(s) also involved (Steinhauer & Tisdall, 1984).

Those whose ego boundaries are adequate have sufficient autonomy to defend against and repel pressure toward enmeshment from others whose boundaries are less complete. The circular relationship between affective involvement, role performance, and control should be obvious from the above discussion. Various subsystems (subgroups) often illustrate different types of affective involvement, so that an enmeshment in one dyad (e.g., parent and child) often reinforces and is reinforced by uninvolvement in another subsystem (e.g., husband and wife). Problem solving (task accomplishment), the types of solutions sought for family problems, and the degree to which family members achieve and support others' achievement of autonomy are markedly influenced by the type of affective involvement typical of a given family. Problem solving is one major area in which families either give or withhold affection and support in response to autonomous behavior. This response not only affects the quality of task accomplishment, but has a major role in reaffirming or denying those personal qualities related to successful separation and individuation (e.g., self-concept, psychological self-esteem, and completeness of boundaries) (Steinhauer & Tisdall, 1984; Winnicott, 1958).

Control. Families use various strategies or techniques to influence members' behavior. Because family roles are reciprocal, members need to influence each other—at times, to sustain ongoing functioning and, at others, to adapt it to meet changing task demands (Spiegel, 1957; Tharp, 1965). Ideally, families exert sufficient control to guarantee security and cohesion, at the same time allowing enough flexibility to support ongoing individuation (Skynner, 1969). The components of control are found in Figure 6.

The *maintenance component* of control governs how family members influence each other to ensure the accomplishment of the instrumental tasks and role requirements of daily life (Epstein & Bishop, 1981; Tharp, 1963). Because task and role requirements are not constant, successful control of maintenance functioning, including minor adjustment on a day-to-day basis, is needed for successful task accomplishment. Without it, roles are not integrated, and the results are frequent role conflict, inefficient task accomplishment, and the ongoing friction and tension that these inevitably evoke.

But periodically changing developmental and environmental circumstances places new and different demands on families (Skynner, 1969). Families vary greatly in their ability to adapt habitual patterns of functioning and problem solving to accommodate the need for change. The less adaptable the family, the more chronic tension and interference with task accomplishment are likely to result from its inability to perceive and adapt appropriately to new or different problems and developmental demands. How family members influence each others' adaptations to demands for change constitutes the *adaptation component* of the control dimension (see also Hoffman, 1965; Leavitt, 1951; Olson *et al.*, 1979).

ESSENTIAL PROCESSES

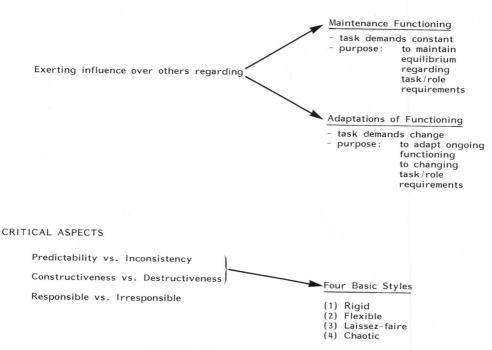

FIGURE 6. The components of control.

Both the maintenance and the adaptation components of control are affected by a given family's style, which may vary in its predictability, constructiveness, and responsibility (Mussen, Conger, & Kagan, 1974). *Predictability* results from the consistency of the style; if extremely high, it leaves little room for spontaneity. If it is extremely low, no one knows what will happen next. *Constructiveness* refers to whether control techniques are educational and nurturant or shaming and destructive to initiative and self-esteem. Whether members influence others by trying to achieve consensus or, alternately, by strongly imposing their will on the weak without regard for their feelings or agreement also affects the constructiveness of a family's control. A third critical aspect of control involves the achievement and internalization of a sense of personal *responsibility* (Winnicott, 1958, 1976). This is so important to personal motivation and initiative that its achievement represents a major developmental task affecting both productivity and relations with others. As this sense of responsibility occurs at the interface between family and individual functioning, it will be described in detail.

The internalization of a sense of responsibility, a prerequisite for self-discipline and initiative, is related to several simultaneously occurring processes. These begin with the absorption through identification of the essential values of the family and the influence of the parents as role models. Although secondary identifications and role modeling do occur, particularly during adolescence, those with the parents begin the gradual internalization and integration of a stable system of inner values essential to the child's capacity for impulse control, self-discipline, and inner-directedness. Children often experience pressure from their peers to behave in ways that contradict or challenge these early internalized values. If familial and societal pressures are mutually consistent, they reinforce each other. If, however, there are inherent contradictions, as when parents try to train a child to be responsible while demonstrating consistent irresponsibility in their own behavior, or when peers' values conflict with those of the parents, the resulting dissonance invites both interpersonal and intrapsychic conflict that confuse and undermine the development of inner controls. Whereas identification is clearly related both to affective involvement (either positively or negatively; Weinrich, 1982) and to role performance (via role modeling), the internalization of a sense of personal responsibility and the capacity for impulse control are prerequisites for responsible and productive social behavior. We consider simplistic and incomplete any model of family functioning that views control entirely as an interpersonal phenomenon and neglects the role of individual responsibility.

A family's predictability and constructiveness vary independently, and combining them defines four prototypical control styles: *rigid, flexible, laissez-faire,* and *chaotic.* A *rigid* style is extremely predictable but low in constructiveness and adaptability. All know what is expected and what will happen if they don't comply. Rigid families are often quite successful in maintenance control, but their rigidity frequently interferes with successful adaptation and the assumption of personal responsibility. Under stress, when change is required, the forced and punitive aspects of this style encourage subversion, passive aggressiveness, displacement of anger outside the home, and multiple power struggles (Mussen *et al.,* 1974), which, in turn, are used to rationalize further rigidity.

A *flexible* control style combines moderate predictability with high constructiveness. It is consistent enough so that members know what to expect of each other, though not at the expense of individuality or spontaneity. A flexible style assists task accomplishment because its supportive and educational tone encourages family members to participate and to identify with the ideals and rules of the family (Hoffman, 1965; Tallman, 1970). Control is benign yet effective, relying on consensus where possible but setting and enforcing limits when necessary. Maintenance functioning is usually relatively efficient, and the capacity for adaptation is a major family asset.

A *laissez-faire* style combines moderate predictability with low constructiveness. Because anything goes, inertia and indecision take the place of organized planning and activity. In such families, members do as they please so long as they avoid bothering others, as little responsibility is assumed or expected. Because of their constant disorganization, role integration is rarely achieved, task accomplishment is haphazard, and communication is frequently insufficient, unclear, and indirect. The breakdown of organization in such families often leads to considerable chronic frustration and ineffective task accomplishment. The lack of parental guidance often results from a low degree of affective involvement. Children raised in such families often demonstrate insecure, attention-seeking behavior and inadequate impulse control, self-discipline, and self-direction. These characteristics frequently cause difficulties when the children begin school and are expected to conform and to produce on demand.

A *chaotic* style is extremely low in both predictability and constructiveness, plunging between being laissez-faire at times and, at others, being excessively but ineffectively punitive and rigid. Changes occur less in response to situational demands than to the whim or mood of powerful family members. Instability and inconsistency typify such families, and the overall effect is destructive. The resulting disorganization typically interferes with both maintenance and adaptational functioning, so that hostility and/or withdrawal is a typical response to the continual frustration, confusion, and unpredictability that these families provide. The security component of affective involvement is not achieved, although a pseudoautonomy, which contributes to premature and stormy detachment from the family, often occurs (Steinhauer, 1972). The circular relationship between the various aspects of control and the parameters of task accomplishment (e.g., problem solving), role performance, and communication is obvious.

Values and Norms. Every aspect of family functioning directly or indirectly reflects that family's values and norms. The way in which roles are defined, the forms of communication considered acceptable, the predominant patterns of affective involvement, and the control style are all shaped by values derived partly from the influences of the parents' families of origin, and partly from the culture and subgroups to which the family belongs (Boszormenyi-Nagy & Ulrich, 1981).

Consider first the values and norms brought into the nuclear family by the parents from their own earlier life experiences. Skynner (1969) emphasized the family's special role as a bridge between the members of one generation and those of the next. Across this bridge are passed values and patterns derived either by identification or through a more-or-less conscious repudiation of the grandparents, mediated by the influences of peers and subcultural groups on the parents during their growing up. These, although originally experienced as external influences, have since been internalized, persisting as intrinsic parental values (Weinrich, 1982).

Second, consider the influences of the subgroups to which the members of the current family belong. Living in neighborhoods with a high rate of delinquency, being exposed to the philosophies of the women's movement, being a teenager in the 1980s, and being deeply religious in a time of changing sexual mores can strongly influence both individuals and families. Should there be major dissonance (i.e., conflict) between subgroup values and those of the family, the likelihood of both intrapsychic and interpersonal confusion, tension, and discord is higher than there is high concurrence.

Third, consider the influences of the culture as a whole. Development occurs within concentric rings of relationships: the individual is part of a family, which, in turn, is contained and shaped by the surrounding society (Erikson, 1963; Rakoff, 1980a; Skynner, 1969). Each successive ring can enhance the possibilities of achievement or of failure during each developmental stage. One's personal identity and sense of self-worth, defined originally by family relationships, are increasingly refined with age, as one moves beyond the protective boundaries of the family and out in society.

Some families are restless movers, whereas others remain essentially detached from the contexts of extended family, place, religion, history, or communal customs. Just as the child must bond to the mother to develop a capacity for intimacy, so failure of the family to feel bonded within the larger community results in restless apathy, growing detachment, alienation or anomie, and a loss of moral and existential significance. Rakoff (1980a,b) suggested that growing up in a family lacking any social context will, even without significant family pathology, predispose to existential depression and suicide (and, the authors would add, potential violence), all symptomatic of the failure to bond to—and therefore, to feel bound by—the values of society (Steinhauer, 1982).

The family's values may be either dissonant or consonant with those of society and particular subcultures (Pearce, 1980). For example, most parents in the 1960s considered marijuana dangerous and immoral, although the youth subculture sanctioned it as harmless and socially desirable. Similarly, liberal attitudes toward abortion, originally confined to well-defined pressure groups and opposed by society generally, have shifted the national attitude toward abortion, resulting in more liberal abortion laws. As a result, there is now higher consonance between the legal (i.e., culturally sanctioned) position on abortion and that of those subgroups that effectively pressed for abortion reform. Individuals and families find this new legal position either dissonant or consonant with their own individually held values.

These multiple influences on values and norms contribute to the development of a family's value system, consisting of ideas and rules. Those values toward which the family aspires constitute that family's ideals, which are either moral-religious or personal-social. To approach these ideals, the family develops rules that define acceptable behavior, that is, ways in which its ideals are to be pursued. The resulting interplay between ideals and rules defines that family's norms, that is, that standard of behavior considered minimally acceptable within the family. The norms are the specific behaviors by which adherence to the family's rules—and therefore, to its ideals—are judged. Thus, a family's value system is derived from a number of complex and interrelated processes that provide many opportunities for dissonance and conflict. The critical dimensions of values and norms are illustrated in Figure 7. These include whether the various influences on the family's value system are dissonant or consonant with each other, whether there is consonance between explicit and implicit rules, and what latitude is allowed members to develop their personal value systems. For example, a family that explicitly demands honesty and integrity may delight in its ability to profit from dishonest business practices or may condone known antisocial behavior (e.g., theft or cheating) as long as this behavior remains undetected outside the family.

Moral and religious values include all definitions of what is morally acceptable resulting from either social (i.e., by a religious denomination or from subcultural

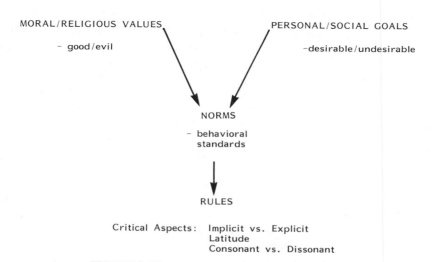

FIGURE 7. The components of values and norms.

influences) or from psychological (i.e., by the internalized value system or super-ego) influences. *Goals and standards* are personally held beliefs, socially or psychologically influenced, that define what constitutes desirable behavior. For example, being successful, hardworking, self-supporting, or ambitious, or being an "A" student may be important or unimportant, depending on the goals of the particular family. Moral and religious values are judged in terms of right or wrong (i.e., in terms of moral validity), but goals and standards are seen as being desirable or undesirable (i.e., in terms of psychological or social desirability).

Family *rules* are both explicit and implicit. Explicit rules are clearly, directly, and openly stated. Certain families, however, have a second set of rules that cover some of the most critical areas of attitude and behavior, and that are never made explicit. These implicit rules may conflict with those that are explicit. For example, an explicit demand that children respect parents may be sabotaged by one parent's covertly encouraging the children to defy the other, with whom there is indirect conflict. *Metarules,* unspoken rules that define which explicit rules are to be considered binding, are an important set of implicit rules. The greater the dissonance between explicit and implicit rules, especially when meta-rules are not clearly sensed and universally accepted, the more the resulting anxiety and confusion (Watzlawick *et al.*, 1967).

Latitude—that is, the scope allowed individuals to determine their own attitudes and behavior—correlates highly with the family's tolerance of individual autonomy. The family with a narrow latitude has rules covering most areas of family life, allowing little individual choice. In extreme cases, such families, termed *pseudomutual* (Wynne *et al.*, 1958), demand the right to define how family members should think or feel, a situation obviously incompatible with autonomy. The family with a broad latitude has fewer rules and tolerates more individual choice, although in extreme situations excessively broad latitude may produce chaos and may undermine family functioning. Most families find a range of latitudes optimal for adaptive functioning, whereas extremes in either direction may be conducive to dysfunction and psychopathology.

A family's *norms* are the sum total of what is and is not acceptable within that family. Derived from the influences discussed above, norms define the minimal standards to which both individuals and the family as a whole are expected to adhere. Even in families that agree that honesty is desirable, family norms may introduce important expectations and qualifications. For example, although "little white lies" to avoid hurting someone's feelings may be acceptable, lies to cover up misbehavior may not. Or lying within the family may be intolerable, although lying to protect a family member in trouble with outsiders, such as neighbors or the police, is expected. In view of these inconsistencies, the family's norms may have to be learned by rote. They are the final word concerning what is considered acceptable behavior.

Although the process model identifies characteristics of each of the previously discussed dimensions that are conducive to healthy or pathological functioning, it is unable to take any such position with respect to values and norms. Except for our stated concern about the effects of dissonance between conflicting psychological and/or cultural influences, we cannot identify patterns within this dimension, independent of specific content, that are inherently healthy or pathological. Nevertheless, understanding a family's values and norms is crucial to understand that family's functioning. Values and norms are diagrammatically represented outside the basic model to emphasize their pervasive direct and indirect influences on all aspects of family functioning (see Figure 1).

DISCUSSION AND CONCLUSIONS

How does the process model of family functioning compare to other models discussed earlier in this chapter?

The process model is a general and comprehensive model of family functioning, intended to be compatible with other major models of family and individual functioning and psychopathology. It does not treat specialized aspects of family functioning in the same depth as some of the experimental models discussed. Klein and Hill (1979), for example, more thoroughly analyzed family problem-solving, and Aldous (1971), Walsh (1982), and Carter and McGoldrick (1980) have discussed the effects of development on family functioning more intensively than does the process model. However, the process model is compatible with all the above models, and its users are encouraged to regard it as a framework around which to organize and integrate other data and theories, rather than as a model complete within itself.

The process model meets both those criteria set forth by Klein and Hill (see pp. 82–83) and those considered essential by practicing family therapists (see p. 86) for a comprehensive model of family functioning. Like the models of Fleck (1980) and Epstein *et al.* (1978), it maintains that any model comprehensive enough to capture the multiplicity of family structure and functioning must include the interaction of many more universal parameters than such two-dimensional models as those of Reiss (1971), Straus (1968), Broderick and Pulliam-Krager (1979), Kantor and Lehr, (1975), and Olson *et al.* (1979). A family model based on only two variables is obviously easier to validate than a more complex one. None of these two-dimensional models, however, meets either Klein and Hill's criteria (1979) or those of the author for comprehensiveness and clinical utility. Despite some differences in organization and labeling, the similarities between those prime parameters of universal family functioning selected by Klein and Hill, Epstein, Fleck, and the author are far more marked than any discrepancies.

The major differences between the process model and the McMaster model lie in the process model's increased emphasis on the interrelationships between the prime parameters of family functioning, those between family and individual pathology, and, through the inclusion in the process model of values and norms as a separate parameter, the pervasive influence on all aspects of family functioning at the interface between family and society.

Fleck's model of family systems parameters (1980) deals with roughly the same prime parameters of family functioning as the McMaster and process models and, like the latter, stresses the ongoing interaction between them. As in the process model, Fleck considered the interface between family and society but was less concerned with the interface between the interpersonal (familial) and intrapsychic (individual) subsystems. Fleck did refer briefly to the problems that occur in trying to relate individual psychiatric diagnoses to classifications of family pathology. He suggested that pinpointing the nature of the family disorder would be useful in deciding on a course of management, but that family pathology is only very weakly correlated with individual psychiatric diagnosis. One also regrets the lack of detailed description of the contents and interrelationships of Fleck's parameters that makes Fleck's model more a theoretical statement of the relationship between key parameters than a comprehensive model of family functioning.

Fleck did, however, avoid suggesting that a straight-line relationship exists between a family typology and the major individual diagnostic categories. To have done so would be to imply, via linear thinking, that common family pathology produces similar pathological reactions in vulnerable children. Yet, we

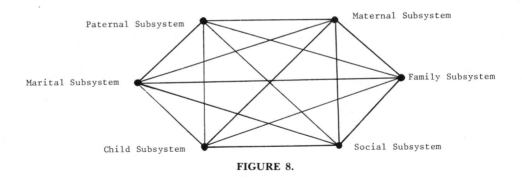

FIGURE 8.

know that this is not so. Clinically, different children react differently to common stresses and are influenced less by the nature of the common stress than by the interacting effects of the age, the sex, and the basic temperament of the child; the child's typical character structure and habitual ways of dealing with stress (including the type and use of defense mechanisms); the characteristic structure and interactional rules of the family; and subcultural influences (Sameroff & Kelly, 1977). A formulation based on linear thinking (e.g., Family Type A ⟶ Disorder Type B) would have a greater chance of being successful if there were only two basic sets of variables involved. However, to understand the pressure either toward or away from (i.e., protecting against) psychopathogenesis within a given family, one must understand and formulate the contributions and interrelationships of at least six sets of variables (see Figure 8):

1. Contributions from father:
   a. Genetic
   b. Psychodynamic
2. Contributions from mother:
   a. Genetic
   b. Psychodynamic
3. Contributions from the nature of the marital subsystem
4. Contributions from the individual (child) subsystem:
   a. Biological factors in the child, including genetic and other biological and constitutional factors.
   b. Psychological factors in the child
5. Contributions from the nature of the family system
6. Contributions from the nature of the social system and any relevant subsystems

The topic of systemic formulation is discussed and illustrated in more detail by Steinhauer (1983).

In summary, the process model is a good starting point for those interested not only in family therapy (i.e., therapy directed toward the alteration of family structure and functioning) but also in systems therapy (i.e., a therapy whose goal is to improve functioning and to relieve distress of the family and its members at intrapsychic, interpersonal, and social levels of equilibrium). Papers on the clinical applications of the model (Steinhauer, 1984) and on its usefulness in providing a theoretical rationale for the systematic selection and integration of individual and family therapies have been published and presented (Steinhauer & Tisdall, 1982). More recently, Steinhauer and Tisdall (1984; Steinhauer, 1985) have pressed the clinical utility of the model further as part of their attempt to develop a comprehensive and client-centered theoretical rationale for treatment selection in both outpatient and community settings.

The test based on the model, the Family Assessment Measure, is already widely used as a research tool, and the recent development of a hand-scored version has, for the first time, made it practical to use clinically, either as one component of a family assessment or to monitor changes in response to therapy (Skinner *et al.*, 1983). A computerized version of the test, being completed, should increase its attractiveness to children and adolescents. Also, for researchers, this version should provide a change and a rest from the pencil-and-paper testing that forms part of extensive test batteries. The test is more fully described in Chapter 11.

As a teaching device, the model has several potential advantages. It breaks down the universal aspects of family functioning into six prime parameters, each of which has a small number of clearly defined critical variables. It serves as a guide to ensuring the comprehensiveness of family assessments and as a method of helping inexperienced family therapists shift from anecdotal data to the underlying themes of pathological structure and functioning from which the data are derived. It can help inexperienced therapists to find their bearings when overwhelmed by sensory and emotional overload and can assist them in setting and measuring progress toward therapeutic goals. The model encourages its users to take a broad and truly systemic approach to case formulation and treatment planning, selection, and management. This approach helps to prevent the common tendency to polarize family and individual therapies as if they were incompatible, thus encouraging students to integrate new and complementary ways of understanding case material with those with which they are already familiar (Steinhauer, 1984). By transcending the doctrinal barriers that have too long insisted that psychologically oriented and systems-oriented approaches to therapy are incompatible, the model encourages a creative, rational, and purposeful selection and combination of treatments based on patients' (or clients') needs, rather than on therapists' bias.

ACKNOWLEDGMENTS

The role of Jack Santa-Barbara in initiating the process model of family functioning and the Family Assessment Measure and in serving as the principal investigator until the spring of 1981 is gratefully acknowledged, as is that of Harvey Skinner, who contributed to the development of the process model and, especially, to the subsequent development of the FAM.

REFERENCES

Ackerman, N. W. (1958). *The psychodynamics of family life*. New York: Basic Books.

Ackerman, N. W. (1961). Prejudicial scapegoating and neutralizing forces in the family group, with special reference to the role of family healer. *International Journal of Social Psychiatry* (Special Ed. No. 2), pp. 90–96.

Aldous, J. (1966). *Lower-class males: Integration into community and family*. Paper presented at Sixth World Congress of Sociology, Evian, France.

Aldous, J. (1971). A framework for the analysis of family problem-solving. In J. Aldous, J. Condon, R. Hill, M. A. Straus, & I. Tallman (Eds.), *Family problem solving: A symposium on theoretical, methodological, and substantive concerns*. Hinsdale, IL: Dryden Press.

Aldous, J. (1974). *The developmental approach to family analysis: Vol. 1. The conceptual framework*. Minneapolis: University of Minnesota Press.

Aldous, J. (1978). *Family careers: Developmental change in families*. New York: Wiley.

Alexander, J. F. (1973). Defensive and supportive communication in normal and deviant families. *Journal of Consulting and Clinical Psychology, 40*, 223–231.

Anthony, J. E. (1978). Theories of change and children at high risk for change. In J. E. Anthony & C. Chilands (Eds.), *The child and his family: Children and their parents in a changing world*. New York: Wiley.

Anthony, J. E., & Koupernik, C. (1973). *The child and his family: The impact of disease and death*. New York: Wiley.

Aponte, H. J., & van Deusen, J. M. (1981). Structural family therapy. In A. S. Gurman & D. P. Kniskern (Eds.), *Handbook of family therapy*. New York: Brunner/Mazel.

Ashby, W. R. (1981). *Foundation of family therapy*. New York: Basic Books.

Bales, R. F., & Slater, P. E. (1955). Role differentiation in small decision-making groups. In T. Parsons & R. F. Bales (Eds.), *Family, socialization and interaction process*. Glencoe, IL: Free Press.

Bales, R. F., & Strodbeck, F. L. (1951). Phases in group problem solving. *Journal of Abnormal Social Psychology, 46*, 485–495.

Barnhill, L. R., & Longo, D. (1978). Fixation and regression in the family life cycle. *Family Process, 17*, 469–478.

Bateson, C., Jackson, D. D., Haley, J., & Weakland, J. (1956). Toward a theory of schizophrenia. *Behavioral Science, 1*, 251–264.

Beavers, W. R. (1977). *Psychotherapy and growth: A family systems perspective*. New York: Brunner/Mazel.

Beck, D. F., & Jones, M. A. (1974). *Progress on family problems: A nationwide study of clients' and counselors' views on family agency services*. New York: Family Service Association of America.

Beels, C. C., & Ferber, A. (1969). Family therapy: A view. *Family Process, 8*, 280–318.

Bell, J. E. (1971). *Family group therapy: A method for psychological treatment of older children, adolescents and their parents* (Public Health Monograph No. 64). Washington, DC: U.S. Department of Health, Education, and Welfare.

Bell, N. W. (1962). Extended family relations of disturbed and well families. *Family Process, 12*, 83–94.

Bell, N. W., & Vogel, E. F. (1960). Toward a framework for functional analysis of family behavior. In N. W. Bell & E. F. Vogel (Eds.), *A modern introduction to the family*. New York: Free Press.

Berger, A. (1965). A test of the double-bind hypothesis of schizophrenia. *Family Process, 4*, 198–205.

Berman, E. M., & Lief, H. I. (1975). Marital therapy from a psychiatric perspective: An overview. *American Journal of Psychiatry, 132*, 583–592.

Birchler, G., Weiss, R., & Vincent, J. (1975). Multimethod analysis of social reinforcement exchange between maritally distressed and nondistressed spouse and stranger dyads. *Journal of Personality and Social Psychology, 31*, 349–360.

Bloch, D. A. (1973). *Techniques of family psychotherapy: A primer*. New York: Grune & Stratton.

Blood, R. O., & Wolfe, D. M. (1960). *Husbands and wives: The dynamics of family living*. New York: Free Press.

Boszormenyi-Nagy, I. (1965). Intensive family therapy as process. In I. Boszormenyi-Nagy & J. Framo (Eds.), *Intensive family therapy*. New York: Harper & Row.

Boszormenyi-Nagy, I., & Ulrich, D. N. (1981). Contextual family therapy. In A. S. Gurman & D. P. Kniskern (Eds.), *Handbook of family therapy*. New York: Brunner/Mazel.

Bowen, M. (1965). Family psychotherapy with schizophrenia in the hospital and private practice. In I. Boszormenyi-Nagy & J. Framo (Eds.), *Family therapy*. New York: Harper & Row.

Bowen, M. (1971). The use of family theory in clinical practice. In J. Haley (Ed.), *Changing families*. New York: Grune & Stratton.

Bowen, M. (1975). Family therapy after 20 years. In D. Freedman & J. Dyrud (Eds.), *American handbook of psychiatry: Vol. 5. Treatment* (2nd ed.). New York: Basic Books.

Bowen, M. (1978). Family therapy and family group therapy. In M. Bowen (Ed.), *Family therapy in clinical practice*. New York: Jason Aronson.

Bower, M. A. (1960). Family concepts of schizophrenia. In D. D. Jackson (Ed.), *The etiology of schizophrenia*. New York: Basic Books.

Bowlby, J. (1949). The study and reduction of group tensions in the family. *Human Relations, 2*, 123–128.

Brim, O. G., Jr., Fairchild, R. W., & Borgatta, E. F. (1961). Relations between family problems. *Marriage and Family Living, 23*, 219–226.

Broderick, C. B., & Pulliam-Krager, H. (1979). Family process and child outcomes. In W. R. Burr, R. Hill, F. I. Nye, & I. L. Reiss (Eds.), *Contemporary theories about the family* (Vol. 1). London: Free Press.

Brody, E. (1974). Aging and family personality: A developmental view. *Family Process, 13*, 23–37.

Bronfenbrenner, U. (1961). Toward a theoretical model for the analysis of parent–child relationships in a social context. In J. C. Glidewell (Ed.), *Parental attitudes and child behavior*. Springfield, IL: Charles C Thomas.

Burns, T. (1973). A structural theory of social exchange. *Acta Sociologica, 16*, 188–208.

Caplan, G. (1978). Family support systems in a changing world. In E. J. Anthony & C. Chilands (Eds.), *The child and his family: Children and their parents in a changing world*. New York: Wiley.

Carter, E. A., & McGoldrick, M. (Eds.). (1980). *The family life cycle: A framework for family therapy*. New York: Gardner.

Chasin, R. & Grunebaum, H. (1980). A brief synopsis of current concept and practices in family therapy. In J. K. Pearce & L. J. Friedman (Eds.), *Family therapy: Combining psychodynamic and family systems approaches*. New York: Grune & Stratton.

Cohen, R. L. (1974). *Social class differences in the problem-solving process: An integration of social organization, language and nonverbal communication*. Unpublished doctoral thesis, University of Minnesota, Minneapolis, MN.

Cromwell, R. C., Olsen, D. H., & Fournier, D. (1965). Tools and techniques for diagnosis and evaluation in marital and family theory. *Family Process, 15*, 1–49.

Daly, M., & Wilson, M. (1978). *Sex, evolution and behavior: Adaptations for reproduction*. North Scituate, MA: Duxbury.

Dell, P. F. (1982). Beyond homeostasis: Towards a concept of coherence. *Family Process, 21*, 21–24.

Duvall, E. M. (1971). *Family development* (4th ed.). Philadelphia: Lippincott.

Epstein, N. B. (1963). *Family psychiatry: Comments on theory, therapeutic techniques and clinical investigation*. Paper presented at Conference on Multiproblems Families, sponsored by the Laidlaw Foundation, Toronto.

Epstein, N. B., & Bishop, D. S. (1981). Problem-centered systems therapy of the family. In A. S. Gurman & D. P. Kniskern (Eds.), *Handbook of family therapy*. New York: Basic Books.

Epstein, N. B., Rakoff, V., & Sigal, J. J. (1962). *Family categories schema*. Monograph prepared in the Family Research Group of the Department of Psychiatry, Jewish General Hospital, Montreal, in collaboration with the McGill University Human Development Study.

Epstein, N. B., Bishop, D., & Levin, S. (1978). The McMaster model of family functioning. *Journal of Marriage and Family Counselling, 4*, 19–31.

Erikson, E. H. (1963). *Childhood and society*. New York: W. W. Norton.

Farber, B. (1964). *Family: Organization and interaction*. San Francisco: Chandler.

Fisher, L. (1976, October). Dimensions of family assessment: A critical review. *Journal of Marriage and Family Counselling*, pp. 367–382.

Fleck, S. (1980). Family functioning and family pathology. *Psychiatric Annals, 10*, 46–57.

Flomenhaft, K. (1980). Introduction: The challenge of family therapy. In K. Flomenhaft & A. E. Christ (Eds.), *The challenge of family therapy—A dialogue for child psychiatry educators*. New York: Plenum Press.

Framo, J. L. (1965). Systematic research on family dynamics. In I. Boszormenyi-Nagy & J. Framo (Eds.), *Intensive family therapy: Theoretical and practical aspects*. New York: Harper & Row.

Framo, J. L. (1981). The integration of marital therapy with sessions with family of origin. In A. S. Gurman & D. P. Kniskern (Eds.), *Handbook of family therapy*. New York: Brunner/Mazel.

Freud, S. (1938). Splitting of the ego in the defensive progress. *Collected Papers* (Vol. 5). New York: Basic Books.

Freud, S. (1946). *The ego and the mechanisms of defense*. New York: International Universities Press.

Geismar, L. L., & LaSorte, M. A. (1964). *Understanding the multi-problem family*. New York: Association Press.

Giovacchini, P. L. (1976). Symbiosis and intimacy. *International Journal of Psychoanalytic Psychotherapy, 5*, 413–436.

Glick, I. D. (1955). Life cycle of the family. *Journal of Marriage and Family Living, 18*, 3–9.

Goodrich, A. W. (1980). Introduction of family therapy into child psychiatry training: Two styles of change. In K. Flomenhaft & A. E. Christ (Eds.), *Family therapy: Combined psychodynamic and family systems approaches*. New York: Grune & Stratton.

Graziano, W. G., & Musser, L. M. (1982). The joining and the partings of the ways. In S. W. Duck (Ed.), *Personal relationships: 4. Dissolving personal relationships*. London: Academic Press.

Greenberg, J. (1978). Effects of reward value and retaliative power on allocation decisions. Justice, generosity or greed? *Journal of Personality and Social Psychology, 36*, 367–379.

Group for the Advancement of Psychiatry. (1970). *Treatment of families in conflict: The clinical study of family process*. New York: Science House.

Grunebaum, H., & Chasin, R. (1980). Thinking like a family therapist. In K. Flomenhaft & A. E. Christ (Eds.), *The challenge of family therapy: A dialogue for child psychiatric educators*. New York: Plenum Press.

Gurman, A. S., & Kniskern, D. P. (1978). Research on marital and family therapy: Progress, perspective and prospect. In S. L. Garfield & A. E. Bergin (Eds.), *Handbook of psychotherapy and behavior change: An empirical analysis* (2nd ed.). New York: Wiley.

Hadley, T. R., & Jacob, T. (1976). The measurement of family power: A methodological study. *Sociometry, 39*, 384–395.

Haley, J. (1964). Research in family patterns: An instrument measurement. *Family Process, 3*, 41–65.

Haley, J. (1967). Cross-cultural experimentation: An initial attempt. *Human Organization, 26*, 110–117.

Haley, J. (1976). *Problem-solving therapy*. San Francisco: Jossey-Bass.

Halverson, C. F., & Waldrop, M. R. (1970). Maternal behavior toward own and other pre-school children: The problem of ownness. *Child Development, 41*, 839–845.

Handlin, J. H., & Parloff, M. B. (1962). The treatment of patient and family as a group: Is it group psychotherapy? *International Journal of Group Psychotherapy, 12*, 132–414.

Hansen, D. A., & Hill, R. (1964). Families under stress. In H. T. Christensen (Ed.), *Handbook of marriage and the family*. Chicago: Rand McNally.

Havens, L. L. (1973). *Approaches to the mind*. Boston: Little, Brown.

Hess, R. S., & Handel, G. (1959). *Family worlds*. Chicago: University of Chicago Press.

Hill, R. (1949). *Families under stress*. New York: Harper & Row.

Hill, R. (1965). Generic features of families under stress. In H. J. Parad (Ed.), *Crisis intervention: Selected readings*. New York: Family Service Association of America.

Hill, R. (1970). *Family development in three generations: A longitudinal study of changing family patterns of planning and achievement*. Boston: Shenkman.

Hill, R., & Rodgers, R. H. (1964). The developmental approach. In H. T. Christensen (Ed.), *Handbook of marriage and the family*. Chicago: Rand McNally.

Hoffman, L. (1965). Group problem solving. In L. Berkowitz (Ed.), *Advances in experimental psychology*. New York: Academic Press.

Hoffman, L. (1975). Enmeshment and the too richly cross-joined system. *Family Process, 14*, 457–468.

Hoffman, L. (1976). Breaking the homeostatic cycle. In P. Guerin, Jr. (Ed.), *Family therapy: Theory and practice*. New York: Gardner.

Holman, T. B., & Burr, W. R. (1980). Beyond the beyond: The growth of family theories in the 1970's. *Journal of Marriage and the Family, 42,* 729–741.

Jackson, D. D. (1957). The question of family homeostasis. *Psychiatry Quarterly Supplement, 31,* 79–90.

Jackson, D. D. (1973). Family interaction, family homeostasis and some implications for conjoint family therapy. In D. D. Jackson (Ed.), *Therapy, communication and change.* Palo Alto, CA: Science & Behavior Books.

Jacob, T., Kornblith, S., Anderson, C., & Hartz, M. (1978). Role expectation and role performance in distressed and normal couples. *Journal of Abnormal Psychology, 87,* 286–290.

Jacobs, R. C., & Campbell, D. T. (1961). The perpetuation of an arbitrary tradition through several generations of a laboratory microculture. *Journal of Abnormal Social Psychology, 62,* 649–658.

Johnston, A. (1967). Sanctions for superego lacunae of adolescents. In K. R. Eissler (Ed.), *Searchlights on delinquency.* New York: International Universities Press.

Kantor, D. (1980). Critical identity image: A concept linking individual, couple, and family development. In J. K. Pearce & L. J. Friedman (Eds.), *Family therapy, combined psychodynamic and family systems approaches.* New York: Grune & Stratton.

Kantor, D., & Lehr, W. (1975). *Inside the family.* San Francisco: Jossey-Bass.

Karpel, M. (1976). Individuation: From fusion to dialogue. *Family Process, 15,* 65–82.

Kelley, H. H., & Thibaut, J. W. (1969). Group problem solving. In G. Lindzey, & E. Aronson (Eds.), *Handbook of social psychology* (Vol. 4, 2nd ed.). Reading, MA: Addison-Wesley.

Keniston, K. (1974). Youth and its ideology. In S. Arieti (Ed.), *American handbook of psychiatry* (Vol. 1). New York: Basic Books.

Kenkel, W. F. (1959a). Influence differentiation in family decision-making. *Society and Social Research, 42,* 18–25.

Kenkel, W. F. (1959b). Traditional family ideology and spousal role in family decision-making. *Journal of Marriage and the Family, 21,* 334–339.

Kenkel, W. F. (1961a). Dominance, persistence, self-confidence, and spousal roles in decision-making. *Journal of Social Psychology, 54,* 349–358.

Kenkel, W. F. (1961b). Husband–wife interaction in decision-making and decision choices. *Journal of Social Psychology, 54,* 255–262.

Klein, C. M., & Hill, R. (1979). Determinants of family problem-solving effectiveness. In W. R. Burr, R. Hill, C. M. Klein, & I. Reiss (Eds.), *Contemporary theories about the family* (Vol. 1). London: Free Press.

Klein, M. (1946). Notes on some schizoid mechanisms. *International Journal of Psychoanalysis, 27,* 99.

Lazarus, R. S. (1966). *Psychological stress and the coping process.* New York: McGraw-Hill.

Leavitt, H. J. (1951). Some effects of certain communication patterns on group performance. *Journal of Abnormal Social Psychology, 46,* 38–50.

Leik, R. K. (1963). Instrumentality and emotionality in family interaction. *Sociometry, 26,* 131–145.

Levinger, G. (1965). Marital cohesiveness and dissolution: An integrative review. *Journal of Marriage and Family, 27,* 19–28.

Lewis, J., Bearer, W., Bassett, J., & Phillips, V. (1976). *No single thread: Psychological health in family systems.* New York: Brunner/Mazel.

Liddle, H. A., & Halpin, R. J. (1978). Family therapy training and supervision literature: A comparative review. *Journal of Marriage and Family Counseling, 4,* 77–98.

Lidz, T. (1970). The family as the developmental setting. In E. J. Anthony & C. Koupernik (Eds.), *The child in his family.* New York: Wiley.

Lidz, T. (1979). Family studies and changing concepts of personality development. *Canadian Journal of Psychiatry, 24*(7), 621–632.

Lidz, T., Fleck, S., Cornelison, A. R., & Terry, D. (1958). The intrafamilial environment of the schizophrenic patient: 4. Parental personalities and family interaction. *American Journal of Orthopsychiatry, 28,* 764–776.

Liebowitz, L. (1978). *Females, males, families: A biosocial approach.* North Scituate, MA: Duxbury.

Mahler, M. S., Pine, F., & Bergman, A. (1975). *The psychological birth of the human infant.* New York: Basic Books.

Maier, N. R. F. (1967). Assets and liabilities in group problem-solving: The need for an integrative function. *Psychological Reviews, 74,* 239–249.

Maier, N. R. F. (1970). *Problem solving and creativity in individuals and groups*. Monterey, CA: Brooks/Cole.

Malone, C. A. (1979). Child psychiatry and family therapy: An overview. *Journal of American Academic Child Psychiatrists, 18*, 4–20.

Marmor, J. (1975). The nature of the psychotherapeutic process revisited. *Canadian Psychiatric Association Journal, 8(20)*, 557–565.

Masnick, G. & Bane, M. J. (1980). *The nation's families: 1960–1980*. Cambridge, MA: Joint Center for Urban Studies.

McCubbin, H. T., & Boss, P. G. (Eds.). (1980). Family stress, coping, and adaption (Special issue). *Family Relations, 29, (4)*.

Millbraith, L. W. (1965). *Political participation*. Skokie, IL: Rand McNally.

Minuchin, S. (1974). *Families and family therapy*. Cambridge: Harvard University Press.

Minuchin, S. (1975). *Families of the slums*. New York: Basic Books.

Minuchin, S. & Fishman, H. C. (1981). *Family therapy techniques*. Cambridge: Harvard University Press.

Mittelman, B. (1948). Concurrent analysis of married couples. *Psychoanalytic Quarterly, 17*, 182–197.

Moore, I. K., & Anderson, A. R. (1971). Some principles for the design of clarifying educational environments. In J. Aldous, T. Condon, R. Hill, A. M. Strauss, & I. Tallman (Eds.), *Family problem solving: A symposium on theoretical, methodological and substantive concerns*. Hinsdale, IL: Dryden Press.

Murdock, G. P. (1960). The universality of the nuclear family. In N. W. Bell & E. F. Vogel (Eds.), *A modern introduction to the family*. Glencoe, IL: Free Press.

Murrell, S. A., & Stachiowiak, J. G.(1965). The family group: Development, structure, and therapy. *Journal of Marriage and the Family, 27*, 13–19.

Murrell, S. A., & Stachiowiak, J. G. (1967). Consistency, rigidity and power in the interaction patterns of clinic and non-clinic families. *Journal of Abnormal Psychology, 72*, 265–272.

Mussen, P. H., Conger, J. J., & Kagan, J. (1974). *Child development and personality* (4th ed.). New York: Harper & Row.

Napier, A. Y., & Whitaker, C. (1978). *The family crucible*. New York: Harper & Row.

Olson, D. H., Sprenkel, D. H., & Russell, C. S. (1979). Circumplex model of marital and family systems: 1. Cohesion and adaptability, dimensions, family types, and clinical applications. *Family Process, 18*, 3–28.

O'Rourke, J. (1963). Field and laboratory: The decision-making behaviors of family groups in two experimental conditions. *Sociometry, 26*, 422–435.

Parsons, T., & Bales, R. F. (1955). *Family, socialization and interaction process*. Glencoe, IL: Free Press.

Pavenstedt, E. (1967). *The drifters: Children of disorganized lower class families*. Boston: Little, Brown.

Pearce, J. K. (1980). Ethnicity and family therapy. In J. K. Pearce, & J. Friedman (Eds.), *Family therapy: Combining psychodynamic and family systems approaches*. New York: Grune & Stratton.

Pearce, J. K., & Friedman, L. J. (1980). *Family therapy: Combining psychodynamic and family systems approaches*. New York: Grune & Stratton.

Rae-Grant, Q., Carr, R., & Berman, G. (1983). Childhood developmental disorders. In P. D. Steinhauer & Q. Rae-Grant (Eds.), *Psychological problems of the child in the family*. New York: Basic Books.

Rakoff, V. M. (1980a). History in adolescent disorders. In S. Feinstein & P. Giovacchini (Eds.), *Adolescent psychiatry*. Chicago: University of Chicago Press.

Rakoff, V. M. (1980b). The illusion of detachment. In S. Feinstein & P. Giovacchini (Eds.), *Adolescent psychiatry*. Chicago: University of Chicago Press.

Rapoport, R. (1963). Normal crises, family structure and mental health. *Family Process, 2*, 68–79.

Reiss, D., & Oliveri, M. E. (1980). Family paradigm and family coping: A proposal for linking the family's intrinsic adaptive capacities to its responses to stress. *Family Relations, 29*, 431–444.

Reiss, I. (1971). *The family system in America*. New York: Holt, Rinehart & Winston.

Rosenblatt, P. C. (1977). Needed research on commitment in marriage. In G. Levinger & H. L. Raush (Eds.), *Close relationships*. Amherst: University of Massachusetts Press.

Rutter, M. (1976). Sociocultural influences. In M. Rutter & L. Hersov (Eds.), *Child psychiatry: Modern approaches*. Oxford: Blackwell Scientific.

Ryder, R. G. (1968). Husband–wife dyads versus married strangers. *Family Process, 7*, 233–238.

Sameroff, A. J., & Kelly, P. (1977). In A. Thomas & S. Chess (Eds.), *Temperament and development*. New York: Brunner/Mazel.

Sarett, P. T. (1975). *A study of the interaction effects of infant temperament on maternal attachment*. Unpublished doctoral dissertation, Rutgers University.

Scherz, F. H. (1971). Maturational crises and parent–child interaction. *Social Casework, 52 (6)* 362–369.

Scott, F. G. (1962). Family group structure and patterns of social interaction. *American Journal of Sociology, 68*, 214–228.

Shapiro, E. G. (1975). Effect of expectations of future interaction on reward allocations in dyads: Equity or equality. *Journal of Personality Social Psychology, 31*, 873–880.

Sheehy, G. (1977). *Passages*. New York: Bantam Books.

Skinner, H., Steinhauer, P. D., & Santa-Barbara, J. (1983). The family assessment measure. *Canadian Journal of Community Mental Health, 2(2)*, 91–105.

Skynner, A. C. R. (1969). A group-analytic approach to conjoint family therapy. *Journal of Child Psychology, 10*, 81–106.

Skynner, A. C. R. (1976). *Systems of family and marital psychotherapy*. New York: Brunner/Mazel.

Skynner, A. C. R. (1981). An open-systems, group analytic approach to family therapy. In A. S. Gurman & D. P. Kniskern (Eds.), *Handbook of family therapy*. New York: Brunner/Mazel.

Slipp, S. (1980). Interactions between the interpersonal in families and individual intrapsychic dynamics. In J. K. Pearce & L. J. Friedman (Eds.), *Family therapy: Combining psychodynamic and family systems approaches*. New York: Grune & Stratton.

Sluzki, C. E., & Veron, E. (1972). The double bind as a universal pathogenic situation. *Family Process, 11*, 397–410.

Solnit, A. (1978). Change and the sense of time. In E. J. Anthony & C. Chilands (Eds.), *The child and his family: Children and their parents in a changing world*. New York: Wiley.

Spiegel, J. P. (1957). The resolution of role conflict within the family. In M. Greenblatt, D. J. Levinson, & R. H. Williams (Eds.), *The patient and the mental hospital*. Glencoe, ILL: Free Press.

Spiegel, J. P., & Kluckhohn, F. L. (1968). Integration and conflict in family behavior (GAP Report No. 27A, Vol. 6).

Sprey, J. (1966). Family disorganization: Toward a conceptual clarification. *Journal of Marriage and the Family, 28*, 398–406.

Steinhauer, P. D. (1964). *Family therapy, what it is and what it is not*. Paper presented at Annual Meeting, Canadian Psychiatric Association.

Steinhauer, P. D. (1968). Reflections on criteria for selection and prognosis in family therapy. *Canadian Psychological Association Journal, 13*, 317–22.

Steinhauer, P. D. (1974). Abruptio familiae: The premature separation of the family. In A. B. Tulipan, C. L. Attneave, & E. Kingstone (Eds.), *Beyond clinic walls*. Tuscaloosa: University of Alabama Press.

Steinhauer, P. D. (1980). Infancy and childhood. In S. Greben, A. Bonkalo, R. Pos, F. H. Lowy, & G. Voinescos (Eds.), *A method of psychiatry*. Philadelphia: Lea & Febiger.

Steinhauer, P. D. (1982, January). Excerpt from Youth in the 80s—What can we expect? In J. R. MacDonald (Ed.), *Working with adolescents: A basic training program for front-line staff and supervisors of children's aid societies in the province of Ontario*. Toronto: Ministry of Community and Social Services.

Steinhauer, P. D. (1984). Clinical applications of the process model of family functioning. *Canadian Journal of Psychiatry, 29*, 98–110.

Steinhauer, P. D. (1985). Beyond family therapy—Towards a systemic and integrated view. *Psychological Clinics of North America, 8(4)*, 923–945.

Steinhauer, P. D., & Dickman, D. (1983). Psychological crises in the child and the family. In P. D. Steinhauer & Q. Rae-Grant (Eds.), *Psychological problems of the child in the family*. New York: Basic Books.

Steinhauer, P. D., & Tisdall, G. W. (1982). *How to mobilize a frozen system: A rationale for choosing between family, individual and combined therapies*. Paper presented at World Congress of International Association of Child Psychiatry and the Allied Professions, Dublin, Ireland.

Steinhauer, P. D., & Tisdall, G. W. (1984). The integrated use of individual and family psychotherapy. *Canadian Journal of Psychiatry, 29 (2)*, 89–97.

Steinhauer, P. D., Levine, S., & DaCosta, G. (1971). Where have all the children gone?—Child psychiatric emergencies in a metropolitan area. *Canadian Psychiatric Association Journal, 16*, 121–127.

Steinhauer, P. D., Santa-Barbara, J., & Skinner, H. (1984). The process model of family functioning. *Canadian Journal of Psychiatry, 29*, 77–87.

Steinhauer, P. D., Tisdall, G. W., Malone, C. A., Broder, E., Gilbert, M., Ridgely, E., Skinner, H. (1984). *Systems psychiatry: A guide to assessment and treatment of children and families.* Postmeeting Institute presented at the Joint Annual Meeting of the Canadian and American Academies of Child Psychiatry, Toronto.

Straus, M. A. (1968). Communication, creativity and problem-solving ability of middle- and working-class families in three societies. *American Journal of Sociology, 73*, 417–430.

Strodbeck, F. L. (1951). Husband–wife interaction over revealed differences. *American Society Review, 16*, 468–473.

Strodbeck, F. L. (1954). The family as a three person group. *American Society Review, 19*, 23–29.

Strodbeck, F. L. (1958). Family interaction, values and achievement. In D. McClelland (Ed.), *Talent and society.* Princeton, NJ: Van Nostrand.

Strodbeck, F. L., & Mann, R. D. (1956). Sex role differentiation in jury deliberations. *Sociometry, 19*, 3–11.

Tallman, I. (1970). The family as a small problem solving group. *Journal of Marriage and the Family, 32*, 94–104.

Tallman, I. (1971). Family problem solving and social problems. In J. Aldous, T. Condon, R. Hill, M. A. Straus, I. Tallman (Eds.), *Family problem solving: A symposium on theoretical, methodological, and substantive concerns.* Hinsdale, IL: Dryden Press.

Tallman, I. (1972). *Social structure and socialization for change.* Paper presented at the Annual Meeting of the National Council on Family Relations, Portland, OR.

Tallman, I., & Miller, G. (1971). Communication, language style, and family problem solving. In R. Hill (Ed.), *Application for continuation grant.* Minneapolis: University of Minnesota Press.

Tallman, I., & Miller, G. (1974). Class differences in family problem solving: the effects of verbal ability, hierarchical structure and role expectations. *Sociometry, 37*, 13–37.

Tannenbaum, P. (1967). The congruity principle revisited: Studies in the reduction, induction and generalization of persuasion. In L. Berkowitz (Ed.), *Advances in experimental social psychology* (Vol. 3). New York: Academic Press.

Taylor, G. J. (1975). Separation-individuation in the psychotherapy of symbiotic states. *Canadian Psychiatric Association Journal, 20*, 521–526.

Tesser, A. (1978). *Self-esteem maintenance processes in interpersonal behavior.* Unpublished research proposal, University of Georgia.

Tesser, A., & Reardon, R. (1981). Perceptual and cognitive mechanisms in human sexual attraction. In M. Cook (Ed.), *The bases of human sexual attraction.* New York: Academic Press.

Tharp, R. (1963). Psychological patterning in marriage. *Psychological Bulletin, 60*, 97–117.

Tharp, R. (1965). Marriage roles, child development, and family treatment. *American Journal of Orthopsychiatry, 35*, 531–538.

Thibaut, J. W., & Kelley, H. H. (1959). *The social psychology of groups.* New York: Wiley.

Turner, F. (1970). *Family interaction.* New York: Wiley.

Vogel, E., & Bell, N. W. (1960). The emotionally disturbed child as a family scapegoat. *Psychoanalysis, 47*, 21–42.

von Bertalanffy, L. (1968). *General systems theory.* New York: George Braziller.

von Bertalanffy, L. (1969). General systems theory—An overview. In W. Gray, F. J. Duhl, & N. D. Rizzo (Eds.), *General systems theory and psychiatry.* Boston: Little, Brown.

Wallach, M. A., Kogan, N., & Bean, D. (1964). Diffusion of responsibility and the level of risk taking in groups. *Journal of Abnormal Social Psychology, 68*, 263–274.

Walsh, F. (1982). *Normal family processes.* New York: Guilford Press.

Walters, L. H. (1982, November). Are families different from other groups? *Journal of Marriage and the Family, 44* (4) 841–850.

Walters, L. H., Miller, B. D., Rollins, B. C., Thomas, D. L., Galligan, R. J. (1982, November). Change and its impact on the variables of interest. *Journal of Marriage and the Family, 44* (4) 841–886.

Watzlawick, P. (1963). A review of the double-bind theory. *Family Process, 11*, 132–153.

Watzlawick, P., Beavin, J. H., & Jackson, D. (1967). *Pragmatics of human communication.* New York: Norton.

Watzlawick, P., Beavin, J. H., Skiorski, L., & Mecia, B. (1970). Protection and scapegoating in pathological families. *Family Process, 9(1)*, 27–39.

Waxler, N. W., & Mishler, E. G. (1978). Experimental studies of families. In L. Berkowitz (Ed.), *Group processes.* New York: Academic Press.

Weick, K. E. (1971). Group processes, family processes, and problem solving. In J. Aldous, T. Condon, R. Hill, M. A. Straus, & I. Tallman (Eds.), *Family problem solving: A symposium on theoretical, methodological and substantive concerns.* Hinsdale, IL: Dryden Press.

Weinrich, P. (1982, July). *A conceptual framework for exploring identity development: Identity structurer analysis and IDEX.* Paper presented at the World Congress International Association for Child Psychiatry and Allied Professions, Dublin, Ireland.

Weiss, R. L. (1975). *Marital separation.* New York: Basic Books.

Weiss, R. L., & Margolis, G. (1976). Marital conflict and accord. In A. R. Ciminero, H. D. Calhoun, & H. E. Adams (Eds.), *Handbooks for behavioral assessment.* New York: Wiley.

Wertheim, E. S. (1973). Family unit therapy and the science and typology of family systems. *Family Process, 12*, 361–376.

Whitaker, C. A., Felder, R. E., & Warkentin, J. (1965). Countertransference in the family treatment of schizophrenia. In I. Boszormenyi-Nagy & J. L. Framo (Eds.), *Intensive family therapy.* New York: Harper & Row.

Williams, J. R., & Gold, F. K. (1972). From delinquent behavior to official delinquency. *Journal of Social Problems, 20(2)*, 209–229.

Winnicott, D. W. (1958). Psychoanalysis and the sense of guilt. In J. D. Sutherland (Ed.), *Psychoanalysis and contemporary thought.* London: Hogarth Press.

Winnicott, D. W. (1965). *The family and individual development.* New York: Basic Books.

Winnicott, D. W. (1976). The capacity to be alone. In D. W. Winnicott (Ed.), *The maturational processes and the facilitating environment.* London: Hogarth Press.

Winter, W. D., Ferreira, A. J., & Bowers, N. (1973). Decision-making in married and unrelated couples. *Family Process, 12*, 83–94.

Wynne, L. C., Rycoff, I. M., Day, J., & Hirsch, S. I. (1958). Pseudomutuality in the family relations of schizophrenics. *Psychiatry, 21*, 205–220.

Zuckerman, E., & Jacob, T. (1979). Task effects in family interaction. *Family Process, 18*, 47–53.

CHAPTER 4

Social Learning Theory and Family Psychopathology

A Kantian Model in Behaviorism?

ELIZABETH A. ROBINSON
AND
NEIL S. JACOBSON

HISTORY AND DEVELOPMENT OF SOCIAL LEARNING THEORY

The foundation of social learning lies in diverse fields: social psychology (Homans, 1961; Thibaut & Kelley, 1959); psychiatry (Sullivan, 1965); and experimental psychology (Skinner, 1957). The superstructure of a cogent theory, however, can be attributed to Bandura (e.g., Bandura, 1969, 1977; Bandura & Walters, 1963). His theoretical work, derived from modeling and aggression studies, was primarily concerned with normal behavior. The challenge of developing social learning as a framework for understanding psychopathology was left to researchers such as Patterson (1969; Patterson & Reid, 1973), Weiss (Weiss, Hops, & Patterson, 1973), and Wahler (1980; Wahler, House, & Stambaugh, 1976), among others. These psychologists built on a methodological groundwork laid by operant behaviorists, including Azrin, Stuart, Goldiamond, Krasner, Ullman, and others who had been applying learning principles to "problems in living." The result was a stimulation of interest in applied research with troubled families in the 1960s and 1970s that was to have a profound impact on the treatment of both childhood disorders and marital dysfunction.

ELIZABETH A. ROBINSON AND NEIL S. JACOBSON • Department of Psychology, University of Washington, Seattle, WA 98105. Preparation of this chapter was partially supported by National Institute of Mental Health grants 5-R01-MH34279 to E. A. Robinson and 5-R01-MH33838-05 to N. S. Jacobson.

The application of social learning to clinical psychology invigorated research efforts to understand pathology, led to the adoption of the family as a unit of analysis, and moved research out of the laboratory and into the home. This new perspective maintained learning theory's tradition of hard-nosed empiricism and adopted its theoretical concern with discrimination learning and hence the situational specificity of behavior. As a result, the studies relied heavily on direct observation of interpersonal interaction. These pioneering efforts by social learning researchers led to the development of strong assessment tools and bold new treatment approaches. The conceptual upshot of this cross-fertilization was the generation of a model that tied theory and research to clinical practice. One benefit of this endeavor was that it provided a healthy constraint on armchair theorizing. A data-based model that required clinical relevance ensured that theory and research would not conspire to generate elegant but irrelevant solutions. Social learning theory constituted an antithesis to the previously dominant views of classical psychoanalytic and phenomenological theories. A love of parsimony was the guideline, and complex notions of causality gave way to simple formulations of cause and effect. Theoretical constructs were to be added as needed—if the most straightforward conceptualization proved inadequate. Enthusiastic rejection of overly complex and undefinable notions characteristic of earlier theories led to heavy reliance on empiricism, augmented with only limited use of basic concepts such as reinforcement, punishment, and stimulus control.

Although social learning theory has proved to be a valuable heuristic since the mid-1960s, it, as most approaches, is not without its shortcomings. In the real rather than the ideal world, it is remarkably easy to lose sight of the fact that clinical success supported by hard data does not necessarily prove theory. An intervention may be highly efficacious, although the reasons by which it operates remain poorly understood. In fact, treatment kudos may actually discourage theoretical rethinking. Failures, on the other hand, force reevaluation of what went wrong and why. Theoretical developments in social learning theory have focused on the conceptualizations of coercion in child pathology and of reciprocity in marital interaction. In addition, questions of generalizability and maintenance of treatment effects have been given considerable attention. Although these issues have been important to the conceptualization and treatment of family pathology, they have not necessarily addressed the larger question of theoretical sufficiency. The emphasis has been on "what" and "how" as opposed to "why." Research questions have been oriented toward describing pathological families and bringing about behavior change rather than toward close scrutiny of the adequacy of the model. As a result, theory development has not always kept pace with clinical strides.

One of the strengths of the social learning approach is its self-correcting nature (Vincent, 1980). It is the purpose of this chapter to reexamine some of the theoretical issues that have been overlooked in the age of technology so that social learning may continue to renew itself. We will do so by first returning to the theoretical forefather of contemporary social learning, Albert Bandura, and then considering specific models of family pathology.

STRUCTURE AND PURPOSE OF THIS CHAPTER

This chapter examines both the explicitly stated constructs and the implicit philosophical assumptions of representative theoreticians and researchers who are currently studying family psychopathology within a social learning framework. It begins with a consideration of social learning in the broadest sense and then discusses two circumscribed areas of theoretical development with particular relevance to families: child psychopathology and marital dysfunction. The following researchers who have focused on a specific aspect of family pathology are included: Gerald Patterson, who in 1982 published a largely theoretical work summarizing his research with children since the mid-1960s, and several prominent marital researchers, including Robert Weiss, John Gottman, Neil Jacobson, Gayla Margolin, and Richard Stuart. Although there are other investigators who could legitimately be covered, only those mentioned will be considered in detail.

Each of the three major theoretical conceptualizations considered in this chapter—Bandura's social learning theory, Patterson's coercive family process, and social learning models of marital discord—is discussed in terms of five basic questions: (a) What are the epistemological presuppositions of the model? (b) What are its structural constructs? (c) What constitutes motivation? (d) How are developmental changes incorporated? (e) How are individual differences explained? This organization, adopted from Rychlak (1981), not only facilitates comparison among the models considered in this paper but also permits social learning theory to be evaluated in terms of the adequacy with which it addresses some of the central issues considered by all theories of personality. In addition, each section begins with the necessary "Background Information" and ends by integrating the major points under the heading "Conclusions."

The theoretical constructs used to address the five basic queries are examined not only for their explicit meaning, but also in terms of their implicit assumptions. To facilitate this comparison, two philosophical models are employed: empiricism and rationalism (cf. Rychlak, 1981). Each of these terms has many meanings, and lest they be misconstrued, let us clarify our intent. First, by the use of *empiricism*, we are referring to the philosophical school, often termed *British empiricism*, to which writers such as John Locke, David Hume, and John Stuart Mill belonged. Their writing is characterized by an adherence to the premise that knowledge originates in experience. We are not using *empiricism* to mean reliance on observation and experimentation. All science is empirical in the second meaning of the word. By the use of *rationalism*, we are referring to the philosophical position that reason is a source of knowledge independent of sense perceptions as this position is found in the work of philosophers such as Emmanuel Kant and René Descartes. We are not defining rationalism as the belief that reason and experience, as opposed to the nonrational, are to be used in the solution of problems. Science is inherently "rational" in the latter sense. Throughout the text, the terms *Lockean* and *Kantian* are used as convenience terms to refer to the philosophical schools of empiricism and rationalism, respectively.

In the history of science, empiricism and rationalism emerge as two conflicting views of the world. The empiricist's position, exemplified by John Locke (1700/1924), holds that the truth about natural phenomena can be known (theoretically, at least) by studying events and objects that occur outside the human being and have an independent reality of their own. This epistemological stance, called *realism*, dominated most scientific thinking between the sixteenth and nineteenth centuries and is the principal assumption underlying the writing of traditional behaviorists such as Skinner (1953) and Wolpe (1958, p. 16). The rationalist's analysis, termed *idealism*, is represented in the writing of Emmanuel Kant (1781/1881) and holds that our sense of the "reality" of our physical environment is speculative at best. Although Kant stated that he *believed* that events and objects in the physical environment did exist independent of his perception of them, he made it clear that his belief was an article of faith and was not subject to verification. For example, we cannot know the nature of a tree directly but only as interpreted by our senses as green, rough-barked, fragrant, and cool. We choose to accept the "truth" of the tree's existence because it is convenient and most probably accurate, but it is important to recognize this belief as an assumption that we cannot show to be true independent of our sensory apparatus. The result of this line of philosophical reasoning is the conclusion that a proper subject of study is the way people construe meaning or interpret events. This position has particular significance for psychology and is reflected in theories such as a structural approach to the study of language (Chomsky, 1968) or a Piagetian formulation of cognitive development (Piaget, 1936/1952, 1937/1954).

Lockean and Kantian models in science diverge in many important respects, but there are three critical differences with particular relevance to our purposes: (a) As discussed above, their epistemological positions differ, with Locke adhering to realism and Kant to idealism. (b) Locke postulated that the individual is a *tabula rasa* at birth, whereas Kant argued that human beings have *pro forma* capacities that exist by virtue of one's being a human being. And (c) the Lockean model of scientific explanation adheres to reductionism. It assumes that all phenomena can be explained in terms of categorically simpler "units" that can then be broken down even further into component parts, until some final, irreducible "unit" is found. Explanation is unidirectional and linear, and simple ideas are used as building blocks to explain more complex concepts. In contrast, the Kantian model is conceptual. Explanation is given in terms of a network of interrelated abstractions. Phenomena can be explained in terms of either more or less abstract conceptualizations, but there is no ultimate unit that can not be broken down.

BANDURA'S SOCIAL LEARNING THEORY

Background

Behaviorism is rooted in the Lockean tradition when it claims that behavior can be explained by observing antecedents and consequences that impinge on the behaving organism. From this vantage, an individual's interpretation of events is unnecessary to the prediction and control of human behavior primarily because inner events are viewed as being a result of environmental contingencies and are not in themselves causal. True to the empirical position, thoughts are seen as determined by the input received by the individual and are in no sense capable of generating something new in the world.

Epistemology

Does social learning theory depart from the tough-minded realism characteristic of the behavioral tradition? It is our position that it does, at least in the implication of its major constructs. The role of awareness in learning and the process of abstract modeling in particular seem to move away from Lockean empiricism and toward a Kantian model in behaviorism.

Bandura has taken seriously the position espoused by Spielberger and De Nike (1966) that most human learning requires an awareness of the operating contingencies. Rather than being an automatic strengthening of the stimulus–response bond, reinforcement is seen as providing the organism with both information about the environment and incentives (Bandura, 1977, p. 21). This is a very important reformulation of the reinforcement mechanism because it is now the individual's *interpretation* of the event and not the event itself that is causal. This hypothesis places the organism squarely in a mediational position between the stimulus and the response and raises some very important questions. For example, what determines the nature of the interpretation made by the individual? What is the most useful focus of psychological study, the events external to the organism or the way in which the individual construes and interprets information? One can take the position that the informational and motivational aspects of an event are determined by past experiences and are best studied through careful monitoring of behavior over a period of time. On the other hand, it is also possible to argue that the internal frame of reference is partly independent of external events and determines behavior in ways that are not entirely predictable on the basis of observed events (Bandura, 1981). If one assumes that the organism is active in shaping information and is not only the recipient of environmental inputs, then one moves away from the Lockean model of traditional behaviorism and toward a Kantian epistemology, and it becomes necessary to study both the environmental events and how the individual construes them.

Abstract modeling is a second construct that implies an epistemological idealism. Concretely modeled events, such as a blow to the head of a Bobo doll, can be easily accommodated by realism, but what about the abstract modeling that occurs when people generate rules from the behavior of others, as in language learning or moral development? Abstract modeling can "create generative and innovative behavior . . . when observers derive the principles underlying specific performances for generating behavior that goes beyond what they have seen and heard" (Bandura, 1977, p. 41). This formulation sounds dangerously close to a Kantian model because it presupposes an active organism capable of bringing to bear its own mental frame of reference. The imitator is a generator of abstractions. By imposing order on the behavior of others, the child learns grammatical forms and moral precepts as an active participant creating something new—the rule—that is greater than the sum of its individual parts. When an ability to generate rules is invoked as causal, then it follows that, in order to understand human behavior, the mechanisms whereby those rules are created must be studied. This position is inconsistent with the philosophy of traditional behaviorism, which holds that cognitions are determined by environmental events. If the structuring of input by the individual determines what is learned, as is hypothesized to be the case in abstract modeling, then it seems essential to broaden the focus of study to include how events are interpreted and organized because behavior is no longer theoretically predictable solely on the basis of observed antecedents and consequences.

The inclusion of awareness and abstract modeling in social learning theory has important implications for the study of the family because it suggests that, until psychology examines how people interpret events within a family structure, researchers will not be able to fully understand or predict dysfunction. Social learning theory seems to be directing research toward questions such as: What generalizations are drawn by the children in this family? Are there common structural patterns within a family system that lead to certain beliefs among its members? What is this wife's understanding of how her behavior will affect the behavior of her spouse? What do parents of problem children believe about the causes of their child's behavior, and how does that belief influence their behavior? These are not easy questions to answer, but there is precedent in related areas of research that suggests possible methodologies. For example, the moral development literature does not ask children what moral principles they adhere to; instead, children are asked to respond to a specific situation and to draw conclusions about culpability. These data allow the researcher to draw his or her own conclusions about the principles that the child is using. Of course, not all investigators agree with the conclusions drawn about moral development, but the important point is that this work presents a jumping-off spot from which to begin to investigate how generalizations are made about family interactions. It is possible to study both an individual's understanding of the environment and the abstractions used to guide behavior while still remaining within the parameters of scientific objectivity.

Structural Constructs

Reciprocal Determinism. The underlying and unifying premise of social learning theory is the notion that psychological functioning is determined by the environment, by the behavior of the individual, and by factors associated with the person. This interplay of forces is represented schematically as

$$
\begin{array}{c}
P \\
\nearrow \nwarrow \\
B \leftrightarrow E
\end{array}
$$

is dynamic and bidirectional, and moves toward a larger causal role for cognitions than has heretofore been afforded in traditional behavioral approaches.

The model is dynamic in that all three components interact, influencing one another in a moment-by-moment sequence of events. By *reciprocal,* Bandura meant that not only does the environment influence behavior, but behavior also influences the environment. For example, the delinquent may seek other like-minded companions, the environmental enthusiast may select work in a national park, and the aggressive child may alter the response pattern of those with whom he or she interacts. In each case, the *behavior* of the actor alters the environment, which, in turn, influences subsequent behavior by the actor.

The influence of the person is not limited to overt instrumental behavior. Bandura has clearly stated that when he refers to person variables, he is considering cognitive factors. From this point of view, the individual's perception of the situation determines, in part, the impact of the environment on behavior. The importance of the "person" variable can be seen in the literature that examines how violent individuals interpret their interactions with others. Aggressive men tend to attribute hostile intentions to others more frequently than do pacific individuals (cf. Berkowitz, 1978; Toch, 1969). If an individual feels threatened, then the environment *is* psychologically threatening, and he or she behaves accordingly. Thus, the person is capable of partly determining the environment, in a cognitive sense, just as his or her behavior can alter the environment in a physical sense.

The critical element that differentiates social learning from other behavioral models is the notion of bidirectional interaction (Bandura, 1983). All three elements of the triad influence one another, and behavior is determined by an individual's cognitions and environment, which are, in turn, determinants of each other. For example, the thought that one is in danger is not independent of the situation, and the threatening environment is not independent of the individual's cognitions. A police officer knocking on the door of a home in a neighborhood with a history of attacks on police and a neighbor knocking on the same door are not experiencing equivalent environments, even though, to all outward appearances, the circumstances are identical. The power of the interaction between cognitions and the environment is demonstrated by the fatal shooting of 5-year-old Patrick Mason by a police officer after the child pointed a toy gun at him in a dimly lit apartment (Associated Press, 1983).

The importance of this model for psychology lies in its potential to shift the focus of study. When two individuals interact, they become part of each other's environment, and the behavior of each partially determines the behavior of the other (Bandura, 1981). Thus, the interactive nature of reciprocal determinism places families and dyads at center stage. If one imagines the *B-P-E* triad as connected with two arrows on each side of an equilateral triangle, then the arrow most studied by behaviorists is the effect of the environment on behavior. The mechanisms by which behavior shapes the environment have been largely neglected in empirical investigations, and the role of personal perception in both behavior and the impact of the environment has been left to other theoretical paradigms. A potential effect of the social learning perspective is to provide an impetus whereby models of complex human behavior, such as family psycho-pathology, may be developed.

Motivational Constructs

Origin of Behavior. Bandura has stated that the origin of human behavior is primarily imitation. The individual is exposed to an infinite variety of models during a lifetime. Learning is moderated by attentional factors, past experience, and a host of other variables, but the essential process remains imitation. Although biology is not denied, it is given a relatively minor part in psychological processes: "Except for elementary reflexes, people are not equippped with inborn repertoires of behavior" (Bandura, 1977, p. 16).

There are two literatures that suggest a *pro forma* view of human nature and that have particular bearing on the social learning position: the structural view of language development (Chomsky, 1968) and the biological position that humans are predisposed to learn certain behavior, such as aggression, more readily than other actions.

Bandura has been interested in the structuralist view of language, and although he has clearly rejected the notion that the specific grammatical forms are genetically determined, he has equivocated when discussing the possibility that human beings are endowed with an information-processing capability that enables the discovery of the structural properties of language. Instead, he has emphasized that, regardless of genetic endowment, there is little language learning in the absence of modeling. Thus, the most fruitful avenue for the study of language learning remains the external environment and not the *pro forma* capacities of the individual organism.

Some researchers have proposed that a propensity to imitate other people is an inborn capacity that human beings evidence in the first hours of life (Meltzoff & Moore, 1983); they have suggested that, although specific behaviors must be learned through exposure to models, the tendency to learn them may be present at birth. If this hypothesis is substantiated, it will push social learning closer toward a Kantian model than is now the case. The human being who is biologically prepared to imitate brings as-yet-unknown structuring capacities and limitations to interpersonal situations. The individual is no longer a *tabula rasa* and her or his *pro forma* capacities raise important questions: What are imitative mechanisms and how do they work? How does experience interact with an inborn capacity? Or more fundamentally, what makes us capable of imitation? Social learning theory has not been applied to animal learning, and there is good reason for the omission: few animals evidence much learning through modeling (Cairns, 1979, p. 335). The apparent tie between human learning and imitation suggests the need for some form of *pro forma* explanation in any theory that relies as heavily on cognitive mediation as does social learning.

The social-learning-theory view of the origin of behavior broadens the existing scope of inquiry in clinical psychology. It departs from the notion that behavior can be understood simply by observing its interaction with external antecedents or consequences, and it shifts to a cognitively mediated position that presses the investigator to evaluate belief, expectation, and interpretation. Bandura (1983) stated that "memory representation of the past involves constructive rather than reproductive processes in which events are filtered through personal meanings and biases and cognitively transformed" (p. 167). When Bandura wrote that memories contain a *constructive* element and are not simply reproductions, he allowed the possibility that individuals can contribute something causally unique to the determination of behavior and suggested that a full conceptualization of human behavior may require an understanding of the processes whereby personal meaning and bias are created.

Reinforcement. The conceptualization of reinforcement in a social learning framework is clearly different from the traditional view. Reinforcement is said to both give information about the environment and provide motivation to engage in certain behaviors rather than others. For example, when Ms. Jones praises 6-year-old Johnny's attempts to tie his shoelace, she is seen as providing the information that learning to tie a shoe is a praiseworthy behavior in our society and that future efforts will probably lead to further approval and warm, loving smiles. With this information in mind, Johnny may increase his rate of shoe tying if he is a normally developing and reasonably well-socialized child.

Social learning's reconceptualization of the informational and motivational aspects of reinforcement has important practical implications for family intervention. Behavioral psychotherapy with children, for example, relies on the use of tangible and social rewards and extinction to alter deviant child behavior. Children are frequently ignored for undesirable behavior (Budd, Green, & Baer, 1976) under the assumption that this procedure will weaken the bond between the stimulus (e.g., the mother's presence) and the response (e.g., a whine). This paradigm makes more common as well as social learning sense, however, if the child is told what's going on before the extinction begins. In this way, he or she will have new information about the contingencies—namely, that the mother will no longer attend solicitously or even angrily in response to whining—and the child should learn more quickly than would be the case without the information. Similarly, praise for the sake of praise is unlikely to have an effect unless the child knows what it is that he or she is doing right. Children are capable of deducing for themselves the kinds of behaviors that are rewarded and those that are discouraged, but learning may be expedited if the contingencies are clarified for the child. The developmental literature is consistent with the social learning theoretical emphasis on awareness when it stresses the importance of reasoning in the successful socialization of young children (Baumrind, 1967; Baumrind & Black, 1967).

Cognitions. Radical behaviorism is said to provide an impoverished model of human behavior because it "has neglected determinants of behavior arising from cognitive functioning" (Bandura, 1977, p. 10). "There are times when personal factors are the overriding regulators of the course of environmental events" (Bandura, 1977, p. 10). Thus, cognitions are given a central function in social learning theory.

Imitation is able to serve as a primary method of learning because human beings are capable of complex cognitive activities; our anticipatory capacity allows us to be motivated by prospective consequences. According to Bandura, the hypotheses that we develop about the relationships between our behavior and the events in our environment account for the well-established relationship between a stimulus and a contiguous response (Bandura, 1982).

Yet, despite their central role in social learning theory, cognitions have rarely been studied in the social learning literature on family psychopathology. For example, the child's perception of the reinforcing or punishing value of the parent's behavior, his or her understanding of the rules, and the motivating properties of incentives are seldom explored in a research paradigm. However, sensitive clinicians take these cognitive factors into consideration when working with a family. Alexander and Parsons (1973) considered both the cognitive factors and the behavioral contingencies in their highly successful "functional family therapy" by combining contingency management with communication training to help clarify expectations and anticipated consequences for all family members. In a similar vein, the social-learning-theory emphasis on cognitions suggests that parent and child perceptions may also be important variables to be studied in interventions planned for young children. A parent may, for example, have little knowledge of child development and may perceive a child's dawdling as "parent baiting" when, in fact, the child is experiencing genuine difficulty.

Developmental Considerations

An important change that occurs as the child matures is the development of the ability to engage in delayed rather than immediate imitation (Mischel & Metzner, 1962). According to Bandura, the very young child is capable only of instantaneous replication of acts that are presented in the here and now and cannot hold the image of a particular behavior in mind for a period of time and reproduce it later. He called the ability to engage in delayed imitation behavior "representational imitation," a process mediated by the child's ability to use language and attained during the second year of life. Imitation is also influenced by the child's ability to pay attention and to create the motor responses necessary for reproducing a particular behavior. Thus, there are developmental constraints imposed on imitative responses.

The idea that identical models and events can affect children differently at various stages of their development raises the as-yet-unanswered question: How does the human developmental framework for interpreting experience interact with behavioral constructs such as reinforcement, punishment, and modeling?

Bandura (1977) suggested that developmental factors diminish in importance after the age of 2; he referred to the, "Final stages of development, which generally begin in the second year of life" (p. 33). This position does not do justice to the considerable body of literature that describes imitation as mediated by the gradual emergence of social, emotional, physical, and intellectual capacities. For example, developmental researchers suggest that children younger than about 6 years of age have difficulty assuming the point of view of another (Flavell, Botkin, Fry, Wright, & Jarvis, 1968), and the interpretation of violent content in television programs seems to be related to the child's level of cognitive understanding (Collings, Berndt, & Hess, 1974). Others report that, after age 7, tangible rewards result in a devaluation of certain activities (Thomas & Tenant, 1978). Thus, it seems that a child's ability to take another perspective, the way in which aggression is symbolized, and the subjective value of a reward are factors that may influence what and when imitation takes place. These are only a few of the potentially powerful influences on behavior that change over the course of development, yet their absence in social learning studies of family pathology raises the possibility that researchers may be "paying lip service" (Cairns, 1979, p. 344) to the concept of the child as a growing, changing organism without meaningfully integrating developmental findings.

Cognition is of central importance in social learning theory in terms of both the acquisition of behavior (what will be attended to and for how long) and its performance: "Most modeled behavior is acquired and retained through the medium of verbal symbols" (Bandura, 1977, p. 33); therefore, the child's developing ability to symbolize events is critical to the understanding of imitation. What conclusion is a 5-year-old child drawing when spanked by a parent, and does it differ systematically from the conclusion that a young adolescent is likely to draw? When and to what extent is reasoning important in encouraging or discouraging imitation, and do children of different ages respond differently to appeals to reason? What does it mean for a 7-year-old to earn tokens for not stealing as opposed to the interpretation placed on this arrangement by a 12-year-old? Theorists like Kohlberg (1968) have suggested that there are qualitative changes in the child's moral reasoning over the course of development. Issues raised by developmentalists need to be considered in both theory and empirical research, but specific theoretical hypotheses within a social learning framework have yet to be explored.

Perhaps developmental concerns are understated in the behavioral tradition because its overriding model of human behavior does not lend itself to the conceptualization of human beings as shaping and interpreting the environment. The behavioral assumption is the *tabula rasa* view consistent with realism rather than a *pro forma* perspective, suggested by contemporary social learning.

Individual Differences Constructs

Personal Efficacy and Outcome Expectation. The specific social learning formulations most capable of explaining why some individuals seem to lead well-ordered, happy, and productive lives whereas others do not are the constructs that deal with an individual's sense of efficacy and his or her expectations regarding the nature of the outcome. To appreciate the potential utility of these variables, it may be helpful to consider them in their historical context. Learning theories tend to attribute pathology and the idiosyncrasies of normal behavior to the unique learning history of the organism. This position simultaneously explains everything and nothing. Just as id, ego, and superego conflicts can explain all behavior *post hoc* but are not open to scrutiny and causal analyses, so specific events in one's past history can be invoked to "explain" current behavior: the validity of neither speculation can be investigated for the real-life behavior of human beings. The social learning formulations of self-efficacy and outcome expectancy are shorthand ways of representing the cumulative effects of past experience without the necessity of recruiting guardian angels as participant observers. The problem with this hypothesis is that it involves one level of inference that is not present in a strictly behavioral paradigm: Cognitive events cannot be measured directly. Nevertheless, the social learning conceptualization has the striking advantage that it can be assessed.

Behavior is said to be mediated by our sense of personal efficacy and our expectations regarding the outcome of the behavior. For example, the mother who believes that, by insisting that her son go to bed at 8:00 P.M., she will dampen his autonomous spirit and negatively influence his self-esteem is less likely to demand compliance than one who believes that obedience to parental authority will help develop self-control (outcome expectation). Similarly, the mother's idea of her personal efficacy—how effective she will be in getting him to bed—also affects her behavior. Will there be a long tantrum resulting in the child's staying up, or does the mother feel that she will be able to accomplish the task with a minimum of duress? Individuals are said to differ in their levels of self-efficacy and outcome expectation.

An individual's sense of efficacy is situation-specific and varies in strength, generality, and magnitude (Bandura, 1977, p. 85). Some expectancies may be weakly held and easily changed, whereas others, based on repeated or intense learning experiences, may be difficult to change. Individuals also differ in the degree of generality they are willing to impute to their sense of efficacy. One person may anticipate difficulty in influencing the behavior of a teenaged daughter, whereas another may generalize to an anticipated lack of impact in general. Finally, one parent may expect to be moderately effective when faced with a full-blown tantrum, whereas another may apprehend helplessness.

A change in feelings of self-efficacy may be an important component of psychotherapy. Success experiences in solving arithmetic problems are associated with an increase in both the expectation of future success and the level of achievement among children with gross deficits and lack of interest in mathematical tasks (Bandura & Schunk, 1981). Similarly, adults evidencing an extreme fear of snakes show gains in feelings of competency following desensitization procedures (Telch, Bandura, Vinciguerra, Agras, & Stout, 1982). These studies indicate that there may be a relationship between feelings of adequacy and behavior change, yet the possible role of self-efficacy in family intervention is yet to be evaluated (cf. Doherty, 1981a,b; Weiss, 1980). For example, do couples who learn conflict resolution skills feel powerful? Do adults who learn to use time-out become confident parents? And if these changes do occur, do they predict maintenance during the follow-up? If efficacy expectations are important mediators of behavior change, it is important to explore the kinds of belief systems that are conducive to change, to identify those that are characteristic of dysfunctional family systems, and to devise treatment strategies that are most likely to influence them.

The more basic consideration is, of course, the origin of different beliefs and expectations among families. Assuming that personal efficacy and outcome expectation are causally related to psychological functioning, why do some families develop problem cognitions whereas others do not? To what extent does the psychopathology of one individual influence the larger group? Is there any interaction between a sense of potency within the family and social factors such as poverty or social status? Social learning theory does not detail the development of cognitions in complex networks such as the family; it only offers a prefatorial theoretical outline. But by emphasizing the importance of people in creating environments for others, social learning theory sets the stage for the development of a family-systems approach to the study of psychopathology and human variation.

Conclusions

Social learning theory moves behaviorism one giant step toward a Kantian model. Its major theoretical concepts—abstract modeling and cognitions as causal—require that psychology study the spectacles through which people view the world. A Lockean system cannot reconcile these precepts, nor can it accommodate the underlying assumption of reciprocal determinism that eschews the unidirectionality inherent in empiricism.

Behaviorism has long been criticized for its adherence to an outmoded philosophy of science (Koch, 1964), but scientists have seldom been goaded into a "scientific revolution" (Kuhn, 1970) by the scolding of their colleagues, particularly if those associates were philosophers. The real impetus to change has come when the existing paradigm has failed to account for unexpected results (Kuhn, 1970, p. 6). Just such novel findings have been accumulating at an accelerating rate since the mid-1960s (cf. Bolles, 1970; Deci, 1975; Lepper, Greene, & Nisbett, 1973; Melzoff & Moore, 1983; Spielberger & De Nike, 1966). In spite of these nagging challenges, behaviorism has held sway as the dominant view in academic clinical psychology since the early 1960s and has brought with it a period of what Kuhn (1970) might call "normal science" (p. 10), characterized by a "strenuous and devoted attempt to force nature to the conceptual boxes supplied by professional education" (p. 5). This theoretical rigidity has not been all bad; it has solved problems. By generating a large body of literature under the coordinating force of common principles, both the theory and its methodology have been fully exploited (Price, 1972, p. 189). Behaviorism has been remarkably fruitful. Gradually, however, previously inexorable positions have bent with the weight of new findings. For example, it was necessary that something be said about such troubling notions as the absence of "learning" without awareness, the rapidity with which children learn rules of grammar, and the sometimes paradoxical effect of extrinsic rewards. Social learning theory has adapted to these new findings and, in doing so, has proposed a fundamental change in our view of the nature of human beings.

The historical reluctance of behaviorists to relinquish empiricism as a philosophy may be tied to the confusion between *conceptual* and *methodological* behaviorism (Mahoney, 1974, Chapter 2). Conceptual behaviorism adopts the Lockean assumptions of reductionism, the reality of the world as perceived by the experimenter, and a faith that directly observable occurrences determine behavior. Methodological behaviorism, in contrast, takes the position that constructs ought to be operationally defined, that measurement should be objective, and that results must be replicable. These are the principles of good science, and they are not tied to a particular paradigm. One can continue to cherish the methodological rigor of behaviorism without adopting a Lockean philosophy of science. Explanation based on "inner events" has earned a bad reputation in clinical psychology, and there is concern that the new "revolution" may be best conceptualized as a step backward, rather than forward (Dember, 1974; Ledwidge, 1978). There is, after all, a familiar ring to the invocation of cognitions as causal mechanisms. It is our considered opinion, however, that these forebodings are not justified if researchers continue to remain faithful to the principles of methodological behaviorism. A shift in perspective is a potentially invigorating influence with the power to infuse science with new questions and new methodologies.

In the next section, we examine the formulation of the application of general social learning principles to specific areas of family psychopathology.

PATTERSON'S COERCIVE FAMILY PROCESS

Background

Coercive family process theory (Patterson, 1982) is a specific formulation of the causes of high levels of aggression in children. The theory is specifically a *performance* theory, which means that its goal is to describe the conditions in the present moment that lead to aggression. In Aristotelean terms, the theory seeks to explain the *efficient* causes of aggression and not its material, formal, or final causes. The explanatory goal of the coercion hypothesis is a relatively conservative one: It attempts merely to describe the ongoing chain of events that sustain aggression.

Epistemology

The epistemological model presented in coercion theory is realism, which is consistent with the operant tradition but diverges sharply from the view of humans promulgated by social learning theory. Although the conceptual framework is labeled a *social learning approach* (cf. Patterson, Reid, Jones, & Conger, 1975), it does not share all of the assumptions of Bandura's social learning theory (1977). Coercion theory is concerned with the temporal sequence of events that constitute the topography of family interaction, and not with the internal structuring of information.

Modeling plays a minimal role in coercion theory. All behaviors are said to be learned through the imitation of others, but imitation is not invoked as a causal mechanism to explain individual differences in aggression. According to coercion theory, our culture does an efficient job of exposing all of us at an early age to a plethora of aggressive models, and so we have, for all practical purposes *acquired* identical repertoires of violence and interpersonal mayhem. The important task is to reveal the factors that determine the *performance* of aggression, hence a performance theory of aggression.

Coercion theory deemphasizes the causal role of cognitions in learning and behavior:

> The findings from recent developments in cognitive psychology strongly suggest that behavior changes occur in complex social interactions without the participants being aware of them. The present writer believes that most changes in behavior have this quality. (Patterson, 1982, p. 92)

Coercion theory holds that determinants of a behavior can be identified through the monitoring of its objectively observable antecedents and consequents. It is therefore not necessary to study the meaning and interpretations that people place on events because behavior can be adequately predicted by the events that lead up to it and by its effects. This position is consistent with that of Skinner (1953) and is a widely accepted underlying premise in many learning theories. The implication of this view is that the truth, in some objective sense, is knowable through observation. Thus, the proper focus of psychology is on external events and not on cognitions. In discussing the role of awareness in learning, Patterson (1982) pointed out that individuals cannot possibly be aware of the 200 or so behavioral events as coded by his observational system in a 5-minute period, and that people often have mistaken ideas about their behavior (p. 90). Although this statement is undoubtedly accurate, the essential question remains: Which is a better predictor, the actual contingencies or the individual's understanding of them? This issue is, as yet, unresolved.

The methodology of coercion theory's empirical investigations is consistent with its epistemological assumptions. Research is based on a detailed functional analysis of family interaction as recorded live by trained observers. The unit of analysis is a 6-second time block during which the behavior of all family members is recorded in sequence as it occurs in the home. This data collection method shares three important assumptions with empiricism: (a) pathological aggression can be adequately understood in terms of events external to the child; (b) the salient aspects of other people's behavior (environment) are apparent to an observer (realism); and (c) the meaning of family interaction is best captured by examining a unidirectional chain of events.

Structural Constructs

Reciprocal determinism is a unifying construct in coercion theory just as it is in social learning, but the meaning of the term is construed differently. In coercion theory, the individual influences his or her environment and is, in turn, shaped by it; thus, behavior and environment interact. This is a different position from that of social learning theory, which defines *reciprocity* as the interaction of behavior, environment, and cognitions.

Coercion theory's conceptualization of reciprocal determinism is fundamentally an operant standpoint. Classic notions of reinforcement and punishment imply an active organism that responds to the contingencies of the environment (Baltes & Reese, 1977). The effect is bidirectional in that behavior effects the environment and the environment effects behavior. In a simple bar-pressing experiment, the rat leans on a lever that delivers a food pellet, altering his environment. This alteration, in turn, effects the rat's future behavior by increasing the likelihood that it will again press the bar. The reciprocal determinism proposed in coercion theory follows the same format. This child's behavior elicits changes in his or her environment, and those changes influence the probability of future behavior.

The principal mechanism in coercion theory is negative reinforcement. The aggressive child is said to be "the victim and architect" of a coercive system (Patterson, 1976): the child's behavior, as well as that of the parents, is maintained because it results in a termination of some kind of unpleasantness. For example, when Ms. Hardy nags until Frank begins to clean up his room, Frank's compliance is rewarded because his mother stops nagging. Conversely, when Mr. Forman gives in to Jane's tantrum and lets her have another ride on the pony, the parent is negatively reinforced for acquiescence because the irritating and embarrassing tantrum stops. This is referred to as a *coercion trap*. Parents and children are participating in a system that has short-term payoffs but that results in the establishment of long-term behavior problems.

A final (third) speculation that gives structure to the theory is the hypothesized relationship between minor, everyday, annoying child behaviors and more serious forms of aggression, such as violence toward others. Coercion theory suggests that the exchange of low-level aversive events is a precursor to high-amplitude aggression on the part of the child (hitting of the parent) or the parent (child or spouse abuse). Families engaging in coercive processes are seen as escalating from a relatively minor aversive behavior, such as whining, to major aggressive episodes. These escalations proceed through a series of reciprocal interactions in which each "round" grows in intensity and increases the probability of the occurrence of an aggressive act.

Physical aggression is a relatively rare event on a moment-by-moment basis even for a problem child. Although somewhat more frequent, overt verbal aggression, such as name calling, personal insults, and angry shouting, are not high-base-rate behaviors during a 1-hour home observation. The scarcity of aggression leaves the researcher interested in a functional analysis in the difficult position of finding enough behavior to adequately evaluate. Coercion theory circumvents this problem by studying a *class* of behaviors termed *aggressive* that are not, at face value, obviously aggressive. These behaviors are called *coercive*, but perhaps a more neutral term would be *aversive*. Included are negativism, noncompliance, teasing, yelling, whining, issuing a negative command, crying, disapproval, dependency, ignoring, humiliating, engaging in a normally innocuous behavior at a high rate (e.g., running back and forth in the living room), and destruction and physical aggression: "Within the family those events will be labeled as aggressive which can be shown to be *both aversive and contingent*" (Patterson, 1982, p. 12). In other words, there must be agreement among adults that the 14 observed behaviors are aversive, and each behavior must also decrease the probability that the event that precedes it will occur again. Although these steps establish an operational basis for the study of punishing events in family interaction, whether they also constitute a basis from which to study aggression is open to discussion. Children who are reported to be aggressive engage in higher than normal levels of annoying behaviors (Patterson & Reid, 1973), but the chain of events that leads to full-scale aggression has not yet been delineated and remains hypothetical.

Thus, the concepts that give structure to a coercion theory of aggression are the interaction of the child and the response of others in his or her family (reciprocal determinism), the salience of negative reinforcement (coercion), and the hypothetical tie between minor aversive behaviors and actual aggression (escalation).

Motivational Constructs

Origin of Behavior. Coercion theory assumes that behavior is initially learned through observation but does not elaborate on the acquisition phase of learning. With regard to performance, Patterson seems to agree with traditional learning theorists that the cause of a behavior is best conceptualized in terms of the stimulus that elicits it and in the consequences that either increase or decrease the strength of the S–R bond: "The connection between the aggressive response of the child and the stimulus which controls its occurrence is maintained by both positive and negative reinforcement" (Patterson, 1982, p. 85).

The designations *stimulus* and *response* are arbitrary conventions and could easily be reversed. In other words, the aggressive behavior can also be considered a stimulus for the behavior of another individual in the family. It is helpful to think of the stimulus as the context in which a behavior occurs. For example, among children brought for treatment, approximately 34% of their aversive behavior follows an aversive behavior of a family member, and 66% occurs after a neutral or positive behavior (Patterson, 1982, p. 98). These percentages are not significantly different from those observed in control families (25% aversive antecedents). It is also important to keep in mind that the stimulus or context is not necessarily the cause of the behavior but is simply its covariant: "One can think of a significant functional relation as denoting control in a statistical sense, but the prediction of experimental or *treatment* manipulations requires that we specify, *how much* control" (Patterson, 1982, p. 179). In fact, stimulus conditions are not good predictors of deviant child behavior: "By itself, information about the density of controlling antecedents would account for only a very small portion of the variance for the child's overall level of coercive performance" (Patterson, 1982, p. 186).

If stimulus conditions do not "cause" behavior, what does? According to coercion theory, the consequences of behavior maintain it. Positive consequences from other family members for deviant behavior are uniformly high (60%–73%; Patterson, 1982, p. 100) for both aggressive and control children. So, although this may explain why children in general engage in obnoxious behaviors at a high rate, it does not explain why some cause problems whereas others remain within the normal range.

Different rates of punishment also fail to distinguish clearly between normal and problem children. A straightforward behavioral analysis predicts that children who are frequently aversive are probably punished for such behavior less often than are other children; however, data suggest that problem children actually experience a greater proportion of negative consequences for aversive behavior than do controls (Patterson, 1982, p. 127). It is possible that, although punished more frequently, aggressive boys are less responsive to parental disapproval than are their normal counterparts, but the groups are equally likely to stop an aversive behavior following a negative reaction (Patterson, 1982, p. 131). There is a slight tendency for problem boys to increase the probability of repeating an aversive behavior over baseline levels in response to punishment, but this "acceleration effect" is small (Snyder, 1977). Thus, the consequences of deviant behavior are only marginally effective in discriminating between normal and aggressive families.

Coercion theory holds that the essential differences between problem and control families are threefold: (a) parents of problem families are likely to engage in behaviors that continue an aversive exchange; (b) they are more likely than other parents to start an aversive episode; and (c) problem children are more frequently negatively reinforced than controls. These ideas are linked to the observation that problem children are more likely than control children to continue an aversive event once it has begun (Patterson, 1982, p. 189).

There is some evidence to support each of these possible causes of child deviance. Mothers (but not fathers) of problem children are more likely than controls to continue an unpleasant exchange by responding with an aversive behavior (e.g., counterattacking) when their child emits an aversive behavior (Patterson, 1982, p. 151). Counterattacks are important because they are likely to lead to further deviance by the child. Similarly, both mothers and fathers in problem families tend to start aversive exchanges more than do control parents, but the differences are small. Only 4% to 5% of the negative exchanges are begun by parents in problem families, as compared to 1% to 2% of aversive sequences in control families (Patterson, 1982, p. 149). Finally, 13% to 16% of the control child's versus 21% to 22% of the aggressive child's aversive behavior is negatively reinforced (Patterson, 1982, p. 152). Although this difference is significant, it does not take into account the discrepant base rates of deviant behavior among aggressive and control families. There is a higher frequency of unpleasant exchanges among the collateral family members of aggressive than among normal children; as a result, the aggressive child's deviant behavior is more likely to be associated with the termination of aversive behavior by chance alone. To fully evaluate the role of negative reinforcement, differences need to be examined while holding constant the base-rate deviance of other family members (Knutson, 1982).

Cognitions. The role of cognition in coercion theory is minimal. Awareness of contingencies is not necessary for behavior change, and other cognitions are seen as being the result of events that transpire in the environment. For example, depression among mothers of aggressive children (Eyberg & Robinson, 1982; Forehand, Wells, McMahon, Griest, & Rogers, 1982) is conceptualized as a consequence of the high rate of aversive interchanges in these mothers' lives: "It is not only how one *perceives* the aversive events in the environment, but their actual density and intensity that determines [*sic*] stress" (Patterson, 1982, p. 72).

There is some speculation that the coercive process results in negative attributions by the parent. The attribution is tied to Schacter's two-factor theory of emotion, which requires both emotional arousal and a cognitive label: "Given a state of physiological arousal for which an individual has no immediate explanation, he will label this state and describe his feelings in terms of cognitions available to him" (Schacter, 1964, p. 53). Thus, when a parent is arguing with a child, he or she may experience a physiological reaction, including responses such as increased heart rate, elevated blood pressure, and a change in skin conductance. Presumably, the parent can identify these feelings as anger, frustration, depression, hopelessness, or a host of other possibilities, depending on the degree of ambiguity in the situation. The Schacter model may help to explain how parents label their own feelings, but it does not clarify parental attributions of a child's or a spouse's motivation. For example, the model does not explain why some parents attribute the cause of the child's disturbing behavior to malevolent intentions ("He throws tantrums because he hates me"), whereas others ascribe the situation to biological causes ("He must be allergic to duck eggs"), and still others believe they are bad parents ("Maybe if I wasn't working and could give him more attention he wouldn't have to act like this"). The source of parental cognitions regarding the behavior of others remains unexplained.

Developmental Considerations

The major developmental concept in coercion theory is the hypothesis of arrested socialization. The level of aggression among problem children is similar to the level displayed by control children several years younger. For example, the amount of aversive behavior displayed by an 11- or 12-year-old brought for treatment is roughly equivalent to that displayed by a 2- to 4-year-old control child (Patterson, 1982, p. 19). Coercive theory suggests that the reason for the delay is the parents' failure to punish: "Presumably his parents are unable or unwilling to impose sanctions which parents of normal children impose for these same behaviors" (Patterson, 1982, pp. 19–20). Thus, the central developmental theme reflects the cumulative effect of the parents' behavior and does not incorporate maturational concepts in the usual sense.

The lack of emphasis on development may be partly a theoretical bias related to the acceptance of two important premises: (a) the same mechanisms that determine behavior are operating for both children and adults, and (b) cognitive processes are not causal. Coercion theory hypothesizes a general learning process that is operative at all age levels (Sameroff, 1975). If one hypothesizes that learning consists of the strengthening of S–R bonds, it is unnecessary to incorporate concepts from cognitive development to explain changes in the structure or mechanism of learning.

Of course, the essential question is: Are developmental considerations necessary to the study of coercive family interaction? Can an adequate model of family psychopathology be devised without taking into account the child's maturational level? A central theme in coercion theory is that consequences shape psychopathologically aggressive behavior, yet evidence suggest that rewards and punishments are moderated by maturational variables. A tangible reward for a preferred motor activity undermines the persistence of older children (age 9) while increasing persistence among younger children (age 7) (Schultz, Butkowsky, Pearce, & Shanfield, 1975). It is not known if there is a similar interaction between age and reward when the behavior in question is not inherently appealing: Do tangible rewards for completing homework assignments result in decrements in self-motivation or self-discipline? Are young children more easily influenced by parental praise than school-aged children? Are certain types of behavior more responsive to praise than others? Are there differences at various ages between arbitrary rewards (points and stars) and natural consequences (first you wash your hands, then you can have dinner), as suggested by Dreikurs (1964)? These are only a few of the as-yet-unanswered questions concerning the possible interaction of developmental concerns and reinforcement.

The effects of punishment may also be sensitive to maturation. Length of time-out seems to be of little importance to a young child: 1 minute seems to be as effective as 15 minutes (White, Nielsen, & Johnson, 1972); but an adolescent may require a longer time-out period to effect behavior change. The older child may have had the opportunity to engage in more reinforced pairings of the stimulus and the response and may require more punishment, or punishment may be qualitatively different for children at various ages. It is conceivable that time-out may serve an information-giving function for the preschool child, who has limited ability to focus on relevant aspects (Pick, Christy, & Frankel, 1972), by dramatically calling the child's attention to activities that are not approved by the parent. For the older child, who presumably knows what parents do not like, time-out may provide an incentive to avoid those behaviors. These possibilities are speculative, and there are undoubtedly alternative theoretical explanations for the affect of age on punishment, but the central point is that knowledge may be advanced by investigating interactions between age and punishment.

From a purely practical standpoint, it seems particularly important to consider the child's cognitive capacity when implementing punishment. Timing, procedures, rationale, and severity may all need to be modified at various ages. In the usual time-out procedure (Patterson, Cobb, & Ray, 1973), the child is told to go to time-out, and if he or she fails to do so, the parent removes an important privilege, such as use of the bicycle or television for an evening. For this procedure to work effectively, the child must evaluate both the short-term and the long-term consequences and come to the conclusion that he or she is better off taking the mild immediate punishment rather than the more aversive consequence that will occur later. Young children are likely to ignore long-term consequences when making decisions (Mischel & Metzner, 1962), and consequently, a 2- or 3-year-old child may have difficulty acting in accord with his or her own best interests. The children treated by Patterson have been school-aged children, but clinicians working with preschoolers use time procedures consistent with the young child's cognitive abilities (e.g., Eyberg & Robinson, 1982; Forehand & McMahon, 1981, Chapter 3).

Lying, stealing, and physical violence have been studied as moral behaviors, and maturational factors have been found to play an important role. The child development literature supports the social learning notion that the generation of behavioral rules (abstract modeling) is an important component in the socialization of children (Bandura, 1977): the older the child is, the more likely it is that his or her behavior will conform to an intellectual understanding of right and wrong (Henshel, 1971). Moral behavior (Hoffman & Saltzstein, 1967), the development of internal controls (Aronfreed, 1968, pp. 321–322), and considerate behavior toward others (Hoffman, 1963) have been tied to the use of induction by parents. Reasoning, in turn, has been shown to interact with behavioral techniques. When children are confronted with complex moral dilemmas, mild punishment plus induction is more effective than severe punishment with the same explanation (Cheyne, 1971; Parke, 1970). Finally, reasoning and induction seem to be influenced by developmental level. Kindergarten children show no effect of explanation about why they should refrain from an activity, whereas third-graders are better able to delay gratification when a reason for doing so is given (Cheyne, 1972).

Studies such as those discussed above suggest that developmental considerations may interact with the application of reward and punishment. Thus, it seems prudent to explore possible interactions between the type of consequence given, the behavior under consideration, and the maturational status of the recipient (Robinson, 1986).

Individual Differences Constructs

Irritability. "Socially aggressive children live in aggressive families. At a microsocial level, what is meant is that members of these families are disposed to react irritably with each other" (Patterson, 1982, p. 192). Coercion theory includes four kinds of irritability: crossover, counterattack, punishment acceleration, and persistence. *Crossover* is an initiation of an aversive (negative) interchange following a positive or neutral antecedent behavior by another family member. Mothers, fathers, and siblings in families with a problem child are all more likely than members of control families to start conflicts (crossover) with the target child, and the target child is more likely than control children to start conflicts with the mother (Patterson, 1982, p. 193).

Counterattack is an aversive response to a negative behavior of another individual. The problem child is more likely than a control child to counterattack when interacting with his or her mother (but not with other family members). Similarly, both mothers and fathers in problem families are more likely than control parents to counterattack.

In *punishment acceleration*, a negative exchange is followed by a behavior that increases the probability that another deviant behavior will follow. For example, disapproval (criticism) is likely to lead to further aversive behavior, whereas no response tends to decrease the likelihood of its continuing (Patterson, 1982, p. 184).

Finally, *persistence* is the tendency to continue a chain of aversive behaviors regardless of the reaction of other family members. All problem family members are more likely than control family members to continue an aversive behavior once they have started.

Bilateral Trait. The irritability of problem children is conceptualized as a *bilateral trait.* Individual differences in aggression are due to the nature of the child and, partly, to the personality of the mother. For both mother and child, the propensity to react irritably is hypothesized to be a generalized "style of interacting with people and a means of coping with problems" (Patterson, 1982, p. 195) that is consistent in various settings and across time. In support of this hypothesis, there is a high degree of consistency in home deviant behavior over a 1-year period ($r = .74$; Patterson, 1974). There is also some cross-setting generality in that children who are aggressive and disruptive at home are also likely to exhibit these behaviors at school (Patterson, Cobb, & Ray, 1972). Although data on continuity support the notion of persistence in level of deviance, the more specific hypothesis—that aggressive children are more likely than others to evidence counterattack, crossover, persistence, and acceleration in their daily interactions—has not yet been tested. Similarly, the irritability of the mothers outside the home has not been investigated.

To assess individual differences, Patterson has suggested using sequential lag analysis (Sackett, 1979), which examines the conditional probability that a behavior will occur at more than one time interval (lag) following an antecedent. For example, the probability of child aversive behavior following a parent aversive behavior can be examined both immediately after the parent's behavior and in subsequent time intervals. This approach has considerable promise for the understanding of human interaction because it allows for the possibility that the effect of one person's behavior on that of another individual may be either immediate or delayed (lagged). These analyses have been conducted with married couples (Gottman, 1979) and are beginning to be applied to family interaction in the home.

The notion of a bilateral trait makes two important theoretical attributions: (a) It focuses investigation on the parent–child dyad rather than on the individual child, and (b) it incorporates the descriptive finding that aggressive children live in aggressive families. It does not, however, offer a causal explanation for aggressive behavior in children. Whether bilateral aggression is determined by temperamental characteristics, poor communication skills, situational stresses, or other factors is not clear.

Conclusions

Coercion theory adopts the operant assumptions that the maintaining conditions of childhood aggression are to be found in the events that immediately precede and those that follow the behavior. Efforts to substantiate that hypothesis have met with mixed success. Parents of problem children—particularly mothers—are more likely to initiate irritable exchanges with their child and are more likely to counterattack if their child is aversive, but even though these differences are statistically significant, they represent small distinctions in an absolute sense. The finding that continues to emerge loudly and clearly is that families seeking treatment exhibit more aggression than do normal families. Given that *more* aversive behavior occurs, it follows that deviance is more likely to follow deviance (counterattack), that deviant behavior is more likely to continue once it has begun, and that more deviance will follow neutral or positive events than will be the case among families who display a lower base rate of negative behavior. The base-rate differences are large—two to four times the rate displayed by normal families—and they have not been adequately controlled for in analysis of irritability. Knutson (1982) made a similar argument for a conservative interpretation of the role of negative reinforcement. All aversive interchanges must end eventually, and negative reinforcement of something will occur; consequently, aversive exchanges will always be associated with negative reinforcement. Negative reinforcement may not be causally related to deviant behavior but may be an artifact of its definition. Thus, the question remains: Are the small but significant observable differences sufficient to explain the large and consistent differences in aversive behavior?

There are a number of possible explanations for the current ambiguity regarding the empirical status of coercion theory. For example, measurement issues must be considered. Although the overall reliability of the Family Interaction Coding System is excellent—possibly the highest reliability of any complex home observation system—those behaviors of greatest import are also the least adequately coded. The reliability of aversive behaviors ranges from 38% agreement for negativism to 91% for disapproval, with an average of 73.8% for all 14 aversive behaviors (Patterson, 1982, p. 59). These figures are not corrected for chance agreement (Cohen's kappa), nor do they reflect the reliability for chains of behaviors necessary to interpret sequential analyses (Hartmann, 1977). Thus, the absence of differences between deviant and normal families may be at least partly a function of measurement error. The problem of obtaining meaningful observational data cannot be underestimated. It is extremely difficult to code the ongoing behavior of an individual as it occurs by means of a system of 29 behaviors, some of which are coded twice, while at the same time monitoring the reaction of all the other family members. The interaction is particularly difficult to record when the family is chaotic and people talk simultaneously, interrupt each other frequently, and engage in rapid escalations.

The reliability increases when behavior subtypes are combined into generic categories such as *aversive, positive,* and *neutral.* However, this procedure is not without cost. It represents one additional level of inference and implies that the events subsumed under them share common reinforcing or punishing properties. By combining disparate events under one label, potential relationships between antecedent and consequent events may be obscured. For example, whining may be maintained by parental attention, whereas the reinforcer for noncompliance may be a failure to follow through on a command.

The circumscribed use of developmental constructs may also restrict the explanatory power of coercion theory (Cairns, 1979, p. 335). The rewarding or punishing effects of certain parental behavior may interact with the child's cognitive understanding of the event: sarcasm may be punishing to a preadolescent but may not be understood by a concrete, preoperational child. Similarly, the child's ability to be affected by reasons for the parent's disapproval may be influenced by his or her understanding of moral precepts.

Finally, we must consider the likelihood that coercion theory is not sufficiently robust to explain family aggression. For example, cognitions do not play a causal role in coercion theory, yet it may not be possible to fully understand pathological family interaction without assessing how people construe events. Parents' perception of the child may be colored by expectations. Similarly, the child's understanding of the contingencies at home may have greater explanatory power than the actual reward and punishment ratios. Twenty years of painstaking research have not put coercion theory on a sound empirical footing. Although future research may prove coercion theory to be fully adequate, other researchers may wish to open new avenues of investigation.

SOCIAL LEARNING MODELS OF MARITAL DISCORD

Background

Although social learning theories of marital discord began in an operant tradition (Liberman, 1970; Patterson & Hops, 1972; Stuart, 1969; Weiss *et al.*, 1973), these models have evolved in the direction of Kantian idealism. That is, more recent formulations of a social learning perspective have invoked mediational processes as explanatory concepts in attempting to account for both marital satisfaction and distress (Berley & Jacobson, 1984; Doherty, 1981a,b; Jacobson & Margolin, 1979; Jacobson & Moore, 1981a; Weiss, 1980). Their invoking of the reciprocal determinism construct thus resembles Bandura's use of the term much more than it does Patterson's. Spouses are viewed as imposing meaning on relationship events by interpreting those events in light of idiosyncratic cognitive and perceptual processes. Most of the major social learning theorists have hypothesized that observable behavior alone will not maximize one's ability to predict important relationship events (Gottman, 1979, 1982a,b; Jacobson & Margolin, 1979; Jacobson & Moore, 1981b; Margolin, Christensen, & Weiss, 1975; Weiss, 1978, 1980). Rather, attempts have been made to account for variance in interactional behavior by asking spouses to report their thoughts and feelings: What impact does his or her behavior have on you? Why do you think she or he does that? What are your thoughts and feelings when he or she behaves in that way? Theories have expanded to hypothesize cognitive and perceptual events as important mediators of marital conflict and accord. However, these internal processes are not viewed as autonomous; rather, they are both determinants of and determined by environmental events as well as overt behavior. When Spouse B responds to Spouse A's initiation of affection by saying to herself, "He's just trying to placate me for losing his job," her affective response may be to get angry, and on a behavioral level, she might slap him. In a sense, both the affection and the cognition could be considered "causes" of the wife's response. But from the perspective of social learning theories, prediction of her response will be enhanced by the information provided by the wife's interpretation.

Although the social learning tradition has moved toward a Kantian philosophical stance, it remains firmly committed to methodological behaviorism. Included in this emphasis is the Pattersonian legacy of using observational data to describe sequences of interaction in distressed and nondistressed couples (Billings, 1979; Gottman, 1979; Hahlweg, Reisner, Kohli, Vollmer, Schindler, & Revenstorf, 1984; Margolin & Wampold, 1981; Revenstorf, Hahlweg, Schindler, & Vogel, 1984; Schaap, 1984). Thus, although internal processes are hypothesized to exert a causal influence on marital behavior, the research methodology of social learning theorists remains firmly anchored in the performance-based interaction analysis following from Patterson's work on coercion theory

Epistemology

The formal characteristics of early social learning formulations of marital dysfunction placed it within a Lockean model. Marital satisfaction was viewed as the outcome of relatively high rates of reinforcing behavior and low rates of punishing behavior (Stuart, 1969). Moreover, early findings from research investigations tended to support the utility of this conceptualization of marital distress, at least in a descriptive sense. Elsewhere, Jacobson (1979) reviewed this early research and concluded that there is strong support for this hypothesis, at least insofar as distressed couples can be discriminated from nondistressed couples based on the frequency of reinforcing and punishing exchanges.

These findings have been fairly robust across a variety of situations and numerous definitions of *reward* and *punishment*. When the two terms are given standardized definitions by the investigators and are applied to marital interaction in the laboratory, distressed couples generally emit higher frequencies of punishing interactions and lower frequencies of rewarding interactions than do their nondistressed counterparts. The same differences emerge when data are collected from tapes placed in the couple's home (Gottman, 1979). When the definition of the two terms is left to the spouses, the results remain largely the same. Once again, whether the database is restricted to laboratory interaction or is broadened to include exchanges in the home, rewarding and punishing behaviors seem to be predictable, given knowledge of spouses' overall level of marital distress.

However, if one looks more closely, even in these early formulations, internal processes played an important role. The importance placed on spouses' cognitions and perceptual processes manifested itself in a number of ways and can be traced to a number of sources.

First, from the beginning, the phenomenon of interest to marital theorists was inherently subjective and depended, therefore, on an assessment of cognitive and perceptual processes, at least as dependent variables. Aggressive behavior as an observable target has no counterpart for those interested in understanding marriage. Although many early theorists attempted to operationalize marriage in terms of overt conflictual behavior, the overt behaviors measured by marital researchers seldom correspond directly to the presenting problems manifested by couples seeking therapy (Jacobson, Follette, & Elwood, 1984). Marital distress, although expressed in the form of verbal behavior, is merely the reflection of an internal state, and it is that internal state that is ultimately of interest to theoreticians. This interest in measuring internal states has sensitized marital researchers, both behavioral and nonbehavioral, to the importance of measuring cognitive, affective, and perceptual processes. We believe that this sensitization has contributed to the consideration of internal processes as independent as well as dependent variables. This interest has been evident in attempts to investigate the reactivity of subjective marital satisfaction (Jacobson, Follette, & McDonald, 1982; Jacobson, Waldron, & Moore, 1980; Margolin, 1981; Wills, Weiss, & Patterson, 1974); in the attention that has been paid to the subjective *impact* of marital communication (Gottman, 1979; Markman, 1979); and in recent efforts to examine the interface between objective observer and subjective spouse recipient (Floyd & Markman, 1986; Gottman, 1979; Weiss, 1984).

Second, social learning models of marriage were heavily influenced by social-psychological exchange theories, and in particular by the seminal work of Thibaut and Kelley (1959). These theories emphasize the salience of spouses' perceptual processes in imposing meaning on the behavior emitted by the partner. As Gottman (1982a) noted, social exchange theories conceptualize how people perceive interaction rather than the interaction itself. For example, social learning theorists have adopted the exchange concept labeled *comparison level for alternatives* (Jacobson & Margolin, 1979; Stuart, 1969). This concept states that people stay in relationships as long as they perceive them as the best available alternative (Thibaut & Kelley, 1959). In other words, the spouse evaluates his or her current relationship, compares it with his or her "perception" of the available alternatives, and then makes a "decision" regarding whether to stay in the relationship. Obviously, various cognitive and perceptual processes are invoked to predict when people will terminate relationships and when they will remain in them.

Third, research findings have seemingly compelled social learning researchers to move in the direction of Kantian idealism. All attempts to account for important interactional phenomena independently of spouses' appraisals and perceptions have been foiled. It has been shown time and time again that spouses have unique access to the meaningful events in their relationship, and that their phenomenal world is, to a large extent, inaccessible to observers.

For example, various researchers have investigated the event-by-event correspondence between observer ratings of behavior and corresponding ratings by the spouses themselves. Typically, the rated dimension is a "positive–negative" dimension. Observer ratings of positivity are simply not very predictive of the ratings provided by the spouses themselves (Gottman, 1979; Weiss, 1984). Thus, the valence of marital behaviors seems to depend substantially on spouses' private appraisal systems. Despite the ability of observers to distinguish between distressed and nondistressed couples on the dimension of "positiveness," observer ratings of "positive" and "negative" behavior may have little to do with the functional impact of the behaviors in question on the spouses themselves.

The picture of marital interaction that began to emerge from this early research was described by Jacobson and Margolin (1979):

> People talk to themselves, they appraise their environments, and they make attributions and interpretations of their world. These self-statements, appraisals, and attributions mediate and moderate the effects of environmental stimuli on behavior, and can serve either as eliciting of discriminative stimuli. Attributions of the part of one's spouse regarding the "intent" or the partner's behavior can moderate the reinforcing effect of that behavior. Emotional reactions can be elicited by specific self-statements, which often serve as interpretations of an environmental event. . . . The inclusions of cognitions as possible mediators of behavior will have important implications for the analysis and treatment of distressed relationships. (p. 12)

Structural Constructs

Reward–Punishment Ratios. All major theoretical statements derived from the social learning perspective adopt the hedonistic conception of marital satisfaction that began with social exchange theory. This is the notion that marital satisfaction is the result of the quality of outcomes for each spouse in the relationship (Azrin, Naster, & Jones, 1973; Gottman, 1979; Jacobson & Margolin, 1979; Jacobson & Moore, 1981a; Stuart, 1969, 1980; Weiss, 1978, 1980; Weiss *et al.*, 1973). A variety of studies, referred to in the previous section, support the social learning hypothesis that nondistressed couples provide each other with higher rates of rewarding behavior and with lower rates of punishing behavior than do their distressed counterparts.

In deciding how to interpret these data, we are faced with dilemmas similar to the ambiguities in interpreting the research with children cited in the previous section. The issue is the distinction between *description* and *explanation*. It seems clear that marital interaction can be described according to the frequency of rewarding and punishing interchanges, and that these descriptions have some discriminative validity. However, this descriptive information is not very interesting in and of itself, and it certainly provides no direct support for social learning theories. Very few theorists of any orientation would be surprised by the finding that distressed couples are relatively "negative," and that nondistressed couples are relatively "positive." The assertion that marital distress is *caused* by particular frequencies of rewarding and punishing exchanges is another matter. These correlational investigations, cited above, should not be confused with the type of longitudinal or experimental design needed to establish a causal relationship between rewarding and punishing events, on the one hand, and marital distress, on the other.

An additional interpretive dilemma that one faces with these correlational investigations involves the definition of terms such as *reward* and *punisher*. In none of the above-cited studies was the term *reward* or the term *punisher* defined empirically. Yet, to be consistent with the operant definition of these terms, the definition must be an empirical one; they both must be defined according to

their effects on the subsequent probability of the particular behaviors to which
they are temporally related. For example, an interactional event emitted by the
wife would be labeled as a reinforcer to the extent that its contingent presentation increased the probability of some particular behavior on the part of the
husband. This determination would have to be made separately for each couple,
and standardized definitions of these terms would be precluded. It is obviously
impossible to adhere to these strict definitional criteria. It is important to remember, then, how these definitions have been compromised, because the departure from the operant definition inevitably leads to a theoretical departure
from an operant model. Some investigators have used standardized definitions
that are applied across couples (Billings, 1979; Birchler, Weiss, & Vincent, 1975;
Gottman, 1979; Hahlweg et al., 1984; Margolin & Wampold, 1981; Revenstorf et
al. 1984; Schaap, 1984; Vincent, Friedman, Nugent, & Messerley, 1979; Vincent, Weiss, & Birchler, 1975). These studies measure behaviors believed by the
investigator to be rewarding and punishing for most couples, and the discriminant validity of these measures tells us that there are some generally identifiable
behavioral signs of marital distress and satisfaction. However, we have already
cited evidence to suggest that these measures are often poor predictors of the
spouses' experience of the same events. Thus, other investigators have eschewed
standardized criteria and have left it to the spouses themselves to label marital
behaviors as either rewarding or punishing.

Reciprocity. In addition to base-rate differences in the frequency of rewarding and punishing behavior, social learning theories have examined the patterning of interactional exchanges over time, as well as the extent to which marital
distress is associated with particular types of exchange sequences. This literature
addresses and attempts to identify contingent relationships between spouses'
behavior. The basic question addressed by these studies is: Is there a lawful
relationship between one spouse's delivery of reinforcing and punishing behavior and the other's? The major finding is that *negative reciprocity* characterizes the
interaction sequences of distressed couples (Billings, 1979; Gottman, 1979; Margolin & Wampold, 1981; Revenstorf et al., 1984; Schaap, 1984). Negative or
aversive behavior in distressed couples tends to occur in sequential chains. For
example, the probability of the wife's behaving negatively, given that the husband has just behaved negatively, is greater than the overall probability that the
wife will behave negatively. Our ability to predict negative behavior on the part
of the wife is enhanced by knowing whether the husband has just engaged in
negative behavior. Thus, it is not simply the frequency of negative behavior that
distinguishes between distressed and nondistressed couples but also the timing
of negative behavior. In nondistressed couples, punishing behavior by one
spouse is less likely to be immediately reciprocated; it appears that spouses (and
in particular, wives) in generally satisfying relationships "edit" their partners'
negative communication by responding to it in such a way that the escalation
process is halted (cf. Gottman, 1979).

The findings for positive reciprocity are less consistent. Collapsing across
levels of marital distress, some studies provide evidence of the existence of
positive reciprocity, and others do not. What has been consistent across studies is

the failure of positive reciprocity to discriminate between distressed and non-distressed couples. Thus, distressed couples are more likely than nondistressed couples to reciprocate immediate negative behaviors, whereas the tendency to reciprocate positive behaviors is equivalent for distressed and nondistressed couples.

Reactivity and the Importance of Immediate Contingencies. The tendency toward negative reciprocity in distressed couples appears to be only one manifestation of a more general characteristic, which has been described as a tendency to be highly *reactive* to immediate events in the relationship. A number of studies have provided evidence that the subjective satisfaction of distressed spouses at a given point in time is highly dependent on the quality of outcomes on that particular day (Jacobson *et al.*, 1980, 1982; Margolin, 1981). In other words, on days when a relatively high frequency of negative events occurs, subjective satisfaction is particularly low in distressed couples; conversely, there is some evidence that satisfaction is particularly high in distressed couples on days when relatively large numbers of positive events occur (Jacobson *et al.*, 1982). This reactivity phenomenon is hard to assimilate within a Lockean model. It states that couples use contingencies differently depending on their level of distress. In other words, it is not just the contingencies that control behavior, but the way in which those contingencies are perceived on a subjective, affective level also determines their salience and potency.

These data suggest that immediate contingencies are more important in the regulation of behavior for distressed relationships. In this regard, they are consistent with the findings regarding negative reciprocity, which similarly suggest that immediate contingency control—at least, for negative behavior—is more characteristic of distressed couples. Along the same lines, Gottman (1982b) reported a study in which the physiological responses of both husbands and wives were recorded during a discussion of how their day had gone. Based on skin conductance measures, "physiological coupling" was negatively and highly correlated with marital satisfaction. Spouses within a distressed relationship shared similar degrees of physiological arousal; such was not the case for nondistressed couples. This is another example of "linkage" between spouses in a distressed relationship, except in this case the linkage is physiological rather than behavioral.

Weiss (1980) coined the term *sentiment override* to describe a process in which subjective satisfaction or sentiment is relatively independent of what is actually transpiring between spouses on a behavioral level. Based on the reactivity literature, sentiment override seems to characterize nondistressed couples. Gottman (1979) suggested a "bank account" metaphor to describe the interaction of satisfied couples. Nondistressed couples, according to this metaphor, have a history of a high ratio of positive (deposit) to negative (withdrawal) behavior. It is suggested that such couples exchange high rates of rewards, but that these rewards are not exchanged in a contingent manner. The high ratio of positive to negative behaviors, combined with the absence of positive reciprocity, describes the interaction of happily married couples.

Jacobson and Moore (1981a) integrated the literature on reciprocity and reactivity with the metaphors provided by Gottman and Weiss, suggesting that happily married couples have learned to behave independently of the immediate consequences of their behavior. Negative behavior is not reciprocated on a behavioral level, nor does it effect satisfaction adversely on an experiential level. Positive behavior may also be under the control of long-term rather than immediate contingencies in generally happy couples. Perhaps immediate reciprocity is unnecessary to maintain behavior after a long history of high rates of rewards in the relationship. Negative behavior may also be benign in its impact because history has taught that it will not occur very often. This independence between marital satisfaction and immediate events may provide an operational definition of trust.

This appears to be a promising area of research, and the findings thus far have sharpened the ability to describe marital interaction. However, it should be pointed out that all of this research remains on a descriptive rather than an explanatory level. No causal links have been established. Both the emphasis on the relative rather than the absolute effects of overt contingencies and the findings of the reactivity research place this area within a Kantian tradition.

Emotional Responsiveness. Based on his own research, Gottman (1982a) hypothesized that

> closeness in marriages is symmetry in emotional responsiveness. It is precisely the absence of this responsiveness, I believe, that leads to high levels of negative affect, which produce emotional withdrawal and bursts of reciprocity. (p. 119)

Although this emotional responsiveness hypothesis has not been proved, it is based on a variety of converging findings. For example, the "editing" process described above as characterizing nondistressed wives is one example of a "responsive" behavior that prevents escalation and maintains closeness. Other research on dominance has suggested that an asymmetrical pattern of dominance is found in distressed couples. Husbands were less emotionally responsive to their wives than their wives were to them.

It is not completely clear what Gottman meant by *emotional responsiveness.* Some of his data would appear to be at variance with his hypothesis, at least insofar as emotional responsiveness is interpreted as including responsiveness to negative behavior. Distressed couples appear to exhibit more predictable, stereotypical interaction patterns, interaction patterns that are readily identifiable to an observer as signs of marital conflict. Their interaction exhibits a greater degree of "temporal structure." In other words, distressed couples actually seem to be more emotionally congruent with one another, although the congruence is in terms of negative affect rather than positive affect. Gottman was obviously referring to positive affect.

Motivational Constructs

Origin of Behavior. Thus far, almost all of the research that has been described is cross-sectional and correlational and thus does not speak directly to the evolution of marital satisfaction. The interaction patterns exemplified in constructs such as reactivity and reciprocity describe the end result of a long interactional history. There has been very little research on the causes of these descriptive patterns. However, there has been a great deal of speculation, and a number of hypotheses have been generated that are potentially testable.

Social learning models of marital distress have hypothesized that a number of skills are required in order for a relationship to succeed. Deficiencies in any one of a number of these skills can lead to marital conflict. This view of marital conflict has been termed by Weiss (1980) a "competency-based" model of marriage. He has speculated that couples need four basic types of skills to maintain a satisfying intimate relationship: objectification skills, which refer to pinpointing and the ability to perceive the same events as occurring; the ability to provide mutually supportive and empathic communication; problem-solving and decision-making skills; and skills in bringing about behavior change. There is some evidence of performance deficiencies in the first three areas in distressed couples, although virtually no evidence that deficiencies in any of these areas bear a causal relationship to marital distress. Distressed couples do appear to exhibit considerable divergence in their perception of events in their relationship (Christensen & Nies, 1980; Christensen, Sullaway, & King, 1983; Elwood & Jacobson, 1982; Jacobson & Moore, 1981b). The research cited above suggests a relative absence of empathic communication in distressed couples. Finally, research to be reviewed below provides evidence of deficiencies in problem-solving skills. Interestingly, there is virtually no evidence that distressed couples are deficient in their ability to bring about behavior change, although this hypothesized skill deficit is the oldest and most widely emphasized cause of marital discord in the social learning literature. The earliest social learning formulations of marital conflict posited that, to compel the partner to change, distressed couples use aversive control strategies, which include punishment and negative reinforcement. This hypothesized deficit was contrasted with the supposed mechanisms used by nondistressed couples, which included an emphasis on positive control (Patterson & Hops, 1972; Stuart, 1969; Weiss et al., 1973).

A number of other researchers and theorists have hypothesized that marital conflict is caused by deficits in communication skills (e.g., Gottman, 1979, 1982a,b). In support of this hypothesis, several performance deficits have been identified in the communicative repertoires of distressed couples. First, there are the studies based on observational coding systems, where communication positiveness is defined by the investigator in a standardized manner. These studies, already discussed, consistently document generally negative communication patterns in distressed couples. Second, studies have compared distressed and nondistressed couples in their "receptive" and "expressive" communication skills (Gottman & Porterfield, 1981; Noller, 1981). Spouses were asked to deliver speeches of a fixed verbal content to their partners and to strangers. Receivers were asked to guess the "intent" of the communication on the basis of nonverbal cues emitted by the sender. The results of two studies uncovered deficiencies in the receptive skills of husbands in distressed relationships. Third, Gottman (1979) reported a study in which a mechanical device allowed interacting couples to produce an ongoing record of the "impact" that each partner's responses had on the other (on a positive–negative dimension), and the "intent" of each partner's own communication to the partner. Both sender "impact" and receiver "intent" were reported with every turn in the conversation. The results were that distressed couples could be discriminated on the basis of lower impact ratings, although differences were not apparent in the reported communicative "intent." The authors interpreted these results as supporting a "communication deficit" explanation of marital discord, because there was a discrepancy between the intent of the communication and its impact on the partner. It should be mentioned that other equally plausible interpretations of these findings exist. The intent–impact discrepancy could result from social desirability. It is not socially desirable to intend to be negative; distressed spouses may have simply distorted their intent ratings. Impact ratings, on the other hand, are not as likely to be altered by social desirability.

A particular type of communication deficit that has received attention from social learning theorists has been conflict resolution interaction. Many current behavioral techniques for treating couples with marital problems are based on the notion that deficits in the ability to resolve conflict bear a causal relationship to marital distress. Gottman's research (1979) has come closest to identifying specific performance deficits in the repertoires of distressed couples. Based on sequential analyses of laboratory interaction, Gottman has identified three stages in a conflict resolution discussion: an agenda-building phase, a middle arguing phase, and a resolution phase. The agenda-building phase characterizes the beginning of the conflict resolution discussion, and its objective is to define the problem from the perspective of each partner. The goal of the arguing phase is for each partner to vigorously present his or her point of view. The goal of the resolution phase is to negotiate a solution to the problem.

Distressed couples are notably different from nondistressed couples during all three phases. During the agenda-building phase, satisfied couples typically enter into "validation loops," whereas distressed couples are more likely to exhibit "cross-complaining." The validation loop involves one partner's expressing feelings about a problem, while the other validates and attempts to understand the concern. Cross-complaining can be distinguished from validation in that the partner responds with countercomplaints rather than validation. Although both distressed and nondistressed couples argue during the middle of the discussion, this phase ends with a proposal for change and subsequent agreement for happy couples. This happy ending is less likely to occur in distressed couples; instead, they are more likely to enter into long chains of unproductive and redundant clarifying and rephrasing of the problem.

All of the studies mentioned thus far that deal with communication deficiencies are cross-sectional. In fact, only one longitudinal study has been conducted to test social learning hypotheses regarding communication deficits. Although longitudinal studies do not directly test causal hypotheses, they do at least allow for the possibility of demonstrating that the hypothesized cause existed before the phenomenon that the study is trying to predict. Markman (1979, 1981) followed couples over a five-year period. At Time 1, they were all "planning to marry." Their communication was examined by means of the mechanical recording device described above to produce "impact" and "intent" ratings. Although impact ratings were uncorrelated with relationship satisfaction at Time 1, they were highly predictive of relationship satisfaction both 2½ and 5 years later. In other words, ratings by one partner of the other's communication predicted subsequent marital satisfaction. This is the only evidence existing in the literature that suggests a communication deficit before subsequent marital conflict. Unfortunately, even here, the predictor was a self-report of a communication problem rather than an objectively verified communication problem. These findings show only that "perceptions" of communication predict subsequent satisfaction and provide another example of the ability to predict that important relationship phenomena will be enhanced by an examination of spouses' internal processes, thus demonstrating the virtues of a Kantian perspective in understanding marriage.

With the exception of Markman's study, there is no evidence that communication deficits of any kind bear a causal relationship to marital conflict. It is quite conceivable that communication deficits represent little more than a manifestation of marital distress rather than a primary cause. In fact, some evidence was provided by Vincent and his associates (1979) that distressed couples are quite capable of altering their communication under certain stimulus conditions so that it is no longer easily distinguishable from that of nondistressed couples. Research such as this suggests that the observed differences reflect not skill deficits but performance deficits that persist even though distressed spouses generally possess the requisite skills in their repertoire. Similar cautions can be raised with respect to the more general notion of skill deficiencies as causes of marital conflict. The notion that marital distress is a function of skill deficiencies remains central to social learning conceptualizations. However, at this point, the notion remains an empirical question.

Jacobson and Margolin (1979) recognized the important distinction between description and explanation and, in that spirit, speculated on possible antecedents to marital conflict. The following variables were hypothesized to exist before and to bear some causal relationship to marital discord:

1. *Inadequate problem-solving skills.*

2. *Reinforcement erosion.* Jacobson and Margolin (1979) hypothesized that a reduction in a partner's reinforcement value for the other over time contributes to marital discord. They suggested that this "erosion" process occurs to some degree in all long-term relationships because of habituation. But couples who have a wide-ranging *repertoire* of reinforcers to provide for one another are less likely to become seriously distressed as a result of the reinforcement erosion process. Couples who are highly dependent on a few restricted classes of reinforcers (e.g., sex) are at higher risk for marital conflict. This one hypothesized antecedent has little to do with *relationship skills*. It suggests that couples may be very skillful yet still be unhappy because there has been a decline in reinforcement value.

3. *Rules.* Theorists from a variety of perspectives have emphasized the im-

portance of rules in the effective functioning of a relationship (Haley, 1963; Jackson, 1965; Weiss, 1978). Ambiguous or nonexistent rules, or rules that the spouses each interpret differently, can produce marital conflict.

Factors External to the Relationship. In their notion of comparison level for alternatives (Thibaut & Kelley, 1959), social exchange theorists have drawn attention to the extent to which relationships depend on exogenous factors, that is, factors external to their own interaction. Both marital satisfaction and marital stability are expected to vary according to each spouse's perception of how desirable that alternatives to the present relationship are. Thus, marital conflict can be caused or preceded by one or both spouses' perceiving themselves as having very attractive alternatives to the present relationship. Similarly, external stresses can disrupt marital stability despite the initial absence of interactional difficulties. Economic hard times, societal and cultural changes, and a variety of other factors can serve as a sociocultural backdrop for marital conflict and can, indeed, cause marital distress.

Although these and other expected antecedents of marital conflict remain speculative, they draw attention to the complexity of the phenomena that marital researchers are trying to predict. Jacobson and Margolin (1979) suggested a multivariate model in which causes are viewed not as dichotomous but as probabilistic. The model that will best predict the development of marital distress will probably be exceedingly complex, despite our desire for parsimony. As the next section will confirm, in the late 1960s and early 1970s researchers found John Locke to be appealing, but it appears that Kant has emerged the winner since that time.

Cognitions. The role of cognitive and perceptual processes in mediating marital satisfaction and distress has been increasingly emphasized by social learning theorists (Berley & Jacobson, 1984; Doherty, 1981a,b; Eidelson & Epstein, 1982; Epstein, 1982; Epstein & Eidelson, 1981; Jacobson, 1984; Jacobson & Margolin, 1979; Margolin *et al.*, 1975; Schindler & Vollmer, 1984; Weiss, 1980). However, the general hypothesis is that systematic differences exist between distressed and nondistressed couples in how marital behaviors are perceived and interpreted. Theoretical speculation has focused on attribution theory (Berley & Jacobson, 1984; Doherty, 1981a; Weiss, 1980), as well as the *cognitive models* popularized by Bandura (Doherty, 1981b; Weiss, 1980); Ellis (Eidelson & Epstein, 1982; Epstein & Eidelson, 1981); Beck (Epstein, 1982); and Meichenbaum (Schindler & Vollmer, 1984).

In addition to theoretical speculation, a number of studies have identified differences between distressed and nondistressed couples that seem related to a general tendency toward cognitive and perceptual distortions in the former. Jacobson, McDonald, Follette, and Berley (1985) found that distressed spouses are more inclined to attribute their partners' positive behavior to external or situational factors and their negative behavior to internal or trait factors. The authors suggested that these attributional tendencies serve to maintain marital distress by discounting positive behavior and holding their partners responsible for negative behavior. Robinson and Price (1980) found that, in comparison with observers, distressed couples underestimated the frequency of the partner's positive behavior, a finding that suggests a tendency to selectively track negative behavior. Eidelson and Epstein (1982) found that distressed couples were particularly likely to endorse unrealistic or irrational relationship beliefs. Several investigators have found relatively low consensus rates among distressed spouses regarding the occurrence of particular behaviors (Christensen & Nies, 1980; Christensen *et al.*, 1983; Elwood & Jacobson, 1982; Jacobson & Moore, 1981b).

Combining the results of the various studies summarized in this section, it seems that at least part of the discrepancy between distressed and nondistressed couples in the exchange of reinforcement and punishment has to do with their perceptions of and cognitions about what they are getting, rather than what they are actually receiving. Marital distress may result as much from cognitive distortions and dysfunctional perceptual processes as it does from actual reduction in the ratio of rewards and punishments.

A number of cognitive operations have been hypothesized as altering spouses' perceptions of the reinforcing and punishing behavior that they are receiving from one another. First, some have suggested a "selective tracking" process, whereby negative behavior is made salient and positive behavior is ignored or at least forgotten (Jacobson & Margolin, 1979; Stuart, 1969; Weiss *et al.*, 1973). Second, regardless of the accuracy of the perceptual scanning or tracking apparatus, behaviors may be reinterpreted so that once positive behaviors are now viewed as either neutral or negative. Third, many theorists have invoked attribution theories to suggest that the motivational inferences regarding the intent of the partner's behavior differ according to the level of distress, whereas others are viewed as conducive to causing, enhancing, or maintaining marital satisfaction (Berley & Jacobson, 1984; Doherty, 1981a,b; Fincham, 1983; Weiss, 1980).

The dimensions hypothesized as varying according to level of distress differ from author to author. However, various theorists share the belief that distressed couples attribute their partners' positive behavior to external, situational, or involuntary factors, whereas nondistressed couples are more likely to attribute such behaviors to internal, traitlike, and voluntary factors. In the former case, positive behaviors are somehow written off so that their impact is not as positive as it would otherwise be, whereas in the latter case positive behavior is accentuated and made more salient. Conversely, negative behaviors in distressed couples are attributed to internal, traitlike, and voluntary sources, whereas in nondistressed relationships, negative behaviors are written off via an external (situational) attribution.

What remains ambiguous in these theoretical speculations, as well as in others cited in previous sections, is the extent to which these processes are put forth as explanations for marital discord. The distinction is seldom raised because distal causal explanation is deemphasized in social learning theories, which have always been more interested in describing present contingencies and in delineating factors that maintain and exacerbate behavior than in describing the historical evolution of behavior. Thus, faulty perceptual and cognitive processes may simply serve to maintain or exacerbate marital conflict that has been caused by other factors, or the processes may have existed before marital conflict. There is very little speculation one way or the other in the literature.

Developmental Considerations

Although social learning theorists have been called to task for ignoring the potential significance of the family life cycle in their theoretical formulations (Knudson, Gurman, & Kniskern, 1979), there has been little noticeable trend toward examining the evolution of marital relationships at different stages. The one major exception has been a focus on the impact of children on marital interaction and satisfaction. There is a general tendency toward a decline in marital satisfaction after the birth of a child (Margolin, 1981; Waldron & Routh, 1981). Moreover, in other respects, nondistressed couples develop characteristics that resemble those of distressed couples after children enter the picture: these couples show a greater tendency toward both immediate reciprocity and negative reactivity (Vincent, Cook, & Messerly, 1980). Jacobson *et al.* (1982) found that nondistressed wives were less reactive to their husband's positive behavior after childbirth. Thus, there is some indication that the period immediately following childbirth is stressful for couples, but with the exception of this work, developmental issues have been virtually ignored.

The delineation and empirical verification of developmental stages within the course of a marriage remains an important area for future investigation. There is no reason to suspect that the period following the birth of the first child is the only aberrant era in an otherwise constant relationship course. Dividing relationship evolution into stages is likely to be fruitful. For example, a number of theorists have suggested that there is something unique about courtship (Jacobson & Margolin, 1979; Weiss, 1980). It is alleged that exchanges are relatively noncontingent during this period, and that "sentiment" overrides the need for some of the skills that are necessary for later relationship stages. Thus, the determinants of marital satisfaction during this early relationship stage are likely to differ from those at a later stage. Moreover, both age and marriage duration are likely to prove significant as predictors of types of variables that mediate relationship satisfaction. As people get older, their repertoires of potential reinforcers change, and these changes can have an impact on both expectations and outcomes. The comparison level for alternatives also changes with age. The pool of eligibles gradually diminishes, and this process occurs more quickly for women in our culture than it does for men. All of these variables are bound to have an effect on the determinants of marital satisfaction.

Individual Differences Constructs

Consistent with many behavioral models, the social learning models of marriage have had very little to say about individual difference variables and their role in explaining the individual difference issues that potentially impinge on attempts to explain marital satisfaction. There are actually two such types of individual differences issues. One is the typical type of interpersonal variable often associated with research on individual differences; the other can be best described as "dyadic individual differences," or individual differences in dyadic combination types. Are certain combinations of people particularly likely to "make it or not make it" together?

The one area of activity that bears on individual differences is the recent work and discussion related to the effects of sex roles and sex-role combinations on marital satisfaction (Burger & Jacobson, 1979; Jacobson & Margolin, 1979; Margolin *et al.*, 1975). There is some evidence that characteristics traditionally associated with the feminine role are important for both marital satisfaction and effective communication (Baucom, 1983; Burger & Jacobson, 1979), although it does not matter which spouse manifests these behaviors (Burger & Jacobson, 1979). Jacobson and Margolin (1979) speculated that, when spouses differ greatly in the importance placed on an intimate relationship as a source of gratification in life, marital conflict is likely. Implicit in this belief is the idea that people bring reinforcement preferences into relationships, and that there are individual differences in the extent to which people depend on the kinds of reinforcers one derives from relationships:

> Some people display characteristic preferences, which transcend any particular relationship, for a relatively high rate of interpersonal contact. Moreover, these people often prefer "intimate contact" such as affection, conversation about feelings, and the like, to simple companionship and shared activities. Finally, these people find the scarcity of these events aversive. There are also people who characteristically prefer relatively low rates of interpersonal contact, a low ratio of intimate contact in simple companionship, and often prefer to be alone. Excessive rates of interpersonal contact are experienced as aversive to these people. When these two types are matched in a marital relationship, the capacity for conflict is great. (p. 28)

Although there is no evidence as yet regarding the usefulness of this individual difference variable in predicting marital satisfaction, Jacobson has collected some unpublished data showing that this affiliation–independence dimension is related to sex and to sex role. Women are more likely to depend on relationships for reinforcement, whereas independent activities are more likely to be the predominant source of life satisfaction for men. Moreover, high femininity scores on sex-role scales are associated with preferences for interpersonal forms of gratification, whereas high masculinity scores are associated with preferences for independent sources of gratification. Finally, highly affiliative women are associated with a negative response to marital therapy; in other words, when women are highly dependent on relationships as a source of gratification, marital therapy is unlikely to lead to relationship improvement.

If these hypotheses regarding affiliation and independence are correct, traditional marriages, where roles are based on sex, would be expected to be high-conflict relationships. However, such relationships would not necessarily be unstable, that is, highly likely to end in divorce. At this point, the data only suggest that this sex-role-reinforcement preference-constellation may prove to be a useful variable in understanding marital satisfaction. However, the early work appears to be promising.

Conclusions

There is no coherent social-learning theory of marriage; rather, there is a set of loosely connected and isolated theoretical statements. Much of the research has been designed to describe interaction processes and to deduce their discriminatory power on dimensions related to marital satisfaction. Thus, marital distress is associated with fewer positive behaviors, a relative abundance of negative behaviors, negative reciprocity, and reactivity to immediate events. Cognitive and perceptual distortions accompany both distress and satisfaction; distressed couples distort in the direction of other-directed blame and self-exoneration, whereas happy couples tend either to ignore or to minimize events that detract from their dyadic self-image of being happily married.

These theoretical notions belong in the social learning camp because of the prominence of mediational constructs. Cognitive variables are not simply viewed as epiphenomena but are seen as exerting primary causal influence, while acting in concert with environmental events. This flexibility allows the social learning perspective to approach complex interactional phenomena that would be eschewed and, in fact, defined out of existence by pure operant models. If social learning theories are to move further in the direction of comprehensively accounting for marital phenomena, they must begin to pay attention to "content" and must diverge from their tendency to be captivated only by functional analyses and temporal delineations of process. Social learning theory must begin to tackle questions such as: What are the important rewarding and punishing stimuli in marriage? There is also a singular need for longitudinal investigations to directly test social learning hypotheses.

CONTRIBUTIONS OF SOCIAL LEARNING THEORIES

Social learning theories have made contributions in three main areas: the conceptual understanding of marital and family discord, the development of assessment instruments, and the evolution of effective treatment techniques.

Although we have been critical of the etiological significance of some social learning theories, there can be no doubt that they have enhanced our ability to *describe* as well as to differentiate between functional and dysfunctional family interaction. Moreover, as performance-based theories, they have helped to uncover current variables in the social environment that maintain faulty marital and family interaction. The work of Patterson and his associates has been seminal in this regard, although recent work in the marital area—especially that of Gottman and his associates—has been extremely important.

At the assessment level, social learning theories have been the primary innovators in the development of observational technology, as well as of methods for analyzing observational data. Although these methods were derived primarily for social learning models and have therefore been closely identified with those models, they are really descriptive tools that could be used in any theoretical framework whose goal is studying couples and families (Robinson &

Eyberg, 1984). In addition to their contributions to observational technology, the social learning investigators have developed other assessment instruments that have increased our understanding of marital and family dynamics. For example, the self-report measures that have been generated in social learning laboratories have a degree of behavioral specificity lacking in most previously generated laboratories. Once again, although this behavioral specificity is particularly suited to a social learning framework, the instruments could be used by researchers of any theoretical persuasion. Finally, social learning theorists have made singular contributions by their use of self-monitoring instruments for use by family members in the home. Unlike self-monitoring devices used by individuals, instruments that can be used by multiple family members can be checked for reliability and thus have a potential for objectivity that renders them extremely useful as barometers of naturalistic family interaction.

Perhaps the most important contribution of social learning theories has been their production of powerful and influential intervention strategies for dealing with difficult clinical disorders. The parent-training model of intervention with families presenting with aggressive children remains the treatment of choice for these disorders at the present time, even though recent evidence questions its efficacy (Bernal, Klineert, & Schultz, 1980; Robinson, 1987). These techniques were derived directly from the operant social-learning model presented earlier. This same model also led to early versions of behavioral marital therapy, which has since been modified to accommodate more recent theoretical explications of social learning constructs such as reciprocity, reactivity, and causal attributions. Although behavioral marital therapy can by no means be construed as a total solution to the problems of distressed couples, it has been subjected to more experimental research than all other approaches to marital therapy combined, and it seems to be viable for a substantial proportion of distressed couples.

FINAL COMMENTS

Social learning theory represents a reconceptualization of some of the basic theoretical presuppositions of behaviorism. The role of thought in Bandura's theory differs fundamentally from a conventional model in three central ways: (a) In reciprocal determinism, cognitions can be the cause, rather than simply the effect, of human behavior. This change in thinking is seen most dramatically in the hypothesized effect of thoughts and feelings or perception of the environment. (b) The proposed role of awareness in learning allows the individual to act outside the *observable* parameters of stimulus, reinforcement, and punishment. (c) Finally, the notion of abstract modeling allows the individual to be a creator of and not simply a perceiver of order. These theoretical innovations suggest a changing philosophical position.

Social learning theory is moving from empiricism toward rationalism. Assumptions about the origin of knowledge, the proper focus of investigation, and the way in which events are related to one another are undergoing profound modification. The sources of important information about behavior now include both the environment and the individual. Thus, the object of study shifts from extrinsic causation, associated with empiricism, to rationalism's emphasis on the participant. This change in perspective does not lend itself to reductionism: instead, it introduces a conceptual model consistent with rationalism in which explanation is based on an interrelated network of abstract concepts. The goal of a science of psychology within this model is to create useful explanatory constructs and to elucidate the causal relationships among them.

The characteristics that make Bandura's theory more than an elaboration of existing behavioral constructs are not yet fully reflected in the family psychopathology literature. The major social-learning statement as applied to children—coercion theory—remains an operant model in both theory and practice. In contrast, the marital dysfunction literature evidences a movement toward a Kantian model. For example, Weiss (1980) offered an intervention strategy that is conceptual and nonreductionistic.

It is likely that the Kantian notions in Bandura's theory will be used with increasing frequency as a model for future family research. A strictly operant model has not proved adequate to explain family pathology. Coercion theory data do not provide overwhelming support for this operant theory, and similarly, early marital research that used a strictly behavioral model also failed to account fully for the behavior of satisfied and dissatisfied couples. Some researchers and theoreticians have indicated dissatisfaction with a noncognitive explanation of behavior (e.g., Mahoney, 1974; Weiss, 1980) and are directing their efforts toward the development of a more complete theoretical statement.

Until the 1950s and the impetus of behaviorism, clinical psychology was essentially in a prescientific period characterized by a plethora of conflicting theories and little empirical research (Kuhn, 1970). Behaviorism, as presented by Skinner, offered a paradigm. In clinical psychology, this simple framework stimulated an outpouring of treatment-related research. The contribution of behaviorism was, however, twofold. It not only offered a causal model but also introduced the rigors of science to clinical psychology. An investigation is "science" and not some other type of activity (e.g., philosophy or theology) when it relies on operational definitions, the generation of testable hypotheses, and the reproducibility of results. No theoretical school has an exclusive claim to the possession of the tools of science. Although the future of clinical psychology may lie in the direction of the development of a Kantian theoretical model, it must also continue to adhere to the basic parameters of science that were ushered in and developed under the Lockean model of behaviorism.

Acknowledgments

The authors thank Thomas Nelson, Ilene Bernstein, Laura Feshbach, and Sheila Eyberg for their useful comments on an early draft of this paper. We are also grateful to Catherine Iiams and Joan Kohlenberg for their help in preparing the manuscript and to Virginia Waters and David Fathi for their library assistance.

REFERENCES

Alexander, J. F., & Parsons, B. V. (1973). Short-term behavioral intervention with delinquent families: Impact on family process and recidivism. *Journal of Abnormal Psychology, 81,* 219–225.

Aronfreed, J. (1968). *Conduct and conscience: The socialization of internalized control over behavior.* New York: Academic Press.

Associated Press. (1983, March 8). *The Herald: Western Sun Edition,* p. 5A.

Azrin, N. H., Naster, B. J., & Jones, R. (1973). Reciprocity counseling: A rapid learning-based procedure for marital counseling. *Behavior Research and Therapy, 11,* 365–382.

Baltes, M. M., & Reese, H. W. (1977). Operant research in violation of the operant paradigm? In B. Etzel, J. LeBlanc, & D. Baer (Eds.), *New developments in behavioral research: Theory, method, and application.* Hillsdale, NJ: Erlbaum.

Bandura, A. (1969). Social learning theory of identificatory processes. In D. A. Goslin (Ed.), *Handbook of socialization theory and research.* Chicago: Rand McNally.

Bandura, A. (1977). *Social learning theory.* Englewood Cliffs, NJ: Prentice-Hall.

Bandura, A. (1981). In search of pure unidirectional determinants. *Behavior Therapy, 12,* 30–40.

Bandura, A. (1982). Self-efficacy mechanism in human agency. *American Psychologist, 37,* 122–147.

Bandura, A. (1983). Temporal dynamics and decomposition of reciprocal determinism: A reply to Phillips and Orton. *Psychological Review, 90,* 166–170.

Bandura, A., & Schunk, D. H. (1981). Cultivating competence, self-efficacy, and intrinsic interest through proximal self-motivation. *Journal of Personality and Social Psychology, 41,* 586–598.

Bandura, A., & Walters, R. H. (1963). *Social learning and personality development.* New York: Holt, Rinehart & Winston.

Baucom, D. H. (1983). A comparison of behavioral contracting and problem-solving/communication training in behavioral marital therapy. *Behavior Therapy, 13,* 162–174.

Baumrind, D. (1967). Child care practices anteceding three patterns of preschool behavior. *Genetic Psychological Monographs, 75,* 43–88.

Baumrind, D., & Black, A. E. (1967). Socialization practices associated with dimensions of competence in pre-school boys and girls. *Child Development, 38,* 291–327.

Berkowitz, L. (1978). Is criminal violence normative behavior? *Journal of Research in Crime and Delinquency, 15,* 148–161.

Berley, R. A., & Jacobson, N. S. (1984). Causal attributions in intimate relationships: Toward a model of cognitive behavioral marital therapy. In P. Kendall (Ed.), *Advances in cognitive-behavioral research and therapy* (Vol. 3). New York: Academic Press.

Bernal, M. E., Klinnert, M. D., & Schultz, L. A. (1980). Outcome evaluation of behavioral parent-training and client-centered parent counseling for children with conduct problems. *Journal of Applied Behavior Analysis, 13,* 677–691.

Billings, A. (1979). Conflict resolution in distressed and nondistressed married couples. *Journal of Consulting and Clinical Psychology, 47,* 368–376.

Birchler, G. R., Weiss, R. L., & Vincent, P. P. (1975). A multimethod analysis of social reinforcement exchange between maritally distressed and nondistressed spouse and stranger dyads. *Journal of Personality and Social Psychology, 31,* 349–360.

Bolles, R. C. (1970). Species-specific defense reactions and avoidance learning. *Psychological Review, 77,* 32–48.

Budd, K. S., Green, D. R., & Baer, D. M. (1976). An analysis of multiple misplaced parental social contingencies. *Journal of Applied Behavior Analysis, 9,* 459–470.

Burger, A. L., & Jacobson, N. S. (1979). The relationship between sex role characteristics, couple satisfaction and couple problem-solving skills. *The American Journal of Family Therapy, 7,* 52–60.

Cairns, R. B. (1979). *Social development: The origins and plasticity of interchanges.* San Francisco: W. H. Freeman.

Cheyne, J. A. (1971). Some parameters of punishment affecting resistance to deviation and generalization of a prohibition. *Child Development, 42,* 1249–1261.

Cheyne, J. A. (1972). Punishment and "reasoning" in the development of self-control. In R. D. Parke (Ed.), *Recent trends in social learning theory.* New York: Academic Press.

Chomsky, N. (1968). *Language and the mind.* New York: Harcourt, Brace & World.

Christensen, A., & Nies, D. C. (1980). The Spouse Observation Checklist: Empirical analysis and critique. *The American Journal of Family Therapy, 8,* 69–79.

Christensen, A., Sullaway, M., & King, C. (1983). Systematic error in behavioral reports of dyadic interaction: Egocentric bias and content effects. *Behavioral Assessment, 5,* 129–140.

Collings, W. A., Berndt, T. J., & Hess, V. L. (1974). Observational learning of motives and consequences for television aggression: A developmental study. *Child Development, 45,* 799–802.

Deci, E. L. (1975). *Intrinsic motivation.* New York: Plenum Press.

Dember, W. N. (1974). Motivation and the cognitive revolution. *American Psychologist, 29,* 161–168.

Doherty, W. J. (1981a). Cognitive processes in intimate conflict: 1. Extending attribution theory. *The American Journal of Family Therapy, 9,* 5–13.

Doherty, W. J. (1981b). Cognitive processes in intimate conflict: II. Efficacy and learned helplessness. *American Journal of Family Therapy, 9,* 35–44.

Dreikurs, R. (1964). *Children: The challenge.* New York: Hawthorn.

Eidelson, R. J., & Epstein, N. (1982). Cognition and relationship maladjustment: Development of a measure of dysfunctional relationship beliefs. *Journal of Consulting and Clinical Psychology, 50,* 715–720.

Elwood, R., & Jacobson, N. S. (1982). Spouse agreement in reporting their behavioral interactions: A clinical replication. *Journal of Consulting and Clinical Psychology, 50,* 783–784.

Epstein, N. (1982). Cognitive therapy with couples. *American Journal of Family Therapy, 10,* 5–16.

Epstein, N., & Eidelson, R. J. (1981). Unrealistic beliefs of clinical couples: Their relationship of expectations, goals and satisfaction. *The American Journal of Family Therapy, 9,* 13–22.

Eyberg, S. M., & Robinson, E. A. (1982). Parent–child interaction training: A treatment outcome study. *Journal of Clinical Child Psychology, 11,* 130–137.

Fincham, F. D. (1983). Clinical applications of attribution theory: Problem and prospects. In M. Hewston (Ed.), *Attribution theory: Extensions and applications.* Oxford: Blackwells.

Flavell, J. H., Botkin, P., Fry, C., Wright, J., & Jarvis, P. (1968). *The development of role-taking and communication skills in children.* New York: Wiley.

Floyd, J. F., & Markman, H. J. (in press). Observational biases in spouse observation: Toward a cognitive/behavioral model for marriage. *Journal of Consulting and Clinical Psychology.*

Forehand, R., & McMahon, R. J. (1981). *Helping the noncompliant child: A clinician's guide to parent training.* New York: Guilford Press.

Forehand, R., Wells, K. C., McMahon, R. J., Griest, D., & Rogers, T. (1982). Maternal perception of maladjustment in clinic-referred children: An extension of earlier research. *Journal of Behavioral Assessment, 4,* 145–151.

Gottman, J. M. (1979). *Marital interaction: Experimental investigations.* New York: Academic Press.

Gottman, J. M. (1982a). Emotional responsiveness in marital conversations. *Journal of Communication, 32,* 108–120.

Gottman, J. M. (1982b). Temporal form: Toward a new language for describing relationships. *Journal of Marriage and the Family, 44,* 943–962.

Gottman, J. N., & Porterfield, A. L. (1981). Communicative competence in the nonverbal behavior of married couples. *Journal of Marriage and the Family, 43,* 817–824.

Hahlweg, K., Reisner, L., Kohli, G., Vollmer, M., Schindler, L., & Revenstorf, D. (1984). Development and validity of a new system to analyze interpersonal communication (KPI: Kategoriensystem für partnerschaftliche Interaktion). In K. Hahlweg & N. S. Jacobson (Eds.), *Marital interaction: Analysis and modification.* New York: Guilford Press.

Haley, J. (1963). Marriage therapy. *Archives of General Psychiatry, 8,* 213–234.

Hartman, D. P. (1977). Considerations in the choice of interobserver reliability estimates. *Journal of Applied Behavior Analysis, 10,* 103–116.

Henshel, A. (1971). The relationship between values and behavior: A developmental hypothesis. *Child Development, 42,* 1997–2007.

Hoffman, M. L. (1963). Parent discipline and the child's consideration for others. *Child Development, 34,* 573–588.

Hoffman, M. L., & Saltzstein, H. D. (1967). Parent discipline and the child's moral development. *Journal of Personality and Social Psychology, 5,* 45–47.

Homans, G. C. (1961). *Social behavior: Its elementary forms.* New York: Harcourt, Brace & World.

Jackson, D. D. (1965). Family roles: Marital quid pro quo. *Archives of General Psychiatry, 12,* 589–594.

Jacobson, N. S. (1979). Behavioral treatments for marital discord: A critical appraisal. In M. Hersen, R. M. Eisler, & P. M. Miller (Eds.), *Progress in behavior modification*. New York: Academic Press.

Jacobson, N. S. (1984). The modification of cognitive processes in behavioral marital therapy: Integrating cognitive and behavioral intervention strategies. In K. Hahlweg & N. S. Jacobson (Eds.), *Marital interaction: Analysis and modification*. New York: Guilford Press.

Jacobson, N. S., & Margolin, G. (1979). *Marital therapy: Strategies based on social learning and behavior exchange principles*. New York: Brunner/Mazel.

Jacobson, N. S., & Moore, D. (1981a). Behavior exchange therapy of marriage: Reconnaisance and reconsideration. In J. P. Vincent (Ed.), *Advances in family interaction, assessment, and theory* (Vol. 2). Greenwich: JAI Press.

Jacobson, N. S., & Moore, D. (1981b). Spouses as observers of the events in their relationship. *Journal of Consulting and Clinical Psychology, 49*, 269–277.

Jacobson, N. S., Waldron, H., & Moore, D. (1980). Toward a behavioral profile of marital distress. *Journal of Consulting and Clinical Psychology, 48*, 696–703.

Jacobson, N. S., Follette, W. C., & McDonald, D. W. (1982). Reactivity to positive and negative behavior in distressed and nondistressed married couples. *Journal of Consulting and Clinical Psychology, 50*, 706–714.

Jacobson, N. S., Follette, W. C., & Elwood, R. W. (1984). Research on the effectiveness of behavioral marital therapy: Methodological and conceptual critique. In K. Hahlweg & N. S. Jacobson (Eds.), *Marital interaction: Analysis and modification*. New York: Guilford Press.

Jacobson, N. S., McDonald, D. W., Follette, W. C., & Berley, R. A. (1985). Attributional processes in distressed and nondistressed married couples. *Journal of Consulting and Clinical Psychology, 9*, 35–50.

Kant, E. (1881). *The critique of pure reason* (J. H. Sterling, Ed. and Trans.). Edinburgh: Oliver. (Original work published 1781)

Knudson, R. M., Gurman, A. S., & Kniskern, D. P. (1979). Behavioral marriage therapy: A treatment in transition. In C. M. Franks & G. T. Wilson (Eds.), *Annual review of behavior therapy* (Vol. 7). New York: Brunner/Mazel.

Knutson, J. F. (1982). Perspective on Chapter 7. In G. R. Patterson, *A social learning approach: 3. Coercive family process*. Eugene, OR: Castalia.

Koch, S. (1964). Psychology and emerging conceptions of knowledge as unitary. In T. W. Wann (Ed.), *Behaviorism and phenomenology*. Chicago: University of Chicago Press.

Kohlberg, L. A. (1968). Moral development. *International Encyclopedia of the Social Sciences*. New York: Macmillan.

Kuhn, T. S. (1970). *The structure of scientific revolution* (2nd ed.). Chicago: University of Chicago Press.

Ledwidge, B. (1978). Cognitive behavior modification: A step in the wrong direction. *Psychological Bulletin, 85*, 353–375.

Lepper, M. R., Greene, D., & Nisbett, R. E. (1973). Undermining children's intrinsic interest with extrinsic reward: A test of the overjustification hypothesis. *Journal of Personality and Social Psychology, 28*, 129–137.

Liberman, R. P. (1970). Behavioral approaches to family and couple therapy. *American Journal of Orthopsychiatry, 40*, 106–118.

Locke, J. (1924). *An essay concerning human understanding* (A. S. Pringle-Pattison, Ed.). Oxford: Clarendon Press. (Original work published 1700)

Mahoney, M. J. (1974). *Cognition and behavior modification*. Cambridge, MA: Ballinger.

Margolin, G. (1981). Behavior exchange in happy and unhappy marriages: A family cycle perspective. *Behavior Therapy, 12*, 329–343.

Margolin, G., & Wampold, B. E. (1981). Sequential analysis of conflict and accord in distressed and nondistressed marital partners. *Journal of Consulting and Clinical Psychology, 49*, 554–567.

Margolin, G., Christensen, A., & Weiss, R. L. (1975). Contracts, cognition, and change: A behavioral approach to marriage therapy. *The Counseling Psychologist, 5*, 15–26.

Markman, H. J. (1979). Application of a behavioral model of marriage in predicting relationship satisfaction of couples planning marriage. *Journal of Consulting and Clinical Psychology, 47*, 743–749.

Markman, H. J. (1981). Prediction of marital distress: A 5-year follow-up. *Journal of Consulting and Clinical Psychology, 49*, 760–762.

Meltzoff, A. N., & Moore, M. K. (1983). Newborn infants imitate adult facial gestures. *Child Development, 54,* 702–709.

Mischel, W., & Metzner, R. (1962). Preference for delayed reward as a function of age, intelligence, and length of delay interval. *Journal of Abnormal and Social Psychology, 64,* 425–431.

Noller, P. (1981). Gender and marital adjustment level differences in decoding messages from spouses and strangers. *Journal of Personality and Social Psychology, 41,* 272–278.

Parke, R. D. (1970). The role of punishment in the socialization process. In R. A. Hoppe, G. A. Milton, & E. C. Simmel (Eds.), *Early experiences and the process of socialization.* New York: Academic Press.

Patterson, G. R. (1965). An application of conditioning techniques to the control of a hyperactive child. In L. Ullman and L. Krasner (Eds.), *Research in behavior modification.* New York: Holt, Rinehart & Winston.

Patterson, G. R. (1969). Behavioral techniques based upon social learning: An additional base for developing behavior modification technologies. In C. Franks (Ed.), *Behavior therapy: Appraisal and status.* New York: McGraw-Hill.

Patterson, G. R. (1974). Interventions for boys with conduct problems: Multiple settings, treatments, and criteria. *Journal of Consulting and Clinical Psychology, 42,* 471–481.

Patterson, G. R. (1976). The aggressive child: Victim and architect of a coercive system. In L. A. Hammerlynck, L. C. Handy, & E. J. Mash (Eds.), *Behavior modification and families: Theory and research* (Vol. 1). New York: Brunner/Mazel.

Patterson, G. R. (1982). *A social learning approach: 3. Coercive family process.* Eugene, OR: Castalia.

Patterson, G. R., & Hops, H. (1972). Coercion, a game for two: Intervention techniques for marital conflict. In R. E. Ulrich and P. Mounjoy (Eds.), *The experimental analysis of social behavior.* New York: Appleton.

Patterson, G. R., & Reid, J. B. (1973). Interventions for families of aggressive boys: A replication study. *Behaviour Research and Therapy, 11,* 383–394.

Patterson, G. R., Cobb, J. A., & Ray, R. M. (1972). Direct intervention in the classroom: A set of procedures for the aggressive child. In F. Clark, D. Evans, & L. Hammerlynck (Eds.), *Implementing behavioral programs for schools and clinics.* Champaign, IL: Research Press.

Patterson, G. R., Cobb, J. A., Ray, R. S. (1973). A social engineering technology for retraining the families of aggressive boys. In H. E. Adams & I. P. Unikel (Eds.), *Issues and trends in behavior therapy.* Springfield, IL: Charles C. Thomas.

Patterson, G. R., Reid, J. B., Jones, R. R., & Conger, R. E. (1975). *A social learning approach to family intervention: 1. Families with aggressive children.* Eugene, OR: Castalia.

Piaget, J. (1952). *The origins of intelligence in children* (M. Cook, Trans.). New York: International Universities Press. (Original work published 1936)

Piaget, J. (1954). *The construction of reality in the child* (M. Cook, Trans.). New York: Basic Books. (Original work published 1937)

Pick, A. D., Christy, M. D., & Frankel, G. W. (1972). A developmental study of visual selective attention. *Journal of Experimental Child Psychology, 14,* 165–175.

Price, R. H. (1972). *Abnormal behavior: Perspectives in conflict.* New York: Holt, Rinehart & Winston.

Revenstorf, D., Hahlweg, K., Schindler, L., & Vogel, B. (1984). Interaction analysis of marital conflict. In K. Hahlweg & N. S. Jacobson (Eds.), *Marital interaction: Analysis and modification.* New York: Guilford Press.

Robinson, E. A. (1985). Coercion theory revisited: Toward a new theoretical perspective on the etiology of conduct disorders. *Clinical Psychology Review, 5,* 597–625.

Robinson, E. A. (1987). *Treatment of conduct problems in childhood: A comparative study.* Manuscript submitted for publication.

Robinson, E. A., & Eyberg, S. M. (1984). Behavioral assessment in pediatric settings: Theory, method, and application. In P. Magrab (Ed.), *Psychological and behavioral assessment: Impact on pediatric care.* New York: Plenum Press.

Robinson, E. A., & Price, M. G. (1980). Pleasurable behavior in marital interaction: An observational study. *Journal of Consulting and Clinical Psychology, 48,* 117–118.

Rychlak, J. F. (1981). *Introduction to personality and psychotherapy: A theory-construction approach* (2nd ed.). Boston: Houghton Mifflin.

Sackett, G. P. (1979). The lag sequential analysis of contingency and cyclicity in behavioral interaction research. In J. Osofsky (Ed.), *Handbook of infant development*. New York: Wiley.

Sameroff, A. J. (1975). Early influences on development: Fact or fancy? *Merrill-Palmer Quarterly, 21*, 267–294.

Schaap, C. (1984). A comparison of the interaction of distressed and nondistressed married couples in a laboratory situation: A literature survey, methodological issues, and an empirical investigation. In K. Hahlweg & N. S. Jacobson (Eds.), *Marital interaction: Analysis and modification*. New York: Guilford Press.

Schacter, S. (1964). The interaction of cognitive and physiological determinants of emotional state. In L. Berkowitz (Ed.), *Advances in experimental social psychology* (Vol. 1). New York: Academic Press.

Schindler, L., & Vollmer, M. (1984). Cognitive perspectives in behavioral marital therapy: Some proposals for bridging theory, research, and practice. In K. Hahlweg & N. S. Jacobson (Eds.), *Marital interaction: Analysis and modification*. New York: Guilford Press.

Schultz, T. R., Butkowsky, J., Pearce, J. W., & Shanfield, H. (1975). Development of schemes for the attribution of multiple psychological causes. *Developmental Psychology, 11*, 502–510.

Skinner, B. F. (1953). *Science and human behavior*. New York: Macmillan.

Skinner, B. F. (1957). *Verbal behavior*. New York: Appleton-Century-Crofts.

Snyder, J. J. (1977). A reinforcement analysis of interaction in problem and nonproblem families. *Journal of Abnormal Psychology, 86*, 528–535.

Spielberger, C. D., & De Nike, L. D. (1966). Descriptive behaviorism versus cognitive theory in verbal operant conditioning. *Psychological Review, 73*, 306–326.

Stuart, R. B. (1969). Operant interpersonal treatment for marital discord. *Journal of Consulting and Clinical Psychology, 33*, 675–682.

Stuart, R. B. (1980). *Helping couples change*. New York: Guilford Press.

Sullivan, H. S. (1965). *Collected works*. New York: Basic Books.

Telch, M. J., Bandura, A., Vinciguerra, P., Agras, A., & Stout, A. L. (1982). Social demand for consistency and congruence between self-efficacy and performance. *Behavior Therapy, 13*, 694–701.

Thibaut, J. W., & Kelley, H. H. (1959). *The social psychology of groups*. New York: Wiley.

Thomas, J. R., & Tenant, K. (1978). Effects of rewards on changes in children's motivation for an athletic task. In F. L. Smoll & R. E. Smith (Eds.), *Psychological perspectives in youth sports*. Washington, DC: Hemisphere.

Toch, H. (1969). *Violent men: An inquiry into the psychology of violence*. Chicago: Aldine.

Vincent, J. P. (1980). The empirical-clinical study of families: Social learning as a point of departure. In J. P. Vincent (Ed.), *Advances in family intervention, assessment, and theory*. Greenwich, CN: JAI.

Vincent J. P., Weiss, R. L., and Birchler, G. R. (1975). A behavioral analysis of problem solving in distressed and non-distressed married dyads. *Behavior Therapy, 6*, 475–487.

Vincent, J. P., Freidman, L. L., Nugent, J., & Messerly, L. (1979). Demand characteristics in observations of marital interaction. *Journal of Consulting and Clinical Psychology, 47*, 557–566.

Vincent, J. P., Cook, N. I., & Messerly, L. (1980). A social learning analysis of couples during the second postnatal month. *American Journal of Family Therapy, 8*, 49–68.

Wahler, R. G. (1980). The insular mother: Her problems in parent–child treatment. *Journal of Applied Behavior Therapy, 13*, 207–219.

Wahler, R. G., House, A. E., & Stambaugh, E. E., II. (1976). *Ecological assessment of child problem behavior: A clinical package for home, school, and institutional settings*. New York: Pergamon Press.

Waldron, H., & Routh, D. K. (1981). The effect of the first child on the marital relationship. *Journal of Marriage and the Family, 43*, 785–788.

Weiss, R. L. (1978). The conceptualization of marriage from a behavioral perspective. In T. J. Paolino & B. S. McCrady (Eds.), *Marriage and marital therapy: Psychoanalytic, behavioral, and systems perspectives*. New York: Brunner/Mazel.

Weiss, R. L. (1980). Strategic behavioral marital therapy: Toward a model for assessment and intervention. In J. P. Vincent (Ed.), *Advances in family intervention, assessment and theory* (Vol. 1). Greenwich, CN: JAI Press.

Weiss, R. L. (1984). Cognitive and behavioral measures of marital interaction. In K. Hahlweg & N. S. Jacobson (Eds.), *Marital interaction: Analysis and modification*. New York: Guilford Press.

Weiss, R. L., Hops, H., & Patterson, G. R. (1973). A framework for conceptualizing marital conflict, technology for altering it, some data for evaluating it. In L. A. Hamerlynck, L. C. Handy, & E. J. Mash (Eds.), *Behavior change: Methodology, concepts, and practice*. Champaign, IL: Research Press.

White, G. D., Nielsen, G., & Johnson, S. M. (1972). Time-out duration and the suppression of deviant behavior in children. *Journal of Applied Behavior analysis, 5,* 111–120.

Wills, T. A., Weiss, R. L., & Patterson, G. R. (1974). A behavioral analysis of the determinants of marital satisfaction. *Journal of Consulting and Clinical Psychology, 42,* 802–811.

Wolpe, J. (1958). *Psychotherapy by reciprocal inhibition*. Stanford, CA: Stanford University Press.

CHAPTER 5

Developmental Perspectives on Family Theory and Psychopathology

BARCLAY MARTIN

A developmental perspective on family theory and psychopathology is not uniquely different from other views. Systems, social learning, and the cognitive-intrapsychic models all have developmental features. The difference between this chapter and others in this section is one of emphasis. Here, our attention will be on change over time. In traditional developmental psychology, the individual has been the unit of study, even when studied in groups; and textbooks in this area tend to follow individual development from infancy to adulthood (or old age, in life-span development) with respect to motor, cognitive, social, and personality functioning. The family has also been taken as the unit of developmental study and has been followed in its course from marriage to old age. In this chapter, we will adopt the latter perspective and focus primarily on the interactional dynamics of the family as they unfold over time and as they relate to psychopathological behavior.

The concept of the family as the unit of developmental study is not especially new but has until recently been advocated more by sociologists (e.g., Aldous, 1978; Duvall, 1971; Rodgers, 1964) than by developmental psychologists. These writers describe family stages (or careers) and the various developmental tasks associated with different parts of the family life cycle. A typical listing of family stages was given by Aldous (1978): (a) newly established couple; (b) childbearing; (c) families with schoolchildren; (d) families with secondary-school children (adolescents); (e) families with young adults; (f) families in the middle years; and (g) aging families. Of course, these stages are somewhat arbi-

---

BARCLAY MARTIN • Department of Psychology, University of North Carolina, Chapel Hill, NC 27514.

trary, with no sharp boundaries, and if there is more than one child, the stages overlap. Nevertheless, in broad outline, there is clearly a changing sequence of circumstances in the life cycle of a family that involves different tasks and challenges.

The term *developmental tasks* has been used to refer both to the individual's development (e.g., the tasks of motor and language development, resolving dependence–independence issues, and achieving sex-role identity) and to family development. From the family perspective, there are a number of "tasks" to be dealt with, many of which are associated with transition periods in the family life cycle. Thus, there are transitions involving the birth of children, having children leave home and eventually becoming once again a two-person family, becoming grandparents, and retirement and old age. The tasks associated with these transitions may create strains in the family system that can result in symptomatic behavior. Issues of togetherness and separation (dependence and independence) are especially important at several transitions. The birth of the first infant can threaten one or both spouses' dependence on the other; entry into school can precipitate a crisis in an already-developed overprotective-parent and over-dependent-child system, and the struggle of adolescents and their parents to accomplish the emotional separation necessary for adult functioning has potential for the development of psychological disorders.

To understand fully the process of development, it is necessary to integrate family systems concepts into the developmental perspective. As we will see, much of the relevant research, even when interactional in focus, usually attends to only one family dyad at a time—most commonly, the mother and child. What has also been neglected until quite recently are the paths of influence among these dyads. The nature of the relationship in each of these subsystems can both affect and be affected by the nature of the relationship in each of the other subsystems so that triadic and higher order systems can come into play. How a mother interacts with her child can be influenced by her interactions with her husband, just as interaction with her husband can be influenced by the nature of her interaction with her child. The same is true for the father. And how the child interacts with one parent can be affected by the interaction with the other parent. When there is more than one child, the complexity of the system increases at a rapid rate and includes, of course, sibling interactions. A child's interaction with other family members is influenced by the number and sex of the other siblings, the ordinal position of the child in the sibling hierarchy, and the age spacing between the siblings. An eldest boy with younger sisters may well develop differently from a youngest boy with older brothers.

Any consideration of family interactional factors related to the development of psychopathology must take into account both multiple variables and their interactions. As an organizational aid to thinking, it may be useful to classify these sources of influence in the following manner:

1. *Characteristics of the individual.* These are present before interaction within the family system begins. For the newborn infant, these would include genetic dispositions toward certain types of temperament, levels of intelligence, or cen-

tral nervous system dysfunctions. For the spouses, these would include all characteristics (personality, attitudinal, intellectual, or whatever) present before their relationship began.

2. *Interactive effects.* As soon as two or more individuals begin to interact, their behavioral dispositions begin to be affected, sometimes to a minor or trivial extent, sometimes to a profound degree. To use a commonplace example, the newborn infant with a "difficult" temperament may evoke in a given parent (because of the parent's preexisting personality or attitudinal characteristics) a response of irritation that may further instigate "difficult" responses in the infant, which, in turn, produce even greater annoyance and disappointment in the parent, and so on. The interactive process proceeds to a disturbed parent–child relationship, perhaps even child abuse, that is different from the point where either participant started.

However, interactional results do not explain everything. There still remain characteristics in both parent and infant that were present before this relationship started, and these can influence future interactions. Some characteristics are readily modifiable by social interactional influences, but others are less malleable. For example, the phenotypic expressions of intellectual abilities or of schizophrenia, but not the underlying genotypes, may be influenced by interactional dynamics. Certain aspects of a Down syndrome child's behavior may be affected by interactional experiences, but the basic deficit in intellectual capacity cannot. Or from the parents' perspective, an attitude of like or dislike for an infant may, in many cases, be changed markedly, in either a positive or a negative direction, by the course of interaction. In other cases, the parental disposition to like or dislike the infant is so strong that this attitude is relatively unaffected by the subsequent interactional history.

3. *Extrafamilial influences.* Individuals, groups, or institutions outside the family can affect family relationships. A family's religious affiliation, economic status, and events beyond its control (for example, economic recessions, racial and other oppressions, and natural disasters) are examples of these external influences. Extrafamilial interactions may be a source of stress or may be supportive and may serve as a buffer against stressful circumstances.

I will conclude this introductory sketch of a developmental perspective with a brief summary of one of the few long-term longitudinal studies of the development of psychopathology, a study that included many of the measures that the above outline would suggest are important. Werner and Smith (1977, 1982) followed from birth to age 18 all of the 698 youth on the island of Kauai, Hawaii, born in 1955. At age 10, 25 of the children were considered in need of long-term mental-health services. A large majority of these children were showing acting-out problems: fighting, destructiveness, truancy, stealing, and so on. A smaller number had chronic nervous habits or anxiety–withdrawal symptoms. As a group, these children tended to come from families rated low or very low in socioeconomic status (SES): 88% compared to 56% for the total population. SES was found to have strong associations with psychological disorders throughout this study; accordingly, a control group matched with the deviant group on SES, sex of child, and ethnicity was selected. Compared to the control group, a higher proportion of children in the deviant group has been low-birth-weight babies, had suffered from moderate to severe perinatal complications, had been rated by their mothers as being "not cuddly, not affectionate" at age 1, and had mothers rated by interviewers as less relaxed, affectionate, energetic, happy, and intelligent when the babies were age 1. At age 2, a higher proportion of future deviant children came from homes rated low in stability, as indicated by such characteristics as illegitimacy of child, absence of father, marital discord, alcoholism, emotional disturbance of parents, and long-term separation of the child from the mother without an adequate substitute caretaker.

These findings suggest that a higher proportion of the deviant 10-year-olds were born with constitutional tendencies to be "difficult" infants. The results also strongly suggest that the mothers, and probably also the fathers, brought characteristics to the relationship with the child that were not entirely reactive to having a "difficult" child; and even with SES controlled, stressful life circumstances were more often present that would be likely to make adequate parenting difficult. Another analysis showed that perinatal complications and/or low birth weight predicted later psychological disorders only within the low SES group and not in the middle-class group. Characteristics associated with the middle-class family environments would seem to have ameliorated the constitutional vulnerabilities.

Not all infants who experienced risk factors of the above types before age 2 developed later mental-health problems. The authors identified a group of *resilient* children, as they were called, who also lived in chronic poverty and had experienced at least four risk factors before age 2, but who had not developed subsequent adjustment problems by either age 10 or age 18. There were no differences between these resilient children and a group of children who had developed serious mental-health problems by age 18 in the percentages who had experienced perinatal stresses, had low birth weights, and had conditions requiring further hospital care after the mother was discharged. The resilient children, however, were more often firstborn, especially the males, had fewer congenital defects, were more often perceived by their caretakers as active and socially responsive infants, elicited and received more attention during their first year of life, less often experienced prolonged separations from their mothers during the first year, less often experienced serious or repeated illnesses in the first 2 years, and had families that had experienced fewer life stresses during the child's first 2 years. This matching does not allow us to separate constitutional characteristics from factors in the social environment. However, the results do suggest that perinatal complications and low birth weight occurring in a context of chronic poverty do not inevitably lead to later mental-health problems. The factors that remain after this matching continue to suggest the importance of infant temperament (and in a small number of cases, congenital defects) and an attentive, available caretaker during the first two years of life. In addition, resilient children continued to be rated as experiencing more emotionally supportive family relationships between ages 2 and 10. The authors speculated that the positive effect for males of being firstborn may have been due to the greater amount of individual attention that these infants could be given in these poor and usually large families.

This study clearly points to the importance of considering multiple variables in any attempt to understand and predict the development of psychopathology. The results might have been even more interesting if the authors had used multiple-regression techniques to reveal which variables made contributions independently of other variables. And of course, quite understandably, the authors did not obtain the repeated measures of family interactional and other variables that would permit us to follow the details of psychopathological development.

In summary, a developmental perspective on family theory and psychopathology stresses the multiple, mutual influence processes that occur over time that eventuate in the individual or interactional behaviors that we label symptoms. This is easy to say but extremely difficult to translate into research that does justice to the concept. No one study can include all the variables, obtain all the repeated longitudinal measures, and perform all the manipulations necessary to provide the complete understanding of even one form of psychopathology. We must for the most part, be satisfied with a piecemeal approach to the larger picture. In the remainder of the chapter, I will selectively survey research findings that illustrate, although incompletely, the direction in which such a developmental perspective is taking us.

THE HUSBAND–WIFE SYSTEM

The first family developmental task is the establishment of the husband–wife relationship. Mate selection has consequences for the remainder of the family life cycle. When mates are chosen because they offer an escape from an unhappy family of origin, because of an unplanned pregnancy, or because of any number of hidden emotional agendas, the marriage is fraught with potential for future strain, and there is ample indication that the presence of marital conflict is associated with psychological disturbance in the children (e.g., Emery, 1982).

Marital instability, as measured by separation or divorce, in one generation is associated with an increased likelihood of marital instability in the next generation, although the relationship is not a strong one (Bumpass & Sweet, 1972; Kulka & Weingarten, 1979; Mueller & Pope, 1977). With socioeconomic level, rural-urban status, and religious affiliation controlled, Mueller and Pope (1977) found that wives whose parents had divorced were, on the average, younger, less educated, and more often pregnant at the time of marriage and had married younger, lower-status males. The authors speculated that the divorced parent (usually the mother) of those women was less able to provide the supervision and control that might have prevented some of these events from happening, for example, marrying at a young age or being pregnant at the time of marriage. This "supervision" hypothesis received some support from the fact that there was no discrepancy in the divorce rates between women from divorced and nondivorced parents when the analysis was limited to daughters who had no siblings. Presumably, a single mother could concentrate whatever supervisory time she had on the only daughter.

Youthful marriages seem to be especially vulnerable to strains and eventual dissolution. In a longitudinal study of women born in the 1920s, Elder and Rockwell (1976) found that women who married early, compared to women who married later, tended to marry husbands with low incomes, had to work outside the home to supplement the family income, had more children, and had them earlier. Four times as many of the early-married women were subsequently divorced.

In the past, there has been a controversy about whether spouse similarity or spouse complementarity on various personality traits is more highly related to marital satisfaction. The weight of current evidence supports the similarity hypothesis (e.g., Barton & Cattell, 1972; Bentler & Newcomb, 1978; Cattell & Nesselroade, 1967; De Young & Fleischer, 1976), although the variance in marital satisfaction accounted for by degree of similarity is small.

Little is known about interactional styles before or early in marriage that predict later marital distress. Markman (1979, 1981) has made a beginning on answering this important question. In a laboratory setting, he had couples who were planning to marry rate the positive or negative impact that their partners' expressions had on them. Couples who were relatively dissatisfied with their marriage 2½ and 5 years later had experienced their partners' expressions as less positive and more negative in the premarital session. These ratings did not predict marital satisfaction after only 1 year of marriage. The results suggest that the interactional patterns contributing to marital dissatisfaction were present before marriage and before the couples considered themselves dissatisfied in the marriage.

We might expect that certain personality characteristics in spouses would be predictive of marital distress. Bentler and Newcomb (1978) found relatively few relationships—and these of a low magnitude—between traits measured in newlyweds and whether the couples were divorced four 4 years later. Perhaps the most promising research on this issue has focused on the personality traits of masculinity and femininity (MF). Although older studies using the bipolar MF scale of the Minnesota Multiphasic Personality Inventory (MMPI) have yielded conflicting results (Newmark & Toomey, 1972; Osborne, 1971; Swan, 1957), more recent research using separate masculinity and femininity scales has produced more consistent findings.

Interestingly enough, and somewhat counterintuitively, two cross-sectional studies have found that couples tend to report less marital satisfaction when the marriage is characterized by traditional sex roles, that is, a masculine man and a feminine wife. Shaver, Pullis, and Olds (1980) obtained questionnaire responses from 2,100 women and found that women in traditional sex-role marriages reported less marital satisfaction and more often feeling fat, sad, depressed, and shy relative to women in marriages in which one or both partners were androgynous or there was a reversal of sex roles, that is, a feminine man and a masculine woman. Antill (1983) interviewed both spouses, also found marital satisfaction to be low for traditional sex roles, and, on the basis of the overall results, concluded that marital happiness is directly related to the femininity of one's partner (male or female). In another cross-sectional study, Burger and Jacobson (1979) did not analyze their data in terms of traditional sex-role pairings but did find that both males' and females' femininity scores were positvely correlated with their respective self-reported marital satisfaction. They also found that femininity correlated positively with a number of behavioral ratings of constructive communication skills.

Baucom and Aiken (1984) pursued this topic further with larger samples of both clinic and nonclinic couples. They predicted that both masculinity and femininity would correlate positively with marital satisfaction in both males and females, with masculinity being associated with active, goal-oriented problem-solving ability and femininity with sensitive, caring, and emotionally supportive behavior. Both characteristics, in other words, should contribute to an effective and satisfying marriage. The results generally supported this expectation. For both sexes, femininity and masculinity were significantly correlated with self-reported marital satisfaction, with femininity showing the higher correlation. In the clinic sample, both husbands and wives showed significant increases in masculinity but not femininity after treatment. This result had also been predicted on the basis that the particular form of behavioral marriage therapy used by these authors had emphasized the learning of active, problem-solving skills. In general, these results suggest that some degree of androgyny in both spouses is associated with marital satisfaction, and indeed, these authors did find a higher proportion of androgynous males and females in the nonclinic sample.

The finding in these studies that the relationship-oriented traits of emotional expressivity, nurturance, and sensitivity (that is, femininity) was an important correlate of marital happiness in *both* partners is important. These aspects of femininity may be what were reflected in ratings of constructive communication skills found by Burger and Jacobson (1979) and in the greater positive and less negative impacts found to be predictive of marital satisfaction by Markman (1979, 1981). If these qualities are indeed important to marital satisfaction, then this may be at least a partial explanation for the lower satisfaction in traditional sex-role marriages. A highly feminine woman, by this definition, is not having her expressive and relationship needs met by a highly masculine man, and her dissatisfaction will eventually affect the husband's marital happiness (Ickes, 1986). One might question how useful the terms *masculinity* and *femininity* are in this context, based as they are on traditional stereotypes of male and female behavior. It might be less confusing simply to study personality correlates of successful marriages, such as interpersonal sensitivity and communication skills, without labeling these traits as masculine or feminine.

Clinicians (e.g., Bowen, 1978; Satir, 1964) have proposed that individuals tend to select mates whose general level of mental health is about the same as their own. Empirical research is not entirely clear on this point. There is evidence that indicates that, when one spouse has a psychological disorder, the other spouse has an increased likelihood of also having some kind of psychological disorder. (See Merikangas, 1982, for a review of this research.) This above-chance concordance could result because prospective mates with equal vulnerabilities to psychopathology select each other, as Bowen and Satir have suggested (the assortative mating hypothesis), or it could result from the interactive dynamics of the marriage, in which, for example, a neurotic spouse may promote the development of a neurotic disorder in the other spouse. Some researchers in the United States and England have found an increasing concordance of psychological disorders (usually neurotic or personality disorders) as a function of the duration of the marriage (Hagnell & Kreitman, 1974; Hare & Shaw, 1965; Kreitman, 1964; Kreitman, Collins, Nelson, & Troop, 1970; Ovenstone, 1973), a finding implying that marital interaction is the source of the concordance. Other investigators have not found an increase in similarity as a function of marriage duration (Agulnik, 1970; Slater & Woodside, 1951), a finding more consistent with assortative mating. Perhaps both factors contribute to the obtained concordances.

Most of the research on this topic is cross-sectional, the samples having been simply grouped according to how long the couples had been married. Hagnell and Kreitman (1974), however, performed an impressive longitudinal study in which the entire population of a semirural area in southern Sweden was interviewed twice, with a 10-year interval between interviews. For the 269 couples married at both Time 1 (1947) and Time 2 (1957), the proportion of couples concordant for psychiatrically diagnosed disorders increased over this time period, and consistent with a trend found by Kreitman (1964), wives were more likely to show an increase in psychological symptoms if their husbands had been mentally disturbed at Time 1 than were husbands if their wives had been mentally disturbed at Time 1. Wives, in other words, were more adversely affected by having a disturbed husband than vice versa.

On the basis of his cross-sectional English data, Krietman (1964) suggested that, in traditional marriages, wives are generally more dependent on their husbands for external social outlets than are husbands on wives, and thus, a wife with a symptomatic husband may have more difficulty in finding satisfying relationships outside marriage than would be true for the husband of a symptomatic wife. The kind of marital relationships typical of semirural Sweden and England in past decades may not be representative of contemporary marital relationships in those countries or in the United States, and accordingly, we should be a bit tentative about concluding that wives are more vulnerable to husbands' psychopathology than vice versa until this finding is supported by more current data.

From a family-life-cycle perspective, the developing marital relationship is of central importance to family health or psychopathology. The presentation to this point has been purposely oversimplified by omitting the impact of children on the marital relationship, an omission that will be remedied in the following sections.

FAMILIES WITH INFANTS

What the Infant Brings to the Relationship

Infants are born with differences in temperament and in sensorimotor as well as cognitive competencies, and of course, some genetically influenced characteristics will not appear until months or years later as a result of maturational processes. The course of interactions with family members can be significantly affected by these biologically based differences. (See Bell and Harper, 1977, for a review of the effects of infant and child characteristics on adults.)

Through parent interviews, Thomas, Chess, and Birch (1968) identified several components of temperament in infants. Characteristics associated with infants they called "difficult" were biological irregularity, especially with respect to sleep, feeding, and elimination cycles; withdrawal and distress to new stimuli such as the first bath or new foods; slow adaptability to change; and generally negative mood states involving a readiness to fuss and cry with high intensity. Other investigators using direct observation have also identified individual differences in temperament, for example, frequency and duration of crying (Beckwith, 1978; Loundsbury & Bates, 1982); ease of soothing when crying (Birns, Blank, & Bridger, 1966; Korner, 1971); state of alertness or wakefulness (Korner & Grobstein, 1967; Osofsky, 1976); responsiveness to stimulation (Birns, 1965; Osofsky, 1976); and cuddliness (Schaffer & Emerson, 1964). However, when longer time periods are considered, the consistency of traits of temperament found in the first month or so of life decreases and in some cases disappears altogether (Bell & Ainsworth, 1972; Thomas *et al.*, 1968).

Buss and Plomin (1975) postulated four main dimensions of temperament: emotionality, activity, sociability, and impulsivity. On the basis of their twin research with young children (average age of 55 months) and an extensive review of other studies, they concluded that a good case could be made for stability over time and for a genetic contribution to individual differences in emotionally, activity, and sociability, but not for impulsivity.

Premature infants often have characteristics such as an aversive high-pitched cry (Zeskind & Lester, 1978) and lessened responsivity (DiVitto & Goldberg, 1979), and their mothers frequently respond either with excessive attempts to stimulate and keep the infants' attention (interrupting and not attending to the infants' signals) or with passivity and nonresponsiveness (Field, 1983). The former is more characteristic of middle-class mothers and the latter of lower-class mothers (Field, 1980; Tulkin & Kagan, 1972). When infants experience either of these maternal styles, they are likely to show gaze aversion and fussiness (Field, 1983).

Evidence is not consistent on the extent to which these difficulties in interaction between mothers and their premature infants continue as the children grow older. Crawford (1982) and Goldberg, Brachfeld, and DiVitto (1980) found that, by 12 to 14 months of age, mother–child interaction for prematures was no

longer different from that for nonprematures on most measures. Crnic, Ragozin, Greenberg, Robinson, and Basham (1983), however, found that the lower
responsiveness and more negative affective tone of both the prematures and
their mothers continued to be present at 12 months of age. Field (1979) and
Field, Dempsey, and Shuman (1981) found that mothers who were more active
and less sensitive to their preterm infants' gaze signals at 4 months gave more
imperatives and were overprotective or controlling during interaction at 2 years.
Their infants showed more behavioral problems, such as hyperactivity, short
attention span, and language production delays, at 2 and 3 years of age. Bakeman and Brown (1980) reported that prematures showed a cognitive deficit
(Stanford Binet IQ) at 3 years but no deficit in social interaction.

In conclusion, individual differences in infants, whether resulting from
genetic differences or prenatal and perinatal difficulties (such as prematurity),
may be associated with some increased risk of disturbed early parent–child
interaction, which may or may not be long-lasting. For some parents and children, however, these difficulties do not go away; instead, they escalate to more
troublesome behavioral problems at a later age (Thomas *et al.*, 1968; Werner &
Smith, 1977), and it is in these children and their families that we have a special
interest.

What the Parent Brings to the Relationship

Although later difficulties may develop in some children primarily because
they begin life with extreme deviations of one kind or another, it is likely that
different parental response to children with the same degree of temperamental
or other deviance accounts for the fact that some of these children show disturbed interaction and others do not.

A study that can serve as a good illustration of the importance of considering both parent and infant variables as well as external life circumstances in
analyzing the development of disordered parent–child relationships is that of
Egeland, Brietenbucher, and Rosenberg (1980). These authors obtained measures on a sample of 267 primiparous women from low socioeconomic back-
grounds (most were on welfare) before birth and during the first year of the
child's life. Thirty-two of the mothers were rated as either abusing or severely
neglecting their infants. A stepwise discriminant-function analysis showed that a
Brazelton nonoptimal score (obtained within the first few days after birth and
reflecting orientation to stimuli, irritability, consolability, and other factors that
may reflect infant temperament); maternal insensitivity to the infant's cues;
maternal personality characteristics of aggressiveness, defensiveness, and sus-
piciousness (obtained before birth); and high life stress—all made independent
contributions to predicting infant abuse or neglect.

Other researchers have assessed maternal characteristics before birth and
found correlations between these measures and maternal and infant characteristics after birth (Heinicke, Diskin, Ramsey-Klee, & Given, 1983; Moss, 1967;
Robson, Pederson, & Moss, 1969; Shereshefsky & Yarrow, 1973). Moss (1967),

for example, found that mothers' acceptance of the nurturing role and their general positive evaluation of babies, measured 2 years before birth, predicted actual responsiveness to their infants at age 3 months. Heinicke *et al.* (1983) found that mothers' responsiveness to infants' needs at 1, 3, 6, and 12 months was predicted by a cluster of maternal variables obtained before birth: an interview-based rating of adaptation and competence, as well as MMPI scales of Ego Strength and Basic Trust.

Some parents are experiencing psychopathological disorders of their own that interfere with adequate care of their child in infancy or childhood. Observational studies have not found striking differences between the parenting behaviors of mothers with and without a history of schizophrenia (Sameroff, Barocas, & Seifer, 1980; Schachter, Elmer, Ragins, Wimberly, & Lachin, 1977), although some trends were found for schizophrenic mothers to be less spontaneous and less expressive. However, several studies suggest that separation from a schizophrenic mother during childhood is related to reduced symptomatology in these high-risk children in adolescence or young adulthood (Rieder & Nichols, 1979; Sobel, 1961; Walker, Cudeck, Mednick, & Schulsinger, 1981), a finding that implies that the mother–child interaction contributes to at least part of the symptom pattern.

Although Sameroff, Seifer, and Zax (1982) found few differences between the parenting behavior of schizophrenic mothers and that of normal mothers, they found striking differences in mothers who were neurotically depressed or who were rated high on chronicity or severity of disorder, regardless of diagnosis. The authors concluded that the long-term emotional nonavailability of the depressed mother is especially detrimental to normal child development. More specifically, they found that children of depressed mothers had the worst obstetric status at birth, were less responsive to people 4 months later, and showed a variety of less adaptive behaviors in the home at 30 months postpartum. At 4 months, the depressed mothers were less spontaneous, happy, vocal, and proximal to their child during home observations. At 30 months, low socioeconomic class was as good a predictor of child impairment as severity of maternal disorder; however, at 48 months, severity of mental illness was the better predictor (Seifer, Sameroff, & Jones, 1981). Grunebaum, Cohler, Kauffman, and Gallant (1978) also found greater impairment in cognitive functioning in 6- to 12-year-old children of depressed mothers than in children of schizophrenic or normal mothers.

Weissman, Prusoff, Gammon, Merikangas, Leckman, and Kidd (1984) compared 107 children of mothers with major depressions (unipolar) with 87 children of normal mothers. Symptoms of disorder were three times as likely to occur in children with depressed mothers, with depression being the most common symptom; 13.1% of the children of depressed mothers were depressed, compared with none of the children of normal mothers. Attention deficit, separation anxiety, and conduct disorders, in that order, were the next most common disorders in children of depressed mothers. Baldwin, Cole, and Baldwin (1982) studied 7- and 10-year-old children who had one parent with a history of psychiatric disorder. They found that high lability of affect in mothers who were patients (some of these mothers had bipolar affective disorders) was *positively* correlated with school competence; whereas mother-patients with high scores on withdrawal, depression, and incongruous affect had children who scored poorly on measures of school competence.

Gaensbauer, Harmon, Cytryn, and McKnew (1984) followed the early development from birth of seven male infants who had a parent (four mothers and three fathers) with a bipolar affective disorder. Compared to seven matched controls, the infants with an affectively disordered parent showed no difference in security of attachment to the mother at 12 months, but by 18 months, they had developed a significantly higher proportion of insecure attachments, mostly of the avoidant type. (These attachment types will be described more fully in a later section.) Reporting on the same families, Davenport, Zahn-Waxler, Adland, and Mayfield (1984) found that the mothers of the children with an affectively disordered parent were less active and more disorganized and tense than control mothers in directly observed interaction. Genetic factors, of course, may also contribute to symptomatology in children of depressed parents, but the results of these studies strongly imply that maternal nonresponsiveness also influences the developing disorder.

Several experimental studies have documented the adverse effects of even a brief period of maternal nonresponsiveness on normal infants (Carpenter, Tecce, Stechler, & Friedman, 1979; Cohn & Tronick, 1983; Tronick, Als, Adamson, Wise, & Brazelton, 1978). Cohn and Tronick (1983), for example, found that normal infants reacted to 3 minutes of maternal "depression" (face relatively expressionless and speaking in flat, uninteresting monotone) with repetitive episodes of protest, wariness, and looking away. The negative reactions of the infants continued for some time after the mothers switched from depressed to normal interaction. If such a brief period of maternal "depression" can produce such a marked change in infant response, it is easy to imagine that the effect of a chronically depressed mother may be severe and long-lasting.

The general point to be made here is that, before the birth of the child, the parents already have behavioral dispositions, in some instances to a psychopathological degree, that can affect their subsequent interactions with the infant.

Father–Mother–Infant: The Interactional Dynamics

The birth of an infant affects the marital relationship. The quality of the marriage affects how the parents respond to the infant. How the parents respond to the infant can modify infant characteristics, which, in turn, can affect the marital relationship. How can we tease out cause and effect in all of this? Short of experimental manipulations, we probably cannot. Correlational research does suggest, however, that all of these sources of influence may exist to varying degrees in a given family system.

Marital Satisfaction and Mother–Infant Interaction. Pregnancy and the birth of the first child is a major transition in the family life cycle. There is some evidence that a couple's satisfaction with their marital relationship decreases somewhat after the birth of their firstborn and decreases even further after the birth of their secondborn (Belsky, Spanier, & Rovine, 1983; Feldman, 1971; Ryder, 1973; Waldron & Routh, 1981). If the spouses are especially dependent on each other for companionship or the gratification of emotional needs, the arrival of children may interfere with this aspect of marital interaction and may accentuate marital dissatisfaction. Feldman (1971) and Luckey and Bain (1970) have reported findings of this kind. However, these average trends toward marital dissatisfaction as a function of the birth of children probably have little implication for the development of psychopathology. More likely, it is the combined or interactive effect of this trend with other circumstances that can produce potentially pathological effects.

The husband's reaction to the wife during the birth–infancy period is such a factor. Thus, mothers who experienced emotional support from their husbands were more likely to have had a positive postpartum adjustment (Shereshefsky & Yarrow, 1973; Wandersman, Wandersman, & Kahn, 1980). Pedersen and his colleagues (Pedersen, 1975; Pedersen, Anderson, & Cain, 1977) reported that maternal feeding competence was negatively correlated with tension and conflict between husband and wife (as reported by fathers), and that the husband's esteem for his wife as a mother was positively related to her skill in feeding. Pedersen, Anderson, and Cain (1979) also found that, the more husbands criticized their wives, the more negatively oriented these mothers were toward their 5-month-old infants. Crnic et al. (1983) found that mothers who reported satisfying intimate relationships with their husbands (or their unmarried partners, in some cases) were rated as more sensitive to infant cues and as showing more positive affect during observed interaction with their 4-month-old infants. The infants of these mothers with satisfying intimate relationships were rated as being more responsive and as showing more positive effect.

These associations are correlational and may be mediated by various causative paths. Crnic et al. (1983) performed a regression analysis and found that the path from satisfying intimacy with the husband to the infant's behavior seemed to go indirectly through the mother's positive affect. When maternal affect ratings were partialed out, intimacy with the husband no longer correlated with infant behavior. There are several causative possibilities involving maternal affect. Husbands may have facilitated the wives' positive affect, or women who have characteristically positive affect before marriage may be more likely to marry emotionally supportive husbands and may also interact more sensitively and positively with infants than do mothers who have characteristically negative affect before marriage. It would take longitudinal research to begin to unravel some of these causative possibilities.

The Attachment Process. Infants of many species show attachment to a specific adult, usually the mother, manifested by tendencies to seek physical contact or proximity, to maintain visual or auditory contact, and to show distress at forced separation. The human infant develops an attachment to its mother sometime between 5 and 14 months of age, with a wide range of individual differences in age of onset (Ainsworth, Blehar, Waters, & Wall, 1978). Ainsworth and her associates have developed a standardized procedure for measuring attachment that relies heavily on the behavior of infants when they are reunited with their mothers after a period of forced separation. Infants' attachment behaviors are classified as *secure, insecure-avoidant,* or *insecure-ambivalent* on the basis, respectively, of proximity-seeking, avoidant, or angry resistant responses to reunion. Classifications of infants of middle-class parents into these categories have been found to be quite stable between 12 and 18 months of age by Connell (as reported in Ainsworth *et al.,* 1978) and Waters (1978), but to be only moderately stable by Thompson, Lamb, and Estes (1982). For infants of mothers living at poverty levels, Vaughn, Egeland, and Sroufe (1979) found much less stability in attachment categories from 12 to 18 months, and changes from secure to insecure attachment were associated with increases in life stress for the mothers.

Research on attachment represents a notable attempt to incorporate the developmental perspective. Because much of this research is longitudinal and also because of its relevance to the development of psychopathology, we will consider this topic in some detail. The style of interaction between mothers and their infants during the first few months of life has been found to be related to these attachment categories assessed at 1 year of age. Thus, mothers of securely attached infants were more responsive to their infants' cries, held their babies more tenderly and carefully, paced the interaction more contingently during face-to-face interaction, and exhibited greater sensitivity in initiating and terminating feeding (Ainsworth *et al.,* 1978).

According to Ainsworth and her colleagues, securely attached infants can use the mother as a secure base from which to explore and manipulate the environment and can thus develop confidence in their competencies. The insecurely (or anxiously) attached infants would seem to be at some risk for future adjustment difficulties. Several studies support this possibility. Matas, Arend, and Sroufe (1978) found that, at 24 months, toddlers assessed as being securely attached at 18 months were more enthusiastic, persistent, and cooperative and showed more positive and less negative affect and less frustration behavior in a free-play situation with their mothers and a problem-solving task with their mothers. These advantages of the securely attached could not be explained in terms of general intelligence; at least, variation on the Bayley Mental Developmental Index was relatively independent of the measures of interactional competence. Following up the same children, Arend, Gove, and Sroufe (1979) reported that the children categorized as securely attached at 1 year of age were more ego-resilient at age 5, as measured both by teacher Q-sort ratings and by a battery of objective behavioral measures. *Ego resiliency* is a term used by the Blocks (e.g., Block & Block, 1979) and is defined as the ability to respond flexibly, persistently, and resourcefully in problem situations. Ego brittleness, or lack of ego resiliency, is characterized by inflexibility and a tendency to become disorganized in the face of novelty or stress. Using different samples, Waters, Wippman, and Sroufe (1979) and Sroufe (1983) reported similar relationships between early secure attachment and interactional competence with peers and teachers at ages 3½ and 4 years, respectively. The early relationship with the mother that has been called *secure attachment* would seem to have important consequences for the later social adjustment of the child.

A systems view would naturally make us curious about attachment to the father. In two studies, the same infants' attachment to both parents was assessed. Lamb (1978) found a small but significant degree of consistency—and Main and Weston (1981) found no consistency—between the three categories of attachment to mother and father. This different tendency to attach to the father and the mother suggests that attachment amounts to more than individual differences in infant characteristics and is, to a substantial extent, an interactional outcome between the infant and each parent. Main and Weston (1981) also found that the positive correlates of secure attachment, as measured by social competence in another situation, were enhanced if the infant was securely attached to both parents, or conversely, that the negative correlates of insecure attachment to one parent were reduced if the infant was securely attached to the other parent.

We have already suggested that both infant and maternal characteristics present at the infant's birth contribute toward the quality of mother–infant interaction in the early months, and by extrapolation, one might expect these same variables to play a role in the later development of attachment. Indeed, there is evidence that infants who are temperamentally difficult in the first few months have a higher likelihood of being classified as insecure-ambivalent in their attachment at 1 year (Ainsworth *et al.*, 1978; Waters, Vaughn, & Egeland, 1980). There was no relationship between early temperament and the insecure-avoidant category. In considering these results along with the relative lack of consistency of attachment behavior to the mother and to the father, we must conclude that, although infant temperament contributes something to the attachment process, much of the variance must be explained in terms of the interactional histories of each parent–child dyad.

Crockenberg (1981) brought together several variables in one study. Measures of infant irritability in the first 10 days, maternal responsiveness in mother–infant interaction at 3 months, and social support assessed by interview at 3 months were all related to infant attachment at 1 year. Social support, which included support from the father as well as from relatives and other people, served as an important moderator variable. High infant irritability in the first 10 days was associated with insecure attachment only within the low-social-support group. It is possible that mothers who had irritable infants but who also had strong social supports may have been able to interact with their infants in ways that prevented the development of insecure attachment. Just how social support mediates this beneficial effect or how lack of social support mediates the more disturbed outcome remains to be studied, although common sense would suggest that a mother who is enjoying supportive relationships would find it easier to be relaxed and attentive to her infant and not so easily frustrated by a "difficult" infant. Recall that Crnic *et al.* (1981) found that social support from a partner was associated with more positive mother–infant interaction at 4 months.

Although security of attachment has been found to have some stability between 12 and 18 months (especially for stable, middle-class families) and to have some predictive correlates to later peer interactions and problem-solving behavior, we should be wary of thinking of security of attachment as a trait in the same sense as we often think of intelligence. First, attachment is defined in the

context of a specific dyadic relationship and can be different in other relationships, and second, attachment is markedly affected by changes in the larger
social systems in which it is embedded. It is still not altogether clear how stable
the Ainsworth categories of attachment are. It is only prudent to remain a bit
cautious about the generality and long-term consequences of a characteristic
assessed on the basis of 5 minutes or so of observed interaction. As in most
behavioral dispositions, there are probably individual differences in the extent to
which infants are consistent from week to week on this characteristic. The likelihood of subsequent maladjustment is probably greatest for infants who consistently show insecure attachment, and as Sroufe (1983) pointed out, the relation of 12-month attachment styles to adjustment 3 to 4 years later is not highly
specific. There are too many opportunities for interactional changes in the life of
the young child.

FAMILIES WITH YOUNG CHILDREN

Developmental Levels of Competence

Infants and children go through developmental processes that affect and
are affected by the family's interactional dynamics. Motor, perceptual, cognitive,
and linguistic competencies change enormously as infants become toddlers and
toddlers become young children and young children become adolescents. The
relationships of family interactional processes to the development of psychopathology cannot be studied without taking into account these changing levels of
competence.

The following example will illustrate this point. Inconsistency in the verbal
and nonverbal channels of communication has been suggested as an important
correlate of family psychopathology since the double-bind theory was first proposed by Bateson, Jackson, Haley, and Weakland (1956). There has been little
support for the double-bind theory of schizophrenia (Olson, 1972), and there
has been mixed evidence for the proposition that incongruities in the verbal and
nonverbal communications of parents are associated with other forms of disturbed child behavior (Jacob & Lessin, 1982). Jacob and Lessin (1982) suggested
that one reason for these inconsistent results may be that investigators have not
taken into account the developmental levels of children with respect to their
ability to comprehend incongruencies. Several studies indicate that the verbal
content of a message is more influential on young children than is tone of voice
or visual cues, but as children get older or become adults, the tonal and visual
aspects of the message become equally or more important. Bugental, Kaswan,
Love, and Fox (1970), for example, compared contradictory messages given in
the visual, verbal-content, and tone-of-voice channels and found that the visual
channel was less influential at lower ages (5–8 years) than verbal or tonal channels and more influential at older ages (13–18 years). Bugental, Kaswan, and
Love (1970) found that conflicting messages in which the speaker smiled while
making a critical statement were interpreted more negatively by children than by
adults.

Any research on the relation of incongruency of communications to behavioral disturbances in children would have to take the level of cognitive development of the children into account, with the expectation being that incongruent messages would be most disturbing when the child is old enough to comprehend the discrepancy. Of course, factors such as the intensity of the nonverbal component may moderate the effects of developmental level; that is, if the nonverbal aspect of the message were intense enough, even a young child might "get the message."

The perception of incongruity is only one example of a changing developmental ability. Changes in cognitive functioning of the kinds that Piaget (Piaget & Inhelder, 1969) described and the changes in physical maturation associated with adolescence are other examples of developmental changes that have implications for the study of family interaction correlates of psychopathology.

The Interactional Dynamics of Warmth–Hostility and Control

The domains of warmth–hostility and control, especially as manifested in parents, were given special prominence in the older researchers (for a review, see Martin, 1975). Because these domains continue to be important in understanding parent–child interaction, we will make some use of them, but, as far as possible, in an interactional context. *Warmth–hostility* (sometimes called *acceptance–rejection*) refers generally to behaviors involving a strong affective component of either like or dislike. These would include tendencies to express appreciation rather than criticism and blame, to seek out and enjoy the company of the other, and to be sensitive to the signals and needs of the other. *Control* (sometimes called *restrictiveness–permissiveness*, or *dominance–submission*) refers to the domain of behavior related to how individuals attempt to influence or exert power over others. In the older research, the measures of warmth–hostility and control tended to be uncorrelated, so that it was possible to conceptualize a two-dimensional space in which a person might show any particular combination of these variables; for example, high controlling behavior could be associated with high warmth or low warmth (Schaefer, 1959).

If we look at these variables interactionally, we find a strong tendency toward reciprocity for measures of warmth; that is, when one member of a dyad is responding with a high rate of friendly behaviors, so, often, is the other member, and likewise for unfriendly, aversive behaviors. This interactional reciprocity holds for children interacting with peers, siblings, or parents, and for spouses with each other (Baumrind, 1967; Hauser, Powers, Noam, Jacobson, Weiss, & Follarsbee, 1984; Jacobson & Martin, 1976; Kogan, Wimberger, & Bobbitt, 1969; Patterson, 1982). In the attachment literature, the combination of sensitive mother and securely attached infant versus insensitive mother and insecurely attached infant would seem to represent the same reciprocity of friendly or unfriendly behaviors. Patterson (1982) suggested one explanation of how this reciprocity develops. He proposed that, in addition to occasional positive reinforcements, negative reinforcements play an especially important role in training family members to exchange aversive behaviors such as yelling and hitting. Participants are reinforced for escalating the intensity of their attacks by the occasional giving-in of the target person; that is, the target person ceases his or her aversive behavior, and this reduction in aversive stimulation negatively reinforces the first person. The reinforcements need only be occasional for the partial reinforcement effect to work, so it is feasible that both members over time are shaped by the negative reinforcement contingencies, until one sees a dyad or a family with high rates of reciprocal aversiveness.

The initial dispositions of the child or the parents should perhaps be added to this formulation. When both mother and child bring to their interactional career negative dispositions, a "difficult" temperament on the part of the child and a nonaccepting attitude or possibly depression on the part of the mother, a pattern of reciprocal negative interchanges is more likely to develop. Other combinations would be likely to lead to intermediate degrees of reciprocal warmth or unfriendliness. An especially cheerful infant or young child may shape a moderately nonaccepting parent toward greater warmth–acceptance, or a nonaccepting parent may influence a moderately cheerful infant toward a more irritable style of response. Or an especially difficult infant may shape a moderately accepting parent toward hostile nonacceptance. Forces outside the dyad, such as the marital relationship or the social support network, could also influence the benign or pathological direction that the interaction takes.

With respect to the concept of control, in any interaction there is some mutual influence, and therefore each person is, in a sense, exerting some control over the other. Issues of control, however, become more salient when one person is trying to get the other one to do something that the other is not particularly inclined to do, as is frequently the case in the socialization process. Depending on the type of controlling attempts used, difficulties in interaction or symptomatic behavior may develop.

Let us consider research by Baumrind (1967, 1971) that illustrates some developmental correlates of both the warmth and control domains. On the basis of observer ratings, Baumrind (1967) selected three groups of children from a larger group of 3- to 4-year-old nursery-school children. Group I was composed of children rated higher than either of the other two groups on each of the following: self-reliance, approach to novel or stressful situations with interest and curiosity, confidence, self-control in situations requiring some appropriate restraint, high energy level, achievement orientation, cheerful mood, and friendly peer relations—clearly a psychologically healthy set of youngsters. Group II children, when compared to Group III children, were more passively hostile, guileful, unhappy in mood, and vulnerable to stress, but they did more careful work. Group III children were more purely impulsive and lacking in self-discipline but also more cheerful; they also recovered from expressions of annoyance more quickly than did Group II children.

Parents of Group I children (friendly, self-radiant), relative to parents in both other groups, were found to exert more general control over the child's behavior and did not succumb to the child's "nuisance value"; they made more demands for mature, age-appropriate behavior; engaged in more open communication with the child, in which reasons were given; more often solicited the child's expression; and used more open rather than disguised means of influence. They were also more nurturant, as indicated by a greater use of positive reinforcement and less use of punishment. Parents of Group III children (impulsive, immature), relative to parents of Group II children (unhappy, withdrawn), generally exerted less control and were less persistent in enforcing demands in the face of the child's opposition. Baumrind (1967) stressed the importance of firm, consistent parental control in a context of nurturance and sensitivity to the child's needs and opinions as a correlate of the psychologically healthy children.

Stayton, Hogan, and Ainsworth (1971), however, argued that parental tactics of control are not so important and suggested that human infants are genetically disposed to acquire self-restraints and to comply with adult demands if provided an ordinary, predictable social environment, and that no specialized training procedures are required. Their finding that young children's internalized controls were correlated with maternal sensitivity to the child's needs but not to frequency of verbal commands or physical interventions was taken as support for this view. Lewis (1981) likewise suggested that Baumrind (1967) had gone too far in emphasizing firm control and that such a view went counter to a body of experimental research on attribution theory. In that research, strong external controls seem to produce a reduction in internalization of standards, whereas the least degree of external control sufficient to elicit compliance is associated with the greatest internalization. Attribution theory, in other words, would suggest that the least degree of parental external control needed to obtain compliance would be associated with more self-controlled and responsible children than would more strict disciplinary practices.

Lewis (1981) reevaluated Baumrind's results (1967) and concluded that the measures of parental control in that study could as well have reflected an absence of parent–child conflict or the child's willingness to obey as much as the parents' willingness to exercise control. Baumrind (1983) conceded that extreme degrees of parental control, especially when not accompanied by those characteristics subsumed under warmth, may well be associated with noncompliance in children, particularly in adolescence. Perhaps Baumrind overstated to some extent the importance of firm control, but Lewis (1981) and Stayton et al. (1971) may have gone too far in the opposite direction in playing down the importance of parental control. Empirical data cannot clearly resolve the issue at this time, although two studies should be mentioned that would seem to suggest that maternal sensitivity is at least as important as maternal control as a correlate of child compliance. Lytton (1977, 1980) found that harmonious mother–child relationships were likely to exist when 30-month-old boys complied with maternal requests *and* the mothers complied with their boys' requests.

Schaffer and Crook (1980) studied children's compliance and maternal control techniques at even earlier ages (15 and 24 months) and found that the mothers' success in obtaining compliance with requests was greatly facilitated by the mothers' sensitivity to the child's attentional state at the time of the request.

> A request for action coming out of the blue has little chance of succeeding; such a request must be part of a sequential strategy, the first step of which is to ensure that the child is appropriately oriented. . . . Thus even the imposition of controls by an adult on

a child represents a dyadic process, in the sense that both the behavior of the adult and the outcome are a function of the child's initial state. By successfully manipulating this state, the parent can avoid the clash-of-wills that is so often portrayed as typical of all socialization efforts, whereby compliance is supposedly extracted from an invariably reluctant child. (p. 60)

What would seem to be left out of this controversy, although not entirely by Lewis (1981), are individual differences in the infant or child. As most parents of more than one child know, some children are easier to socialize than others. The principle derived from attribution theory has a key qualification; namely, internalization is maximum when the *minimum* control necessary to produce compliance is used. Some infants probably require higher minimums to gain compliance in the first place. Does that mean that these infants will develop less internalization of parental requests? Possibly. The harmonious mother–child interaction described in these studies is reminiscent of the kind of early infancy interaction that predicts secure attachment at 12 months of age, which was also found by Crockenberg (1981) to be affected by infant temperament. One might speculate, for example, that Baumrind's Group I children would have shown secure attachments to one or both parents at 1 year of age and possibly had easygoing temperaments in the first months of life.

An ongoing longitudinal study conducted at Berkeley by the Blocks has some relevance to the dynamics of warmth–hostility and control (Block & Block, 1979). Let us consider only that aspect of their study that focuses on the variable of ego control, defined at the overcontrolling end of the dimension as involving excessive inhibition of impulses, feelings, or desires, and at the undercontrolling end of the dimension as involving excessive impulsivity and inability to delay gratification. They related parental child-rearing attitudes measured when the children were 3 years of age to measures of ego control obtained when the children were 11. Their findings indicated that more extreme attempts at parental control, when accompanied by low parental acceptance, are associated with the later development of overcontrolling children, an important qualification of Baumrind's possible overemphasis on control.[1]

The Blocks' results may have some relation to the attachment literature. Arend *et al.* (1979) found that children categorized as insecure-ambivalent in their maternal attachment as infants were rated as more undercontrolling at ages 4 to 5, and children who had been categorized as insecure-avoidant were rated as more overcontrolling. This finding should be replicated before we make too much of it, but it does suggest that characteristic styles of ego control have their roots in early parent–infant interactions. Furthermore, this research may have implications for the development of that class of symptoms called *internalizing* (overcontrol) and those called *externalizing* (undercontrol). Perhaps an insecure-avoidant attachment is a common precursor of the later development of the system involving an overly dependent child and an overly protective mother that

---

[1]Dr. Jack Block kindly sent me the results for the 11-year testing that are referred to here and that had not been published at the time of the writing of this chapter.

has been shown to be associated with separation anxiety (e.g., Waldron, Shrier, Stone, & Tobin, 1975). Only longitudinal research will tell.

An especially interesting subgroup of mothers studied by Sroufe, Jacobvitz, Mangelsdorf, DeAngelo, and Ward (1985) are those who are seductive and do not maintain clear intergenerational boundaries with their male children. A key characteristic in these mothers' seductive behavior is that it seems determined by the mothers' needs rather than being solicited by the children. These authors found these mothers to be consistent in this kind of behavior from 24 to 42 months, and when these young boys had sisters, the mothers showed derisive hostility toward them. A significantly higher percentage of these mothers (42%) reported a history of being sexually abused in their families than did control mothers (8%). Although disturbed sexuality in the boys was noted only anecdotally in this report, the authors have made a significant beginning in studying the developing family dynamics for disturbed sexual behavior.

In summary, the processes involved in warmth and control are most profitably viewed in interactive terms. Harmonious interactions between parent and child are more likely to result when parental control efforts are sensitive to and moderated by the infant's or child's state, in other words, when accompanied by many of the qualities summarized as warmth. When parental control efforts are severe and insensitive to the child's state, or at the other extreme, when few or no efforts are made at control, there is again a mutual control process, but one that may be associated with over- or undercontrolling tendencies in the child. Characteristics that both parent and child initially bring to their relationship influence the future course of the interaction.

The Sibling Configuration

The presence of more than one child further complicates the interactional dynamics of the family, and the basic question for our present purpose is whether vulnerability to psychological disorder is increased for certain positions in the sibling configuration. With family size and socioeconomic level controlled, research has not shown strong tendencies for adult psychopathology to be related to sibling position (Wagner, Schubert, & Schubert, 1979). With respect to children, however, there is some suggestive evidence that firstborns, especially males, and perhaps middleborns are more vulnerable to psychological difficulties than are siblings in other positions.

Firstborns. Four studies of children indicate that, with family size controlled, firstborn males are more likely to have psychological problems than are later-born males (Fishbein, 1981; Lahey, Hammer, Crumrine, & Forehand, 1980; Tuckman & Regan, 1966). In their two studies, Lahey *et al.* did not find that firstborn girls were more likely to have adjustment difficulties. One other study that included boys and girls, not analyzed separately by sex, also found firstborns to have more problems (Shrader & Leventhal, 1968). In the second study of Lahey *et al.* (1980), firstborn boys showed more symptoms of both an acting-out, aggressive form and the more internalizing, anxiety type.

There are two discordant findings in the literature. Recall that Werner and

Smith (1982) found more firstborn males among their resilient children. Families in this subsample lived in chronic poverty, and it is possible that being firstborn under these conditions assures at least some degree of parental attention, which might have outweighed any detrimental factors associated with being firstborn. The other discrepant finding was reported by Belmont (1977). She had access to information on 400,000 19-year-old Dutch men who had undergone military examinations. Fewer firstborns (excluding only children) relative to lastborns received psychiatric diagnoses, regardless of family size. Firstborns were also found to score higher on measures of intelligence and to fail less often in school. Belmont (1977) did find that only children were diagnosed as having psychiatric disorders more often than were either first- or lastborns. As this study involved the whole population of Dutch males born between 1944 and 1947, we cannot set the results aside as a sampling quirk. Perhaps the major difference between this study and the four American studies is that psychopathology was assessed in adults (19-year-olds) rather than children, but whether and how that difference accounts for the difference in the findings is not clear.

Some factors associated with being firstborn may facilitate psychological strength and competence. The most obvious factor is that the undivided attention given to firstborns in the first year or two of life may stimulate the development of cognitive competence (Zajonc & Markus, 1975). A number of studies have shown that mothers respond differently to firstborns both in infancy and in early childhood. Cohen and Beckwith (1976, 1977) and Jacobs and Moss (1976) reported that mothers of firstborn premature infants were more responsive than mothers of later-borns, and at 3 months of age, the firstborns showed more attention-seeking behavior (Jacobs & Moss, 1976).

However, the undivided attention may be a mixed blessing, and there is research that suggests that firstborns are at risk of becoming overly attached to their mothers, with accompanying fearfulness and separation anxieties. Lasko (1954) observed mothers and their children repeatedly over a period of years so that it was possible to compare the *same* mothers' treatment of first- and later-borns when the children were the *same* age. She found that mothers attempted to accelerate the verbal and intellectual development of their firstborn children during the first two years more than they did with their later-borns. However, by the age of 3 or 4, with other siblings around the home, the firstborns were treated less warmly, and disciplinary friction developed between mother and child. Even so, the mothers continued to press for accelerated development. The general trend of these findings has been supported by Cushna (1966) with 16- to 19-month-olds, Hilton (1967) with 4-year-olds, and Rothbart (1971) with 5-year-olds. Cushna (1966) also found firstborns to be more disturbed by their mothers' leaving home.

That the birth of the secondborn is a stressful experience for many firstborns is well documented (Dunn & Kendrick, 1982; Nadelman & Begun, 1982). Dunn and Kendrick (1982) reported some especially suggestive findings that indicate that the temperament and sex of the firstborn and the mother's relationship with the firstborn before and after the second child's birth are related to the later friendliness between the siblings. For example, when there had been a relatively high frequency of joint play and attention between mother and first-born daughter before and immediately after the birth of the second child, the firstborn girl was much *less* likely to behave in a friendly way to her sibling 14 months later. These mothers also gave a high frequency of attention to their secondborns, and one interpretation of the finding is that the firstborns reacted with hostility on having to share this attention.

The age spacing between firstborns and secondborns may be an important factor. Lasko (1954) reported that both first- and secondborns were more distressed by the birth of a younger sibling for intermediate age spacings (2–3 years) than for either shorter or longer spacings. For male adolescent firstborns (excluding only children), Kidwell (1981) also found a curvilinear relationship between the spacing of the next younger sibling and perceived parental support. Parents were perceived as least supportive if the next younger sibling was 2 to 4 years different in age and most supportive if the next younger sibling was either 1 year or 5 years different in age. Kidwell suggested that the 2- to 4-year spacing accentuates the feeling of having to share the parents' time and other resources. For a 1-year spacing, the child essentially has always had to share parental attention and does not know the difference; for the 5-year spacing, he or she has had a long period of unshared attention.

These findings with samples of normal children are at least suggestive of how firstborns may develop a greater vulnerability to symptomatic behavior. One consistent theme is a relatively intense emotional involvement between mother and child. We might speculate that such an involvement would be associated with greater emotional dependency in the firstborns and also with greater interpersonal friction between parent and child as each attempts to resolve conflicting tendencies toward overinvolvement, on the one hand, and separation and autonomy, on the other hand. The birth of siblings 2 to 4 years younger could accentuate these conflictual tendencies. Why firstborn males might become symptomatic more than firstborn females is not clear from the current evidence. There is some indication that mothers put greater demands on firstborn males than on firstborn females (Cushna, 1966). Another possibility is that males may lag, relative to females, in the maturation of certain cognitive abilities, and this lag could accentuate interactional difficulties if parents do put greater achievement pressures on firstborn males.

Middleborns. Although some studies have found lower self-esteem in middleborns than in either first- or later-borns, overall the results are inconsistent. (See Nystul, 1974, and Schooler, 1972, for reviews.) Kidwell (1982), however, showed that, with family size controlled, the age spacing of the siblings is an important moderator variable. In her study of a national sample of 2,200 adolescent males, middleborn subjects reported lower self-esteem than either first-borns or later-borns, an effect that was greatly accentuated when the average age spacing to the nearest older and younger siblings was 2 years. At smaller or larger average age differences, the middleborns were only slightly lower in self-esteem. Achieving status, affection, and recognition from parents may be more difficult for middleborns, especially with age spacings of the order of 2 years. Relatively speaking, less distinction would probably be made between siblings when the age difference was of the order of 1 year, and thus, there would be no relative deprivation of attention for the middleborns; and at fairly large age spacings, it may be easier for parents to provide equal amounts of attention to all children. Further analyzing this same sample, Kidwell (1981) also found that male adolescents, all sibling positions combined, perceived their parents as more punitive the fewer the number of years between the subject and his closest sibling. In addition, with all sibling positions combined, males perceived greater parental punitiveness when the closest sibling was a female, with the perceived punitiveness being a curvilinear function of nearness in age, a spacing of 2 to 3 years showing the most perceived punitiveness.

It should be kept in mind that the overwhelming majority of children in any one position in the sibling configuration do not develop psychological disorders. Multiple factors contribute to the development of psychopathology, and research to date suggests that sibling position accounts for a very small proportion of the variance. Nevertheless, Kidwell's research indicates that, when factors such as sibling spacing and sex of sibling are combined with position in the birth order, we are more likely to find some correlations with psychological disorders. Even here, we find some contradiction between research done primarily with preadolescents, which suggests that firstborns and only children were more vulnerable to difficulties, and the research on adolescents, which indicates that middleborns may be more at risk, at least in terms of self-esteem. Without taking into account the constitutional and family interaction dynamics, it is likely that position in the sibling configuration, even with age spacing and sex of siblings included, will remain a weak correlate of psychopathology.

FAMILIES WITH ADOLESCENTS

The major task of adolescence is the gradual achievement of psychological independence. Hoffman (1985a) developed a questionnaire measure of several components of psychological separation from parents. Two of these are most relevant to this discussion: emotional dependence, defined as excessive need for approval, closeness, and emotional support from the parent; and conflictual dependence, defined as excessive guilt, anxiety, mistrust, resentment, and anger in relation to the parent. In a correlational study with college students, Hoffman (1985a) found that greater conflictual dependence on father and on mother (measured separately) was related to poorer personal adjustment, especially with regard to love relationships. Greater emotional dependence was found to be related to a greater frequency of academic problems.

There is some evidence that suggests that psychological separation is more likely to be difficult when marital conflict between the parents is high. Both Offer and Offer (1975) and Westley and Epstein (1970) reported that adolescents who came from homes where parents had a healthy relationship had a relatively smooth separation process, generally devoid of turbulence, and developed strong positive identities. This association between marital characteristics and the separation process may result if a parent who is dissatisfied in the marriage becomes overly involved with a child, or if marital distress results from more general maladjustment in one or both parents and this maladjustment leads to disturbed parent–child relations.

In a subsequent study, Hoffman (1985b) found that perceived interparent conflict, mother symptoms, and father symptoms (all reported by the college-aged children) were related to both mother and father conflictual dependency in both sexes. Partial regression analyses, however, indicated that, for female subjects, only mother symptoms significantly related to conflictual dependency on the mother with the other two parent variables partialed out, whereas both interparent conflict and father symptoms were independently associated with conflictual dependency on the father. For male subjects, with the other two parent variables partialed out, mother symptoms were related to conflictual dependence on the mother, and the father symptoms were related to conflictual dependence on the father. Interparent conflict made no independent contribution. These findings require further exploration with independent assessment of parental attributes.

Issues of control loom large in the separation process in adolescence, and Steinberg (1981), in a longitudinal design, showed that conflictual interaction between male adolescents and their parents is more closely associated with changes in physical maturity than with chronological age or formal reasoning abilities. It was found in direct observation of these middle-class families that, as the male adolescent matured physically from the beginning of puberty to the pubertal apex, there was increasing conflict, indicated by mutual interruptions between adolescents and their mothers, and adolescents deferred to their mothers less often. Following the pubertal apex, conflict with the mothers decreased. A different pattern was seen for the adolescent–father interaction. Father assertiveness and adolescent deference increased throughout the period under study.

Similar findings were reported by Jacob (1974), who compared directly observed measures of conflict and dominance in 11- and 16-year-old sons and their parents for middle- and lower-class samples. For both classes of families with preadolescent sons, there was relative equality between parents, both of whom were more dominant than their son. For both classes of families, the adolescent sons were more dominant at the expense of the mother. The relative dominance of middle-class fathers remained the same regardless of the child's age. The relative dominance of lower-class fathers was less with their adolescent than with their preadolescent sons. These social class differences should alert us to the importance of controlling for social class in family interactional research as well as to more substantive questions about the meaning of these differences in middle- and lower-class family dynamics.

The increasing overt conflict that males have with their mothers during adolescence is documented in both of these studies, but the longitudinal study of Steinberg (1981), with its reliance on physical characteristics as a marker of developmental stage rather than on chronological age, suggests that conflict with the mother, after reaching a peak, decreases as adolescence proceeds, although there is no return to the preadolescent levels of deference to the mother.

The relevance of these findings to the development of psychopathology is indirect. As is true of most normal developmental processes, it is only when other factors, of the kinds we have previously considered, are present that this transition in the individual and family life cycle has potential for pathological development. Two factors likely to be of special importance are the quality of the marital relationship and the past history of how control issues have been handled between parent and child. Neither of these variables was included in these studies.

In a cross-sectional analysis, Hauser, Powers, Noam, Jacobson, Weiss, and Follansbee (1984) showed that adolescent ego-development, as measured by Loevinger's sentence-completion test, was correlated with directly observed family-interaction measures. The interaction measures were grouped into those that were thought to *enable* other individuals to be more autonomous and differentiated (enabling ego development) and those thought to *constrain* autonomy and differentiation. Enabling involved cognitive (focusing, problem solving, curiosity, and explaining) and affective (acceptance and empathy) factors. Constraining also involved cognitive (distracting, withholding, and indifferent) and affective (excessive gratifying, judging, and devaluing) aspects. Adolescents at the lower stages of ego development, relative to those at highter levels, showed more constraining and less enabling behavior toward their parents, and their parents showed less enabling and more constraining behavior toward them. This correlation of positive with positive and negative with negative is, of course, one more instance of the reciprocity found in many studies. What is needed are longitudinal studies and the measure of additional situational and organismic variables that will help us to understand how the "constraining" interactions develop. Hauser *et al.* (1984) did provide us with potentially meaningful categories of directly observed interaction, and they planned to follow some of these families longitudinally—a promising start.

THE MARITAL RELATIONSHIP AND CHILD SYMPTOMS

The importance of the marital relationship has been emphasized throughout the foregoing sections. In this section, we will look at additional research on marital interaction correlates of disturbed behavior across a wide age range of children.

Marital Conflict

Chess, Thomas, Korn, Mittelman, and Cohen (1983) reported that a rating of marital conflict obtained for the parents in their New York Longitudinal Study when the children were 3 years old correlated significantly with a rating of poor adult adaptation obtained when the children were 18 to 22 years old. The prediction held for both male and female children. In cross-sectional research with both clinical and nonclinical samples, marital conflict is most commonly associated with conduct disorders in boys (Block, Block, & Morrison, 1981;

Chawla & Gupt, 1979; Emery & O'Leary, 1982; Oltmanns, Broderick, & O'Leary, 1977; Porter & O'Leary, 1980; Rutter, 1971; Whitehead, 1979). (See Emery, 1982, for a review.) Rutter (1971), for example, studied a sample of London families in which one or both parents had been under psychiatric care. When marriages were rated as "good," none of the boys showed antisocial behavior, compared with 22% when the marriage was "fair" and 39% when the marriage was "very poor." The quality of the marriage would seem to have outweighed the effect of having one parent who had experienced a psychiatric disorder. In addition, Rutter found that the association between marital conflict and the son's antisocial behavior was strongly affected by whether the son had a good relationship with one or both parents. When the marital relationship was "very poor" and the son had a good relationship with one or both parents, 38% were antisocial; when the son had a poor relationship with both parents and the marital relationship was "very poor," almost 90% were antisocial. Research has also shown that the relationship between marital conflict and antisocial behavior in sons is stronger when the conflict is overt than when it is more covert or the marriage is characterized by apathy (Porter & O'Leary, 1980; Rutter, Yule, Quinton, Rowlands, Yule, & Berger, 1974).

One can advance a number of explanations for the obtained association between severity of marital conflict and conduct disorders in boys. Parents who engage in overt conflict with each other may also be the kind of people who engage in more harsh and punitive disciplinary practices with their children, a well-established correlate of antisocial behavior in children (Martin, 1975), and these parents provide clear models of aggressive behavior. If parents who engage in more dramatic displays of overt conflict tend also to be generally more impulsive and erratic in their behavior, they may well be more inconsistent in their disciplinary tactics than parents who show less overt conflict. Inconsistency of discipline has also been found to characterize parents of antisocial children (Martin, 1975).

Perhaps causality works the other way. An aggressive, acting-out child may produce tensions between the parents. One bit of data, however, does not support this direction of cause and effect. Oltmanns, Broderick, and O'Leary (1977) found that marital satisfaction did not increase after problem behavior in children had been successfully decreased by a therapeutic intervention. Another possibility, suggested largely by family therapists (e.g., Minuchin & Fishman, 1981), is that children may develop behavior problems in order to draw attention to themselves and to distract the parents from their conflicts. Of course, if this action were successful, we should not find a strong association between child problems and overt marital conflict. Yet another possibility proposed by family therapists is that a parent who is dissatisfied with the marriage may substitute a child for the spouse, and the resulting overinvolvement may engender behavior problems. The few empirical data available argue against this idea. Gilbert, Christensen, and Margolin (1984) did find weak interparent alliances in the distressed families, as therapists have noted, but they also found weak alliances and quite negative interactions between the mothers and the target children, the dyad that is usually expected to reflect a relationship that substitutes for the marriage. Christensen and Margolin (1981) also found a positive correlation between maternal ratings of relationship satisfaction with the spouse and relationship satisfaction with the target child in distressed families: the correlation should be negative according to the "substitute relationship" theory. Although some of these clinically derived dynamics may be true in specific instances, they do not seem to be so common as to emerge in these rather small studies.

The relationship of marital conflict, by itself, to anxiety–withdrawal disorders has not been so clearly demonstrated. There are two studies of nonclinical samples (Block, Block, & Morrison, 1981; Whitehead, 1979) in which marital conflict was found to be related to aggressive, acting-out behavior in boys and, to a lesser degree, to more anxious, withdrawn behavior in girls. However, studies of clinical samples have not found either conduct disorders or anxiety–withdrawal disorders to be associated with marital conflict in girls (Emery & O'Leary, 1982; Gassner & Murray, 1969).

Interaction of Marital Conflict and Parent Dominance

There is evidence that, when marital conflict is accompanied by opposite-sex parent dominance, children of both sexes are at risk for developing the more internalizing types of disorders (Gassner & Murray, 1969; Hetherington, Stouwie, & Ridberg, 1971; Klein, Plutchik, & Conte, 1973; Schwarz & Getter, 1980). Let us consider some theoretical background for this "triple-interaction hypothesis," as Schwarz and Getter (1980) referred to it, which involves marital conflict, parent dominance, and sex of child.

Under normal circumstances, in our culture, children show a relative tendency to model their behavior on, and thereby to identify with, the same-sex parent. This tendency can be complicated and can perhaps be thwarted in certain circumstances. Thus, in addition to imitating the same-sex parent, there is a tendency to imitate the more dominant parent, especially when the dominant parent is rated high on warmth (Hetherington, 1965; Hetherington & Frankie, 1967). Mixed-identification tendencies may result from having a warm, opposite-sex parent who is dominant, but these tendencies do not necessarily increase the risk of psychopathology. However, children may also identify with a dominant parent even when this parent is hostile and lacking in warmth, providing that the nondominant parent is also low in warmth and parental conflict is high. This situation was found by Hetherington and Frankie (1967), who interpreted their results as supporting the psychodynamically derived concept of identification with the aggressor. Does an identification with the aggressor increase the risk of psychopathology regardless of whether the parent is of the same or the opposite sex? The answer has not yet been determined by empirical research. However, when the dominant parent is of the opposite sex and there is high marital conflict, the child may be placed in an especially difficult position with respect to modeling and imitative tendencies. Thus, a son whose dominant father is in overt conflict with a weak, passive-aggressive wife can follow the expected tendency to identify with his father, both because the father is the same-sex parent and because he is dominant. By contrast, a daughter in the same situation may tend to identify with her mother because she is of the same sex, but the daughter may also have a conflicting tendency to identify with the father because of his dominance and power. Overt marital conflict is an important feature in this line of reasoning. The father's disparagement of the mother and possibly his disparagement of the daughter, if she behaves like the mother, may make it hard for the daughter to identify with the mother. Conflict may then develop within the daughter over whether to be like the mother or like the father. This conflict, as well as the partial identification with a weak, disparaged mother, may then be accompanied by anxiety, low self-esteem, depression, and other neurotic symptoms.

The previously listed studies provide support for this line of thinking. For example, Gassner and Murray (1969) found neurotic children of both sexes seen at a child guidance clinic to come more often than did normal children from families in which marital conflict was high and the opposite-sex parent was dominant (both assessed by the revealed-differences technique). Schwarz and Getter (1980) used self-report questionnaires to measure all variables on college subjects and found the predicted triple-interaction effect, with neuroticism as the dependent variable. Hoffman (1985b), however, failed to find this triple interaction in a study of college subjects. Klein, Plutchik, and Conte (1973) studied families coming for family therapy and found that sons had more behavior problems (of all kinds) when their mother was dominant and their father was passive; the opposite held for the girls. Marital conflict was not measured in this study.

Finally, research by Hetherington et al. (1971) further suggests the importance of parent dominance and marital conflict, at least for boys. In this study, adolescent delinquents were segregated into three types: neurotic delinquents, who showed signs of conflict, anxiety, or guilt about their antisocial behavior; socialized-aggressive delinquents; and conduct-disordered delinquents (or unsocialized delinquents). A pattern of maternal dominance and marital conflict, as measured by the revealed-differences technique, was high for the neurotic male delinquents, and paternal dominance with relatively low marital conflict was characteristic of the socialized-aggressive delinquents. Neurotic female delinquents were also associated with high maternal dominance but with low marital conflict. This latter finding should warn us that the pattern of high marital conflict and opposite-sex parental dominance is not associated with all forms of child deviance. We should also be a bit cautious in assuming that these variables are always validly measured by the relatively brief interaction obtained in the revealed (or unrevealed, in some cases) differences technique. Jacob (1974) has shown that some of the specific measures used in the conflict and dominance indices obtained by this technique are related to social class. Nevertheless, it may reasonably be concluded at this time that marital conflict and opposite-sex parental dominance form a pattern of some significance for anxiety–withdrawal symptoms in children.

Except for the work of Chess et al. (1983), all researches in these last two sections on marital conflict and parent dominance are cross-sectional. From a developmental perspective, we will need to learn how these aspects of family structure and associated symptoms in children emerge over time.

THE OVERALL FAMILY LIFE CYCLE

It is a popular veiw that transitions from one stage in the family life cycle to another create strains and represent high-risk occasions for the development of psychological disorders. We have already seen that there is some evidence of a decrease in marital satisfaction associated with the birth of children (e.g., Feldman, 1971). Let us consider some other transition points further along in the life cycle.

Tensions occur in many contemporary families when the wife is freed of the responsibilities of taking care of infants and preschool-aged children, begins to feel dissatisfied in the role of housewife, and decides to embark on a career of her own—a decision that may involve going back to school, taking a full-time job, or other endeavors that require a major renegotiation of family duties. The final physical and psychological separation of children from the family can be an especially trying time for some families. Those who take a family systems view of schizophrenia tend to attribute great importance to the inability of the "identified patient" to make a successful transition from a highly conflicted dependence on the family to adult independence, and they suggest that this is why the onset of schizophrenia so often comes in late adolescence or young adulthood (Haley, 1973). Other transitions are also thought to be important as precipitators of family disturbance. When the last child leaves, couples are faced only with each other, and they may discover that the children have served as a distraction from some basic marital dissatisfactions. Taking care of elderly parents, adapting to the role of grandparent, and adjusting to retirement are other transition points that must be faced by most couples.

That these transition periods are high-risk occasions for family dysfunctioning is an intuitively appealing idea. Research on samples of normal families, however, has provided only weak support for this proposition. By far the largest body of research has dealt with marital satisfaction as a function of transitions in the family life cycle, and there is fairly consistent evidence of a weak curvilinear relationship over time; that is, marital dissatisfaction decreases with the advent and presence of children and increases after the last child has left home. (See Rollins & Galligan, 1978, for a review.) Anderson, Russell, and Schumm (1983) reported further evidence supporting this curvilinear trend, and consistent with this trend, other investigators have found that families with children report less marital satisfaction than those without children (Glenn & McLanahan, 1982; Spanier & Lewis, 1980). The presence of children may adversely affect the marital relationship in various ways, for example, by interfering with marital companionship, by lessening the spontaneity of sexual relations, and by provoking jealousy and competitiveness in the parents. On the other hand, some couples with a poor marital relationship may stay together "for the sake of the children," in which case the presence of children would not necessarily contribute to the marital distress.

In contrast to most research on this topic, which has been cross-sectional, Menaghan (1983) performed a short-term longitudinal study in which before and after measures were obtained for eight groups of families undergoing different transitions in the family life cycle, two groups undergoing two transitions simultaneously, and one group not going through any transition during the same time period. Overall, there were few differences in measures of marital satisfaction as a function of the life transitions. The two significant findings revealed that marital satisfaction increased when the youngest child left home and that marital satisfaction decreased in the double transition in which the oldest child entered adolescence and the youngest child began school. Also of interest in this study was the finding that a measure of skill in coping with marital issues obtained at Time 1 significantly predicted the extent to which marital satisfaction was affected by the transitions: the more adequate the coping skills, the less the decrease in marital satisfaction.

Although there has been some speculation that women find the point at which their youngest child leaves home to be especially stressful (e.g., Bart, 1971), the so-called empty nest syndrome, the research reviewed earlier suggests that just the opposite may be the case, at least with respect to marital satisfaction. Harkins (1978) compared three groups of mothers: those with the youngest child still at home, those with a child who had left home within the last 18 months, and those whose youngest child had been gone for over 2½ years. Mothers whose child had just left home reported greater psychological well-being than mothers in either of the other two groups. These results suggest that the positive effects of the "empty nest" may be transitory.

Again, we must ask what is the relevance of the research on life cycle stages and transitions to the development of psychopathology. First, in the normal populations used in these studies, relationships between life stages or transitions and indications of psychological distress were weak. Many families undoubtedly experience considerable satisfaction from children, despite the average trends indicating that the presence of children creates strains in some marriages. These transitions become relevant to psychopathology only when other factors are present. When the genetic and psychosocial histories of the individual family members and the interactive history of the family system result in increased vulnerability, then these transition periods may precipitate psychopathological reactions, as suggested by Menaghan's finding (1983) that parents with good marital coping skills were least negatively affected by the transitions.

THE DEVELOPMENTAL PERSPECTIVE: AN OVERVIEW

A developmental perspective directs our attention to change over time and to the common as well as the unique tasks that confront the individual and the family at different points in the life cycle. To understand the course of family development, we must consider what the participants have brought to the relationships as well as the subsequent interactional and systems dynamics. Each spouse in a young married couple has brought to the relationship his or her own personality, including psychopathological tendencies in some cases, and by the time the first child arrives, the couple has already formed certain interactional styles. The new infant brings a unique genotype that can be expressed in traits of temperament, anxiety-proneness, cognitive deficits, vulnerabilities to schizophrenia and affective disorders, and so on.

These individuals—parents and one or more infants—embark on an interactional journey in which all parts of the family system impinge on all other parts. The marital relationship would seem especially important in affecting the interaction between parents and children. For example, emotional support from the husband is associated with greater maternal sensitivity to the infant's cues. In older children and adolescents, there is evidence that the pattern of high interparent conflict and dominance of the opposite-sex parent can lead to conflicting identification tendencies and to associated psychological symptoms.

The characteristics of parent and infant that lead to persistent manifestations of those behaviors called *insecure attachment* may be of considerable importance in creating a vulnerability to future disturbances in the child. At the same time, we must guard against attributing too much importance to what happens in the first 2 years of life in the development of later psychological problems. It is often the case, as in the children of Kauai, that undesirable features of infant temperament or parenting that were present during the first year or so of the child's life are highly correlated with continuing undesirable familial characteristics in later childhood. It may well be that factors that put the child at risk during the early years can be ameliorated by a change to a more benign environment in later years.

In the years of childhood and adolescence, the ways in which warmth and hostility are expressed and in which issues of control are handled may be importantly associated with the extent and type of psychopathology that develops. Child temperament and parental styles of child rearing interact to produce harmonious or disharmonious parent–child relations. Research rather strongly suggests that parental characteristics of warmth (affection, sensitivity, acceptance of individuality, and openness of communication) and a degree of control that is intermediate between excessive overcontrol and total permissiveness are associated with harmonious relationships. But lest we give parents too much credit for this happy outcome, we should not forget that it is much easier to be warm toward and exert control over some children than others: child temperament is an important factor.

In a developmental perspective, certain features of family structure should also be included, especially the sibling configuration. Firstborn and middleborn males, depending on the age spacing to the nearest siblings and the sex of the siblings, may be somewhat more at risk for childhood disorders.

Few of the above variables, in themselves, are highly correlated with the development of psychopathology. It is only in combination that certain initial dispositions of the family participants and certain types of developing interactions have a high probability of leading to psychopathology. In the developmental perspective, we attempt to trace these interactional dynamics over time, and thus far, we have made only a modest beginning in filling the empirical gaps in the family life cycle.

ACKNOWLEDGMENTS

I wish to thank Nancy J. Martin, John Weisz, and the editor for their helpful comments on a draft of this chapter.

REFERENCES

Agulnik, P. L. (1970). The spouse of the phobic patient. *British Journal of Psychiatry, 117*, 59–67.

Ainsworth, M., Blehar, M., Waters, E., & Wall, S. (1978). *Patterns of attachment.* Hillsdale, NJ: Erlbaum.

Aldous, J. (1978). *Developmental change in families.* New York: Wiley.

Anderson, S. A., Russell, C. S., & Schumm, W. R. (1983). Perceived marital quality and family life-cycle categories: A further analysis. *Journal of Marriage and the Family, 45*, 127–140.

Antill, J. K. (1983). Sex role complementarity versus similarity in married couples. *Journal of Personality and Social Psychology, 45*, 145–155.

Arend, R., Gove, F. L., & Sroufe, L. A. (1979). Continuity of individual adaptation from infancy to kindergarten: A predictive study of ego-resiliency and curiosity in preschoolers. *Child Development, 50*, 950–959.

Bakeman, R., & Brown, J. V. (1980). Early interaction: Consequences for social and mental development at three years. *Child Development, 51*, 437–447.

Baldwin, A. L., Cole, R. E., & Baldwin, C. P. (1982). Parental pathology, family interaction, and the competence of the child in school. *Monographs of the Society for Research in Child Development, 47(5,* Serial No. 197).

Bart, P. (1971). Depression in middle-aged women. In V. Gornick & B. K. Moran (Eds.), *Women in sexist society.* New York: Basic Books.

Barton, K., & Cattell, R. B. (1972). Real and perceived similarities in personality between spouses: Test of "likeness" versus "completeness" theories. *Psychological Reports, 31*, 15–18.

Bateson, G., Jackson, D., Haley, J., & Weakland, J. (1956). Toward a theory of schizophrenia. *Behavioral Science, 1*, 251–264.

Baucom, D. H., & Aiken, P. A. (1984). Sex role identity, marital satisfaction, and response to behavioral marital therapy. *Journal of Consulting and Clinical Psychology, 52*, 438–444.

Baumrind, D. (1967). Child care practices anteceding three patterns of preschool behavior. *Genetic Psychology Monographs, 75*, 43–83.

Baumrind, D. (1971). Harmonious parents and their preschool children. *Developmental Psychology, 4*, 99–102.

Baumrind, D. (1983). Rejoinder to Lewis's reinterpretation of parental firm control effects: Are authoritative families really harmonious? *Psychological Bulletin, 94*, 132–142.

Beckwith, L. (1978). Caregiver–infant interaction and the development of the high risk infant. In G. P. Sackett (Ed.), *Observing behavior: Theory and application in mental retardation* (Vol. 1). Baltimore: University Park Press.

Bell, R. Q., & Harper, L. V. (1977). *Child effects on adults.* Hillsdale, NJ: Erlbaum.

Bell, S. M., & Ainsworth, M. D. S. (1972). Infant crying and maternal responsiveness. *Child Development, 43*, 1171–1190.

Belmont, L. (1977). Birth order, intellectual competence and psychiatric status. *Journal of Individual Psychology, 33*, 97–103.

Belsky, J., Spanier, G. B., & Rovine, M. (1983). Stability and change in marriage across the transition to parenthood. *Journal of Marriage and the Family, 45,* 567–577.

Bentler, P. M., & Newcomb, M. D. (1978). Longitudinal study of marital success and failure. *Journal of Consulting and Clinical Psychology, 46,* 1053–1070.

Birns, B. (1965). Individual differences in human neonates' responses to stimulation. *Child Development, 36,* 249–256.

Birns, B., Blank, M., & Bridger, W. H. (1966). The effectiveness of various soothing techniques on human neonates. *Psychosomatic Medicine, 28,* 316–322.

Block, J. H., & Block, J. (1979). The role of ego-control and ego-resiliency in the organization of behavior. In W. A. Collins (Ed.), *Minnesota Symposia on Child Psychology* (Vol. 13). Hillsdale, NJ: Erlbaum.

Block, J. H., Block, J., & Morrison, A. (1981). Parental agreement–disagreement on child-rearing orientations and gender-related personality correlates in children. *Child Development, 52,* 965–974.

Bowen, M. (1978). *Family therapy in clinical practice.* New York: Aronson.

Bugental, D., Kaswan, J., & Love, L. (1970). Perception of contadictory meaning conveyed by verbal and nonverbal channels. *Journal of Personality and Social Psychology, 16,* 647–655.

Bugental, D., Kaswan, J., Love, L., & Fox, M. (1970). Child vs. adult perception of evaluative messages in verbal, vocal, and visual channels. *Development Psychology, 2,* 367–375.

Bumpass, L. L., & Sweet, J. A. (1972). Differentials in marital instability: 1970. *American Sociological Review, 37,* 754–766.

Burger, A. L., & Jacobson, N. S. (1979). The relationship between sex role characteristics, couple satisfaction and couple problem-solving. *American Journal of Family Therapy, 7,* 52–60.

Buss, A. H., & Plomin, R. (1975). *A temperament theory of personality development.* New York: Wiley.

Carpenter, G. C., Tecce, J. J., Stechler, G., & Friedman, S. (1970). Differential visual behavior to human and humanoid faces in early infancy. *Merrill-Palmer Quarterly of Behavior and Development, 16,* 91–108.

Cattell, R. B., & Nesselroade, J. B. (1967). Likeness and completeness theories examined by sixteen personality factor measures on stably and unstably married couples. *Journal of Personality and Social Psychology, 7,* 351–361.

Chawla, P. L., & Gupt, K. (1979). A comparative study of parents of emotionally disturbed and normal children. *British Journal of Psychiatry, 134,* 406–411.

Chess, S., Thomas, A., Korn, S., Mittleman, M., & Cohen, J. (1983). Early parental attitudes, divorce and separation, and young adult outcome: Findings of a longitudinal study. *Journal of the American Academy of Child Psychiatry, 22,* 47–51.

Christensen, A., & Margolin, G. (1981, August). *Correlational and sequential analyses of marital and child problems.* Paper presented at the meeting of the American Psychological Association, Los Angeles.

Cohen, S. E., & Beckwith, L. (1976). Maternal language in infancy. *Developmental Psychology, 12,* 371–372.

Cohen, S. E., & Beckwith, L. (1977). Caregiving behaviors and early cognitive development as related to ordinal position in preterm infants. *Child Development, 48,* 152–157.

Cohn, J. F., & Tronick, E. Z. (1983). Three-month-old infants' reaction to simulated maternal depression. *Child Development, 54,* 185–193.

Crawford, J. W. (1982). Mother–infant interaction in premature and full-term infants. *Child Development, 53,* 957–962.

Crnic, K. A., Ragozin, A. S., Greenberg, M. T., Robinson, N. M., & Basham, R. B. (1983). Social interaction and developmental competence of preterm and full-term infants during the first year of life. *Child Development, 54,* 1199–1210.

Crockenberg, S. B. (1981). Infant irritability, mother responsiveness, and social support influences on the security of infant–mother attachment. *Child Development, 52,* 857–865.

Cushna, B. (1966, September). *Agency and birth order differences in very early childhood.* Paper presented at the meeting of the American Psychological Association, New York.

Davenport, Y. B., Zahn-Waxler, C., Adland, M. L., & Mayfield, A. (1984). Early child-rearing practices in families with a manic-depressive parent. *American Journal of Psychiatry, 141,* 230–235.

De Young, G. E., & Fleischer, B. (1976). Motivational and personality trait relationships in mate selection. *Behavior Genetics, 6,* 1–6.

DiVitto, B., & Goldberg, S. (1979). The development of early parent–infant interaction as a function of newborn medical status. In T. Field, A. Sostek, S. Goldberg, & H. H. Shuman (Eds.), *Infants born at risk.* Holliswood, NY: Spectrum.

Dunn, J., & Kendrick, C. (1982). Siblings and their mothers: Developing relationships within the family. In M. E. Lamb & B. Sutton-Smith (Eds.), *Sibling relationships.* Hillsdale, NJ: Erlbaum.

Duvall, E. M. (1971). *Family development.* Philadelphia: Lippincott.

Egeland, B., Breitenbucher, M., & Rosenberg, D. (1980). Prospective study of the significance of life stress in the etiology of child abuse. *Journal of Consulting and Clinical Psychology, 48,* 195–205.

Elder, G. H., & Rockwell, R. C. (1976). Marital timing in women's life patterns. *Journal of Family History, 1,* 34–55.

Emery, R. E. (1982). Interparental conflict and the children of discord and divorce. *Psychological Bulletin, 92,* 310–330.

Emery, R. E., & O'Leary, K. D. (1982). Children's perceptions of marital discord and behavior problems of boys and girls. *Journal of Abnormal Child Psychology, 10,* 11–24.

Feldman, H. (1971). The effects of children on the family. In A. Michel (Ed.), *Family issues of employed women in Europe and America.* Leiden: Brill.

Field, T. (1979). Interaction patterns of high-risk and normal infants. In T. Field, A. Sostek, S. Goldberg, & H. H. Shuman (Eds.), *Infants born at risk.* New York: Spectrum.

Field, T. (1980). Interactions of preterm and term infants with their lower- and middle-class teenage and adult mothers. In T. Field, S. Goldberg, D. Stern, & A. Sostek (Eds.), *High-risk infants and children: Adult and peer interactions.* New York: Academic Press.

Field, T. (1983). Early interactions and interaction coaching of high-risk infants and parents. In M. Perlmutter (Ed.), *The Minnesota Symposia on Child Development* (Vol. 16). Hillsdale, NJ: Erlbaum.

Field, T., Dempsey, J., & Shuman, H. (1981). Developmental follow-up of pre- and postterm infants. In S. L. Friedman & M. Sigman (Eds.), *Preterm birth and psychological development.* New York: Academic Press.

Fishbein, H. D. (1981). Sibling set configuration and family dysfunction. *Family Process, 20,* 311–318.

Gaensbauer, T. J., Harmon, R. J., Cytryn, L., & McKnew, D. H. (1984). Social and affective development in infants with a manic-depressive parent. *American Journal of Psychiatry, 141,* 223–229.

Gassner, S., & Murray, E. J. (1969). Dominance and conflict in the interactions between parents of normal and neurotic children. *Journal of Abnormal and Social Psychology, 74,* 33–41.

Gilbert, R., Christensen, A., & Margolin, G. (1984). Patterns of alliances in nondistressed and multi-problem families. *Family Process, 23,* 75–88.

Glenn, N. D., & McLanahan, S. (1982). The effects of offspring on the psychological well-being of older adults. *Journal of Marriage and the Family, 44,* 63–72.

Goldberg, S., Brachfeld, S., & DiVitto, B. (1980). Feeding, fussing, and play: Parent–infant interaction in the first year as a function of prematurity and perinatal medical problems. In T. M. Field, S. Goldberg, D. Stern, & A. M. Sostek (Eds.), *High-risk infants and children.* New York: Academic Press.

Grunebaum, H., Cohler, B. J., Kauffman, C., & Gallant, D. (1978). Children of depressed and schizophrenic mothers. *Child Psychiatry and Human Development, 8,* 219–228.

Hagnell, O., & Kreitman, N. (1974). Mental illness in married pairs in a total population. *British Journal of Psychiatry, 125,* 293–302.

Haley, J. (1973). *Uncommon therapy.* New York: Norton.

Hare, E. H., & Shaw, G. K. (1965). The patient's spouse and concordance on neuroticism. *British Journal of Psychiatry, 111,* 102–103.

Harkins, E. G. (1978). Effects of empty nest transition on self-report of psychological and physical well-being. *Journal of Marriage and the Family, 40,* 549–556.

Hauser, S. T., Powers, S. I., Noam, G. G., Jacobson, A. M., Weiss, B., & Follansbee, D. J. (1984). Familial contexts of adolescent ego development. *Child Development, 55,* 195–213.

Heinicke, C. M., Diskin, S. D., Ramsey-Klee, D. M., & Given, K. (1983). Pre-birth parent characteristics and family development in the first year of life. *Child Development, 54,* 194–208.

Hetherington, E. M. (1965). A developmental study of the effects of sex of the dominant parent on sex-role preference, identification, and imitation in children. *Journal of Personality and Social Psychology, 2,* 188–194.

Hetherington, E. M., & Frankie, G. (1967). Effects of parental dominance, warmth, and conflict on imitation in children. *Journal of Personality and Social Psychology, 6,* 119–125.

Hetherington, E. M., Stouwie, R., & Ridberg, E. H. (1971). Patterns of family interaction and child rearing attitudes related to three dimensions of juvenile delinquency. *Journal of Abnormal Psychology, 77,* 160–176.

Hilton, I. (1967). Differences in the behavior of mothers toward first and later born children. *Journal of Personality and Social Psychology, 7,* 282–290.

Hoffman, J. A. (1985a). Psychological separation of late adolescents from their parents. *Journal of Counseling Psychology, 31,* 170–178.

Hoffman, J. A. (1985b). *Presenting problems and family dynamics of college students.* Unpublished doctoral dissertation, University of North Carolina, Chapel Hill.

Ickes, W. (1986). Sex-role influences on compatibility in relationships. In W. Ickes (Ed.), *Compatible and incompatible relationships.* New York: Springer-Verlag.

Jacob, T. (1974). Patterns of family conflict and dominance as a function of child age and social class. *Developmental Psychology, 10,* 1–12.

Jacob, T., & Lessin, S. (1982). Inconsistent communication in family interaction. *Clinical Psychology Review, 2,* 295–309.

Jacobs, B. S., & Moss, H. A. (1976). Birth order and sex of sibling as determinants of mother–infant interaction. *Child Development, 47,* 315–322.

Jacobson, N. S., & Martin, B. (1976). Behavioral marriage therapy: Current status. *Psychological Bulletin, 83,* 540–566.

Kidwell, J. S. (1981). Number of siblings, sibling spacing, sex, and birth order: Their effects on perceived parent–adolescent relationships. *Journal of Marriage and the Family, 43,* 315–332.

Kidwell, J. S. (1982). The neglected birth order: Middleborns. *Journal of Marriage and the Family, 44,* 225–235.

Klein, M. M., Plutchik, R., & Conte, H. R. (1973). Parental dominance–passivity and behavior problems of children. *Journal of Consulting and Clinical Psychology, 40,* 416–419.

Kogan, K. L., Wimberger, H. C., & Bobbitt, R. A. (1969). Analysis of mother–child interaction in young mental retardates. *Child Development, 40,* 799–812.

Korner, A. F. (1971). Individual differences at birth: Implications for early experience and later development. *American Journal of Orthopsychiatry, 41,* 608–619.

Korner, A. F., & Grobstein, R. (1967). Individual differences at birth: Implications for mother–infant relationship and later development. *Journal of American Academy of Child Psychiatry, 6,* 676–690.

Kreitman, N. (1964). The patient's spouse. *British Journal of Psychiatry, 110,* 159–173.

Kreitman, N., Collins, J., Nelson, B., & Troop, J. (1970). Neurosis and marital interaction: 1. Personality and symptoms. *British Journal of Psychiatry, 117,* 33–46.

Kulka, R. A., & Weingarten, H. (1979). The long term effects of parental divorce in childhood on adult adjustment. *Journal of Social Issues, 35,* 50–78.

Lahey, D. B., Hammer, D., Crumrine, P. L., & Forehand, R. L. (1980). Birth order × sex interactions in child behavior problems. *Developmental Psychology, 6,* 608–615.

Lamb, M. E. (1978). Qualitative aspects of mother and father infant attachments. *Infant Behavior and Development, 1,* 265–275.

Lasko, J. K. (1954). Parent behavior toward first and second children. *Genetic Psychology Monographs, 49,* 96–137.

Lewis, C. C. (1981). The effects of parental firm control: A reinterpretation of findings. *Psychological Bulletin, 90,* 547–563.

Loundsbury, M. L., & Bates, J. E. (1982). The cries of infants of differing levels of perceived temperamental difficultness: Acoustic properties and effects on listeners. *Child Development, 53,* 677–686.

Luckey, E. B., & Bain, J. K. (1970). Children: A factor in marital satisfaction. *Journal of Marriage and the Family, 32,* 43–44.

Lytton, H. (1977). Correlates of compliance and the rudiments of conscience in 2-year-old boys. *Canadian Journal of Behavioral Sciences, 9*, 242–251.

Lytton, H. (1980). *Parent–child interaction: The socialization process observed in twin and singleton families.* New York: Plenum Press.

Main, M., & Weston, D. R. (1981). The quality of the toddler's relationship to mother and to father: Related to conflict behavior and the readiness to establish new relationships. *Child Development, 52*, 932–940.

Markman, H. J. (1979). Application of a behavioral model of marriage in predicting relationship satisfaction of couples planning marriage. *Journal of Consulting and Clinical Psychology, 47*, 743–749.

Markman, H. J. (1981). Prediction of marital distress: A 5-year follow-up. *Journal of Consulting and Clinical Psychology, 49*, 760–762.

Martin, B. (1975). Parent–child relations. In F. D. Horowitz (Ed.), *Review of child development research* (Vol. 4). Chicago: University of Chicago Press.

Matas, L., Arend, R. A., & Sroufe, L. A. (1978). Continuity of adaptation in the second year: The relationship between quality of attachment and later competence. *Child Development, 49*, 547–556.

Menaghan, E. (1983). Marital stress and family transitions: A panel analysis. *Journal of Marriage and the Family, 45*, 371–386.

Merikangas, K. R. (1982). Assortative mating for psychiatric disorders and psychological traits. *Archives of General Psychiatry, 39*, 1173–1180.

Minuchin, S., & Fishman, H. C. (1981). *Family therapy techniques.* Cambridge: Harvard University Press.

Moss, H. A. (1967). Sex, age, and state as determinants of mother–infant interaction. *Merrill-Palmer Quarterly, 13*, 19–36.

Mueller, C. W., & Pope, H. (1977). Marital instability: A study of its transmission between generations. *Journal of Marriage and the Family, 39*, 83–93.

Nadelman, L., & Begun, A. (1982). The effect of the newborn on the older sibling: Mothers' questionnaire. In M. E. Lamb & B. Sutton-Smith (Eds.), *Sibling relationships.* Hillsdale, NJ: Erlbaum.

Newmark, C. S., & Toomey, T. (1972). The *MF* scale as an index of disturbed marital interaction. *Psychological Reports, 31*, 590.

Nystul, M. S. (1974). The effects of birth order and sex on self-concept. *Journal of Individual Psychology, 30*, 211–214.

Offer, D., & Offer, J. B. (1975). *From teenage to young manhood.* New York: Basic Books.

Olson, D. (1972). Empirically unbinding the double bind: Review of research and conceptual reformulations. *Family Process, 11*, 69–94.

Oltmanns, T. F., Broderick, J. E., & O'Leary, K. D. (1977). Marital adjustment and efficacy of behavior therapy with children. *Journal of Consulting and Clinical Psychology, 45*, 724–729.

Osborne, D. (1971). An MMPI index of disturbed marital interaction. *Psychological Reports, 29*, 852–854.

Osofsky, J. D. (1976). Neonatal characteristics and mother–infant interaction in two observational situations. *Child Development, 47*, 1138–1147.

Ovenstone, I. M. K. (1973). The development of neurosis in the wives of neurotic men: 2. Marital role functions and marital tension. *British Journal of Psychiatry, 122*, 711–717.

Patterson, G. R. (1982). *Coercive family process.* Eugene, OR: Castalia.

Pedersen, F. (1975, September). *Mother, father, and infant as an interactive system.* Paper presented at the meeting of the American Psychological Association, Chicago.

Pedersen, F., Anderson, B., & Cain, R. (1977, March). *An approach to understanding linkages between the parent–infant and spouse relationships.* Paper presented at the meeting of the Society for Research in Child Development, New Orleans.

Pedersen, F., Anderson, B., & Cain, R. (1979, March). *Parent–infant interaction observed in a family setting at age 5 months.* Paper presented at the meeting of the Society for Research in Child Development, San Francisco.

Piaget, J., & Inhelder, B. (1969). *The psychology of the child.* New York: Basic Books.

Pond, D., Ryle, A., & Hamilton, M. (1963). Marriage and neurosis in a working-class population. *British Journal of Psychiatry, 109,* 592–598.

Porter, B., & O'Leary, K. D. (1980). Marital discord and childhood behavior problems. *Journal of Abnormal Child Psychology, 8,* 287–295.

Rieder, R., & Nichols, P. (1979). Offspring of schizophrenics: 3. Hyperactivity and neurological soft signs. *Archives of General Psychiatry, 36,* 665–674.

Robson, K. S., Pedersan, F. A., & Moss, H. A. (1969), Developmental observations of diadic gazing in relation to the fear of strangers and social approach behavior. *Child Development, 40,* 619–627.

Rode, S. S., Chang, P. N., Fisch, R. O., & Sroufe, L. A. (1981). Attachment patterns of infants separated at birth. *Developmental Psychology, 17,* 188–191.

Rodgers, R. (1964). Toward a theory of family development. *Journal of Marriage and the Family, 26,* 262–270.

Rollins, B. C., & Galligan, R. (1978). The developing child and marital satisfaction of parents. In R. M. Lerner & G. B. Spanier (Eds.), *Child Influences on marital and family interaction.* New York: Academic Press.

Rothbart, M. K. (1971). Birth order and mother–child interaction in an achievement situation. *Journal of Personality and Social Psychology, 17,* 113–120.

Rutter, M. (1971). Parent–child separation: Psychological effects on the children. *Journal of Child Psychology and Psychiatry, 12,* 233–256.

Rutter, M., Yule, B. Quinton, D., Rowlands, O., Yule, W., & Berger, M. (1974). Attainments and adjustment in two geographical areas: 3. Some factors accounting for area differences. *British Journal of Psychiatry, 125,* 520–533.

Ryder, R. G. (1973). Longitudinal data relating marriage satisfaction and having a child. *Journal of Marriage and the Family, 35,* 604–606.

Sameroff, A. J., Barocas, R., & Seifer, R. (1980, March). *Rochester longitudinal study progress report.* Paper presented at the Risk Research Consortium Conference, San Juan, Puerto Rico.

Sameroff, A. J., Seifer, R., & Zax, M. (1982). Early development of children at risk for emotional disorder. *Monographs of the Society for Research in Child Development, 47, (199).*

Satir, V. (1964). *Conjoint family therapy.* Palo Alto, CA: Science & Behavior Books.

Schachter, J., Elmer, E., Ragins, N., Wimberly, F., & Lachin, J. M. (1977). Assessment of mother–infant interaction: Schizophrenic and non-schizophrenic mothers. *Merrill-Palmer Quarterly, 23,* 193–206.

Schaefer, E. S. (1959). A circumplex model for maternal behavior. *Journal of Abnormal and Social Psychology, 59,* 226–235.

Schaffer, H. R., & Crook, C. K. (1980). Child compliance and maternal control techniques. *Developmental Psychology, 16,* 54–61.

Schaffer, H. R., & Emerson, P. E. (1964). Patterns of response to physical contact in early human development. *Journal of Child Psychology and Psychiatry, 5,* 1–13.

Schooler, C. (1972). Birth order effects: Not here, not now! *Psychological Bulletin, 78,* 161–175.

Schwarz, J. C., & Getter, H. (1980). Parental conflict and dominance in late adolescent maladjustment: A triple interaction model. *Journal of Abnormal Psychology, 89,* 573–580.

Seifer, R., Sameroff, A. J., & Jones, F. H. (1981). Adaptive behavior in young children of emotionally disturbed women. *Journal of Applied Developmental Psychology, 1,* 251–276.

Shaver, P., Pullis, C., & Olds, D. (1980). Report on the LHJ "Intimacy Today" survey: Private research report to the *Ladies' Home Journal.* Also described in Ickes, W. (Ed.). (1986). Compatible and incompatible relationships. New York: Springer-Verlag.

Shereshefsky, P. M., & Yarrow, L. J. (1973). *Psychological aspects of a first pregnancy and early postnatal adaptation.* New York: Raven.

Shrader, W. K., & Leventhal, T. (1968). Birth order of children and parental report of problems. *Child Development, 39,* 1165–1175.

Slater, E., & Woodside, M. (1951). *Patterns of marriage.* London: Cassell.

Sobel, D. E. (1961). Children of schizophrenic patients: Preliminary observations on early development. *American Journal of Psychiatry, 118,* 512–517.

Spanier, G. B., & Lewis, R. S. (1980). Marital quality: A review of the seventies. *Journal of Marriage and the Family, 42*, 825–839.

Sroufe, L. A. (1983). Infant–caregiver attachment and patterns of adaptation in preschool: The roots of maladaptation and competence. In M. Perlmutter (Ed.), *The Minnesota Symposia on Child Development* (Vol. 16). Hillsdale, NJ: Erlbaum.

Sroufe, L. A., Jacobvitz, D., Mangelsdorf, S., DeAngelo, E., & Ward, M. J. (1985). Generational boundary dissolution between mothers and their preschool children: A relationship systems approach. *Child Development, 56*, 317–325.

Stayton, D. J., Hogan, R., & Ainsworth, M. D. S. (1971). Infant obedience and maternal behavior: The origins of socialization reconsidered. *Child Development, 42*, 1057–1069.

Steinberg, L. D. (1981). Transformations in family relations at puberty. *Developmental Psychology, 17*, 833–840.

Swan, R. J. (1957). Using the MMPI in marriage counseling. *Journal of Counseling Psychology, 4*, 239–244.

Thomas, A., Chess, S., & Birch, H. G. (1968). *Temperament and behavior disorders in children.* New York: New York University Press.

Thompson, R. A., Lamb, M. E., & Estes, D. (1982). Stability of infant–mother attachment and its relationship to changing life circumstances in an unselected middle-class sample. *Child Development, 53*, 144–148.

Tronick, E., Als, H., Adamson, L., Wise, S., & Brazelton, T. B. (1978). The infant's response to entrapment between contradictory messages in face-to-face interaction. *Journal of American Academy of Child Psychiatry, 17*, 1–13.

Tuckman, J., & Regan, R. A. (1966). Intactness of the home and behavioral problems in children. *Journal of Child Psychology and Psychiatry, 7*, 225–233.

Tulkin, S., & Kagan, J. (1972). Mother–child interaction in the first few years of life. *Child Development, 43*, 31–41.

Vaughn, B., Egeland, B., & Sroufe, L. A. (1979). Individual differences in infant–mother attachment at twelve and eighteen months: Stability and change in families under stress. *Child Development, 50*, 971–975.

Wagner, M. E., Schubert, H. J. P., & Schubert, D. S. P. (1979). Sibship-constellation effects on psychosocial development, creativity, and health. In H. W. Reese & L. P. Lipsitt (Eds.), *Advances in child development and behavior* (Vol. 14). New York: Academic Press.

Waldron, H., & Routh, D. K. (1981). The effect of the first child on the marital relationship. *Journal of Marriage and the Family, 43*, 785–788.

Waldron, S., Shrier, D. K., Stone, B., & Tobin, F. (1975). School phobia and other childhood neuroses: A systematic study of the children and their families. *American Journal of Psychiatry, 132*, 802–808.

Walker, E., Cudeck, B., Mednick, S., & Schulsinger, F. (1981). The effects of parental absence and institutionalization on the development of clinical symptoms in high risk children. *Acta Psychiatrica Scandinavica, 63*, 95–109.

Wandersman, L., Wandersman, A., & Kahn, S. (1980). Social support in the transition to parenthood. *Journal of Community Psychology, 8*, 332–342.

Waters, E. (1978). The reliability and stability of individual differences in infant–mother attachment. *Child Development, 49*, 483–494.

Waters, E., Wippman, J., & Sroufe, L. A. (1979). Attachment, positive affect, and competence in the peer group: Two studies in construct validation. *Child Development, 50*, 821–829.

Waters, E., Vaughn, B. E., & Egeland, B. R. (1980). Individual differences in infant–mother attachment relationships at age one: Antecedents in neonatal behavior in an urban, economically disadvantaged sample. *Child Development, 51*, 208–216.

Weissman, M. M., Prusoff, B. A., Gammon, G. D., Merikangas, K. R., Leckman, J. F., & Kidd, K. K. (1984). Psychopathology in the children (ages 6–18) of depressed and normal parents. *Journal of the American Academy of Child Psychiatry, 23*, 78–84.

Werner, E. E., & Smith, R. S. (1977). *Kauai's children come of age.* Honolulu: University Press of Hawaii.

Werner, E. E., & Smith, R. S. (1982). *Vulnerable but invincible.* New York: McGraw Hill.

Westley, W. A., & Epstein, N. B. (1970). *The silent majority.* San Francisco: Jossey-Bass.

Whitehead, L. (1979). Sex differences in children's responses to family stress: A re-evaluation. *Journal of Child Psychology and Psychiatry and Allied Disciplines, 20,* 247–254.

Zajonc, R. B., & Markus, G. B. (1975). Birth order and intellectual development. *Psychological Review, 82,* 74–88.

Zeskind, P. S., & Lester, B. M. (1978). Acoustic features and auditory perceptions of the cries of newborns with prenatal and perinatal complications. *Child Development, 49,* 580–589.

CHAPTER 6

Paradigm and Pathogenesis

A Family-Centered Approach to Problems of Etiology and Treatment of Psychiatric Disorders

DAVID REISS
AND
DAVID KLEIN

During the last 15 years, David Reiss and his associates have explored ways in which the family develops and maintains its own, distinctive convictions about reality. They have focused their work on differences among families in their conceptions of the safety or danger in the world, the families' belief about whether the world treats the family as a group or as isolated individuals, and the novelty or familiarity that the families experience in their environment. These explorations have been guided by an evolving theory of family process; currently, the most familiar concept in this theory is the notion of the family's *paradigm*, which refers to the underlying assumptions about reality that, in any family, are presumed to be shared by all members. The research has used a variety of objective and quantitative methods for studying the family. The best known of these methods are laboratory, problem-solving procedures, although questionnaires, field observations, and structured interviews have also been used. This approach has aimed at understanding the family process in clinical families as well as in those who have never sought help for psychological distress or problems in relationships among members. In the course of this work, a number of important clinical phenomena have been analyzed: family correlates of psychopathology, the processes by which families engage in treatment programs, families' support networks, and families' response to stress.

Although many of the theoretical ideas, as well as substantive findings, are

DAVID REISS • Department of Psychiatry and Behavioral Sciences, Center for Family Research, George Washington University Medical Center, Washington, DC 20037. **DAVID KLEIN** • Department of Sociology, University of Notre Dame, Notre Dame, IN 46556.

now becoming well known in clinical fields, only a handful of investigators in this country and abroad—aside from Reiss and his colleagues, whose work remains very active—are pursuing this line of thinking and analysis. Thus, in contrast to other chapters on theory, it falls to the "author" of this approach to also be an author of the chapter reviewing the work. However, authors are poor critics of their own work. They may be effective in sensing its potential but may require help in placing it in perspective. Thus, a second author has joined in writing this chapter. The second author has followed the work, as a constructive critic, almost from its inception and enters the work more actively now to help in placing it in perspective, to help delineate its strengths and limitations. These delineations, although scattered throughout the chapter, are brought together and most clearly described in the concluding section.

This chapter has four sections. In the first, we lay out some of the major theoretical notions concerning the family's construction of reality. We focus on the concept of the *paradigm* and also briefly summarize other related concepts. In the second section, we summarize some of the evidence on which these ideas are based. In a third section, we explore the relevance of these ideas to psychopathology in individuals as well as to family stress, crisis, and therapy. Finally, in the fourth section, we take a critical look at this approach to analyzing the family process: What has it yielded? What are its strongest potentials? And what are its principal liabilities?

THE FAMILY'S CONSTRUCTION OF REALITY

Let us begin with three brief vignettes.

THE O'HARA FAMILY

The O'Hara family consists of a father and a mother in their late 70s and three grown sons, now successful businessmen, who, years ago, moved away from the parental home. The O'Haras have had a dramatic and, in some ways, distinguished past. The father's grandfather made and lost a fortune drilling some of America's earliest oil wells in Pennsylvania. The father's father was a hardy farmer and a lawyer well known for a mixture of compassion and toughness. The father himself was a newspaper editor who had successfully run for Congress but had been defeated after one term. A fundamental theme in the O'Haras was achieving preeminence through a special blend of physical toughness, the willingness to take risks (even to risk all, as in drilling oil wells, raising crops, and running for election) and, following success, sympathetic compassion for the "less fortunate." When the three sons were boys, the family developed a ritual response to the father's return home (often after prolonged absences required by his political activity). The boys would briefly arm-wrestle with the father, and the mother would sit, as an audience at a fight between gladiators, cheering them on. A crucial component of this brief but often-repeated ritual was that the fight would look tough but that that father would be careful to inflict no real pain or injury. Now, when the sons return home, the ritual is still repeated, but it is now the sons who are careful to inflict no pain on the aging father.

THE BRADY FAMILY

The Brady family was seen in treatment for over a year as part of a comprehensive treatment program for a son, Fred, aged 27, who had become depressed, socially withdrawn, and—finally—immobilized by frightening and disorganized somatic delusions; he felt that his body was empty, falling apart, decaying. He became suicidal. Fred was the only child of a father, a successful internist, who had died 20 years previously and a mother who was in her late 60s. Shortly after the father's death, the father's younger brother came to live with Fred and his mother and never left. The uncle was a shy, timid clerk in the local branch of a national chain of retail stores. The trio continued to live in the same apartment as had Fred and his mother when his father was alive. The father's medical books, photographs, and many other possessions were left in place. The trio felt themselves to be a doctor's family and occasionally referred to the dead father in the present tense. Clearly, they were preserving an important, shared illusion about themselves. Their shared hope that Fred would soon matriculate in medical school was an extension of this illusion. One support for this illusion was the mother's role as a specialist in obtaining information for the family from the outside world. She was the only one in the family who watched TV news and read the papers. She also answered all incoming phone calls whenever she was home. Indeed, these were trivial examples of the mother's role as the family's regulator of the selection and interpretation of information. In virtually every aspect of the family's life, it was the mother who selected the relevant outside data and provided the interpretations. For example, after many months in the hospital, Fred received a partial discharge enabling him to begin his first job as a technician's helper in a hospital laboratory. He never did well in this job, but the mother focused exclusively on the medical aspects of this work and presented the job to the family and the therapist as evidence that Fred might soon return to college, go to medical school, and become a doctor. Fred and his uncle acquiesced, quite willingly, in mother's highly filtered selection and interpretation of signals. These provided them both with a continuous sense of the family's vigor, prestige and permanence.

THE RAMOS-ANTHONY-COOPER FAMILY

The Ramos-Anthony-Cooper family needs three names to describe a fact that also reflects the deep and pervasive division within it. It is a family of three women living together: 24-year-old and 26-year-old daughters and a twice-divorced mother, aged 51. Maureen Ramos is the youngest daughter. Her last name is that of her biological father, whom her mother divorced when she was 5. Mary Anthony is the older daughter, whose last name is that of her estranged husband. Molly Cooper is the mother, whose last name is that of her second husband, divorced 10 years previously. The family does not feel itself a connected, integral unit—in sharp contrast to the O'Hara and Brady families. Maureen is constantly preoccupied with her fantasies and is given to wandering; the content of her fantasies or wanderings is unknown to the other two. Mary is sexually promiscuous, has been illegitimately pregnant at least twice, and has been involved in petty crimes. She is known to the other two by her bad reputation, but her feelings, the specifics of her impulsive behavior, and, indeed, much of her life are entirely her own. The mother deals with her two daughters as if they were two external burdens. She longs to establish them in a psychiatric treatment program to remove the pressure of their burden, yet, constantly lonely, she is comforted by their presence, which seems to forestall complete isolation. In fact, all three women feel that their home is barren, lonely, and ungiving. They rarely bring friends there. Among themselves, the roles are clear: the mother is the stoic; Maureen is the withdrawn introvert, becoming periodically psychotic; and Mary is the irresponsible floozie. Although their roles are clear, their alliances are constantly shifting, and two—any two—often team up against the third.

The differences among these three families could be described from many points of view. Reiss and his group have focused on differences in the way the family, as a group, experiences its personal or experiential world and their own place in that world. The O'Haras see the world as rough, full of risks, but masterable, in the end, by families who are tough and clever enough. There is a distinct sense that the men in the family not only have the capacity to conquer the forces of the world but that, for generations, the O'Hara men have taken great risks, have sized up adversity with cunning, and have wrested victories of enormous proportions. The Bradys also have a distinct sense of lineage, but it is organized around a more fragile, distant, and stereotyped conception of the world and their place in it. Indeed, the family has no clear and vivid conception of the world itself, of its pitfalls, its treacheries, its opportunities. Rather, its sense of position and prestige is organized around an increasingly hollow memory of times past. Indeed, current realities are a gauzy haze filtered entirely through mother's brittle and restrictive optimism. However different from one another, the O'Haras and the Bradys are alike in regarding themselves as a unitary group. More to the point, they are deeply convinced that the world perceives them as a group. The success (or failure) of one O'Hara reflects on all the others. As the "doctor's family," the Bradys are convinced that the world should bestow on them a special and protected niche. In sharp contrast is the Ramos-Anthony-Cooper family. They have no conception of themselves as a group, and more specifically, they cannot imagine that the outside world perceives them as a group. Indeed, the family conveys a clear sense that the universe is divided into at least three wholly separate and clearly bounded compartments: one for each member of the family. None of them knows what the other two do in their workaday world because none of them can imagine that the peformance of one of the others, and the reactions it elicits from those outside the family, has the slightest bearing on her own life.

These three families can be described or understood as differing in their underlying *paradigm*. This concept is a metaphor borrowed from the philosophy of science (Kuhn, 1962), and it is applied to families to emphasize shared, un-spoken, and unquestioned assumptions that family members hold in common about their social environment. These are not assumptions about any particular situation, event, relationship, or circumstance but abiding conceptions of the environment in which these more discrete events are embedded. Thus, for the O'Haras, any particular event—an election, an oilfield, or a news article—may be more-or-less understandable, more-or-less masterable. What the family believes—without question—is that these events exist within a matrix of laws, principles, artifices, maneuvers, and manipulations that all have the essential attribute of ultimately being understandable, predictable, and masterable even if—at the moment—they cannot be understood, predicted, or mastered. Thus, the concept of the paradigm refers to the hidden or unseen or as-yet-to-be-experienced potential that resides in each situation. The paradigm determines how a family searches and explores new experiences and how it interprets what it learns. Thus, because the Ramos-Anthony-Cooper family sees their experienced world as compartmentalized, the family will always explore new situations as individuals. Except under extreme circumstances (described later), experience does not alter the paradigm. Rather, the paradigm determines what experience will be sought and how it will be understood.

Paradigms can be thought of as almost infinite in variety. Indeed, each family has its unique atmosphere or character. Moreover, paradigms can be thought of as relatively stable or enduring, under usual circumstances, over long periods of time, thus helping to explain the repeating patterns of family life. Indeed, much of the way in which the family typically interacts with outsiders, as well as the interaction within its own home, can be understood with reference to its paradigm. For example, the Bradys' careful arrangement of the relics of the father's practice reflects its enduring paradigm of privileged removal from a distant world. Despite their great variety, three dimensions or attributes of the paradigm have been useful in summarizing or representing some of the contrasts among families.[1]

Configuration expresses the degree of patterning and lawfulness that the family perceives in its environment. It reflects the degree to which the family

---

[1]The names for these three dimensions—*configuration, coordination,* and *closure*—are not similar to other terms used to describe dimensions of family experience in other research and, at this juncture in the development of family studies, need an extra word of explanation. The terms were first used in a 1971 paper (Reiss, 1971b). They were derived by comparing performance among three sets of families: those without serious psychopathology, those with an adolescent suffering a severe character disorder, and those with an adolescent with acute schizophrenia. Each of these terms was originally intended to describe—in a single word—two components of each concept: the problem-solving behavior that was measured to position a family along a dimension, as well as the experience—within the family group—that such behavior was thought to reflect. Thus, *configuration* alludes to the patterned arrangement of the cards as well as the subjective experience of families that the world has a pattern or order. Reiss and his group have resisted changing the terms in favor of apparent synonyms used by other family classificatory systems unless there are empirical data to suggest some equivalence. For example, *coordination* might be thought of as synonymous with the term *cohesion* and *closure* with the term *adaptability*. The alternate terms are used in the widely known circumplex model of Olson and his colleagues (Olson, Sprenkle, & Russell, 1979). However, recent data suggest that there is no equivalence between *closure* and *adaptability* and, at best, a marginal overlap between *coordination* and *cohesion*. Likewise, *coordination* is not an antonym of *conflict* in the classificatory system proposed by Moos and Moos (1976). Oliveri and Reiss (1984) showed that there is no correlation between measures of these two concepts. Supplementary terms for these dimensions are possible. For example, in Table 1, we have proposed the terms *mastery, solidarity,* and *openness* when the concepts are applied to coping. These alternate terms are useful for linking the three basic terms to styles of coping but are less apt, for example, when the same terms are applied to patterns of kin relationships. Supplementary terms have also been introduced to describe the ineffable assumptions about animate and inanimate reality that, according to theory, lie at the core of the family paradigm (configuration = coherence; coordination = integration; and closure = reference; see Reiss, 1981). Family studies are made complex by the profusion of terms, and this model contributes its fair share. Yet, complexity would be replaced by inaccuracy if terms were treated as synonymous (and thus the less popular ones dropped from scientific parlance) without supporting evidence.

believes there are stable, discoverable, noncapricious laws that underlie the critical phenomena in their experienced world. The O'Haras' paradigm would be judged high on this dimension. In the end, they feel that they can figure things out. Even the capriciousness and maneuvers of the business and political worlds have their underlying principles and can be learned by a clever family and used to their advantage. Families high on configuration feel that every circumstance has the potential for mastery even if it is, as yet, unmastered. For the Bradys and the Ramos-Anthony-Cooper family, there is no sense of mastering the current world as it is. For example, not one member of the Brady family has any inkling of how one gains entry into medical school nor even a sense that the pathways to entry can be discovered and fully mapped.

Coordination refers to the family's conception of how it is regarded by the social environment. Again, the O'Haras are hypersensitive to how the behavior of one—in the eyes of the community—reflects on them all. They stick together because they regard it as an immutable fact that they are regarded as a group by their social world. In a different spirit, so do the Bradys. In sharp contrast, the Ramos-Anthony-Cooper family can recognize no image of itself, as a group, in the eye of the community. Their paradigm would be regarded as low in coordination.

Closure refers to the balance between openness to new experience (delayed closure) and being dominated by tradition (early closure). The Bradys' sense of order and stability comes not from a grasp of the patterns and principles of their current world, but from their cleavage to a simple, highly structured image of the past—smoothed and refined, without fundamental change, as the years pass. In contrast, there is no living past in the life of the Ramos-Anthony-Cooper family. They respond by impulse. From the perspective of the observer, the life of this family is dominated by the immediate and peremptory passions of the moment: sex, anger, or cravings for nurturance. From the family's perspective, each shift in each other and in the world that they inhabit beckons for action, demands immediate engagement or withdrawal. Each member is enslaved by the immediate stimulation of her private universe.

These concepts about the family have their origins in a rich tradition of observation and theory in psychology, sociology, and the clinical sciences. In psychology, Fritz Heider (1958) delineated the "naive psychologies" constructed by everyone. Heider was fascinated with how human social behavior is dominated by our understanding of the psychology of others. In the same tradition, George Kelly (1955) developed an entire psychology of "personal constructs." He saw each individual as organizing his or her personal universe with categories and systems for anticipating and explaining actions and their consequences. More generally, Piaget (1952) argued that the basic unit of mental life was the schema, a flexible, developing, and differentiated subjective representation of the personal world that both controls behavior and can be modified by the results of behavior.

It remained for the philosopher-sociologists Berger and Luckmann (1966), however, to clarify that personal theories, constructs, and schemata cannot be built by individuals in isolation. Individuals serve as reference points for each other's personal schemata. Durable, personal visions of reality must be reinforced and, indeed, shared by others, Berger and Luckmann argued. Indeed, these personal conceptions are structured and sustained through the patterns, norms, and institutions of social interaction. Berger and Luckmann were concerned with social interaction, social institutions, and groups quite generally.

For small therapeutic groups, Bion (1959) provided graphic descriptions of partly conscious and unconscious fantasies—called *basic assumptions*—developed by all members; many of these centered on the leader and her or his relationship to specific members. With respect to families, Lyman Wynne (1958) described— in poignant terms—how families of schizophrenics construct an experiential "rubber fence" around themselves. They struggle to maintain a conception of themselves as harmonious and untroubled families with an indefinite, flexible capacity to exclude from this family self-conception any experience, in themselves or in the outer world, that would contradict this view. Hess and Handel (1959) recognized that intensely subjective "family worlds" characterize the lives of all families, not just clinical ones. Each family has its unique convictions about both its internal workings and the possibilities inherent in the world in which it lives.

The concept of the family paradigm represents a theoretical condensation of many of these lines of inquiry about individuals and about groups. The theory of family paradigms extends this previous work by emphasizing the role of the family in current society and in the development of personal constructs, by relating a broad range of normal, healthy family phenomena to the concept of shared constructions of reality; by specifying particular dimensions along which family paradigms differ; by developing specific methods for assessing these dimensions and their ramifications for families; by accounting for the origins and stability of family paradigms, as well as for their change; and by applying systematically these concepts of shared personal constructs to clinical problems. Most of this work has been summarized elsewhere (Reiss, 1981). Only the last point is relevant to this chapter and will be summarized in the third section.

EVIDENCE FOR THE FAMILY PARADIGM

Entirely by happenstance, a rather eccentric laboratory, problem-solving method, called the *card-sort procedure*, has emerged as a good estimate of aspects of the family paradigm. Although Reiss and his group are exploring a number of other approaches to assessing a family's paradigm, the card-sort procedure remains the most thoroughly investigated effort to operationalize the concept of the paradigm. The card-sort procedure asks each member to sit in an isolated booth in contact with other members by a telephonelike device. Each member is asked to sort one deck of cards (each card containing a patterned sequence of symbols) as an individual and a second deck in concert with his family. The procedure permits measurement of the subtlety of pattern that a family recognizes in the symbols of the cards, the degree to which they work together in the second phase of the task, and the degree to which, either as individuals or as a family group, they change their sorting schemes as new evidence becomes available.

As detailed elsewhere (Reiss, 1981), this procedure was developed for entirely different purposes: to explore the relationship between family interaction and the thought disorder of schizophrenic patients. In the course of early work, it was discovered that most families regularly developed "mistaken" conceptions about what the researcher expected of them. Usually, these conceptions were expressed in the family's "misunderstanding" of experimental instructions. These "misunderstandings," however, turned out to be a gold mine in disguise. For example, all the members of one family regularly misheard the researcher as instructing them that they *must* agree on all phases of the task's solution (when no such instruction had ever been given). This family turned out to be terrified of the whole research procedure, which they viewed as a covert effort to split and thereby humiliate the family. Their "misunderstanding," then, served to enforce family cohesiveness in the face of this perceived threat. Reiss and his group hypothesized that all families had their own intensely personal views of what the research staff was really up to. Even those who trusted the staff seemed to do so on the basis of their own convictions; there was hardly adequate information available to the family for them to test systematically the trustworthiness of the staff. The critical notion was that these misunderstandings, which expressed the family's subjective view of the research project, were vividly portrayed by their task performance, a performance that was easy to measure with precision. An intriguing possibility, still being pursued, is that these perceptions by the family of the research staff are not unique to the research situation but express latent tendencies in the family to construe idiosyncratically all novel or ambiguous circumstances.

This possibility has been pursued in several steps. First, it was important to know if the procedure did yield several dimensions or clusters of behaviors that, on their face, seemed to express theoretically sensible dimensions of the paradigm. This, in fact, has been a repeated finding in the Reiss group (Oliveri & Reiss, 1981b) and in a Hebrew version of the task conducted in Israel (Shulman & Klein, 1982). The pattern-recognizing behavior seems to reflect configuration, the shared pacing reflects coordination, and the ability to respond to new information reflects (delayed) closure. These dimensions are stable for at least 6 to 9 months (Oliveri & Reiss, 1984) and are unrelated to intelligence, education, social class, family size (Oliveri & Reiss, 1981b), a wide variety of individual perceptual styles (Reiss & Oliveri, 1983c), and several personality measures, such as Hogan's measure of empathy and Rotter's internal-locus-of-control scale (unpublished data). Taken together, these data suggest that the card-sorting procedure measures at least three dimensions that are stable over time and that are not simply reflections of individual members' skills or some major social or family structural variables.

Second, it was important to know whether these dimensions did reflect aspects of the family's experience of its personal world. Three studies addressed this inquiry. A projective test, requiring the family to arrange figures of a family, strangers, and geometric figures, suggested that, in the card sort, configuration did indeed express a sense of comfort and mastery, and that (delayed) closure did reflect openness to experience (Oliveri & Reiss, 1982). A second study assessed how the subject families perceived other families in a therapeutic multiple-family group (Reiss, Costell, & Berkman, 1980). The card-sorting configuration was correlated with a detailed and subtle grasp, by the subject families, of the dynamics of relationship in the other families. This coordination was correlated with a view shared by all members of these families. A third study measured the family's view of an inpatient psychiatric service into which an adolescent member had recently been admitted (Costell, Reiss, Berkman, & Jones, 1981). The configuration on the card sort predicted the subtlety of the family's perception of emotional details in the ward's social system, and the coordination predicted the similarity of the family's conception—subtle or coarse—of the social system.

Third, it was important to know that the dimensions of the paradigm, as measured by the card sort, could predict actual transactions of the family with its social community. One critical component of any family's social community is the family's extended kin. Indeed, each of the three dimensions is correlated with theoretically predictable ties to extended kin (Oliveri & Reiss, 1981a). For example, delayed closure, as a measure of openness to diverse experience, correlated with the number and diversity of kin to whom the subject families felt closely tied. The data strongly suggested that it was the paradigm of the subject family that determined its ties to kin rather than the reverse (Reiss & Oliveri, 1983a).

The important role that these processes play in the life (and death) of the family was recently revealed in a startling series of findings (unpublished data). The Reiss group has studied families of patients with end-stage renal disease, patients who require thrice weekly hemodialysis to remain alive. During a year of follow-up observation, delayed closure in families predicted a relative absence of severe medical complications in the renal patient. Paradigm dimensions also predicted the death or survival of the patient. Surprisingly, both high coordination and delayed closure predicted early death of the renal patients. The explanation here seems to depend on the family's social construction of the illness. High-closure families cannot avoid recognizing the immediate and obvious: this illness cannot be mastered. They are overwhelmed by a current reality—in this case, a tragic one—that death is inevitable and inexorable. High-coordination families sense that this death will deprive the family of a piece of itself. Thus, for families high in both delayed closure and coordination at the onset of end-stage renal disease, the illness is indeed terrifying for both family and patient. For families low on both dimensions, the illness is less stressful, and survival, paradoxically, is more likely.

THE FAMILY-CENTERED APPROACH TO PSYCHOPATHOLOGY

Theory is a tool. It is at once a repository and a guide for the future. As a repository, good theory is a condensation of previous ideas, containing propositions grounded in empirical observations and integrating ideas in a systematic way. As a guide to the future, theory specifies the limits of knowledge, forming the most pressing questions and suggesting the methods and techniques for answering those questions. Above all, as both repository and guide, good theory is an intellectual seduction. Good theory is intriguing and beckons searching minds to engage in interactive processes.

One feature of theory that intrigues searching minds is a fascinating phenomenon. We have begun this chapter with three very brief clinical vignettes. Our own understanding of three different families has been helped by our theory of paradigms. It has alerted us to a quality of experience in family life to which other theories are inattentive. We cannot imagine a reader reaching this far in the chapter without being at least a bit intrigued by the phenomena in these case descriptions.

A second source of attraction in good theory is explanation. Good theory relates many things that look different from each other. The searching mind loves and struggles with explanation in an endless dialogue. Its love arises from its wish for order, a deep and profound unseen order that only the intellect— and not the senses—can grasp. At the same time, the searching mind struggles against explanation; it is constantly vigilant against explanation, knowing that, at its core, it is a seductive product of another mind, and not a reality. A searching mind fights off an explanation with counterexplanation. In this struggle between explanation and counterexplanation lies a major building block of exciting science.

Family theories about psychopathology fall heir to the requirements of good theories everywhere. They must address intriguing phenomena and they must explain. In this brief chapter, we have tried to give a sense of what family phenomena are addressed by a theory of paradigms. An intrigued reader is referred elsewhere for a more complete account (Reiss, 1981). What of explanation? Paradigm theory, as an emerging general theory of family process, addresses many interrelated phenomena related to psychopathology. An assessment of its explanatory power rests on a brief survey of the many "loose ends" in psychopathology and related topics that it has attempted to tie together. In all, we have identified four closely interrelated areas addressed by paradigm theory: (a) the pathogenesis of psychiatric disorder; (b) the stability of family patterns over time and their transmission across generations; (c) family coping with routine challenges and severe stress; and (d) the engagement of families in treatment programs and the mechanisms by which their enduring patterns are changed in naturally occurring circumstances or in treatment.

Regarding pathogenesis, a particularly economical approach to research in this area is to identify a variable that is correlated with a particular syndrome, say, schizophrenia, and then to follow these steps to explore its role: (a) Determine, in cross-sectional studies, whether or not the variable is uniquely associated with schizophrenia or whether it is associated, more generally, with many illnesses requiring hospitalization. (b) If it is a relatively specific correlate, determine, from longitudinal studies, whether it predicts the course of the illness in a high-risk population. (c) Scrutinize the existing data, and design new studies to make sure that the variable in question is not an epiphenomenon but is directly linked to the illness (e.g., it is not a proxy for educational level or genetic loading or family size). (d) "Manipulate" the variable to determine its effect on pathogenesis or clinical course; this means "experimentally" changing the variable in families of high-risk individuals to reduce incidence of the illness and making comparable changes in families with an established illness to determine their effects on relapse rates. A strategy of this kind may be termed *variable-centered*. It has been pursued, productively, for example, for the variable "expressed emotion" and its relationship to schizophrenia (see Chapter 11 for a full description of this research).

However, even when this kind of research program has fully traversed the four steps described above, and the "expressed-emotion" (EE) research comes as close as any to achieving just that, many questions are left unanswered. For example, what family processes produce high EE in the first place? Is high EE always a maladaptive process, or does it serve some function for the family (other than the patient)? If we manage to change just that aspect of interaction, does that change pose some risk to the family? How is that risk to be conceived and assessed? When it comes to modifying EE, how is that to be done: by a direct frontal attack on the behavior itself or by a treatment plan that takes account of its origins and functions in family life? Does EE, defined as it is behaviorally, have the same functions in all families (two-parent versus one-parent, one ethnic group as opposed to others, etc.)? Questions of this kind would require, at the least, placing the "variable-centered" strategy in a larger "family-centered" context. Indeed, one can argue that there are advantages to pursuing both a variable-centered and a family-centered approach.

The "family-centered" strategy does not separate pathogenesis as a biopsychological phenomenon from other clinically relevant aspects of family life. The "family-centered" strategy focuses on how families function, attempting to understand pathogenesis as only one aspect of family process. The paradigm model leads to a family-centered research strategy. Thus, in addition to pathogenesis *per se*, we have laid out three other pertinent areas: family stability, family coping and the health and illness of the family system, and the family's engagement in treatment. We believe that a richer understanding of the role of a particular family process in pathogenesis will be best understood in relation to these three additional areas.[2]

---

[2]It could, quite logically, be argued that a fifth area is crucial here: the *origin* of family patterns. That is, a complete family-centered theory should account not only for the relationship between family process and pathogenesis, for the stability of the key family processes, and for how these processes serve adaptive or coping functions and how they influence treatment, but for the very origins of those processes and the mechanisms by which they emerge. Reiss and his colleagues have focused, quite explicitly, on this problem, and some of the work is described later in this chapter. They have considered three possibilities. First, a family's paradigm may emerge from the individual styles of apprehending the universe that are typical of its members. A recently published study (Reiss & Oliveri, 1983) suggests that this is not a fruitful area in which to search for origins. A second possibility is that these patterns are transmitted across generations. A study currently under way is exploring that possibility. A third possibility is that the family's paradigm represents a residue of a particularly calamitous experience or period of time in the family's unique history of development. Reiss (1981) has provided detailed case histories to show how this might be the case. An extended discussion of origins of paradigms, however, seems somewhat tangential to the main thrust of this

Stability

Pathogenic factors in the family are of interest because they are, presumably, enduring. Why do they endure? Perhaps because they serve some adaptive function. Steinglass and his colleagues (Steinglass, Weiner, & Mendelson, 1971) have argued, for example, that alcoholic behavior in families endures because it serves a positive, adaptive function for the family. But the adaptive advantages of a family process suggest only one possible mechanism to account for its endurance. Indeed, the analysis of the stability of a process can be aided by a concept of how family patterns in general are conserved across time and how they are, in many cases, transmitted across generations.

Coping

The adaptive consequence of a family process is related to pathogenesis in a second way. If a family process appears to play a pathogenic role for one member, might it also, at the same time, serve some hidden but important adaptive role for the family or one of its members? For example, Walsh has presented evidence of the possible adaptive significance of mothers' overinvolvement with their children. From one perspective, there is evidence that a mother's overinvolvement may place her child at risk for schizophrenia (Summers & Walsh, 1978). However, Walsh has reported that, in almost half the families in a comparable sample, there was a death of a grandparent at about the time of the child's birth (Walsh, 1978). Thus, it is plausible that the mother's symbiotic ties to her infant represent an attempt to cope with a recent loss.

A related question about the pathogenic family factor is: does it relate to the mechanisms by which the family mobilizes outside resources in the face of stress? For example, using an analysis of the social networks of schizophrenic patients, Hammer (Hammer, Makiesky-Barrow, & Gutwirth, 1978) argued that the communication deviance *internal* to families of schizophrenics may reflect the isolation of the entire family from its social community. In other words, communication deviance may be understood as secondary to a broader defect in family coping, the inability of the whole family to form supportive ties to its social community.

Both these questions raise a third: Is it possible that a family process that is pathogenic for one member serves a positive or adaptive function for another member? Or to phrase the question more broadly, what does the presence of a pathogenic factor imply about the functioning or health of the whole family system? This question requires a conception of health and illness in family systems and a way of relating assessments of health and illness on this level to more specific pathogenic factors viewed from the perspective of the individual patient or the person at risk for psychopathology.

---

chapter. We focus here on the aspects of the model that are most apposite to clinical understanding and decision making. Although the ultimate origins of a family's paradigm are of great theoretical significance, their relevance to pathogenesis is less clear.

Treatment and Change

Our primary interest in identifying pathogenic processes is to alter them to prevent or treat mental illness. An understanding of the relationship between these treatment-related processes, on the one hand, and family coping and stability, on the other, will certainly help in planning and testing rational intervention programs. However, we cannot assume that families will enter willingly into such programs or that, once engaged, they will undergo the requisite changes. Effective treatment programs for pathogenic processes will be best achieved if we understand how they are related to family mechanisms of engagement in or withdrawal from treatment and to family mechanisms favoring or resisting change.

Paradigm theory is a family-centered approach to pathogenesis. As such, it has attempted to relate pathogenesis to stability, coping, and change in family life. It is a new theory, elaborated and explored by a very small team of investigators. It has addressed each of these areas only partially. Below, we address how far has it come, what promises or limitations are already apparent in the work so far reported, and what we may reasonably expect of this approach in the future.

PARADIGM THEORY AND PATHOGENESIS

The design of research on the family's role in the pathogenesis of psychopathology has dramatically improved in the last 15 years. Four advances in particular have enabled investigators to begin to disentangle the central conundrum of cause and effect: Does aberrant family process induce psychopathology, or is it a response to pathology shaped by other factors, or is there a reciprocal relationship between the two? The principal advances have been (a) the use of pseudofamilies to attempt to partial out parent and child effects (the influence of parents on children with whom they interact for the first time in the study—that is, strangers—versus the influence of children on stranger parents) (Liem, 1976); (b) the use of longitudinal designs to determine the temporal ordering of family process and psychopathology (Doane, West, Goldstein, Rodnick, & Jones, 1981); (c) the use of adoption studies, particularly "cross-fostering" approaches, to tease apart the influence of environment and heredity (Wender, Rosenthal, & Kety, 1974); and (d) the availability of powerful new econometric or structural statistical techniques for testing causal models from both cross-sectional and longitudinal data (Kenny, 1979). The paradigm approach has not, as yet, been wedded to these new tools, although one major longitudinal study exploring the temporal ordering of variables in the model is now under way. The paradigm approach has been restricted to cross-sectional studies, studies that compare families with at least one member who has serious psychopathology with families in which the members are free of major psychopathology. The major areas of psychopathology studied in this way are schizophrenia, certain character disorders, and alcoholism. These studies have not sought to clarify the causal nexus of psychopathology. Rather, the paradigm approach has been used to delineate graphically differences among groups of families, differences that may be either the cause or the effect of psychopathology or both. That is, paradigm theory has been useful in the necessary first step in the analysis of pathogenesis: the clarification of the familial correlates of psychopathology, correlates whose position in the causal nexus must still be established.

The Original Studies of Schizophrenia and Character Disorder

At the outset of their work, the Reiss group sought to delineate the critical features of families whose adolescent or young-adult member showed serious psychopathology. The first pilot study contrasted three small groups of families: one of normals; a second of hospitalized impulse-ridden character disorders, who would meet current DSM-III criteria for severe conduct disorder (mostly undersocialized and aggressive) or antisocial personality disturbance; and a third group of families of recent-onset schizophrenics involved in their first or second hospitalization.

Three procedures were used. The first was a hypothesis testing procedure that required the family to form a series of hypotheses in order to discover the underlying pattern in a pattern recognition task (Reiss, 1967). The second, a forerunner of the current card-sort procedure, tested the family's ability to organize information given to them but, in contrast to the hypothesis-testing procedure, did not require them to seek additional information (Reiss, 1968). A third task—presenting a communication problem requiring the family to use a simple, artificial language—assessed the families' effectiveness and strategy in sharing simple information about patterned and structured stimuli (Reiss, 1969). The findings were quite striking, even in this small sample. The families of normals exceeded both other groups in their ability to seek and organize the information available from the experimenter. However, the families of schizophrenics were every bit as good as the families of normals in transmitting information among their members; their deficit was selective: an ability to search for information in the outer world. Families of character disorders showed deficits in both areas. These differences were clearest in the behavior patterns of the families. A large range of measures of verbal interactional style showed few differences among the three groups.

From the outset, Reiss focused on uncovering the subjective experience of the members of these families. What would it be like to be a member, for example, of a family that could not organize or make sense of the external world but in which members were hypersensitive to subtle changes in each other? Reiss suggested that, in these families, each member would come to depend on the action of other members as a principle source of order and predictability; the outside world, by comparison, would be distant, chaotic, and capricious (Reiss, 1970). In families of character disorders, where there was a deficit in processing information from the outer world and from other members, the experience of family membership would be a bewildered loneliness: each member would feel caught up in a isolated, unpredictable world.

These efforts to reconstruct the feelings of family membership fit with some important informal observations in these first studies: the particular misunderstandings of the experimental instructions. For example, talk among members of several families of schizophrenics suggested that they believed the laboratory puzzles had no real solution and that the experimenter had some hidden, undiscoverable intent in requesting the family to participate. Likewise, discussion in some families of character disorders suggested that they viewed the study as a form of intelligence test, pitting one member against the rest to see who was smarter. They had no sense that the family was being observed as a group.

These results and their interpretations, in combination with informal observations, gave birth to the first notions about paradigm. Reiss formulated two hypotheses. First, the families' information-processing styles or deficits were not primary but secondary to their experience of the laboratory. That is, families of schizophrenics entered the laboratory with a conviction that the motives of the staff were undisclosed, undiscoverable, and perhaps sinister. Their information-processing styles were then understandable and, from their perspective, were even an adaptive response: in their view, there was no sense in exploring an outer world because the exploration would never pay off; the inner world was all the family could count on. This formulation would certainly be apt for the Brady family described at the beginning of this chapter. Reiss's second hypothesis was that the family's view of the laboratory was not a product of the unique stresses of a research setting. Rather, it was typical; it was a fair sample of the family's usual experience of novel settings. Thus, the family's response in the laboratory might predict its response in other novel, strange, or ambiguous settings. This second hypothesis has been explored in detail, and the results will be summarized later in the chapter.

Reiss took two follow-up steps after these initial studies. First, he sought to replicate and expand the findings themselves. The three procedures were combined into one, a procedure very much like the current card-sort procedure. The family's effectiveness in processing information outside the family was more clearly conceptualized and operationalized into the dimension of *configuration* (discussed earlier). Skill in processing information within the family was clarified and operationalized as *coordination*. A new dimension was extracted from the original findings and called *closure;* as explained earlier this variable assesses the balance between the family's openness to new experience versus its dominance by tradition (early closure) (Reiss, 1971c,d). This dimension, too, was measurable by the new card-sort procedure. A somewhat larger sample—divided into the same three groups—was recruited. Findings confirmed the first study (Reiss, 1971d). In addition, they suggested premature closure in families of schizophrenics—a dominance by tradition that was central, for example, in the Brady family.

A second step was a beginning effort at disentangling cause and effect in these findings. One distinct possibility, at least for families of schizophrenics, was that their performance in a pattern recognition task reflected a neurologically based thought disturbance. This would be clearest, of course, for the identified patient; many investigators have documented the perceptual and cognitive deficits in these patients (Draguns, 1963; Epstein, 1953; Goldstein & Salzman, 1967;

Payne, Carid, & Laverty, 1963; Salzman, Goldstein, Atkins, & Babigian, 1966; Silverman, 1964). Subtler deficits have also been identified in close relatives (Phillips, 1965; Reiss & Elstein, 1971; Rosman, Wild, Ricci, Fleck, & Lidz, 1964; Wild, Singer, Rosman, Ricci, & Lidz, 1965). When combined with the patients' deficits, these alone might account for the findings. For example, it was possible that a family whose members had information-processing deficits could be more effective when dealing with information being exchanged among members. In this instance, the pacing and style of information transfer among members, parameters entirely under the family's own control, could be accommodated to their deficits. Indeed, Mishler and Waxler (1968) presented evidence of just such a process in families of acute schizophrenic patients. This process alone might account for the relatively good performance of these families on internal communication tasks. In contrast, information from the experimenter would be harder to deal with because its content and pacing could not be expected to accommodate to the deficits of family members; thus, families of schizophrenics would perform poorly on tasks of this kind.

Three studies were performed to rule out this important cognitive-based counterexplanation. First, Reiss and Salzman (1973) produced a short-term information-processing deficit by giving a high dose of secobarbital to an adolescent member in a group of families, some containing a psychiatrically hospitalized adolescent and others with a healthy child. Both groups showed, on the pattern-recognition card-sort, that they could compensate for the loss of cognitive capacities in one member rather than suffer deficits in group effectiveness as a result of his or her incapacity. A second study used a computerized version of the hypothesis-testing task to show convincingly that the information-processing deficits in the family were a product of interaction among the family members and were unrelated to the skills of its individual members (Reiss, 1971a). The computer presented the family with three different versions of the same hypothesis-testing task. The information-processing requirements were identical; they differed only in the degree of contact that members had with each other. It was only in the high-contact condition that families that had showed deficits in the card-sort procedure showed them as well in the computerized procedure. A final study in this series performed an extremely comprehensive evaluation of the attentional capacities and the perceptual styles of each family member and sought to determine whether, singly or in combination, they bore any relationship to problem-solving performance in the card-sort procedure (Reiss & Oliveri, 1983c). The results strongly suggested virtually no relationship between individual perceptual capacities and family problem-solving. Taken together, these findings indicate that a family's performance on the card-sorting task is unrelated to the attentional, perceptual, and cognitive capacities of its individual members. Rather, it is a true reflection of family-level processes that are replicable correlates of specific psychopathological syndromes.

The Association between Low Coordination and Alcoholism

Attracted as much by the methods as the theory, two other groups have used the card-sorting procedure to study families of adult alcoholics. In contrast to the Reiss studies, the identified patient in these samples was a parent rather than a child.

In one study, Steinglass (1979) was interested in variation among alcoholic families. He tested the hypothesis that alcoholic families have difficulty integrating a broad variety of interaction patterns into the stream of their everyday life. Rather, they swing between two states: a "wet" state, which allows certain interaction patterns and styles to emerge, and a "dry" state, in which these themes and patterns are buried behind an entirely different interactional facade. According to this hypothesis, families come to depend on the wet state for the expression of certain feelings (such as angry assertiveness) and for the accomplishment of certain tasks (such as independent problem-solving). However, these never become integrated into or available in the dry state. In this sense, alcoholic behavior serves a limited but important adaptive function for such families. Steinglass recruited a small sample of alcoholic families but found that they did not cycle frequently enough between "wet" and "dry" states to perform the repeated measures on the same sample that were most crucial to his hypothesis. Rather, his sample was divided between families that were wet for most of the period of study and those that, despite a serious history of alcoholism before the study, remained dry. Steinglass found that the wet families were considerably lower on coordination than the dry families.

In the second study, Davis, Stern, Jorgenson, and Steier (1980) compared 50 families of male alcoholics with 50 normal families on the card-sort procedure and a series of other measures. They found that the alcoholic families, particularly the families of severe alcoholics, had low coordination scores. Indeed, among a very large set of scores measuring the family's contact with extended kin, three discussion tasks originally described by Minuchin, Montalvo, Guerney, Rosman, and Schumer (1967), and a detailed questionnaire on the work experience of the husbands, coordination was the most sensitive discriminator between alcoholic and nonalcoholic families.

These data may be consistent with the earlier Reiss findings concerning problem-solving patterns in families with character disorders (DSM-III conduct disorders and antisocial personality disturbances). The mean age of patients in the two Reiss studies was 19. The ages of the identified patient—the adult alcoholic in the Steinglass and Davis studies—were well into middle age. Both groups—the character disorders and the alcoholics—had low coordination. In the Reiss findings, the families of character disorders also had low configuration scores. Steinglass compared the configuration scores of his entire alcoholic sample ("wet" and "dry") with results from the character disorder and normal samples that Reiss had collected and found his group of alcoholics to be very low on this dimension. Moreover, the families of the most severe alcoholics in the Davis study were also quite low on configuration. Is there a connection between these two sets of data? Recall that the identified patients—the character disorders—in the Reiss studies were adolescents, whereas the alcoholics were middle-aged adults (mostly men) in the Steinglass and Davis studies. At least two additional studies suggest that the different studies may have been examining families of identified patients with the same underlying disorder. In an earlier study, Robins (1966) demonstrated that children with severe conduct disturbances often mature into adults with serious alcohol disturbances. More recently, Jessor and Jessor (1975) has shown the same continuity between poor internalized controls and conduct disturbance in early adolescence and significant alcoholic behavior in later adolescence.

Taken together, then, the Reiss, Steinglass, and Davis data suggest that a fundamental disturbance of impulse control—manifested as delinquency in adolescents and alcoholism in adulthood—is associated with low coordination, and probably with low configuration, in the immediate family. It is possible, of course, to use Mishler and Waxler's terms (1968) from an etiological, responsive, or situational perspective to understand these findings. From an etiological perspective, it may be that low coordination and low configuration induce impulse disorders in adolescents. If those adolescents "end up" in similar families as adults, their underlying control problems are further perpetuated as alcoholism. Conversely, from the responsive perspective, impulse-control disorders in either adolescents or adults may induce low coordination and low configuration in families. Equally plausible is the situational explanation: Families of adolescents with conduct disturbances and families of alcoholics are embarrassed by the behavior of their stigmatized member; thus, in a testing situation, out of extreme chagrin, they can neither concentrate nor cooperate.

The Dispersal of Normal Subject Families

An interesting feature of the Davis, Stern, Jorgenson, and Steier (1980) findings was the dispersal of normal subject families. They found that on all three dimensions—configuration, coordination, and closure—normals were rather evenly distributed from low to high values. This finding was confirmed in several additional samples studied by Oliveri and Reiss (1981b). How can these findings be reconciled with Reiss's original findings, in which normal families tended to be high in configuration, coordination, and delayed closure (the "environment"-sensitive type) (Reiss, 1970, 1971d)? Equally important, how can this finding help us understand the role of the family paradigm in pathogenesis?

Reconciliation of the earlier findings with the current findings may be possible from a close examination of differences in sampling procedures. The initial Reiss study (1971d) used a very small sample of normal families that had been recruited in concert with a much larger study of Mishler and Waxler. The families were drawn from two colleges and three churches, and the majority of children and adults had matriculated in or graduated from college. In the second set of Reiss's studies, the families were sampled from a broader variety of community institutions (1971); however, the adolescent in the family was given a searching psychiatric diagnostic interview to rule out detectable psychopathology. In both studies, the families were paid a small fee. The two samples recruited by Oliveri and Reiss (1981b) were sampled by a less exclusive method. PTAs in a number of suburban high schools were asked to recruit families largely by "internal advertising." That is, they publicized the study and a more generous payment for participation; no effort was made to screen out psychopathology in either adults or adolescents. As the Davis group recruited its sample, it made some effort to rule out serious psychopathology through the use of the Michigan Alcoholic Screening test, a questionnaire on psychiatric treatment, and the Hopkins Symptom Checklist. Apparently, only serious disturbance, as revealed by these inexact screening instruments, was enough to exclude a family from the normal sample. Thus, it seems likely that the correlation between "environment sensitivity" and "normality" in the earlier Reiss studies may have arisen from a more carefully selected normal group. In the first instance, college and church participation, coupled with generally high educational achievement, may have signaled families that were particularly oriented toward collaborative mastery of complex social worlds. In the second, the psychiatric interviewer may have been particularly sensitive to the same profile of competence in the adolescent interviewee.

These considerations may explain why the original Reiss studies showed normals as environment-sensitive. It does not fully explain the dispersal of the nonclinical samples in the Oliveri and Reiss and the Davis studies. For example, in the earlier studies, the families of schizophrenic patients showed high coordination, low configuration, and a tendency toward premature closure. The Oliveri and Reiss and the Davis *et al.* (1980) studies found many families of this kind in their nonclinical samples. Despite the absence or inexactness of their screening methods, it is extremely unlikely that there were any schizophrenic patients among the adults or adolescents in these studies. Taken together, these data suggest that the character of the family's paradigm alone is not a correlate of psychopathology *per se*. That is, any particular paradigm may be associated with either psychological health or psychological illness in its members. However, in the presence of a particularly vulnerable member, or overwhelming stress, a particular paradigm may give particular form and shape to a pathological syndrome. For example, a vulnerable child growing up in a high-coordination, low-configuration family may become schizophrenic and, in a low-coordination, low-configuration family, may have a conduct disturbance in adolescence and may become an alcoholic in adulthood.

These considerations clarify further the essential definition of the concept of the paradigm. The paradigm describes, nonevaluatively, variation in a set of coordinated meanings and assumptions in family life. Intrinsically, no paradigm is more adaptive or more health-promoting than another. Psychopathology arises, according to this view, only under two special circumstances: when the paradigm itself begins to disintegrate (see the section below on "Paradigms and Coping" or when one or more individuals is particularly vulnerable—perhaps for biological reasons—to pathological development.

PARADIGM THEORY AND FAMILY STABILITY

We have drawn on data from four separate studies to suggest that the paradigm may play a necessary but not sufficient role in the pathogenesis of specific psychopathological syndromes. For that reason alone, it is important to inquire whether family paradigms are relatively stable over time, and if so, what factors are responsible for their stability. Beyond the specific role of family paradigms, however, our inquiry about the stability of family patterns may be of importance in explaining the stability of other patterns in family life that play a significant role in pathogenesis. In other words, the mechanisms that sustain the paradigm may operate to sustain other family structures and patterns.

First, what is the evidence that paradigms are stable over time? On empirical grounds this issue is just beginning to be explored by the Reiss group. For example, using a small sample of families, Oliveri and Reiss, (1984) compared performance on one form of the card-sort procedure with that on an alternative form six to seven months later. The results were consistent, with considerable to moderate stability across time. The Pearsonian correlations for Time 1 versus Time 2 were .72 ($p < .0001$) for configuration; .86 ($p < .0001$) for coordination; and .43 ($p < .04$) for closure. The average coefficient for all three dimensions was .67, which compares favorably with the average correlation of Time 1 and Time 2 correlations for all 11 scales of the Famijy Environment Scale ($r = .69$) (Moos & Moos, 1976). This scale, a widely used family-assessment questionnaire, was applied to the same sample without the use of an alternate form (thus, the estimates of reliability were inflated because, on the second test, subjects could simply remember at least some of their responses from the previous test). It must be emphasized that this simple test–retest design probably significantly under-estimates the stability of the underlying paradigm, as the Pearsonian coefficients are a result of both the reliability of the procedure and the underlying stability of the variables.

Paradigm theory has postulated that the paradigm, except under extraordi-nary circumstances, is stable across far greater reaches of time: certainly for many years and, in interesting cases, across generations. Paradigm theory has begun to explore three different mechanisms that may account for this stability, and empirical studies are under way to document both the extent of the stability and the mechanisms presumed to underly it.

The Memorial Function of Family Behavior

The first mechanism currently being explored is family behavior itself. Par-adigm theory is among the first theories to develop a morphology of actual family behavior and to inquire systematically into its role in conserving underly-ing structures. Following from the work of Steinglass (1979), Bossard and Boll (1950), Wolin, Bennett, and Noonan (1979), Kantor and Lehr (1975), and Howell (1973), the theory distinguishes between two forms of behavior: pattern regulators and ceremonials. Paradigm theory proposes that each form plays a role complementary to the other in maintaining the family's paradigm.

Pattern regulators are a series of highly routinized behavior patterns in every family that have two primary functions. First, they regulate space: the spatial relationship between the family and the outside world and within the family itself. In the Brady family, Fred's mother took charge—as a pattern of routine barely noticeable to the family itself—of the family's ties to the outer world by answering all incoming phone calls and by being the only newspaper reader. Likewise, the family's traffic pattern required detours around the father's old desk and books, leaving them as a sacrosanct family shrine. These behaviors illustrate the second function of pattern regulators: the regulation of the family's experience of time. In the Brady family, these behaviors reflected the domination of the past, a past in which the father and his medical status loomed large. Indeed, the mother's patterns of separating the family from its present world reinforced this preeminence of the past in the family's life. Pattern regulators are usually simple, highly repetitive behaviors engaged in throughout the day. Although they have an important family function, they often directly involve only one or two members. In many instances, the family is unaware of them, although they may be conspicuous to an experienced outside observer. The work of Steinglass (1979) has demonstrated that behavior of this kind can be objectively, quantitatively, reliably, and validly measured.

A second class of behaviors, termed *ceremonials,* is quite different. They are episodic in nature and are engaged in by all family members. Not only are the ceremonials fully conscious and self-aware, but they are often so engrossing that, for the moment, they blot out all other experiences. Beyond that, families often prize ceremonials as the loftiest expression of family ideals and values; ceremonials of this kind are termed *consecration ceremonials.* A very simple ceremonial is illustrated by the arm wrestling in the O'Hara family. This behavior consecrated the family's sense of its own toughness as well as its view that the world belongs to those who can fight for it. The same little sequence had its degrading aspect as well. For its full expression, the arm-wrestling ceremonial required the mother to witness it, appreciatively but passively. This muted role for her was a subtle denigration. Mrs. O'Hara had a history of episodic and severe depression, which did not meet the family's image of itself as tough and resilient. Even more, a long history of suicide on the mother's side struck at the family's sense of invulnerability and was never mentioned.

Paradigm theory suggests that pattern regulators and ceremonials play complementary roles in conserving the family's paradigm. Ceremonials consecrate some aspects of the family's past and denigrate others to shape a family's sense of itself. In subliminal fashion, pattern regulators convert this subjective identity into the family's shared vision of reality. Paradigm theory posits that both forms of behavior are crucial to the family's maintenance of its paradigm. The ceremonial serves a central function: hidden in its myriad of details are symbolic residues of the family's past as well as a symbolic expression of its convictions about the present. Moreover, ceremonials have a preemptory quality: most families struggle to maintain the central ceremonials of their lives and are willing to lay aside most other activities in their favor. In complementary fashion, pattern regulators transform—for the family—subjective and relative beliefs and values into unshakable convictions. In the Brady family, an annual memorial service in the father's memory would have kept thoughts of him alive. However, traffic patterns and Mrs. Brady's processing of information, both subliminal to the family, conspired to give the Bradys an unassailable conviction that, *in fact,* nothing much had changed for the family since the father's death.

The memorial functions of ceremonials and pattern regulators are just beginning to be explored. The most notable work is by Wolin *et al.* (1979). They have been particularly interested in the relationship between family ceremonials and alcoholism. Following Bossard and Boll (1950), they posited that ceremonials are a primary vehicle by which enduring themes of family life are conserved, not just across the years within a single generation, but from parents to children across generations. They reasoned, then, that if alcoholic behavior in the parent became part of the central family ceremonials (for example, vacation ceremonials or the ceremonial practice of Christmas or Thanksgiving in the home), then the children were much more likely to become alcoholics themselves or to marry an alcoholic; either outcome would express their effort to replicate all aspects of ceremonial life in their family of origin. Wolin and Bennett studied a group of families in which at least one parent was alcoholic. In half of these families, alcoholism had become fully integrated into the main ceremonials of family life, such as annual family reunions, Christmastime celebrations, and religious ceremonies in the home. The remaining families had excluded alcoholic behaviors from these same ceremonies. As predicted, the children in the first group were much more likely to develop alcoholism.

The Family and Its Social World: Organizations and Neighbors

The family must rely on more than the momentum of its own behavior to conserve its paradigm. Indeed, the paradigm is not the exclusive possession of the nuclear family alone. A family's paradigm is, in part, embedded in a set of assumptions about and meanings given to broader social communities. The paradigm is a mechanism by which the family is bonded to its broader social world. Thus far, paradigm theory has considered three components of the family's social world: its kin, its community, and formal organizations, such as schools and places of employment. Extended kin, community, and organization are—according to paradigm theory—governed by their own organizing social constructions. These social constructions have many features in common with the paradigm and have unique features as well. We will consider kinship systems in the next section; we briefly describe communities and organizations here.

Just as a paradigm helps to organize a family around enduring assumptions, so, too, do shared constructions in community life. Paradigm theory refers to these shared constructions as *maps*, following the work of Suttles (1972). The term *map* can be deceiving unless its metaphorical and allusory aspects are grasped. The term refers to a shared experience, by members of a community, of the fundamental layout of the community. We propose that, although the map is experienced primarily in spatial terms, it represents both important experiences in the history of the community and a shared sense of the community held by most of its members.

A detailed explication of the concept of the community map has been published elsewhere (Reiss, 1981). By way of summary, we specify that communities differ in their own rootedness in history (contrast a new suburban subdivision with an ancient cathedral town of Western Europe); in the extent to which their members live their whole life in the community or just come there for limited functions of sleeping and recreation (contrast a small New England village with a condominium community organized for "young singles"); in the extent to which it feels secure or embattled (contrast a prosperous and snug Berkshire town with the black community of Stamps graphically described by Maya Angelou, 1970); and in the extent to which the community feels that it controls its own fate (as in a Vermont town run by its own town meeting) or feels dependent on and totally subordinate to a larger governmental authority (for example, "Spanish Harlem" in New York City or a company coal town in West Virginia). In the experience of its citizens, these differences are represented by a shared conception of space and its properties: who may go where (blacks in Stamps traveled into the white areas at their own peril); who controls critical zones in the community (Hispanics in Harlem feel that the schools are dominated by a white power trust downtown, and West Virginia coal-town residents feel that the "outside" coal company controls "everything in town"); and the symbolism and prestige of particular structures (no man, woman, or child in the town of Chartres fails to grasp the extraordinary blend of history and culture of the town's principal structure). These attributes of the community serve to organize and sustain comparable attributes of the paradigms of the families that constitute the community.

Careful empirical studies of the relationship between community maps and family paradigms have not, as yet, been attempted, although clearly this is an area of great importance for understanding both the stability of the family's paradigm and the family's role in psychopathology. For example, the high rate of psychopathology in migrant families can be understood, in part, with reference to the break up of communities in the old world and the failure of migrant families (with paradigms nourished by their former communities) to "fit" into new communities, with their strange, discordant maps (Howe, 1976). However, empirical research has begun on another form of fit between the family and the social world, that between the family and formal organizations. In contemporary society, the most important formal organizations for the family are the school, the place of employment, the church, the voluntary association (for example, the Elks), and the service organization (such as a psychiatric hospital). Sometimes, the family as a unit participates in the organization (as in some religious congregations). Sometimes, the family may be regarded as sending an "ambassador" (the child has an ambassadorial role in the school setting, as does the breadwinner in the place of employment). As the work of Melvin Kohn (1969) and others have shown, the "ambassador" can serve to transmit influences from home to organization and vice versa.

Following the work of Silverman (1970), paradigm theory proposes a term for the social constructions that regulate formal organizations: the *organizational objective*. For the life of the organization, the organizational objective is the analogue to the paradigm and the map. All organizations have tasks and, in a broad sense, a product. At its core, an organization is structured by the shared definitions—among its members—of what, precisely, that task might be. Close inspection of variations among organizations in how the task is conceived of provides clues to variations in organizational structure and values and in the interaction patterns among the members. Reiss, Costell, and Almond (1976) carried out such a study of two psychiatric hospitals, giving a detailed questionnaire to virtually all patients and staff. The questionnaire sought to delineate each respondent's conception of what mental illness "really is" and of what, as a consequence, the fundamental task (the organizational objective) of the organization should be.

From this work, two major dimensions—orthogonal to each other— emerged that can distinguish among organizational objectives. The first is called *belief in the technical order*. Psychiatric hospitals can be organized around the belief that mental illness is a breakdown in a complex, discoverable *mechanism*. The mechanism may be neurochemical, psychological, or both. The fundamental premise, however, is that this mechanism is discoverable by properly trained experts and that, as research progresses, defects in the mechanism can be treated—also by competently trained professionals. Somatotherapy and psychotherapy by highly trained professionals, then, become the treatment of choice, and the hospital is organized to place these therapies at the center. Its practitioners (usually M.D.'s) are given the most authority and prestige; the rest of the staff and patients are subordinated in a relatively hierarchical arrangement. A contrasting dimension is called *belief in the moral order,* which reflects a view that mental illness arises first and foremost from a breakdown in human relationships, not a failure of an arcane mechanism. At its core, the concept is moral: People have an intrinsic, unquestionable importance to one another. This concept is not an object of research but a universal given of experience. In this view, so-called sociotherapy (which would now include some, but not all, forms of family therapy) is the treatment of choice. The primary qualification for the practice of this form of therapy is personal openness, warmth, and a capacity to engage others. These skills do not reside uniquely in certified professionals but may be possessed by a broad variety of professional staff as well as patients. Psychiatric hospitals high on this dimension are not hierarchically organized. There is a dedifferentiation of authority levels as expressed, in extreme form, in the therapeutic community.

These two dimensions—describing differences among organizations—bear clear conceptual relationships to dimensions of the paradigm: belief in the technical order is parallel to configuration; belief in the moral order is similar to coordination. Paradigm theory has proposed that these dimensions may predict a good or poor fit between an institution and a family. Thus, a low-coordination family entering a high-coordination psychiatric hospital may feel as estranged as a migrant family entering a community with a discordant map. We present evidence, in a subsequent section, that this estrangement places the family at a high risk for retreating from the hospital or dropping out altogether, thereby producing a therapeutic calamity.

The Family and Its Kinship World

A third sector of the family's social universe is its own extended kin. Research on the relationship between a nuclear family and its kin suggests that the ties are active, meaningful, and very useful even if family and kin are separated by great distances (Adams, 1968). Paradigm theory, in accord with these data, sees the kinship world as a vibrant social community that plays an ongoing role in family life in general and in the sustenance of the paradigm, in particular. Briefly, paradigm theory has focused on three different aspects of family–kin ties that stabilize the family's paradigm. The first two factors concern the unidirectional influence of the extended kinship system on the family paradigm. The third factor is posited as more reciprocal: The family has both the initiating and a receiving role.

The first important characteristic is the extent to which the kinship group is organized to protect itself, the extent to which it defends its own interests and its continuity even if this defense conflicts with the broader needs or requirements of the community. This form of kinship system—which jealously guards its material possessions as well as its value orientation—has been called "factional" by Bernard Farber (1981). An example may be found in the organization of traditional Jewish kinship systems, where the transmission of property and values from parents to children is a central preoccupation of family life. It is sustained by traditional Jewish inheritance laws, which, after a surviving spouse, make the children the primary or sole inheritors. This system of kinship organization contrasts sharply with "communal" forms of kinship organization. The primary value in these kindreds is the short-term satisfaction or relationship among members. The primary value is not the transmission of values and property from the older to the younger generation but the promotion of affable and useful relationships among peers. Inheritance patterns do not focus on the children as exclusively; sibs, nephews, and nieces and even aunts and uncles may be inheritors. The ultimate effect of this kinship organization is to promote ties of kin not to each other but to the broader community in which the kindred lives. Paradigm theory specifies that it is the factional kindred—bounded and even defended from the broader community—that exerts the most force on the evolution and maintenance of the paradigm of the nuclear families within it. Reiss and Oliveri (unpublished data) have developed a measure, based on Farber's work, that can distinguish factional from communal kindreds. They are currently testing the basic hypothesis: Paradigms will be more similar among nuclear families within a factional kinship system than among those within a communal system.

However, this hypothesis is only a partial one. It states that factional kinship systems exert more influence on the paradigm and play a greater role in sustaining or stabilizing it. However, it does not clarify any specific influences of the kinship system on the paradigm. For example, we cannot say that paradigms in factional kinship systems are more likely to be high in coordination or, for that matter, in configuration. Unpublished data from a study currently in progress suggest just the opposite: that the full range of variation in the paradigm can be found in both factional and communal kinship systems. Paradigm theory posits a second factor of kinship organization that accounts for a more specific relationship. This component of the theory has been more fully described elsewhere (Reiss, 1981). Briefly, it focuses on what Nagy and Sparks (1973) called the "loyalty code": hidden but powerful rules of obligation that regulate the relationships among all members in a kindred. These obligations do not focus simply on the connections between nuclear parents and children, as in the distinction between factional and communal kindred. Rather, they refer much more broadly to (a) the intensity of material and emotional obligations among all kin; (b) whether some kin can be exempted from these obligations and under what conditions; (c) how emotional or material debts can be paid off; and (d) how much the family's myths and accounts of its own history shape its current conceptions of obligations. Paradigm theory has suggested that it is the nature of these hidden loyalty codes that have more specific influences on the paradigm. For example, in kindreds where loyalty obligations are intense and universal, and no one is exempted, there are more likely to be nuclear families with paradigms high in coordination. Likewise, where a child's obligation to her or his parent can be paid off by success or accomplishment in the outside world, the paradigms will be high in configuration.

A third aspect of kinship plays a reciprocal role in stabilizing and sustaining the paradigm. This aspect concerns the nature of the relationships that the family develops with its extended kin. This aspect of family–kin relationships has been carefully conceptualized and studied by Oliveri and Reiss (1981a) and by Reiss and Oliveri (1983a). Very briefly, they presented evidence that, despite the strong influences of kin on the nuclear family, the nuclear family itself still, on its own initiative, prefers particular members or segments of its kin. Families differ a great deal in how they attach themselves to the wider kin group. Oliveri and Reiss (1981a) focused on three dimensions describing this variation: (a) the breadth and diversity of kin with whom members of the same nuclear families had important ties; (b) the extent to which all members of the nuclear family formed strong ties to the same (or different) kin; and (c) the extent to which a nuclear family formed close ties with that part of its kinship system where kin were closely bound together or where kin were, emotionally speaking isolated from one another. Variations along these three dimensions were closely linked to the three dimensions of the paradigm. For example, families whose paradigm showed delayed closure, suggesting an openness to a breach of experience, had a greater breadth and diversity of ties to kin (often, for example, choosing kin from both the maternal and the paternal wings of the family). Reiss and Oliveri (1983a) presented data that supported a reciprocal mechanism in these ties: Families with a particular paradigm form ties consistent with that paradigm, but these ties serve to reinforce or stabilize the paradigm itself. Thus, delayed-closure families pick a broad and diverse set of kin with whom to have important relationships, and this diversity and breadth, in turn, sustain the delayed-closure characteristics of their paradigm.

The preceding description of factors that stabilize the family paradigm not only summarizes an important part of paradigm theory but also suggests how paradigm theory can lay the groundwork for clinical practice. For the clinician, it provides a systematic guide to understanding both family vulnerability and therapeutic change. With respect to vulnerability, this section has highlighted the factors that are required to sustain a family's paradigm. A family without a sustained and nourished paradigm is subject to a variety of uncertainties, internal conflicts, and crises. Thus, paradigm theory suggests specific environmental factors that may contribute to disequilibrium in families, in family–kin ties, and in the relationship of the family to its immediate community, and to problems in the articulation of organizational and family life. In addition, paradigm theory offers the family therapist a systematic guide to strategies for the therapeutic restructuring or strengthening of family paradigms. That is, paradigm theory points to the kind of fit between family and social environment that would support positive therapeutic outcomes. In this connection, it holds promise for clarifying the ecological perspective in family therapy, aimed at enhancing the interrelations of the family and its social environment. The strength of paradigm theory is in its specificity: it clarifies that specific kinds of families fit best with specific kinds of social "ecologies." It provides theoretically derived dimensions for assessing both family and ecology, as well as an emerging set of methods for measuring those dimensions.

PARADIGMS AND COPING

In the previous section, we presented both theory and data exploring factors that maintain paradigm stability. We have focused on two sets of factors. The first is a complementary relationship between two types of family behavior: pattern regulators and ceremonials. The second is the intricate, many-stranded bond between the family and its social world. These concepts provide the foundation for paradigm theory's hypothesis concerning family coping. In broad strokes, these conceptions of stability give us tools to understand stress and coping *as they occur in families*—rather than in individuals. They also provide a frame for conceptualizing relative levels of health and illness of the family as a system. In brief, family coping is directed at any event or chain of events that either disrupts pattern regulators and ceremonials or disarticulates the family from the particular bonds to its social world required to sustain its paradigm, or both of these.

As a first line of defense, families attempt a series of coping strategies aimed at restoring the integrity and stability of their paradigm. It follows that families with different paradigms use different coping strategies and that a knowledge of a family's paradigm will enable us to predict, quite specifically, its coping strategies in the face of stress. As we will show, paradigm theory also posits that successful coping, in and of itself, reinforces the family paradigm; successful coping with stress, then, is really a third mechanism for stabilizing the paradigm.

Finally, if coping fails, the family progressively disintegrates through a series of recognizable stages. At each stage, major opportunities for self-healing are available to the family, but if these mechanisms fail, the family retreats to the next lowest level until either dissolution or paradigm change is the only viable alternative. In this section, we will summarize paradigm theory's approach to coping and will present briefly its three stages of health and illness of family systems. The topic of change, in extreme family crisis, belongs to the subsection on "Treatment and Family Change."

Family Stress

A major conundrum in conceiving of and studying a family's response to stress is defining and measuring the events and circumstances that are stressful to families. A variety of previous attempts, reviewed in Hansen and Johnson (1979) and in McCubbin, Joy, Cauble, Comeau, Patterson, and Needle (1980), have all stumbled on the same obstacles. A stressful event, according to all these approaches, must be ultimately defined only by its impact on the family. That is, we have no way of anticipating whether an event will be stressful to a family until it occurs and we can ask the family how they feel about it and watch how they respond. From both a research and a clinical perspective, this is an obvious predicament.

Paradigm theory has taken a different tack. It posits a two-stage process. The first concerns the *likelihood* that an event or circumstance will be stressful for a family. The second concerns the direct assessment of the *magnitude* of stress engendered by a particular event in a particular family. The first stage entirely bypasses the usual dilemma of relying on the family's perceptions or responses to define stressful events or circumstances. The second stage provides a theory-guided approach to assessment of the magnitude of stress that is broader than most previous efforts.

To estimate the likelihood that an event will be stressful, Reiss and Oliveri (1983b) took a community-based perspective. Following from the work of Goffman (1974), and using the basic conceptual tools of paradigm theory, Reiss and Oliveri proposed that social communities (for example, hospital communities, professional or workplace communities, or neighborhood communities) provide a frame for understanding the meaning and potential threat in virtually any event or circumstances. For example, the work of Scotch (1963) showed that traditional Zulu communities regarded childbirth as a nonstressful blessing that demonstrates a woman's fertility in a traditional culture in which fertility was highly valued. In sharp contrast, urban Zulus were threatened by childbirth because it increased considerably the strain on their marginal capacities to adjust to a strange, new world.

Not only does the community provide a frame for judging the threat in any event, it provides a frame of expectations for each family of what coping—if any—they are responsible for in responding to the event. For example, the communal healing rights of the traditional Navaho clarify that it is the community's, not the family's, responsibility to support and heal the physically ill. In an effort to explore this hypothesis about stress empirically, Reiss and Oliveri studied a group of 48 families from a hemogeneous suburban community and found very high agreement among them in their rating of the threat to families inherent in a large list of events and in the family's accountability for the event. The very high levels of agreement suggested that there was, indeed, a common community frame for evaluating events.

Paradigm theory offers a guide to the systematic assessment of the magnitude of stress engendered by a particular event or circumstance for a particular family. This approach is based on a proposal that an event will be stressful to the family in direct proportion to its impact on organizing and governing structures—in this case, its paradigm. A knowledge of those factors that sustain the family's paradigm leads logically to a scheme for evaluating those factors that threaten it. Thus, it follows that an event is stressful if it interferes with pattern regulators or ceremonials, on the one hand, or the family's bond to its social world (kin, community, organization, etc.), on the other. For example, chronic illness seems to have such a devastating impact on families at least in part because it profoundly distorts and circumscribes the family's daily patterns and ceremonial life. Likewise, migration or natural disasters have their impact, in part, through disrupting the family's bonds to its social world.

Family Coping

Once a family endures significant stress, its first line of defense, according to paradigm theory, is a collective response that, to borrow a rather inadequate term from the genre of individual studies, may be called *coping*. Following from the work of Dewey (1910), Brim (1962), Argyris (1965a,b), and Aldous (1971), paradigm theory has proposed that a family's response to any event or circumstance may be divided into three phases. First, the family defines the event and searches for additional information: Is the event a routine or a problem one? Is it the family's fault, or does it come from outside? Does the family have a responsibility to deal with the event? Then, the family makes an initial response and or fashions several trial solutions. Finally, the family comes to a closing position: If the event has been conspicuous, this process includes the integration of the event and the family's responses to it into the family conception of its own history. These shared memories of the family's response to stress may serve as a guide for future action. These phases may overlap and may occur in any order.

Paradigm theory has proposed that a family's coping responses to stress are determined by its cognitive and emotional appraisal of the event or circumstance, of the efficacy of its own responses, and of the relationship of the event to the family's conception of its own development (Reiss & Oliveri, 1980). This process of appraisal is similar to those we have already described as shaped by a family's paradigm. Thus, the three dimensions of paradigm—configuration, coordination, and closure—should each determine how the family copes in each of the three phases of their response. Table 1 summarizes these proposals. For example, families high in configuration feel a sense of volition, confidence, and potential mastery in ambiguous situations, including stressful ones. They are likely to own up to their responsibility to deal with most stressful events based on a conviction that the family, through its own efforts, can master them. With this basic objective, they will vigilantly search for information, will initiate many trial solutions, and, once they have coped with the event, will take credit for their own success. This process leads to an enrichment of the family's conception of its own vigor, imaginativeness, and competence. Families high in coordination will, in the first phase, see the event as relevant to all members. In these families, members will quickly integrate their own coping efforts with those of others, and

TABLE 1. Hypothesized Influence of Family Paradigm Dimensions on the Three Aspects of the Family's Response to Stressful Events[a]

Paradigm dimensions		Definition of the event and search for additional information	Phases of family coping	
			Initial responses and trial solutions	Final decision or closing position and family's commitment to this
Configuration: Mastery	High	1. *Owning up.* Family takes responsibility for event and/or coping.	2. *Exploration.* Family's initial responses are designed to seek information and outside resources or are in response to information and outside support.	3. *Response to outcome.* The family is proud of accomplishment or feels it has learned something of value in failure.
	Low	Family feels victimized and blames outside forces.	Initial reactions are unrelated to information or explanation.	The family feels fortunate if successful or victimized if not.
Coordination: Solidarity	High	4. *Family identity.* Readily perceived as family issue; information exchanged quickly.	5. *Organization or response.* Organized, integrated response by all family members; roles are clear.	6. *Consensus on decision.* Decision was reached with clear consensus and family remains committed to it.
	Low	Slowly or not perceived as family issue; information exchanged slowly; events are seen as happening to individual members.	Individuals act on own; overt or covert conflict possible.	The consensus was forced on the family by a single individual; the status of agreement is unclear, or no consensus is reached.
Closure: Openness	High (delayed)	7. *Reference to the past.* Focuses on current experiences; past family history unimportant.	8. *Novelty of responses.* First responses include trying something new; individual experiences, intuitions, and guesses are encouraged.	9. *Self-evaluation.* As a result of coping, family alters conception of itself in some way.
	Low	Past determines current perception and action; little interest in raw experience; more interest in convention or tradition.	First responses mostly typical or familiar.	As a result of coping, family confirms conception of itself.

[a]From "Family Paradigm and Family Coping: A Proposal for Linking the Family's Intrinsic Adaptive Capacities to Its Responses to Stress" by D. Reiss and M. E. Oliveri, 1980, *Family Relations, 29,* 441. Copyright 1980 by National Council on Family Relations. Reprinted by permission.

consensus will loom large in the family's closing position. Finally, delayed-closure families will, in the initial phase, focus on current experience rather than using the past as an orientation. They will continually develop new repertoires of responses to crisis rather than depending on previous patterns. Integrating their experience of stress will lead to change in their conceptions of themselves, in contrast to early-closure families, which see in their response to stress a confirmation of their previous conceptions about themselves.

Oliveri and Reiss (unpublished results) have begun to explore this model empirically. They have already shown that it is possible to use standardized, structured family interviews to reconstruct, in detail, the three phases of the family's response to a stressful event. Coders can reliably identify the kinds of coping responses summarized in Table 1. Finally, on a completely blind basis, it has been possible to successfully postdict many of the details of the family's coping response from knowledge of their paradigm as determined by the card-sort procedure. For example, families that scored high on configuration in the laboratory can be distinguished from those that scored low in their detailed reports of how they coped with a stressful life event. High-configuration families become more fully engaged in actual coping responses, more thoroughly organize themselves as a group, altered their responses based on new information, and regard their efforts to cope with a difficult event as an experience from which they can learn something valuable.

Failures of Coping and Stages of a Family's Collapse

What constitutes successful family coping? Paradigm theory argues that a central measuring-rod is the state of the paradigm itself. When daily routines and family ceremonies are restored, and the family rearticulates with its social community, the paradigm returns to its protected status and occupies its typical background position in family life, affording each member a shared conviction in a lively and vivid external reality. Thus, a simple answer is: Coping is successful when family behavior and social bonds are restored. What happens if coping is not successful? Paradigm theory, following from the concepts of Kantor and Lehr (1975), has proposed a series of three stages. In each stage, the family attempts to restore the ordinary routines of daily life and its critical bonds with its social world. If these efforts fail, the family descends to a more serious stage of group dysfunction. The theory is still very schematic—barely a scaffolding for future theoretical and empirical work. The three stages are called *emergence of rules*, the *explicit family*, and *rebellion and action*. Each is defined by typical family behavior and dysfunction, by the major strategies available to the family for self-healing, and by the status of the paradigm.

Emergence of Rules. Ordinary family coping blends imperceptibly into this stage. When stress is chronic and the family's initial coping strategies are unsuccessful, coping responses begin to harden. Rather than becoming flexible and responsive to the demands of the stressful event or circumstance, behaviors become more entrenched and established. The responses become constraints that each member places on the others. They may be explicit and carefully designed or haphazard, implicit, and partially concealed. In either case, these rearrangements burden each family member with additional imperatives or requirements; therefore, following Ford and Herrick (unpublished 1972 paper), we refer to them as *rules*.

All rules that are developed when a family is in an early stage of crisis probably have two objectives: adaptation and constraint. Rules can permit a family to come to grips with the stress. Consider, for example, the James family. It consisted of two parents, a daughter (Marilyn, aged 16), and a son (aged 10). When they were traveling in a foreign country where only the daughter knew the language, they developed a simple rule: "Each time we deal with an official, Marilyn must be with us." This simple rule allowed the family to adapt to an unfamiliar and potentially difficult situation.

A rule of a different quality was formulated in the Michaels family. This was a well-to-do family consisting of a father, a mother, the father's mother, and two boys, 9 and 11 years old. The father was killed in an automobile crash. After the period of acute grief, several rules began to emerge. The first was motivated by the family's heightened fear that yet another member would be killed in some sort of accident: "Neither child is allowed to go out of the house unless accompanied by an adult."

The Explicit Family. Some rules are adaptive. They solve problems and then disappear. Others are not adaptive; they beget other rules, as in the Michaels family. The adults did not recover from their depression and remained drained and without energy. A second rule soon developed: "Everyone in this household should make his or her own breakfast." As the days wore on, yet another rule—more implicit than the previous ones—developed: "The children should not make demands on the adults for anything." From the adults' perspective, any demands by a child were an oppressive intrusion. From the children's perspective, any request led to frustration. All family interaction constituted a burden. Indeed, the family itself came to be experienced as an opaque burden, disowned by its members. The paradigm had been transformed from a background assumption giving meaning and vitality to the full range of external experience; it was becoming an externalized and disowned tyrant.

Just as the stage of family rules provides an opportunity for family reorganization and self-healing, so does the stage of the explicit family. The emergence of rules can, as it did in the James family, constitute the basis of an adaptive strategy. The emergence of the explicit family begins a process in which each individual partitions himself or herself from the family. This is an illusory partition, of course, because each member is projecting aspects of himself or herself onto a reified entity termed "my family." Nonetheless, this illusory partition frees each individual for action. As we will see in the next stage, some of this action may be destructive, but some of it may be constructive in crucial ways.

Rebellion and Action. This stage is a continuation and exaggeration of the last, but it is more grotesque and dangerous. Each member has participated in the creation of an illusory family, which takes on its own vivid reality. It is illusory because many members are disowning it as if they had no part in its creation, but a few others may be taking it within themselves, holding themselves fully responsible for its major characteristics. The family is not just explicit but is experienced, in some sense, by all members as tyrannical. The usual mode of experiencing at this stage, however, is not for each member to feel that the family as a whole is a tyrant. Often, one spouse feels that the other has become an oppressive burden. Usually, the least accepted part of one spouse projects the least accepted aspects of itself onto the other in what Wynne (1965) called the "trading of dissociations." A similar process from parent to child has been delineated as "projective identification" by Zinner and Shapiro (1972). Often, an individual or a subgroup in the family is scapegoated and hounded out of the family.

Two major possibilities seem to lie before a family at this stage. Perhaps the more expectable one is that the family continues to disintegrate. A scapegoated child may be extruded, and the marital couple may break up. What is perhaps more interesting, however, is the possibility of self-healing at this stage. Paradigm theory proposes that some families reaching this crisis point can make major qualitative changes. At this point, the family is particularly open to new, outside influences. These experiences may include a fresh and novel involvement with large segments of the social world, leading, ultimately, to new visions of the possibilities inherent in that world. Or outside influences may enter the family through new relations with outside individuals. The deepening crisis has, in effect, opened the family in this way. The old paradigm is in tatters. As the family's ceremonials and more routine patterns have been disrupted, its sense of itself and of the cardinal realities of its world has weakened. Members are no longer integrated with one another in the subtle and implicit task of reaffirming family convictions and of maintaining the family's usual distance from or closeness to the outside world. Members shift more radically from feeling a part of the family to feeling enclosed in the outside world itself. In this unstable state, individuals may attempt quick alliances with others who are brought into the family in an effort to produce some change.

Treatment and Family Change

We have argued that an advantage of the family-centered approach is that it embraces in one perspective concepts of pathogenesis and treatment. Thus, it is particularly important to review, however briefly, the contributions of paradigm theory to concepts of treatment. Some years ago, W. Ross Ashby (1975) made the influential distinction between first- and second-order change in living systems. Applied to families, first-order changes are relatively modest alterations of family patterns to adjust to short-range events and circumstances. Second-order changes are more profound shifts in long-term patterns of reactions, perceptions, experience, and interaction patterns. This distinction is applicable to the concepts about treatment that paradigm theory has explored.

In the previous section, we considered an instance of first-order change in families: the accommodations and coping strategies that they develop in the face of stress. These are temporary and situation-dependent and, in most instances, return the family to its previous balance. More closely related to the therapeutic process are analogous first-order changes: the family's approach to engagement in or disengagement from the therapeutic encounter is a stressful event for the family. The family's response to this encounter calls into play a variety of coping responses that are, in turn, determined by its paradigm. As in more ordinary coping, the family's responses to the encounter are a mixture of their experience of the encounter and their initial efforts to respond. Thus, as in ordinary coping, it is reasonable to expect that both the family's actual responses in a therapeutic encounter and its experience of that encounter will be shaped by its paradigm.

Reiss, Costell, and their associates sought to examine this hypothesis empirically with a detailed laboratory and field study of 32 families entering an inpatient, family-oriented treatment program for troubled adolescents (Costell *et al.*, 1981). The families were tested on the card-sort procedure, and detailed measurements of their engagement with the ward therapeutic community were made during the following weeks. Reiss and Costell used paradigm theory to generate a number of predictions about engagement as perceived by trained observers, other families, and the subject families themselves.

In this work, the families were grouped into types according to their scores on two of the dimensions: configuration and coordination. Closure was not studied. Following from earlier work, families high on both coordination and configuration were termed *environment-sensitive* because their dominant style was to work collaboratively to explore the full range and subtlety of their social world. Paradigm theory predicted that these families would form strong relationships with other families, would be highly regarded by them, would feel integrated into the ward community, and would be sensitive to subtle emotional cues and variations in the ward's social atmosphere; the findings confirmed these predictions.

Consensus-sensitive families were those low on configuration and high on coordination. These were families that used consensus to protect themselves from the outer social world, from which they felt estranged and threatened. It was expected that these families would be insensitive to subtle cues in the environment and would draw tight boundaries around themselves (as measured by seating position and sociometry). These predictions were confirmed. However, these families showed a greater sense of involvement in the treatment program and were more highly valued by other families than the theory predicted.

Achievement-sensitive families were high on configuration and low on coordination; in general, these were highly competitive families whose members sought to establish themselves firmly in the outer social world but did so competitively with other members of their family rather than cooperatively, as did environment-sensitive families. Paradigm theory correctly anticipated that these families would be unable to develop a shared view or evaluation of the ward community (as measured by a special Q-sort procedure), but that each member would be sensitive to subtle emotional cues in the ward atmosphere. Contrary to predictions, this group also felt estranged from and uninvolved in the treatment program.

Paradigm theory predicted the largest problems for a fourth group, the *distance-sensitive* families. These families, low in both coordination and configuration, consisted of members isolated from one another who also felt awash in a dangerous, incomprehensible social world (recall the Ramos-Anthony-Cooper family at the start of this chapter). Indeed, these families were hardly noticed by other families, their attendance at therapy sessions was poor, they felt the ward to be a dangerous place, and they felt estranged from both other families and the staff. Although none formally dropped out of the program, they seemed to be the group in greatest danger of doing so.

Overall, in these studies, the role of coordination played a particularly conspicuous part and led to a revision of some of paradigm theory's assumptions in this area. According to a revised view, in a family-oriented inpatient service, presumed to be high on the dimension of belief in the moral order, highly coordinated families fit into the social community quite well: they were valued by other families, and they felt safe and integrated into the community. Configuration played a less important role than anticipated. Initially, paradigm theory failed to take the social constructions of the treatment community into account in making its predictions about the engagement of different types of families. It now seems plausible that, had the inpatient service been high on belief in the technical order, the theory might have selected as the "best fitting families" those higher in configuration. With respect to family therapy, in particular, these results can be stated differently. High-coordination families have a clear conception of themselves as an integrated group. In all settings, they *expect* to be treated as a group. They feel particularly comfortable, then, in settings that *do* treat them as a group. It follows that high-coordination families will enter family therapy by making only first-order changes; that is, their successful engagement in family therapy does not require major shifts in paradigm. From the outset, low-coordination families must make a profound second-order change to be successfully engaged in family therapy at all. As a consequence, they pose an immediate challenge to the therapists and may not stay in treatment long enough for them to perform their magic.

These distinctions among families raise the question of second-order change in families as it occurs naturally or in the course of family therapy. In the previous section, we presented paradigm theory's conception of second-order change: Paradigm shifts occur only when the family has passed through the stages of paradigm collapse, that is, first, the emergence of rules, then the explicit family, and finally, rebellion and action. Each member must go through a process of divesting himself or herself of the old paradigm. The family must be seen as an external thing and then as a dangerous tyrant that is, in the end, attacked or defended against with outside help. It is at this juncture that paradigm theory significantly overlaps clinical practice. For example, in his powerful interventions with families of anorexic adolescents, Minuchin seemed to engender—through therapeutic artifice—this form of sequential crisis.

A CRITICAL ASSESSMENT OF FAMILY PARADIGM THEORY

The greatest achievements of any science are its discoveries. Of nearly equal importance are the attempts to disconfirm, discredit, or overturn those discoveries. Earlier, we referred to the interplay of explanation and counterexplanation. More generally, we would argue that knowledge advances to the extent that crucial doses of both commitment and skepticism are attached to lines of inquiry. This dualism is at the core of Popper's critical philosophy of science (1959). According to Popper, science advances by a series of conjectures and refutations. The most worthy ideas are those that have been tested and have not yet been rejected, those that have tentatively passed the scrutiny of the critical intellect.

The first step in the process of refutation is to identify those aspects of an idea that appear to be most vulnerable to criticism. The second step is to design research aimed at the disconfirmation of those aspects. At this juncture, we believe that five features of family paradigm theory may be most vulnerable to criticism: (a) the specification of paradigm dimensions and types; (b) link between cognition and behavior in the theory and the role of awareness; (c) the collectivistic assumption rooted in the idea that paradigms are shared by family members; (d) the tension between paradigm change and stability; and (e) the fusion of theoretical traditions. We do not wish to argue that these vulnerabilities have already weakened the credibility of the theory. Rather, we discuss them to raise issues that remain unresolved and that might well lead to critical research and eventually to refinements of the theory or to its replacement by a more adequate alternative.

Dimensions and Types of Family Paradigms

Research to date using the card-sort procedure has yielded three paradigm dimensions, as described earlier in this chapter. Comparisons across families have produced sufficient variation in scores on these dimensions so that the scores may be broken into categories or arrayed along a continuum, depending on one's research purpose. If scores on each dimension are randomly distributed or are equally likely for some other reason, and if the dimensions are truly independent, as the past experience of the Reiss group suggests, then there should be a great variety of family paradigms, each based on a unique clustering of scores on the three dimensions. Early studies by the Reiss group pointed not toward a large number of paradigm types but to three prevalent types. To some extent, the isolation of these three has been a matter of analytical economy and not a denial of the possible existence of other combinations of scores on the dimensions. Dichotomizing and cross-classifying the three cardinal dimensions yields eight types of families, and in some studies, an "achievement-sensitive" pattern has been isolated among families who score high on configuration but low on coordination (Reiss, 1981).

It seems clear to us that further research is required to establish the range and prevalence of different paradigms based on the three dimensions of configuration, coordination, and closure. It may turn out that some combinations are rare because of skewed or unequal variances in measures, requiring a revision of the assumption that the dimensions are empirically independent. For example, there is already the interesting suggestion that the dimensions serve different functions for different families. Among other unexpected findings, the families of schizophrenics have been shown to exhibit negative correlations between their configuration and coordination scores, whereas families of "normals" show positive correlations (Reiss, 1971b). This finding could mean that coordination impedes configuration in the families of schizophrenics and enhances configuration in normals. Thus, when subject populations are more narrowly defined, the paradigm dimensions may lose their independence from one another.

Furthermore, if we view the history of psychopathology as having produced a catalog of qualitatively distinct syndromes with some taxonomic features, then the question arises: Which particular paradigm is associated with which particular pathology? Although the Reiss team has begun to examine these connections, we suspect that the search will be facilitated as greater paradigm variety and precision are built into the theory to match the current complexity of conceptual schemes for identifying psychopathogenic disorders. It is possible that more than a small number of paradigms will need to be identified.

To date, the primary research tool used to measure family paradigms has been the card-sort procedure. Compared with most techniques commonly used in social and clinical research, the card-sort procedure is relatively dependent on a mechanized technology. The partitioned booth and the electronic communication and recording devices are not especially complicated, compared with other laboratory setups for the study of human social behavior, but they do not have the flexibility of survey methods or the semistructured interviews often used in case studies. Moreover, social scientists are now fascinated by either the technical feats of large-scale survey research or the charms of "naturalistic" observations. The laboratory is suspect because it cannot use random samples and is patently artificial. The result is that few researchers outside the Reiss group have used the procedure, and consequently, independent corroboration or refutation of findings by other research teams has been slow to develop.

Perhaps the most critical issue raised by this situation is whether research on family paradigm theory has, to date, been method-dependent. A theory is most compelling when different research teams and different methods fail to disconfirm the theory. It is conceivable, for example, that family paradigms have more than three dimensions but that the card-sort procedure is sensitive enough to detect only the three that have so far been identified. Family paradigm theory can be viewed as a serendipitous emergent from repeated use of a particular research technique. Now that the theory has taken shape, it is time for other research strategies to be used to assess the degree of its methodological dependence. Not only might such an assessment yield insights about paradigm dimensions thus far unrecognized, but it might also shed light on the circumstances under which the various dimensions are salient.

It seems possible, for example, that a property like family coordination is activated only in peculiar situations, such as when some problem is articulated and when the family feels compelled to respond but the situation appears ambiguous (Reiss, 1981). There is already considerable research evidence that coordination is task-specific (Klein & Hill, 1979). Some problems can be solved by individuals working alone, whereas others require information to be shared. Furthermore, coordination can take many forms. At one extreme, it requires that family members be as similar as possible in skills, and at the other, it calls for a strict division of labor according to individual differences in skill level and areas of assumed competence. If coordination is such a rich and multidimensional concept, we will need measures that capture this complexity.

Is it possible that unobtrusive measures of routine family interaction will yield patterns suggestive of paradigms? Other researchers have cautioned that, when subjected to naturalistic observation, families virtually "melt away" (Patterson, 1982, p. 48). It may not be so much that interviews and passive observations are "too cumbersome and subjective for . . . quantitative effort(s)" (Reiss, 1981) as that they reveal a sort of family reality different from the one hypothesized by paradigm theory.

Another possibility suggested by the above considerations is that families have repertoires of paradigmatic thought and action. Different paradigmatic stances may be evoked in different situations, and if the card sort procedure is situation-specific, it may have limited value in capturing the range of repertoires in a given family. For example, we mentioned earlier that there may be a "wet" and a "dry" paradigm in alcoholic families. It would also seem consistent with other clinical and developmental research to expect that certain forms of pathogenesis are associated with paradigmatic rigidity (limited and inflexible repertoires). The family that resists change in the face of a novel situation may be as much at risk of psychopathology as one that loses its sense of orderliness in the environment.

Cognition, Behavior, and Awareness

The core concept of the family paradigm refers to patterns of cognition, to what we called "underlying assumptions about reality" earlier in this chapter. *Cognition* here does not refer to a narrow rationalistic and dispassionate notion of pure reason. Instead, paradigm theory defines shared experiences as being assumptions, constructs, fantasies, sets, or expectations (Reiss, 1981). To put it slightly differently, a paradigm is a deep-seated and persistent attitude or a set of assumptions about the family's social and physical world (Reiss, 1981).

If we keep this definition in view, a curious anomaly arises. The card-sort procedure measures overtly observable patterns of behavior (or performance) and not beliefs, assumptions, or any of the other terms in the definition of a paradigm. The Reiss group has been willing to assume that behavioral indicators can be used, at least indirectly, to tap phenomena that are essentially mental. This assumption has not been adopted naively. The cognition–behavior linkage has been controversial throughout the history of the social and behavioral sciences and has occupied a great deal of attention. The Reiss group has moved cautiously here and has generally taken the position that it is inadvisable to ask family members about their paradigms because these paradigms may exist beyond the realm of awareness or consciousness. Moreover, the Reiss group has begun to explore the relationship between behavior in the card sort and more direct assessments of assumptions, attitudes, perspectives, and feelings in family life (Costell *et al.*, 1981; Oliveri & Reiss, 1982; Reiss, Costell, Berkman, & Jones,

1980). Our collective heritage of clinical wisdom certainly suggests that people are not always aware of their own motives and beliefs or, at least, are not always able or willing to articulate them.

The issue of correspondence between cognition and behavior probably needs to be addressed more directly, however, and to be applied to tests of family paradigm theory. If families cannot describe their paradigms, what advantage is gained by casting these paradigms in essentially cognitive terms? How can families have assumptions about reality and not be able to express them? Take the dimension of configuration, for example. We defined it earlier in this chapter in terms of perception and belief about the lawfulness of the experienced world. Research is only now emerging on the measurement of configuration in terms of self-description about these perceptionor beliefs (Costell *et al.*, 1981). Hence, family paradigm theory appears still to be vulnerable to the criticism that there is a lack of fit between conceptualization and operationalization. The core concepts are defined cognitively but, for the most part, measured behaviorally.

One way to rectify this problem would be to design interviewing strategies to directly measure perceptions and beliefs and to compare the results with those obtained from behavioral indicators such as the card-sort procedure. Another approach would be to explore those conditions in which self-reports about paradigm dimensions can be trusted as reliable and valid. The development of rapport or the strategy of persuading clients or subjects that the interviewer shares their paradigm or at least respects it may be required to discover otherwise concealed beliefs and assumptions.

Our use of vignettes at the beginning of this chapter suggests that much can be learned about family paradigms by directly observing family interaction, supplemented by in-depth interviewing. The descriptive vignette is not just a sensiziting tool. We expect it to add to the credibility of paradigm theory, in part because the research methods that produce it are acceptable. What remains to be examined in how the O'Hara family, for example, would perform on the card-sorting task. If the family comes out scoring high on configuration, we will have increased confidence in *both* methods. If not, at least the problem of method-dependence will have to be confronted. It must be emphasized that the vignettes provided in this chapter are the result of detailed clinical knowledge of the families described, knowledge acquired over weeks and months of working with these families. To some extent, the process of clinical discovery in these cases represented, in informal ways, the interviewing strategies that we are recommending here. In fact, work is beginning in this direction. The Reiss group has reported on the blind and systematic classification of abbreviated clinical vignettes and the relationship of this classification to families' performance on the card sort (Costell & Reiss, 1982). The blind classifications were made with a high degree of success and fit with expectations derived from paradigm theory.

Whether observations and reports of family activity, ritual, and talk directly measure paradigms or merely the shadowy representations of them, this everyday world is of considerable importance to family members themselves. With more concerted attention to this everyday world of family life, we may be able to release our current dependence on the deliberately artificial card-sort procedure. We suspect that the search for independently developed research techniques for cross-validation purposes will not lead us to acceptable instruments and scales already in existence. The paradigm concept is complex and subtle enough so that it will probably be necessary to start afresh with the goal of developing protocols that have demonstrable content and construct validity.

The problem in this case and its possible solutions are not different in principle from those in any other situation where cognitive-behavioral consistency is an issue. Because the investigator or therapist is part of the environment around which the subject's paradigm is organized, one's ability to penetrate the shroud of that paradigm is always laden with uncertainty. But the opposite is also true. That is, the subject is comprehensible only from the paradigmatic stance of the observer.

The upshot of these considerations may be that paradigms are real only to the extent that they are treated as real. This conclusion may be viewed as a defeat for science because there is no objective way to deny the existence and influence of paradigms. Families may be analyzed as if they possess paradigms whether or not families believe that they have them. More positively, however, we may conclude that human understanding is facilitated if research and therapeutic processes are seen as dialogues between paradigms. The traditional scientific paradigm places heavy emphasis on the qualities of high configuration, high coordination, and delayed closure. That is, nature is viewed as being sensible and controllable once its lawful principles are discovered, the scientific community is expected to operate as a cohesive and cooperative venture rather than as a collection of isolated individuals, and scientific ideas are not viewed as ultimate truths but as tentative conjectures modifiable in the face of new experience. If families differ from each other in significant ways over the content of their paradigms, we should expect scientists or scientific communities to differ as well, at some level, over their own paradigms. When scientists study families, therefore, there is no assurance that the former's paradigm corresponds to the latter's. This is why we draw attention to the idea that knowledge of human affairs—and specifically, of family life—depends on a dialogue of some sort between the investigator's paradigm and the subject's paradigm.

If there is merit in this stance, it suggests that the study of family paradigm theory will advance to the extent that paradigm content becomes the focus of interchanges between researcher and subject as well as between clinician and client. This development would represent a shift away from the idea that family paradigms can be apprehended only by studiously recording the interaction patterns of family members in controlled settings, without engaging in and sharing with them expressions of perception, belief, and feeling.

There is one other interesting aspect of this rather broad area of concern. Let us suppose that it really is the case that family members typically cannot articulate their paradigms because crucial features escape awareness. Then, we may ask, is it not one of the purposes of paradigm theory to *increase* the awareness of paradigms? Who is the likely beneficiary of this new knowledge? Researchers and clinicians will benefit because they will "see" the family in ways previously unfamiliar to them. The families of patients in psychiatric hospitals or the participants in and consumers of paradigm research may also begin to "see" themselves in a new way. In general, then, the pervading assumption of a lack of awareness must be tempered and must be viewed as frail and subject to alteration. We may even speculate that "paradigm sensitivity" helps to distinguish normal or functional families from pathological or dysfunctional ones. Part of the treatment process, in the case of diagnosed disorders or of preventive education in the case of enrichment programs, may eventually center on giving families the tools to comprehend, assess, and increase control over their own constructs of the environment and their relationship to it.

The Shared Nature of the Family Paradigm

The idea that cognitions are shared by members of a group with a common experience has a long heritage. Almost a century ago, Emile Durkheim invoked the concept of "collective conscience" to capture this idea (Nisbet, 1974). Group psychology, cultural anthropology, and the symbolic interaction perspective in sociology have traditionally advanced the idea that shared understandings are, if not inevitable, at least often characteristic of social life and functional for its survival. Despite these precedents, a host of issues is raised by an emphasis on this shared quality as an essential feature of the family paradigm:

1. Why should family life be conducive to shared orientations toward reality? The gender and age differentiation built into most families suggests at least the possibility of different orientations toward reality. It is not farfetched to draw the conclusion from decades of research on family dynamics that family disorganization is the result of fundamental and unresolved disagreements among members about what the family's paradigm is or ought to be. Whatever their origins and consequences, conflicts over orientations do seem to arise in families. Kuhn (1962) saw science as developing through intervals of normal and revolutionary activity. Therefore, at the very least, we should expect that there are periods in the course of family life when a previously established paradigm becomes unglued, when one or more members are pressing for change while others resist. Families may have rituals and thematic aspects that persist over time, but there is no assurance that these endure unchanged. The Reiss team has provided some evidence, discussed above, that family paradigms exhibit short-term stability. Attention may now profitably turn to an exploration of developmental continuities and discontinuities with an eye on the processes by which paradigm conflicts are managed.

As articulated to date, paradigm theory has been sensitive to the implications of viewing constructs as shared. It acknowledges the possibilities of alienation and estrangement. It speculates that the number diagnosed as pathological may be cut off from the paradigmatic stance shared by all other members. It specifies the "crisis" as the occasion when paradigms are most vulnerable to fragmentation (Reiss, 1981). We have even suggested earlier in this chapter that psychopathology may result when a family paradigm disintegrates, regardless of what specific paradigm prevailed before.

We view the theory as vulnerable not because if fails to admit the possibility of conflict, disorganization, or other manifestations of individual differences within a family, but because none of the research evidence so far marshaled in support of the theory gives clues about what families look like when their paradigms are under stress, are in disarray, or are being challenged by one or more members. The card-sort procedure and the scores derived from it lead to the placement of every family studied, whether clinical or nonclinical, in *some* paradigm. It is simply not possible, given the current coding conventions, to detect disputes over paradigms or to conclude that a particular family has no regnant, consistent, and fully shared set of assumptions about reality.

2. If it is the case that family paradigms *are* shared, how do they attain this status? One possiblity is that mating patterns are assortative, so that interpersonal attraction and eventual marriage are based, at least in part, on similarity between paradigms acquired in the families of orientation. Children are born, therefore, into a world where the paradigmatic qualities of their parents are more-or-less given to them in stylized form. What is not assured is that socialization into the prevailing family paradigm is complete or automatic. Very young children have not participated in and could not be expected to participate in the card-sorting task developed by Reiss and his team. If a family has and maintains a fairly distinctive paradigm, however, we should expect certain child-rearing practices to be used during the socialization process. Hence, one direction in which the study of family paradigms may move concerns the processes by which relatively naive members are indoctrinated by others into the pathways of the paradigm. Some psychopathological diagnoses in children may be the result of a failure, for whatever reason, of parents to bring the children into conformity with the paradigmatic stance that the parents view as essential or natural.

3. Even if a paradigm is shared by the members of a family and this state of affairs is viewed as the product of assortative mating and effective socialization, we should expect the prevalence of paradigms to be linked to historical and cultural contexts. For example, it would appear consistent with existing theories of social change that contemporary life, compared with traditional forms in times past, places a relatively heavy emphasis on high configuration, low coordination, and delayed closure. That is, the conditions of modern society reward people who attain a sense of mastery over their environments, who have a clear sense of themselves as autonomous individuals even though they may be able to cooperate with others, and who are deliberate and rational and open enough to novel experiences so that they can adjust in the face of the complex and rapidly changing stimuli in their environments.

Because the functional requirements of social life are not uniform through historical time or across cultural settings, further comparative research is needed to determine which features of family paradigms are universally shared and which are not. From this perspective, it is plausible to argue that some forms of psychopathology result from the inability of some families to fully participate in the cultural ethos that surrounds them. Their paradigms being out of step with prevailing values, they come to be labeled and treated as pathological.

There is nothing in paradigm theory that explicitly denies the importance of cultural or historical context. To date, however, it has mainly had an ancillary role, as in the anecdotal distinction between Puritan families and Great Plains families (Reiss, 1981). Hence, our critique may be read as a call for more research on this topic and as an anticipation that some facets of the theory will need to be loosened up or prefaced by culture-specific contingencies.

4. At what level are family paradigms shared by family members? A family that scores very low on the coordination dimension, for example, may share little beyond a sort of "do-your-own-thing" philosophy. Under such circumstances, it may be difficult to characterize the family on the other dimensions. Because the family lacks a sense of itself as a group, we may expect great variation among members on the configuration and closure dimension. It seems possible in principle, therefore, for families to share one facet of the paradigm without sharing the others.

At least two levels of analysis are suggested by this line of thinking. One reflects the surface features of thought and action. In the routine course of family living, what the family members do and say is apt to suggest some unitary theme that organizes their life. The other level reflects the deep structure of consensus. Family members may act in concert but may have jointly decided to become so. Although difficult to describe, this difference in levels is illustrated by the notion that people in groups can agree to disagree. The implication for research and clinical practice is that one must be sensitive to the level at which the paradigm is operative so as not to be misled by the more accessible surface manifestations.

The idea of levels has occupied attention in the most comprehensive statement of paradigm theory. First, paradigms are characterized as "framing assumptions" or "metarules" (Reiss, 1981). Parents may argue bitterly over who should pick up their child's toys in the front yard, but at the metalevel, they share a concern about not antagonizing the neighbors. Second, and perhaps more important, family paradigms have been distinguished from "ordinary constructs" and "crisis constructs" (Reiss, 1981). Here we wish to draw attention only to the distinction between "ordinary" and paradigmatic levels. It is the former level that is thought to be characteristic of routine family interaction and to be detectable with, for example, the card-sort procedure. Underlying this surface level is thought to be a more abstract version whose cardinal dimensions are "coherence," "integration," and "reference." Without examining these concepts in detail here, we simply wish to pose the challenge that remains to those who wish to pursue them further. Why does the theory need multiple levels? If research to date measures only ordinary constructs, how would one go about establishing the existence of the underlying and more paradigmatic level? Furthermore, can it be demonstrated that there is a homology between dimensions across levels so that, for example, the reference dimension is translated into or applied to assumptions by families about closure? This represents a frontier area in the increasingly comprehensive theory of family paradigms, so our decision to treat it as a source of vulnerability refers mainly to its new and speculative status.

5. The card-sort procedure aggregates the measurable responses of individuals or compares those responses across individual members of the family.

The methods by which one takes the performances of individuals and combines them into a measure of group performance is still a matter of some debate in the field of family studies, as well as in small-group research generally. This issue involves, in part, the decision about which family members are sampled to participate, and the card-sorting technology has developed only to the point where it can accommodate three or four members at a time, an advance over most research designs, which are, at best, dyadic. Still, a methodological problem remains. We are pretty much restricted to describing group properties in terms of the means and variances of responses elicited from individual members of the group. Regardless of the level at which some phenomenon like a paradigm is shared, we are basically dependent on similarity of response across members of the family in order to make statements about the group as a group.

One way to move beyond this atomistic view that a group characteristic is the arithmetical combination of its individual elements is to take the interaction sequence as the unit of analysis. In its most elemental form, the application of this idea to the study of family paradigms would involve the recording and coding of what Member Y does in response to what Member X does. In other words, instead of focusing on the similarity between the members in their cumulative performance, we might define the features of a family paradigm in terms of the degree to which the actions of one family member are predictive of the actions of another family member. Evidence of the existence of a particular paradigm would then be based not on the shared quality of beliefs and perceptions but on the regularity of exchanges of describable types between members of the family or even between members of the family and representatives from outside the family.

We are saying, in effect, that, to the extent that family paradigm theory can shift its fundamental criterion away from similarity of behaviors and toward regularity of interactions, it may be able to overcome one methodological vulnerability. So, for example, the dimension of configuration may be based not on the mean score of family members on a measure of mastery, but on the degree to which one or more family members are able to induce high configurational behaviors in other family members. The investigation of structured sequences of interaction has taken hold in the more behavioristic wing of family process research (Gottman, 1979; Patterson, 1982), and it may profitably be borrowed to explore aspects of paradigm theory.

6. The boundaries of membership in social groups are often difficult to establish, and this is certainly the case with families. Social scientists have invented labels for categories of family relationship, such as nuclear versus extended, and many of these designations are part of common linguistic practice. The relationships among unmarried cohabitants, in-laws, and ex-relatives precipitated by divorce, as well as between adoptive parents and children, contain many familylike qualities, and categories of some intense friendships are given familistic names like *blood brothers*.

Sensitivity to the expansive and precarious nature of family boundaries leads to the speculation that family paradigms are often only partly shared. That is, they may be shared by some members and not by others. There may be factions or coalitions at work, organized according to gender, age, or genealogy. We suspect that, as more members of families serve as participants and informants in research on family paradigms, the theory will need to be revised from its present emphasis on one completely shared paradigm per family to a view that accommodates multiple paradigms and subsystem diversity. This revision would be congenial to the idea of paradigm conflict that we introduced earlier. The focus of research attention might then move toward an examination of how families cope with competing orientations toward reality, which they are apt to see not just in other families but in their own.

Stability and Change

Two threads run through the theory of family paradigms that appear to be contradictory, producing an uneasy tension in the theory at this point in its development. One of these threads is the argument that certain processes operate to conserve a family paradigm once it is established. Briefly restated, the stability argument is that certain instituted practices, such as "ceremonials" and "pattern regulators," function to reinforce the main themes in a family's paradigm. In addition, a paradigm is stabilized in the course of a family's contact with its environment. Captured under the rubric of a *cycle hypothesis,* the basic idea here is that, by selecting specific environments and gaining a reputation in them, a family's paradigm, or at least its ordinary construct, is validated and preserved (Reiss, 1981).

The idea that families select environments that fit with their preexisting paradigm can be illustrated by examining treatment programs in psychiatric hospitals. Reiss (1981, p. 326) has discussed the possibility that, based on prior knowledge or on a trial-and-error-process, families may present themselves to and perform well in those programs of treatment that fit well with the family's own paradigm. This idea takes good advantage of the more general notion that communities, organizations, and other social units *outside* families have their own paradigms, so that, whenever a family encounters its environment, there is a potential problem of fit that must somehow be resolved on both sides.

Unfortunately, we do not yet have clear-cut empirical data to assess this process or to characterize those paradigms that exist outside families. In the major study of family–hospital relationships so far conducted by the Reiss team, all family paradigms were about equally represented (Reiss, 1981). Either self-selection did not occur in this instance or else it occurred sometime *after* the families participated in the card-sort procedure. In the major study of hospital paradigms, two paradigmatic dimensions emerged from a factor analysis of responses to a questionnaire completed by psychiatric staff members (as well as by patients). These two dimensions, "belief in the moral order" and "belief in the technical order," suggest the possibility that whole staff may be classified according to whether one, both, or neither set of beliefs predominates (Reiss, 1981, p. 320). The problem here is that the factor analysis is based on patterns of covariation among individuals. Instead of being in a position to conclude that the two hospitals studied have a paradigm, perhaps one being more technically oriented than the other, we are able to conclude only that there is a great deal of variation among staff members in each hospital with regard to such beliefs. The beliefs may still be paradigmatic, but they do not appear to be shared by the members of either hospital.

A new round of studies with different designs may help us to clarify the ways in which family paradigms interact with nonfamily paradigms and to ascertain whether the latter can even be said to exist. An assessment of family paradigms at intake and at termination of treatment, using the card-sort procedure, would assist in testing the self-selection hypothesis. Such studies could be set up so that dropouts and other case failures are compared with families designated as treatment successes. The design should also permit an assessment of whether successful treatment itself helps to produce a change in a family's paradigm.

Further tests of the validity of the card-sort procedure can also be built into these studies. Instead of using a questionnaire to measure hospital paradigms, analogous to the card-sort procedure could be administered to groups of hospital staff. Staff—family comparisons would then be based on a methodology common to both kinds of groups. This approach would also be a way to examine the closure dimension, as it was not incorporated in the first set of hospital studies (Reiss, 1981). Finally, if data from questionnaires like those in the study already conducted are to be used in the future, it would be desirable to get card-sort measures from the same sample of persons or groups. This procedure would permit an assessment of whether the two methods are measuring the same phenomenon. The study of family—environment transactions in general is still in its infancy (Larzelere & Klein, 1987), so it is not surprising that interesting research designs far surpass the accumulated body of research evidence.

So far, we have drawn attention only to the stability argument and to some possibilities for further research based on a few of the preliminary studies already conducted to assess this argument. The other major thread in paradigm theory, however, is that paradigms are not inevitably stable and that they dissolve or change under particular circumstances. The basic line of reasoning here is that crises precipitate disorganization and reorganization of the paradigm, and the manner in which these occur is fairly elaborate as well as conditional (Reiss, 1981).

We recognize two problems here. The first is that, although the postulated processes following a crisis are quite plausible in theory, they are extremely difficult to demonstrate empirically. As we mentioned above in our critical discussion of the assumption that paradigms are shared, the card-sort procedure simply does not permit the researcher to "see" conflict between paradigms in a family or a collapsed and nonparadigmatic state, even if one or the other is thought to exist. Hence, either the procedure itself or its coding conventions will have to be revised, or else, some entirely new procedure will have to be devised to measure the duration, depth, regions, and other facets of the disorganization and reorganization process.

The other problem is not methodological but theoretical. Given that there are forces leading to stability as well as forces leading to disorganization and change, how do we know which of these forces are going to be stronger? In the face of a crisis or severe stress, we suspect that some families will become disorganized, and others will not. Some families will be able to cope effectively on the basis of their precrisis paradigm, and others will not. Some families will become quite incapacitated, and others will work their way back to health with the aid of a new paradigm. We may hypothesize that, *if* certain mechanisms fail, a particular outcome is likely. Paradigm theory is vulnerable, however, because it does not yet contain within it statements about what antecedent conditions lead to change and what other conditions lead to stability. Instead, we are left on the verge of an unsatisfactory tautology, to the effect that, if a family's paradigm no longer works, it will change.

We suspect that the reason that paradigm theory is not yet able to handle this issue has to do with its own evolution. In the first place, it was not conceived as a theory with a focal dependent variable. Its purpose has been not to explain one particular phenomenon, but to posit an idea, the family paradigm, which can act as the fulcrum of many theoretical arguments. Hence, paradigms are readily imagined to have a host of causes and consequences. The first priority in developing the theory has been to demonstrate that paradigms are important because they have several interesting consequences. So, with several promising and some surprising results, the idea of the paradigm has been used to predict problem-solving behavior, psychiatric disorders, perceptions of specific extra-familial groups, and so on. Attempts have been made to show that family paradigms are better predictors than rival variables, such as the skill level of the individual family members (Reiss, 1981), although the rivals are quite large in number and more research of this kind remains to be conducted (Klein & Hill, 1979).

It is only recently that Reiss and his team have turned to the casually prior questions of what creates a paradigm in the first place and what variables account for their stability or change. It is not surprising, then, that the answers should be tentative and not yet well specified. Scientific theories are living, dynamic constructs in the very same sense that family paradigms are. They resist change, respond to crisis, and most especially are social constructions. Therefore, we surmise that it will be just a matter of time and further collaborative effort before the issue of stability versus change receives the attention now due it.

The Fusion of Theoretical Traditions

A salutary feature of paradigm theory is that it draws on multiple theoretical traditions. It is not parochially confined to the viewpoint of a single intellectual community, academic discipline, or orthodoxy. This lack of confinement means that a wide variety of scholars and practitioners should find appealing at least some of the concepts, hypotheses, and nuances of perspective that lace the theory and its associated program of research. It is also possible, however, that the very liberality and eclectic nature of the paradigm approach is a source of ambiguities. We will illustrate this point below by focusing on two of the intellectual traditions that have energized much of the thinking of the Reiss team.

One tradition that has helped to shape paradigm theory is the Gestalt perspective in psychology (Franklin, 1982). This tradition, of course, has contributed much over the years to the study of perception, cognition, and problem solving in individuals and groups. Its methods have tended to be experimental whenever possible, and its epistemology has been positivistic in thrust. The abstract concepts of form, contrast, and emergent structural wholes guide much of the work conducted under the umbrella of this frame of reference.

In many respects, paradigm theory has the feel of a Gestalt-inspired orientation toward family life. Not only has Reiss (1981) explicitly acknowledged this heritage at several points, but the very idea of the paradigm is reminiscent of a classical Gestalt structure. Furthermore, the experimental methods used by Reiss and his team are generally in keeping with the research designs in Gestalt psychology and its intellectual successors in social psychology. In particular, the card-sort procedure can be viewed as a way of eliciting information about mental processes and their organization at the level of the social problems and especially the family group.

There is a second intellectual tradition with traces in paradigm theory. This is the phenomenological approach in sociology, as elaborated by Peter Berger and others, which Reiss (1981) has also cited favorably at several points. This approach takes a special interest in showing how images of reality are constructed or created by social actors engaged in conversation and other forms of interaction.

Now, in some ways, at least, Gestalt psychology and phenomenological sociology can be viewed as being complementary or even as being in virtual agreement about key assumptions and outlook. There are two respects, however, in which the two perspectives clash. One of these points of confrontation involves the conceptual apparatus, and the other involves epistemology.

In their treatment of a phenomenological sociology of the family, McLain and Weigert (1979) highlighted such concepts as finite provinces of meaning, intentionality, typification, plausibility structures, the natural attitude, and interpretation activities. The challenge to paradigm theory in its present state is to take this conceptual apparatus of phenomenology and ask how it fits with concepts currently used to describe and understand family paradigms. We suspect that this mapping operation would reveal that there is much more in the phenomenological lexicon that remains to be considered for incorporation. There appears, for example, to be much more emphasis on how families interpret their own actions and construct identities in phenomenology than in paradigm theory (Reiss, 1981). A parallel sort of mapping operation could be used to expropriate relatively recent ideas from the Gestalt side, such as attribution (Franklin, 1982).

As this dual process of borrowing and translating from both traditions proceeds, we expect three things to happen. First, the extent to which paradigm theory can be deductively linked to broader theoretical traditions will become more apparent than it now is. Second, paradigm theory will grow in complexity as new concepts are introduced. Third, some problems of fit will emerge. For example, what on the Gestalt side is likely to match the notion of plausibility structures on the phenomenology side?

We hesitate to predict what the outcome of such confrontations may be. All we are suggesting at this point is the potential value of keeping paradigm theory in touch with its various guiding orientations and of anticipating the prospect of conceptual ambiguities as these traditions are translated into the terminology of paradigm theory. Eventually, it may become necessary for paradigm theorists to cast their lot with one tradition and to abandon others on the basis of the inadequacy of these traditions' core concepts.

The other major point of confrontation between Gestalt psychology and phenomenological sociology concerns their epistemologies and, ultimately, the methods of research and demonstration that they view as acceptable. Whereas the Gestalt approach is essentially positivistic in the Popperian sense, phenomenology is decidely antipositivistic. We will only illustrate the difference here.

From a Gestalt perspective, it is legitimate for the scientist to view himself or herself as a detached observer who is objectively discovering patterns that reside in the world. Whether social actors have a complete understanding of what they are doing or why poses no analytical problem. How these actors collaborate to form a gestalt may be the object of investigation, but the observer's comprehension of the process does not depend on being a part of that process. So, for example, the researcher's understanding can in some way be construed as superior or more compelling than what the actors themselves would say is their own understanding.

In contrast, from a phenomenological perspective, it is impossible, or at least undesirable, for the researcher to be detached from the object of inquiry. The key criterion for validity in phenomenology was described by McLain and Weigert (1979) as the "postulate of adequacy." In effect, a scientific description or explanation of human behavior is valid only to the degree that the human subjects under study concur that it makes sense to them and fits their own understanding.

It is, of course, possible to attack both of the epistemologies sketched here, but we are not concerned with how reasonable either one is at this point. Rather, we wish to note the dilemma that these different views create for paradigm theory. To date, the theory has been more positivistic, in line with the Gestalt tradition. Hence, for example, the problem of awareness that we examined earlier has not yet led to studies of the phenomenological validity of paradigm concepts or hypotheses. The argument instead, crudely put, has been that families generally lack awareness of those very structures that the observer can comprehend and analyze.

At the same time, however, the theory of family paradigms explicitly acknowledges that environments impose on—or at least, shape—the paradigmatic features of family life. Furthermore, the theory has treated as a crucial part of the families' environment the researcher who is trying to understand them. It is in the confrontation between scientist (or therapist) and subject (or client) that the family's paradigm comes into view. So, in principle, at least, the observer's understanding of a family depends to a considerable extent on a family's understanding of the observer. In this respect, at least, the theory of family paradigms has remained faithful to a phenomenological epistemology.

Paradigm theory is vulnerable to the extent that the theoretical traditions on which it builds rely on incompatible epistemologies. We have suggested that the theory has selectively borrowed and adapted its conceptual apparatus from at least two traditions but has been much more epistemologically aligned with only one of these traditions. Although phenomenological methods of knowing have received some rhetorical attention in discourse on paradigm theory, they have yet to inspire research based on the "principle of adequacy." We believe that paradigm theory is a fertile ground for addressing epistemological issues in family research. As this mission progresses, we may find that the theory is fully capable of having it both ways, or we may discover the necessity of retrenchment and alignment with only one of these alternatives.

CONCLUSION

In sum, paradigm theory holds promise as a coherent approach to both studies of basic family process and an understanding of pathogenesis. However, very specific and important items are on the agenda for future work. From a substantive point of view, work is beginning on measurement of the levels of family disorganization and on their relationship to both family and individual functioning. Also, major investigations are currently under way to explore the origin of the paradigm—particularly its intergenerational transmission. From a methodological perspective, the card-sort procedure needs to be supplemented with more direct assessment procedures that on the one hand, go more directly to the phenomena of beliefs and assumptions and, on the other, embrace interaction as it unfolds over time and in more natural settings. From a theoretical perspective, a formalization of theory may now be in order. The theory, particularly its fuller explication in Reiss's book (1981), contains many terms and a plethora of conceptions and connections. Simplification and clarification via causal modeling (and the necessary specification of core causal statements or propositions) would be an interesting test of the central logic of the theory. Likewise, the theory needs to be exposed to a broader range of family phenomena, including divorce, remarriage, family therapy and its impact, and cultural and class variations among families. Work on this priority agenda will help to determine whether paradigm theory reflects only a narrow band of intriguing experiences in family life or is approaching a more general model of the family process.

REFERENCES

Adams, B. (1968). *Kinship in an urban setting*. Chicago: Markham.
Aldous, J. (1971). A framework for the analysis of family problem solving. In J. Aldous, T. Condon, R. Hill, M. Strauss, & I. Tallman (Eds.), *Family problem solving: A symposium on theoretical, methodological and substantive concerns*. Hinsdale, IL: Dryden.
Angelou, M. (1970). *I know why the caged bird sings*. New York: Random House.
Argyris, C. (1965a). Explorations in interpersonal competence: 1. *Journal of Applied Behavioral Science, 1*, 58–83.

Argyris, C. (1965b). Explorations in interpersonal competence: 2. *Journal of Applied Behavioral Science, 1*, 147–177.

Ashby, W. R. (1952). *Design for a brain.* New York: Wiley.

Berger, P. L., & Lukmann, T. (1966). *The social construction of reality.* New York: Doubleday.

Bion, W. (1959). *Experience in groups.* New York: Basic Books.

Bossard, J. H. S., & Boll, E. S. (1950). *Ritual in family living.* Philadelphia: University of Pennsylvania Press.

Brim, O. G. (1962). *Personality and decision processes studies in the social psychology of thinking.* Palo Alto, CA: Stanford University Press.

Costell, R., & Reiss, D. (1982). The family meets the hospital: Clinical presentations of a laboratory-based family typology. *Archives of General Psychiatry, 39,* 433–438.

Costell, R., Reiss, D., Berkman, H., & Jones, C. (1981). The family meets the hospital: Predicting the family's perception of the treatment program from its problem-solving style. *Archives of General Psychiatry, 38,* 569–577.

Davis, P., Stern, D., Jorgenson, J., & Steier, F. (1980). *Typologies of the alcoholic family: An integrated systems perspective.* Philadelphia: University of Pennsylvania, Wharton Applied Research Center.

Dewey, J. (1910). *How we think.* New York: D. C. Heath.

Doane, J., West, K. L., Goldstein, M. D., Rodnick, E. H., & Jones, J. E. (1981). Parental communication deviance and affective style. *Archives of General Psychiatry, 38,* 679–685.

Draguns, J. G. (1963). Responses to cognitive and perceptual ambiguity in chronic and acute schizophrenics. *Journal of Abnormal Social Psychology, 66,* 24–30.

Epstein, S. (1953). Overinclusive thinking in a schizophrenic and a control group. *Journal of Consulting Psychology, 17,* 387–388.

Farber, B. (1981). *Conceptions of kinship.* New York: Elsevier North Holland.

Franklin, C. W., II. (1982). *Theoretical perspectives in social psychology,* Boston: Little, Brown.

Goffman, E. (1974). *Frame analysis.* Cambridge: Harvard University Press.

Goldstein, R. H., & Salzman, L. F. (1967). Cognitive functioning in acute and remitted psychiatric patients. *Psychological Report, 21,* 24–26.

Gottman, J. M. (1979). *Marital interaction: Experimental investigations.* New York: Academic Press.

Hammer, M., Makiesky-Barrow, S., & Gutwirth, L. (1978). Social networks and schizophrenia. *Schizophrenia Bulletin, 4,* 522–545.

Hansen, D. H., & Johnson, V. A. (1979). Rethinking family stress theory: Definitional aspects. In W. R. Burr, R. Hill, F. I. Nye, & I. L. Reiss (Eds.), *Contemporary theories about the family.* New York: Free Press.

Heider, F. (1958). *The psychology of interpersonal relations.* New York: Wiley.

Hess, R. D., & Handel, G. (1959). *Family worlds.* Chicago: University of Chicago Press.

Howe, I. (1976). *World of our fathers.* New York: Simon & Schuster.

Howell, J. T. (1973). *Hard living on clay street.* New York: Anchor Books.

Jessor, R., & Jessor, S. L. (1975). Adolescent development and the onset of drinking: a longitudinal study. *Journal of Studies on Alcohol, 36,* 27–51.

Kantor, D., & Lehr, W. (1975). *Inside the family.* San Francisco: Jossey-Bass.

Kelly, G. A. (1955). *The psychology of personal construits* (Vols. 1, 2). New York: Norton.

Kenny, D. A. (1979). *Correlation and causality.* New York: Wiley.

Klein, D. M., & Hill, R. (1979). Determinants of family problem solving effectiveness. In W. R. Burr, R. Hill, F. I. Nye, & I. L. Reiss (Eds.), *Contemporary theories about the family* (Vol. 1). New York: Free Press.

Kohn, M. L. (1969). *Class and conformity.* Homewood, IL: Dorsey Press.

Kuhn, T. S. (1962). *The structure of scientific revolutions.* Chicago: University of Chicago Press.

Larzelere, R. E., & Klein, D. M. (1987). Methodological implications of the family as an object of study. In M. B. Sussman & S. K. Steinmetz (Eds.), *Handbook on marriage and the family.* New York: Plenum Press.

Liem, J. H. (1976). Intrafamily communication and schizophrenic thought disorder: An etiologic or responsive relationship? *The Clinical Psychologist, 29,* 28–30.

McCubbin, H. I., Joy, C. B., Cauble, A. E., Comeau, J. K., Patterson, J. M., & Needle, R. H. (1980). Family stress and coping: A decade review. *Journal of Marriage and the Family, 42,* 855–871.

McLain, R., & Weigert, A. (1979). Toward a phenomenological sociology of family: A programmatic essay. In W. R. Burr, R. Hill, F. I. Nye, & I. L. Reiss (Eds.), *Contemporary theories about the family* (Vol. 2). New York: Free Press.

Minuchin, S., Montalvo, B., Guerney, B., Jr., Rosman, B. L., & Schumer, F. (1967). *Families of the slums.* New York: Basic Books.

Minuchin, S., Rosman, B., & Baker, L. (1978). *Psychosomatic families.* Cambridge: Harvard University Press.

Mishler, E. G., & Waxler, N. E. (1968). *Interaction in families.* New York: Wiley.

Moos, R. H., & Moos, B. A. (1976). A typology of family social environments. *Family Process, 15,* 357–371.

Nagy, I., & Sparks, G. M. (1973). *Invisible loyalties.* Hagerstown, MD: Harper & Row.

Nisbet, R. A. (1974). *The sociology of Emile Durkeim.* New York: Oxford University Press.

Oliveri, M. E., & Reiss, D. (1981a). The structure of families' ties to their kin: The shaping role of social construction. *Journal of Marriage and the Family, 43,* 391–407.

Oliveri, M. E., & Reiss, D. (1981b). A theory based empirical classification of family problem solving behavior. *Family Process, 20,* 409–418.

Oliveri, M. E., & Reiss, D. (1982). Families schemata of social relationships. *Family Process, 21,* 295–311.

Oliveri, M. E., & Reiss, D. (1984). Family concepts and their measurement: Things are seldom what they seem. *Family Process, 23,* 33–48.

Olson, D. H., Sprenkle, D., & Russell, C. (1979). Circumplex model of family and marital systems: 1. Cohesion and adaptability dimensions, family types and clinical application. *Family Process, 18,* 3–28.

Patterson, G. R. (1982). *Coercive family process.* Eugene, OR: Castalia.

Phillips, J. E., Jacobson, N., & Turner, W. J. (1965). Conceptual thinking in schizophrenics and their relatives. *British Journal of Psychiatry, 111,* 823–839.

Piaget, J. (1952). *The origins of intelligence in children* (2nd ed.). New York: International Universities Press.

Popper, K. R. (1959). *The logic of scientific discovery.* New York: Basic Books.

Reiss, D. (1968). Individual thinking and family interaction: 3. An experimental study of categorization performance in families of normals, character disorders and schizophrenics. *Journal of Nervous and Mental Disorders, 146,* 384–403.

Reiss, D. (1969). Individual thinking and family interaction: 4. A study of information exchange in families of normals, those with character disorders and schizophrenia. *Journal of Nervous and Mental Disorders, 149,* 473–490.

Reiss, D. (1970). Individual thinking and family interaction: 5. Proposals for the contrasting character of experiential sensitivity and expressive form in families. *Journal of Nervous and Mental Disorders, 151,* 187–202.

Reiss, D. (1971a). Intimacy and problem solving: An automated procedure for testing a theory of consensual experience in families. *Archives of General Psychiatry, 25,* 442–455.

Reiss, D. (1971b). Varieties of consensual experience: 1. A theory for relating family interaction to individual thinking. *Family Process, 10,* 1–28.

Reiss, D. (1971c). Varieties of consensual experience: 2. Dimensions of a family's experience of its environment. *Family Process, 10,* 28–35.

Reiss, D. (1971d). Varieties of consensual experience: 3. Contrast between families of normals, delinquents and schizophrenics. *Journal of Nervous and Mental Disease, 152,* 73–95.

Reiss, D. (1981). *The family's construction of reality.* Cambridge: Harvard University Press.

Reiss, D., & Oliveri, M. E. (1980). Family paradigm and family coping: A proposal for linking the family's intrinsic adaptive capacities to its responses to stress. *Family Relations, 29,* 431–444.

Reiss, D., & Oliveri, M. E. (1983a). The family's construction of social reality and its ties to its kin network: An exploration of causal direction. *Journal of Marriage and the Family, 45,* 81–91.

Reiss, D., & Oliveri, M. E. (1983b). Family stress as community frame. *Marriage and Family Review, 6,* 61–83.

Reiss, D., & Oliveri, M. E. (1983c). Sensory experience and family process: Perceptual styles tend to run in but not necessarily run families. *Family Process, 22,* 289–308.

Reiss, D., & Salzman, C. (1973). The resilience of family process: Effect of secobarbital. *Archives of General Psychiatry, 28,* 425–433.

Reiss, D., Costell, R., & Almond, R. (1976). Personal needs, values and technical preferences in the psychiatric hospital: A replicated study. *Archives of General Psychiatry, 23,* 795–804.

Reiss, D., Costell, R., Berkman, H., & Jones, C. (1980). How one family perceives another: The relationship between social constructions and problem solving competence. *Family Process, 19,* 239–256.

Reiss, D., Costell, R., Jones, C., & Berkman, H. (1980). The family meets the hospital: A laboratory forecast of the encounter. *Archives of General Psychiatry, 37,* 141–154.

Robins, L. N. (1966). *Deviant children grown up.* Baltimore: Williams & Wilkins.

Rosman, B., Wild, C., Ricci, J., Fleck, S., & Lidz, T. (1964). Thought disorders in the parents of schizophrenic patients: A further study utilizing the object sorting test. *Journal of Psychiatric Research, 2,* 211–221.

Salzman, L. F., Goldstein, R. H., Atkins, R., & Babigian, H. (1966). Conceptual thinking in psychiatric patients. *Archives of General Psychiatry, 14,* 55–59.

Scotch, N. A. (1963). Sociocultural factors in the epidemiology of Zulu hypertension. *Journal of Public Health, 53,* 1205–1213.

Shulman, S., & Klein, M. M. (1982). The family and adolescence: A conceptual and experimental approach. *Journal of Adolescence, 5,* 219–234.

Silverman, D. (1970). *The theory of organizations.* New York: Basic Books.

Silverman, J. (1964). Scanning control mechanism and cognitive filtering, in paranoid and non-paranoid schizophrenia. *Journal of Consulting Psychology, 28,* 385–393.

Steinglass, P. (1979). The alcoholic family at home: Patterns of interaction in dry, wet and transitional stages of alcoholism. *Archives of General Psychiatry, 38,* 578–584.

Steinglass, P., Weiner, S., & Mendelson, J. H. (1971). A systems approach to alcoholism: A model and its clinical application. *Archives of General Psychiatry, 24,* 401–408.

Summers, F., & Walsh, F. (1978). The nature of the symbiotic bond between mother and schizophrenic. *American Journal of Orthopsychiatry, 47,* 136–148.

Suttles, G. D. (1972). *The social construction of communities.* Chicago: University of Chicago Press.

Walsh, F. (1978). Concurrent grandparent death and birth of schizophrenic offspring: An intriguing finding. *Family Process, 17,* 457–463.

Wender, P. H., Rosenthal, D., Kety, S. S., Schulsinger, F., & Welner, J. (1974). Crossfostering: A research strategy for clarifying the role of genetic and experiential factors in the etiology of schizophrenia. *Archives of General Psychiatry, 30,* 121–128.

Wild, C., Singer, M. R., Rosman, B., Ricci, J., & Lidz, T. (1965). Measuring disordered styles of thinking: Using the object sorting test on parents of schizophrenic patients. *Archives of General Psychiatry, 13,* 471–476.

Wolin, S. J., Bennett, L. A., & Noonan, D. L. (1979). Family rituals and the recurrence of alcoholism over generations. *American Journal of Psychiatry, 136,* 589–593.

Wynne, L. C. (1965). Some indications and contraindications for explorative family therapy. In I. Boszormenyi, I. Nagy, & J. L. Framo (Eds.), *Intensive family therapy.* New York: Harper & Row.

Zinner, J., & Shapiro, R. (1972). Projective identification as a mode of perception and behavior in families of adolescents. *International Journal of Psychoanalysis, 53,* 523–530.

PART III

METHODOLOGICAL ISSUES AND STRATEGIES

CHAPTER 7

Research Issues and Strategies

Andrew Christensen and Angela Arrington

The investigation of family interaction and psychopathology presents a number of challenges. Any study in this area faces special difficulties because of the nature of the family, of psychopathology, and of their interaction. Families present methodological problems because they are an unusual unit of analysis. Most researchers examine the individual as the central unit of analysis, but studies of the family must focus on larger units, such as the dyad, the triad, and the entire family system. Systems for measuring and categorizing the person, although far from satisfactory, do have a history and tradition that gives the researcher options from which to choose. For example, the DSM-III provides a taxonomy of individual disorders that, despite its inadequacies, has some consensual validity across practitioners and researchers in the field. Nothing comparable exists for families or for interactional pathology.

The investigation of paychopathology presents special problems because it is a nonmanipulable phenomenon that often has a long developmental history. Our lack of knowledge about the phenomenon as well as our ethical guidelines prohibits the induction of psychopathology, except in analogue situations, which may bear little relation to naturalistic phenomena. We may give hallucinogenic drugs to research participants for brief periods of time to assess possible analogues of schizophrenia, but we could not subject participants to the kind of extended personal and familial stresses that may precipitate psychotic reactions. Furthermore, the developmental nature of most psychopathologies means that one must study subjects over substantial periods of time to learn the etiology and course of the phenomena.

Familes share these two characteristics with psychopathology in that they are also nonmanipulable phenomena with a developmental course. We can not create families by assigning members to them or by taking members away from them (although some researchers assign persons to "artificial" families; see the

ANDREW CHRISTENSEN and ANGELA ARRINGTON • Department of Psychology, University of California at Los Angeles, Los Angeles, CA 90024.

section following on "Comparisons across Relationships"). Furthermore, each family has a history that determines, in part, its unique way of perceiving and behaving in the world. Thus, investigations of family interaction and psychopathology present methodological limitations on experimentation and methodological pressures for longitudinal research.

However, pshychopathology has one additional characteristic, not shared by families, that has important methodological implications. Fortunately for society but unfortunately for the researcher, any particular psychopathology is relatively rare. Therefore, the attempt to study family interaction and psychopathology requires the researcher to be highly selective in the families chosen for participation. This need for selectivity is a special problem when we wish to examine families before and during the course of a disorder. Because we cannot predict well who will be psychopathological, a developmental study of any particular pathology may generate few data on that pathology, as most subjects may not develop it.

In this chapter, we will address the special methodological problems that pertain to the study of family interaction and psychopathology. First, we discuss some general problems of unitization as they relate to the study of the family. Then, in the second section, we discuss attempts at generating taxonomies of families. We move from measurement to design in the third section and discuss strategies for isolating the different causal possibilities in the family, for example, whether some phenomenon is caused individually or interactionally. The last two sections continue the focus on design strategies but consider the special difficulties of understanding psychopathology: the fourth section examines developmental research strategies, including longitudinal designs, and the last section examines the *ex post facto* design, perhaps the most common approach to studying psychopathology.

THE PROBLEM OF UNITIZATION

An adage encourages us to "Cut nature at its joints." Presumbly nature is organized into a pattern of subunits. If we are to understand its functioning, we must discern these "natural units." We must create our conceptual distinctions along the same boundaries as those created by nature. We must divide up the world at the same joints at which nature stuck it together.

In the study of the human body, this task of division is simplified by structural differences between subunits. The heart looks different from the brain. Under a microscope, the boundary between cells can be observed. Indeed, there are actual joints in the body that facilitate our analysis and classification. In the study of human behavior, we are not so fortunate. Certainly, there are structural features that could aid in analysis and classification. Walking bears certain structural similarities to running. Masturbation bears certain structural similarities to sexual intercourse. But a classification system based on structural features would be limited indeed. Writing an angry memo to the boss and writing a love letter would fall into the same category. Staring in wonder and gaping in fear would be in the same group.

In the study of human behavior, the primary criterion for unitization and classification must be based solely on usefulness in understanding, prediction, and control. We do not have a structural anatomy, either behavioral or physiological, on which to base these distinctions. This absence of a useful anatomy adds a great deal of trial and error to the study of human behavior. Without a structural basis for our hypothesizing, we are apt to propose a larger number of units than are necessary. Consider the area of traditional personality assessment. A large variety of units of personality have been proposed and tested, but it is still not clear which ones are essential and which ones are unnecesary. In contrast, the area of cognitive assessment has been noticeably more successful. Measuring units of IQ does clearly serve the purpose of understanding, prediction, and control. Although future efforts will hopefully refine the concept and its measurement, it is likely that the intelligence quotient or some derivative will remain an important unit in the study of human behavior.

Unitization in Marital and Family Research

To this point, our discussion of the problem of unitization has focused implicitly on the analysis of individual human behavior. The problems are magnified when one shifts the focus from the individual to a social group such as the family. All the problems of dissecting human behavior remain. In addition, one has the additional complexity of analyzing and classifying the behavior of two or more people in interaction with one another. In dealing with this complexity, an analysis of different types of units may be helpful.[1]

Unit and Object of Study. At the outset, an investigator must decide on the *unit of study,* the entity or "thing" that will be investigated. Historically, most behavioral research has focused on the individual as the unit of study. Individuals were observed or were questioned about themselves as a means of understanding their functioning. Most of the existing measurement devices assume that the individual is the unit of study.

With the advent of scientific interest in marital and family behavior, investigators proposed a different unit of study. Dyads, triads, and entire family systems, not individuals, were the "thing" under investigation. However, it was not always clear how to go about investigating these larger units, so researchers often retained the individual as the unit of study, although the *object of study,* or what the investigator wished to learn about, was a larger unit. Thus, investigators interviewed wives to learn about marriage. Researchers distributed questionnaires to parents to learn about families. In these studies, data were actually

---

[1]In making these distinctions, we borrowed from Fiske's excellent analysis of unitization in personality research (1978). Our analysis is an attempt to extend, and in some cases, to modify, his distinctions so that they are applicable to the marital-family area.

collected on an individual (the unit of study) but conclusions were drawn about the system (the object of study) of which the individual was a member. Researchers select a unit of study that is different from their object of study for obvious reasons of convenience and expense. However, such a strategy assumes that individuals can and will accurately represent the larger system. Existing data comparing the reports of family members and data comparing reports with objective indices cast considerable doubt on this assumption (see Sullaway & Christensen, 1983, and Yarrow, Campbell, & Burton, 1968, for reviews).

The distinction between different units of study is perhaps deceptively simple. When we study individuals, we typically observe them behave or we question them about themselves. If we want to study a larger unit, such as a dyad, a triad, or a family system, we simply question or observe not one member, but all of the members. And herein lies the complexity: those procedures may reveal data on two or more individuals but little information on the relationship between them. If we questioned or observed how often husband and wife criticize each other, we would learn about these two people but not about their relationship. To learn about the relationship, we would need to question or observe what happens when each one criticizes the other.

Unfortunately, the procedures used by many investigators of relationship units tend to emphasize individual behavior. Observational analyses focus on rates of behavior for each individual present. For example, in a 10-minute observational sample, Dad makes 10 criticisms, Mom 6, and Johnny 4. Although we would want to label these triadic data because they represent what each individual does in the presence of the other, the data tell us nothing about who criticized whom, what each person did to elicit criticism, or what each person did in reaction to the criticism.

As a contrast to the great majority of studies, which examine only individual rates of behavior, consider the pioneering work of Gottman (1979) and Patterson (1982). Like other researchers, Gottman has studied marriage by observing and coding individual behaviors of husband and wife, and Patterson has studied families by observing and coding individual behaviors of parent and child. But in contrast to other investigators, Gottman and Patterson have coded behaviors sequentially and have examined the probabilistic ordering of behaviors between people. They have examined the likelihood that a particular behavior by one family member will lead to or follow a behavior by another member. For example, Gottman (1979) showed that clinical couples seeking marital therapy show greater evidence of negative reciprocity than couples not seeking treatment. That is, clinical couples are more likely than are nonclinical couples to respond to their partner's expression of negative affect with negative affect of their own. Patterson (1982) presented data demonstrating the frequent occurrence of negative reinforcement arrangements in families with behavior problem children. An aversive intrusion by one member is met by a counterattack, which leads the intruder to withdraw; on the basis of this sequence, the connection between intrusion and counterattack is strengthened.

In self-report data on relationships, as well as in observational data, investigators have focused on the individual. Questionnaires typically seek information on one person's behavior, thoughts, or feelings. Typical items ask the respondents to rate some state in themselves (e.g., their satisfaction with the relationship), to rate the occurrence of their behavior (e.g., how often they criticize their spouse), or to rate the occurrence of behavior by another family member (e.g., how often the child exhibits temper tantrums). Although these data tell us what a particular individual does or experiences in the context of a relationship, they tell us nothing about the interaction between participants. They don't indicate how the other responds when one member feels this way or acts this way, what the other does to elicit these reactions, or how these actions or feelings are different from or similar to those of the other. In short, typical self-report measures tell us little about interaction between participants.

In contrast, consider recent work by Peterson (1979) and by Christensen and his associates (Christensen, Sullaway, & King, 1982; Sullaway & Christensen, 1983). Although these investigators used a self-report methodology, they examined the interaction in dyadic relationships. Peterson had married couples decide on the most important interaction of the day and separately write accounts of it, indicating the conditions under which the exchange took place, the way in which the interaction started, and the sequence of behaviors, thoughts, and feelings. Observers then coded these written accounts using a complicated system designed to categorize the interpersonal message, the affect, the construal, and the response expectation for the major acts in the exchange. Peterson (1979) examined the frequencies of two act sequences across disturbed, average, and satisfied couples and found several interesting differences. For example, a pattern of aggression and injury, in which one partner expresses anger and disapproval that leads to hurt and withdrawal by the other, was more common in disturbed couples, and a pattern of aggression and retaliation, in which anger and disapproval were reciprocated, was more common in satisfied couples.

Christensen and his associates (Christensen *et al.*, 1982; Sullaway & Christensen, 1983) had couples independently respond to items that described common interaction patterns in close relationships. Each item described a general pattern and possible examples of the pattern. For example, an item that described what these authors labeled the "demand–withdraw" pattern states the following:

Sometimes A wants more of B's attention and B reacts by withdrawing from A. Possible examples:
   a. A might try to get more contact with B by being unusually affectionate, or outgoing, or demanding. B may react by initiating less contact, by replying with very short answers, or by being preoccupied. A then tries harder to get attention.
   b. When A asks for more attention, B sometimes feels "crowded." A may feel hurt or confused by B's lack of response.

Members of dating or married couples independently completed questionnaires containing items about interaction patterns. The questionnaires assessed the frequency with which the pattern occurred and the roles that each member took in the pattern. The results indicated modest agreement between partners on the extent of pattern occurrence and significant correlations between relationship dissatisfaction and pattern occurrence for several of the patterns, including the one above.

Our discussion here of the ways of examining relationships versus individual units of study has clearly been biased toward molecular, interactional analysis. One could also examine relationship units by ratings of conditions or states of the relationship, for example, by ratings of warmth, trust, and satisfaction in the relationship, made by the members or by external observers. The advantages and disadvantages of these two approaches—broad ratings versus specific behavioral data—will be discussed in a later section.

Unit of Observation. Whatever the thing being examined (what we have called the *unit of study*), data will be collected on some aspect of that unit. It is not possible to gather data on everything about the unit of study; the investigator must focus, implicitly or explicitly, on some aspect of the unit in some situation or situations during some time period. In observational research, these decisions are made explicit. The particular coding system specifies the aspects under investigation, and the observational task specifies the situation and time period. For example, a researcher studies dominance by having family members discuss for 10 minutes what they could do if they, as a group, received a prize of $1 million. The researcher videotapes the interaction, trains observers in a coding system that specifies behavioral manifestations of dominance, and has the observers code the interaction with this system. Thus, the unit of observation has been clearly specified. Of course, the researcher may try to generalize far beyond this circumscribed unit when discussing the results.

In contrast, most verbal-report research leaves the unit of observation unspecified. Respondents are often asked to rate some feeling, thought, or behavior without reference to a particular time period or situation. Presumably, the respondent is to report an average over the entire relationship across all situations. Occasionally, questionnaire and interview schedules will specify the time period or situation with phrases such as "during the last week" or "when you and your partner discuss problems." The particular questionnaire and interview items specify the aspect of the relationship under investigation. Often this aspect is relatively unambiguous, as in questions about frequency of sexual intercourse or in a question about whether the respondent has ever considered separation or divorce. However, items that ask about general qualities, such as trustworthiness or dominance, may not specify the researcher's focus clearly. For example, the respondent may interpret the question on trustworthiness as dealing solely with sexual fidelity, whereas the investigator intended the broader meaning of general integrity. The respondent may interpret dominance as being equivalent to dictatorialness, whereas the researcher meant less extreme activities, such as greater control over major decisions. In observational research, the training of coders and the calculations of reliability serve as checks on whether the researcher has clearly specified the aspect under study. In verbal report research, such checks are usually missing, and the researcher simply assumes that the respondents know what he or she is referring to. Ideally, in both observational and verbal report research, the unit of observation would be clearly specified.

Unit of Measurement. For any unit of observation, a variety of measurement possibilities exist. The measurements may consist of ratings on 7-point scales, checks by lists of adjectives, or code names in successive 10-second blocks of time, to name some common examples. In choosing a unit of measurement, the investigator needs to consider three important dimensions. First, the measurement may be structured or unstructured. Most research has used structured measurement, in which the participant responds to questions by selecting from a list of answers generated by the investigator, or in which the observer categorizes observations by selecting from a list of codes determined by the investigator. However, occasionally, the investigator provides open-ended questions for the participant or the observer. A good example from the verbal report literature is Peterson's research (1979), discussed above, in which spouses wrote accounts of their most important interaction. An example from the observational literature is the Royce and Weiss (1975) study of behavioral cues in the judgment of marital satisfaction. Untrained observers rated the marital satisfaction of couples interacting on videotape and then listed the behavioral cues used in making their judgments. The tapes were later scored for the actual occurrence of these cues, and a model of the judges use of cues in making ratings was generated.

Structured measurements are most appropriate when the investigator knows what the possible responses are and is clear on which possibilities he or she wishes to investigate. An unstructured measurement approach is most appropriate when the investigator wants to see what is "out there," when the investigator wants to get an unconstrained view of the participant's reaction. Structured approaches are limited in that the investigator will get only what she or he asks for and may get it even if it doesn't exist apart from the questionnaire or interview. For example, a question on a participant's attribution of an event will elicit ratings on the scales provided by the investigator (e.g., a scale on internality versus externality); of course, no ratings will be generated on dimensions not assessed by the investigator, and the existing scales will usually elicit ratings even if the participant never previously thought about the cause of the event. Thus, we find out what the participant thinks when confronted with the question, but we do not know what the participant thought about the event before, during, or after its actual occurrence. In contrast to structured measurements, unstructured devices may generate data that are not of interest to the investigator or that are too brief, sketchy, and inconsistent across subjects to be of use to the investigator. Furthermore, unstructured measurements must be translated into structured measurements before data analysis. Observers must code the responses to open-ended questions in order to make numerical analysis possible. This extra and expensive step often prevents the researcher from using unstructured formats, even when they are appropriate.

A second consideration in choosing the unit of measurement is whether it should be categorical or dimensional. The most important criterion in this decision is, of course, the nature of the phenomena to be investigated. For example, the assessment of gender requires categorical measurement, whereas the assessment of height requires dimensional measurement. Even in these clear cases, the alternative approach is possible and, for some investigations, may be desirable.

One could scale maleness and femaleness on the basis of secondary sex characteristics; one could arbitrarily classify certain heights as tall, medium, and short. In most measurement in marital and family research, the phenomenon does not clearly indicate categorical versus dimensional classification, so the investigator must make the decision on other grounds.

A dimensional measurement requires a more complicated judgment than does a categorical measurement. In the latter, the observer needs only to assess whether the event or attribute is present or absent. In the former, the observer must, in addition, assess the frequency of the event or the degree of the attribute. Furthermore, the dimensional judge must relate these observations to an underlying scale, a process that requires the judge to rely on implicit norms. Consider, for example, a question to parents on physical punishment of children. If the question were "Do you ever spank your child?" the parent would need only to determine if this event had ever occurred. If the question were "How often do you spank your child per month?" the parent would need to determine not only whether the event had ever occurred, but its rate. If the question were "How often do you spank your child? Never, rarely, occasionally, frequently, often," the parent would have to, in addition, translate the rate into the qualitative dimension implied by the series of adjectives. In most dimensional assessment in marital and family research, quantitative dimensions like the one above are not possible, for example, in a rating of satisfaction or trust in the relationship. Thus, the respondent must determine the events that indicate the dimension, must determine the frequency of these events, and must translate them into the levels on the given dimension. Often, the normative group is unspecified. For example, in most satisfaction ratings, it is unclear whether the respondents are comparing themselves to all other relationships, to their friends' relationships, or to the variability in their own relationship. The complexity and ambiguity of these kind of judgments make them vulnerable to error.

In observational research, dimensional measurement is completed after a longer period of observation than categorical measurement. For example, in a study of family interaction, a dimensional measurement system might require the observer to watch the entire interaction and then rate it on a 9-point scale of warmth, whereas a categorical system might require the observer to indicate the occurrence of each positive comment throughout the interaction. Because of this difference, categorical measurement is more appropriate for assessing the process of family interaction. A rating of warmth will not provide information on the process of that warmth, for example, that Mom and Dad exchange compliments and the children react with embarrassment and make jokes to each other. However, a categorical system with the proper codes could capture this interactional sequence.

Cairns and Green (1979) argued that dimensional ratings, although not as appropriate to assessing interactional process, are better in assessing stable characteristics of individuals. The rater can observe the entire segment of interaction and sort out stable sources of variance in the person from relational, contextual, and temporary sources. In contrast, the categorical observer simply records each appropriate behavior, no matter what its source of variance. For example, in an observation of children at play, the dimensional rater would note which children initiate aggression (e.g., by taking another child's toy) and which children merely respond to aggression (e.g., by yelling at the child who took the toy) and would thus rate them differently on a scale of aggressiveness. A categorical rater would simply count aggressive acts and might reveal no differences between initiators and responders. Although Cairns and Green (1979) noted the greater complexity of the dimensional rater's task and its vulnerability to error, they summarized data to show that this kind of measurement leads to better future prediction than categorical measurement, which is better at elucidating moment-to-moment dynamics.

A third consideration when choosing the unit of measurement is the size of the unit (Hartup, 1979). Most variables of interest to marital and family researchers can be assessed at varying levels, ranging from the molecular to the molar. For example, family aggression could be studied by ratings of overall aggression, by separate ratings of verbal and nonverbal aggression, or by ratings of specific aggressive behaviors, such as hitting, yelling, or teasing. Unit size is not independent of our second consideration, as dimensional measures tend to be more molar than categorical measures. However, as the example above on aggression illustrates, variations in size are possible for both types of measurement.

Typically, our interest is in the molar. Ideally, science tries to understand as large a class of phenomena as possible with its explanatory concepts. Futhermore, the criteria to which we predict in social science are often molar constructs. For example, we want to learn more about families, so we can create conditions that lead to "productive family life," "bright and adaptive kids," and "satisfactory interpersonal relationships." All these end goals represent broad conditions that are a function, in part, of social judgment, but they cannot be dismissed as too vague and broad for scientific consideration. If we are able to intervene in a family so that a boy increases his eye contact with adults, lowers the volume of his voice by several decibels, and reduces his rate of hitting, but his teachers and neighbors still see him as a "disruptive brat," certainly the treatment would be considered a failure.

Despite the importance of molar constructs, assessment at this level carries risks. First, an implicit assumption is made that the molar construct refers to an identifiable class of phenomena that share similar properties. What if verbal and physical aggression are different—elicited by different events, producing different responses, and showing little covariation? An assessment of the molar construct of aggression would fail to make such a distinction and might lead to weak and confusing results as a consequence. Second, assessment at the molar level forces the participant or the observer to make broad interpretations that may not be consistent across participants and observers or with the investigator. As the size of construct being assessed increases, observers must become more than simply recorders of what they see and hear. They must become theorists, deciding what events are indicative of the construct, and psychometricians, deciding how to combine the data into one estimate.

A study by Christensen, Sullaway, and King (1983) illustrates the tension between molar and molecular assessment. These investigators had members of married and dating couples independently complete items taken from the Spouse Observation Checklist (Patterson, 1976; Weiss & Margolin, 1977), a list of about 400 pleasing and displeasing behaviors. The items were also rated on a number of dimensions, such as molarity and importance to the relationship. The more molar items were rated as more important to the relationship but achieved lower agreement between partners. Thus, items that were methodologically more desirable (e.e., had greater consensual validity) were substantively less important. It should be noted that all these items referred to relatively specific behaviors; none referred to broad dimensions such as trust and respect.

Unit of Data Analysis. Often, the units of measurement are not what finally appear in the data analysis. Although the unit of data analysis (the final score that represents the dependent variable) is always a function of the unit of measurement, there may not necessarily be a direct correspondence between the two. For instance, units of measurement are often combined to create a composite, such as when items on a questionnaire or codes in an observational scheme are added together to form a total scale score. Similarly, in some cases, the unit of measurement is based on information gathered from individuals, but these units are combined in such a way as to create data purported to be representative of a larger unit of functioning. For example, the satisfaction ratings of a husband may be added to those of his wife to create a marital satisfaction score, or family members' individual ratings of family closeness may be averaged to yield a measure of family cohesiveness. In this way, the investigator who uses individuals as the unit of study hopes to represent dyads or larger systems as the object of study.

Despite the popularity of using summed scores, there are a number of problems that result from extending the logic of summing scores on a questionnaire to summing individual scores in order to get a measure of larger unit functioning. One of these problems is that the assumption behind the former procedure (summing questionnaire items) is that, though each individual item is only moderately correlated with the construct of interest (e.g., IQ), summing across items will cause any random measurement error to cancel out, thus producing a "truer" measure of the construct. This approach assumes, of course, random measurement error. But in a case where family members are asked individually to estimate a dimension such as family cohesiveness, all members may be biased in a similar direction (for instance, to "fake good" because of social desirability concerns). As the measurement error in this case would not be random, a summing procedure would produce a highly biased estimate of family cohesiveness.

Additionally, a summing procedure implicitly assumes that the whole is equal to the sum of the parts. Yet, a close examination of this proposition as it would apply to family studies makes it appear unlikely. For instance, a summing (or averaging) procedure could produce results that would equate a couple in which one spouse is very satisfied and the other unsatisfied with a couple in which both partners are moderately satisfied (the average "marital satisfaction" score would be the same). Most clinicians and researchers would conceptualize these two cases in very different ways, and the unit resulting from an averaging procedure would not capture these distinctions. Clearly, then, the whole is *not* equal to the sum of the parts, and more accurate (and probably more complex) models relating subsystem functioning to system functioning must be adopted and applied to the creation of appropriate units of data analysis.

In this section, we have explained the problem of unitization in behavioral research. In the absence of a structural anatomy, a large array of units is possible that must be subjected to empirical effort to test their usefulness in understanding, prediction, and control. In order to conduct research, a behavioral scientist must establish a unit of study, namely, an entity or a thing to be investigated. In marital and family research, these units of study can be conceptualized as individuals, dyads, triads, and family systems. Because of a variety of methodological and practical considerations, the investigator's object of study may differ from the unit of study; for example, an investigator may study individual parents in order to draw conclusions about their children. Once the unit of study has been established, the investigator must establish the unit of observation, the particular time period, the situation, and the aspect of the unit of study that she or he wishes to examine. Within this unit of observation, several different units of measurement are possible, ranging from the structured to the unstructured, from the categorical to the dimensional, and from the molar to the molecular. These units of measurement may then be combined to form a unit of data analysis, which is then subjected to statistical comparisons.

TAXONOMIC ISSUES

Although all family typologies share at least one goal—the attempt to categorize some aspect of family or subsystem functioning—there is a tremendous amount of variability among the existing systems. A flavor of this variability can be acquired through a brief description of a few of the typologies that have been proposed since the early seventies.

Benjamin's model of the structural analysis of social behavior (SASB; 1974) finds its roots in early attempts by Leary (1957) and others (e.g., Chance, 1959; Lorr & McNair, 1963) to systematically describe the important dimensions of interpersonal behavior. Similar to these earlier efforts, the Benjamin typology has the benefit of exhaustive empirical validation and refinement using techniques such as autocorrelation, circumplex analysis, and factor analysis (see Benjamin, 1974). The SASB model is best described as a circumplex, the circular ordering of relevant characteristics around two axes or dimensions, in this case affiliation and interdependence. The affiliation dimension characterizes the positive (intimate) or negative (hostile) quality of the behavior in question. The interdependence dimension involves issues of dependence and autonomy. Each quadrant of the circumplex is further subdivided into nine sections, which include issues such as approach–avoidance, need fulfillment, attachment, logic-communications, attention to self-development, balance in relationships, intimacy–distance, and identity. Such a model permits a systematic analysis of the varieties of interpersonal behavior in a mathematically logical framework. The system is further subdivided into three planes named "other," "self," and "intro-ject." The behaviors in each of the three planes of the model are connected via a three-digit code to their "complements," the behaviors they are most likely to elicit. In addition, the Benjamin model also provides a means for prescribing "antidotes" to specific behaviors, defined as the opposite of the complement. For instance, the antidote to "withdrawn" behavior is defined as "friendly invita-tion."

Although this system is actually a typology for any form of interpersonal behavior, Benjamin (1979) applied it on a conceptual level to a number of family-related phenomena, including differentiation failure and double-bind communication. Benjamin (1977) also convincingly showed the model's utility in developing a family treatment plan and in evaluating outcome. Nonetheless, beyond the exhaustive validation efforts directed toward the creation of the model, little empirical work has been published that specifically relates aspects of family functioning to the model, although Benjamin (1977) reported the find-ings that clinical families show fewer complementary responses as defined by the model than nonclinical families.

Olson's circumplex model of marital and family systems (Olson, Russell, & Sprenkle, 1980, 1983; Olson, Sprenkle & Russell, 1979) represents another ty-pology based on a circular ordering of relevant constructs along two dimensions. However, in contrast to the Benjamin model, the Olson model was developed through a conceptual clustering of psychological and sociological constructs that have evolved over the years to characterize families. As a result of this clustering process, two dimensions, cohesion and adaptability, were identified as integral in classifying families. The location of families on a 4-point scale along each of these two dimensions yields 16 family types. The 4 family types centrally located on the circumplex are defined as normal, and the 4 most extreme types are viewed as dysfunctional. It is hypothesized that, in general, families with moder-ate levels of adaptability and cohesion will produce more adequate functioning, both in the system itself and in individual family members. Recent work with a number of different populations conducted by Olson and his colleagues has confirmed this hypothesis and has demonstrated the model's ability to dis-tinguish clinical from nonclinical populations as well as to differentiate along the spectrum of normal families (Olson *et al.*, 1979, 1980; Russell, 1979; Sprenkle & Olson, 1978). It should also be noted that Olson and his colleagues were careful to point out that families located at the more extreme ends of either continuum may be functional if all family members are comfortable with the resultant behavior. They further noted that families located at the ends of either con-tinuum are common within certain subcultural groupings. The Olson group is currently engaged in attempts to describe the functioning of families at critical stages in the family life cycle.

Closely related to the Olson model is the Beavers model (Beavers & Voeller, 1983), which also proposes two important dimensions in the attempt to under-stand and categorize family functioning. Although both models similarly define a cohesion continuum, there are differences in how the adaptability dimension is hypothesized. Whereas the Olson model essentially proposes a curvilinear relationship between family functioning and adaptability (too much or too little ability to change is seen as a problem), the Beavers model posits a linear relationship between family functioning and adaptability, which is defined as the adaptive flexibility of the system. Therefore, in this model, the more adaptively flexible the system, the more competent it is and the more likely it is to ensure healthy family functioning. The Beavers model produces nine family types that vary in their ability to produce healthy, pathology-free individuals.

Reiss's typology (1971, 1981), which attempts to describe the family's shared consensual experience of its environment, hypothesizes essentially three types of families. Each type is uniquely characterized by its orientation toward the extra-familial environment as defined by its ability to use cues from both the external world and the family members in problem-solving interactions. The "consensus-sensitive" family views problem solving as an opportunity to demonstrate family cohesiveness at all costs, while simultaneously ignoring or underutilizing cues from the external environment, thus permitting no dissent among family members. Reiss (1971, 1981) hypothesized that the schizophrenogenic family falls into this category. The "environment-sensitive" family uses both extrafamilial and intrafamilial cues in its problem-solving attempts. In addition, it fully shares perceptions and hypotheses about the problem among members, thus agreeing on the family-generated final solution. It is suggested that "normal" families fall within this category. Last, the "interpersonal-distance-sensitive" family also effectively uses extrafamilial information, while neglecting to share observations and problem-solving suggestions among individual members because such a practice is construed as weakness. In this case, problem solving is viewed as an individual task associated with the display of autonomy from the system.

Categorization in this system is achieved by assessing family performance along three dimensions: configuration, coordination, and penchant for closure. Research by Reiss and his colleagues (e.g., Reiss, 1981) has somewhat confirmed the hypothesis that each family type relates to specific sorts of individual outcomes. Specifically, families with a delinquent child performed in laboratory tests as interpersonal-distance-sensitive families, families with no pathological children appeared as environment-sensitive families, and families with a schizophrenic offspring appeared as consensus-sensitive families.

The Moos and Moos family social environment typology (1976) represents a cluster-analytically derived taxonomy that assesses family social environment by measuring three factors: interpersonal relationships among family members, the direction of personal growth emphasized in the family, and the organizational structure of the family. Six distinct clusters of family social environment were empirically derived: expression-oriented, structure-oriented, independence-oriented, achievement-oriented, moral–religious-oriented, and conflict-oriented. Surprisingly, disturbed families were found to be primarily represented in the expression-oriented and structure-oriented categories, a finding indicating that emphases on expressiveness or structure are two important discriminating features of families.

Wertheim's family typology (1973, 1975) is based on an examination of change processes in the family, as assessed through three theoretical dimensions. Consensual morphostasis is defined as the stable, balanced distribution of power, consensually validated by all family members. In contrast, forced morphostasis is evidenced by intrafamilial power imbalance with no apparent consensual validation. Last, induced morphogenesis is related to the family's ability to respond to change agents from outside the system. Assessing families at two points (high and low) along each of these three dimensions yields eight distinct family types, two of which are conceptualized as normal and the remaining six of which are believed to contain members with varying degrees of psychopathology.

Although certainly not an exhaustive list, these typologies represent many of the recently developed taxonomic systems available. The tremendous variety among them is evidence of the number of conceptual and practical decisions confronting each individual typologist. In addition, many of the conceptual and measurement issues explored earlier in the chapter are germane to the consideration of taxonomic systems. These issues can be better conceived of in the context of a series of questions important in considering both the development and the use of any typological framework.

How Is the Typology Developed?

Although there is a tremendous amount of overlap, taxonomies are essentially either empirically or conceptually constructed. Conceptually constructed typologies are usually based on clinical observations of family functioning and/or theoretical speculation. An example of such a derivation process can be found in the Olson typology, where dimensions were developed based on the logical clustering of concepts found in the family systems literature. Systems derived in this fashion are often easily adapted to both research and clinical endeavors because the constructs and terminology used are generally familiar to theorists and practitioners alike. On the other hand, empirically derived taxonomies are developed through a process of testing, refinement, and modification, and their taxonomic structure becomes apparent through statistical analyses such as cluster analysis. Because of their empirical background, such taxonomies are often atheoretical, in contrast to conceptually derived systems, and are consequently attractive to researchers from a variety of different perspectives. However, such classification networks may be less useful in clinical endeavors because their application may require a vocabulary and a conceptual framework unfamiliar to many practitioners. (See Skinner and Blashfield, 1982, for additional reasons that cluster-analytically derived classification systems have not been widely adopted by practicing clinicians.)

It should be noted, however, that, although distinct in theory, these derivation processes are often complementary in practice because many typologists strive to create systems that are both scientifically valid and relevant in applied settings. For instance, the development of a conceptually derived typology is often followed by a series of attempts at empirical validation (e.g., Olson *et al.*, 1979, 1980; Russell, 1979; Sprenkle & Olson, 1978). Nonetheless, the initial process of taxonomic derivation is primarily empirical or conceptual, and this distinction, as noted, has important implications for the system's usefulness in various contexts.

What Is the Form of the Typology?

Typologies can take a number of forms, based on conceptual notions and statistical findings about the relationship among classifications. The least complex typology form is simple, unordered classification, in which the relevant types represent distinct and unrelated categories. The Moos and Moos (1976) family-social-environment typology is an example of this form, in which each group in the taxonomy reflects a different family-group orientation. Unordered classification implies no conceptual link among distinguished types. Ordered classification, however, suggests some underlying relationship among categories. Most family-related typologies are of this sort, simply because both abnormal and normal functioning are assumed to exist on the same continuum, so that similar explanatory constructs apply. For instance, closeness is a dimension that is applicable to all families and that may also explain the variability among them.

Ordered classifications of families may assume any number of forms, although the most common are unidimensional and circumplex models. Unidimensional models are essentially concerned with one differentiating aspect of functioning that is conceptualized as a continuum. Reiss's typology (1971, 1981), which appears to be concerned with a dimension related to family cohesiveness or intrusiveness, is one such system. These systems have the advantage of being both efficient and conceptually comprehensible at a glance.

More conceptually complex are the circumplex models, which suggest a circular ordering of constructs. The Benjamin (1974) and Olson, Sprenkle, and Russell, (1979) models are two good examples of such a structure. Classification in these frameworks is determined by the crossing of levels on two relevant dimensions. The additional complexity achieved by such a process can be seen as both having an advantage (a finer differentiation ability) and creating a problem (it is more burdensome in application), depending on the needs of the researcher. The validity of the circumplex model in elucidating interpersonal behavior has been continually demonstrated (Wiggins, 1982), and as a result, such a model shows much promise for classifying aspects of family behavior.

What Is the Function of the Typology?

Taxonomic systems can have a number of important, though often implicit, functions associated with them that become important in evaluating their utility. A *descriptive* function is common to all typologies in that they attempt to describe some aspect of family or subsystem functioning. However, purely descriptive taxonomies do not attempt to define normality or abnormality within the context of the framework and thus do not attach value-laden terms to particular categories. Although many family taxonomies are superficially descriptive, normality or abnormality is often implied in the context of category specification.

Most family typologies are actually *diagnostic* in function in that their aim is not only to describe functioning, but also to differentiate between healthy and pathological systems in the process. Typologies vary in their ability to make these distinctions in a clear-cut manner. Although some systems, such as Olson's (Russell, 1979; Sprenkle & Olson, 1978) and Reiss's (1981) have had some success in differentiating normal from abnormal systems, only research on a wide variety of populations (across racial, ethnic, and class lines) can confirm a taxonomy's functioning in this area.

Typologies that function in a *predictive* fashion seek to characterize some aspect of future functioning, either of the system being typed or of some other related system. For instance, the Benjamin system has built within it predictions about the reactions of one member of a dyad to the interpersonal behavior of the other dyad member. However, most of the predictive functioning of family typologies is reflected in the attempt to link family categorization to individual pathology. Despite a small number of exceptions, few family typologies have reliably linked family type with specific forms of individual pathology. For instance, Olson, Russell, and Sprenkle (1980) have found that the same pathology (substance addiction) can be found in a number of their family system categories. Coming years should witness a proliferation of research attempting to demonstrate the predictive function of family typologies.

Last, the *prescriptive* function of taxonomies represents a direct connection between these systems and the clinical realm. Such a function is reflected in an attempt by some taxonomies to provide information that would directly suggest intervention goals and/or strategies to be used with dysfunctional family systems. Normally, such an attempt requires treatment outcome research indicating the accuracy of prescribed interventions. For example, Benjamin (1977) effectively used the concept of "antidotes" within the framework of her model to successfully prescribe treatment of a child's disruptive and defiant behavior. Similarly, Olson, Russell, and Sprenkle (1980) discussed the usefulness of his circumplex model in setting realistic treatment goals in family therapy and in evaluating its outcome. For instance, they suggested that therapists move families no more than one level on each dimension closer to the center of the circumplex configuration. Research relevant to the prescriptive use of other typologies will most likely appear in the near future.

What Are the Various Units of Interest in the Typology?

A complex array of unitization issues confronts researchers in the development and application of family-related typologies. For one, the previously discussed distinction between the object and the unit of study is germane to the study of taxonomies. Whereas the object of study relates to the system being typed, the unit of study is the system that is actually measured in order to generate the information necessary to carry out the categorization process. These two units are not necessarily the same. For instance, in Olson's framework attempts are made to type the entire family system (object of study) by summing on a questionnaire administered to individuals (unit of study), whereas in the

Reiss taxonomy, families are often typed based on family behavior in the laboratory setting (the object and the unit of study are the same).

Additionally, both the object and the unit of study can range in size and complexity. Although typologies that deal with the family unit as the object of study may seem most relevant to family research, those that are concerned with smaller subsystems are also important. The Benjamin system is primarily dyadic in nature, as are any number of taxonomies that deal with marital and parent–child relationships. Thus, decisions about which typology to use have implications for the level of focus permissible. Family system typologies that characterize the functioning of the system in its entirety (molar analysis) often ignore fine details related to internal aspects of the system (molecular analysis). Taxonomies related to subsystem functioning provide detailed information in this regard, often to the exclusion of larger unit (family) implications. Unfortunately, little attempt has been made to generate typologies relevant to all levels of analysis. More important, little effort has been made to address potential contradictions in typological status for different subsystems within the same family and to explore the subsequent conceptual implications. For instance, some systems refer to family "enmeshment" or a similar concept but make no provisions for a system in which the children are enmeshed with one parent, yet the marital dyad is estranged.

The unit of measurement used by family typologies is almost always structured (as by their very nature typologies limit the range of concepts of interest) and dimensional (as the ability to differentiate stable, enduring characteristics is of primary importance). The unit of measurement used by these systems does range, however, in size and complexity. Molar analysis in this regard refers to global, abstract concepts as the focus of study such as *expressiveness* or *power,* and molecular analysis, predictably, involves more discrete, concrete behaviors, such as the factors assessed in the Benjamin model. Clearly, both forms of analysis play an important role in the attempt to organize family functioning. Typologies using global constructs are efficient in their attempt to be reductive and economical. Classification systems relying on molecular analysis are potentially more descriptive and, as Benjamin (1979) noted, are appropriate for the study of interactive processes and behavior sequences.

As in much other research, in these taxonomies the unit of observation, in terms of situation and time period, is rarely specified. In most cases, taxonomies attempt to classify families across specific situations. Most systems would assume, for instance, that a family displaying evidence of enmeshment in the face of family conflict would also display this behavior when involved in recreational pursuits.

The time period of observation is also rarely detailed. Although a typology clearly attempts to characterize family functioning across a spectrum of time, the limits of time periods of relevance are unclear. For instance, most systems desire to type some enduring aspect of family behavior that extends beyond the moment at which the family is assessed via questionnaires or laboratory tasks, yet probably not across the entire family history because family-life-cycle phases may drastically alter family norms and, consequently, family behavior. Thus, the family typologist is interested in behavior across a wide range of situations, but a more limited range of time periods. Yet, these factors remain unspecified in most frameworks, and thus in the measurement techniques used to generate the information needed to determine typological status.

What Is the Content of Assessment in the Typology?

A number of seemingly different dimensions are presented by the varying typologies that claim to characterize some aspect of family functioning. Nonetheless, there appear to be some striking similarities in the concepts tapped by these dimensions, although they may seem to be superficially distinct. Wiggins (1982) suggested the existence of two essential, independent dimensions in assessing interpersonal behavior: affiliation and dominance. These dimensions can be easily retitled as *closeness* and *power*, two constructs that figure prominently, at least in part, in most of the typologies presented here. Additionally, Wertheim's notions concerning morphogenesis are similar to the factors composing Olson's adaptability dimension: the family's ability to change under stress. In fact, Olson and his colleagues (1979) convincingly demonstrated the underlying similarity of a large number of formal and informal typologies and indicated their relationship to Olson's cohesion dimension. Although typologies have distinctive features, the similarities in content assessed between models, given the tremendous variability in derivation process and measurement technique, suggest the existence of several unique, independent concepts that differentiate among families. Although it is premature to fully define these dimensions at present, their content seems to assess issues of family closeness, power, and flexibility. Further work in this area should clarify these issues, their meaning, and their interrelationships.

Summary

Attempts to devise broad-based family typologies serve a number of different purposes. Taxonomies can contribute conceptual clarity to an area of study by providing an organizational framework for understanding research findings as well as for generating further hypotheses to be tested. Typologies can also be developed to serve a number of communication functions in a given field of study. For one, the classification inherent in a taxonomic system acts as a "shorthand" method of providing a larger amount of information about a unit's functioning and of decreasing the number of data needed to characterize the unit and thus serves a reductive function. Additionally, by standardizing the terms used to describe systems and their behavior, a common vocabulary is developed that bridges the gaps between researchers of different theoretical camps as well as those between researchers, theorists, and practitioners (Olson, 1981). Aside from systematizing the vocabulary of the field, the widespread use of taxonomic frameworks provides a method of comparing the contrasting findings across research studies by standardizing the concepts of interest as well as the system of measurement. The last, and perhaps most important, purpose of family taxonomies concerns the differentiating function inherent in the typological structure. Thus, effective taxonomies offer researchers a method of differentiating among families, a particularly relevant capacity given the relative failure of research efforts to reliably differentiate healthy from dysfunctional family systems (Jacob, 1975).

Nonetheless, disadvantages also accompany the widespread adoption of typologies. Any classificatory system risks the possibility of oversimplification, a potential by-product of its reductive function. More important, although any conceptual framework generates hypotheses to be tested, it also, by necessity, structures and limits which hypotheses can be developed and explored. For instance, a typological system based on a dimension of power distribution in families can produce (and handle) only predictions concerning power in families. In fact, some other dimension such as closeness may also be important in predicting some criterion event (for example, child psychopathology), but the previously described system does not allow the consideration of such issues.

In addressing many of the past problems encountered in the attempt to develop classification systems for individual psychopathology, Skinner (1981) suggested a paradigm for the development of typological structures. Skinner essentially suggested a three-step process, the first step of which is "theory formulation," which involves the proposal of the typological structure, a discussion of etiology, and the specification of the populations to which the typology applies. The second step involves "internal validation," which is the specification of operational definitions of constructs, the empirical verification of the typological structure by means of clustering techniques, and the demonstration of reliability, coverage, homogeneity, and robustness across different samples. Last, "external validation" must take place, including the exploration of the framework's predictive validity, its clinical validity, and its generalizability across populations.

If we bear the above procedure in mind, as well as the problems in the specific development of family typologies discussed earlier, there are a number of important directions that future work in the area of family taxonomies should explore. For one, empirical work seeking to validate existing typologies and/or to provide normative data about relevant classifications and categories should consciously use broad-based samples that include families with a variety of demographic characteristics, most particularly along the dimensions of socioeconomic status and ethnicity. Additionally, family-life-cycle stages must be considered, and normative data must be generated about the effects that these and other environmental changes may have on family system functioning. Last, more exhaustive work must be completed that links family typological classifications to specific forms of individual and subsystem psychopathology, thus exploring the full potential contribution that taxonomic frameworks can make to the area of abnormal psychology.

CAUSALITY IN THE FAMILY

In the preceding sections, we discussed broad issues of family assessment. We considered problems of unitization and classification from both methodological and substantive perspectives. Now we consider design rather than assessment issues. How can the investigator create research designs that sort out the causal relationship between family interaction and psychopathology?

First, the researcher must locate these two phenomena. Psychopathology could affect one or more members of the family. Dysfunctional interaction could occur within a particular dyad in the family (such as the marital dyad), within a particular triad in the family (such as the mother–father–target-child triad), within the full family, or in some combination of these relationships.

Once the psychopathology and dysfunctional interaction have been located, the investigator must examine the relationship between the two. The psycho-pathology may be causing the dysfunctional family interaction, or the dysfunc-tional interaction may be causing the psychopathology. For example, the investi-gator may diagnose the child as autistic, may determine that the parent–child interaction is dysfunctional, and may conclude that the child's psychopathology has led the parents to act in more and more deviant ways with the child.

This description of the researcher's task is overly simplistic in that it fails to consider two major characteristics of family influence, namely, mutuality and reciprocity. By *mutuality,* we mean that interpersonal events are always jointly determined. For an interpersonal event to occur, one person (P) must exhibit a behavior that the other (O) observes. P must produce a potent act, and O must possess the necessary receptivity or vulnerability to receive it. If P does not speak loud enough, then O will not hear; if O is deaf, then even P's shouts will not be heard. Thus, an interpersonal act can be attributed to (or blamed on) one or the other person. For example, O might accuse P of a personal insult, but P could respond that O is supersensitive. Each statement might contain some measure of truth. However, a more comprehensive and objective explanation would point toward both the potency of P's act and the receptivity or vulnerability of O to that act. In this sense, all interpersonal events are mutually determined: both parties contribute to their occurrence (Kelley, Berscheid, Christensen, Harvey, Huston, Levinger, McClintock, Peplau, & Peterson, 1983).

So far, we have discussed only a one-way act, in which P does something to O (P → O). In most cases, O will reciprocate with an act that has an impact on P (O → P). Thus, the interaction of P and O is characterized by a "back-and-forth" causality. This reciprocity demonstrates a second way in which the interaction between P and O is jointly determined.

The qualities of mutuality and reciprocity do not necessarily imply that the contributions of P and O are equal. An interpersonal act may be more attributa-ble to O's vulnerability than to the potency of P. The reciprocal causation during P's and O's interaction may have greater impact on P than on O. Thus, we might determine that O is primarily reacting to P rather than causing P's reactions or, at a more molar level, that P's psychopathology is contributing more strongly to the dysfunctional interaction between P and O, rather than the reverse.

How can a researcher complete an analysis of interpersonal causation that determines the comparative contributions of each of the participants and their interaction? Three methods are possible, but all require data beyond those pro-vided by the current interaction between the participants. The first method is to gather information on how P and O interact with others in similar situations. Consider, for example, a case of sexual dysfunction in which the husband has erectile problems, the wife has difficulty achieving orgasm, and each is critical of the other. Clearly, it is a reciprocally determined problem: the husband's criticisms and erectile difficulties lead to the wife's lack of orgasm; the wife's criticisms and orgasmic difficulties lead to the husband's erectile problems. The wise therapist would undoubtedly treat their sexual difficulties as mutually determined. However, for purposes of scientific analysis, we might be interested in knowing whether the problems were equally determined by husband and wife, or whether one made a primary contribution. The first methodology would require that we obtained information on the husband's and the wife's sexual functioning with other partners, current or past. If we discovered, for instance, that the wife had always functioned adequately in other sexual relationships, being interpersonally loving and physically orgasmic, but that the husband had never functioned adequately, always being interpersonally critical and physically dysfunctional, then we could confidently conclude that the primary cause of the current dysfunction is the husband's inabilities. We should note that the interaction remains reciprocal: the wife is affected adversely by the husband's behavior, which probably serves to maintain his inadequacy. But the reciprocal causation is not equally powerful.

A second methodology would require historical knowledge of the couple's sexual history. If we discovered that the husband had been physically competent and interpersonally loving at the beginning of their sexual relationship but had gradually developed erectile problems and had gradually become less supportive, while wife had been interpersonally cold and physically inorgasmic from the beginning, we would conclude that the primary cause of the current dysfunction is wife's inadequacy. We would still add, of course, that the problem is reciprocally maintained.

A third methodology would require therapeutic manipulation of the partners. If we were able to independently train the husband in social and sexual skills, so that he would be interpersonally loving and physically competent with his wife, and she responded in kind, we would hypothesize that the husband's incompetence had led to the wife's inadeqaucy. If we further knew that independent training of the wife would have no effect on the husband's performance, we would conclude that the husband had more to do with the problem than the wife.

Our examples were chosen for their clarity rather than for their realism. It is doubtful that many sexually dysfunctional couples would have such clear patterns of response or that the information required could be obtained easily. However, these three methodologies are the major methods for disentangling the dynamics of interpersonal causation. We shall call them (a) *comparisons across relationships*, (b) *comparisons across time in the same relationship*, and (c) *treatment manipulations*.

Comparisons across Relationships

Unlike our example above, in which data on other sexual relationships besides the marriage were available, in most actual cases the relationships necessary for comparison do not exist, or data from them are not obtainable. Therefore, investigators have tried to create temporary relationships of interest and to conduct the appropriate comparisons (e.g., Birchler, Weiss, & Vincent, 1975; Haley, 1968; Liem, 1974; Waxler, 1974). For example, Liem (1974) had parents of schizophrenic children and parents of normal children interact with their own child, with a schizophrenic stranger child, and with a normal stranger child. Comparisons on the data generated by these interactions were used to determine the relative effects of parent and child in creating communication problems. The methodological weaknesses of these studies are obvious. Comparisons between the parents' own child and a stranger child are confounded by length of relationship. Comparisons between a stranger normal child and a stranger schizophrenic child are based on brief and usually artificial interactions and cannot be generalized to interactions between long-term intimates. However, for examining the immediate effects of interacting with a pathological individual, these designs are useful.

A second strategy takes advantage of cases in which nature crudely approximates a design like that above. The familiar adoption study examines children at genetic risk for a disorder with children not at genetic risk for the disorder, when both have been adopted by nonrelatives. In those rare cases in which one or both monozygotic twins are adopted and raised separately, one can compare the same "genetic person" across relationships.

A third strategy does not involve deliberate manipulation of relationships or capitalization on the manipulations of nature; rather, it compares genetically different individuals in relationships that are different but are assumed to be similar. The familiar twin study assumes that relationship factors are as similar for dizygotic twins as they are for monozygotic twins. Because genetic factors are identical in the latter but only similar in the former, a comparison of concordance rates indicates different influences of individual factors (i.e., genes) versus relationship factors.

Comparisons across Time

An ideal way to sort out causal influences in the family is to study the members before their formation of a family, in addition to studying their current functioning as a family. Evidence that pathology precedes the family formation would implicate individual factors, whereas evidence that pathology develops after the family formation would implicate relationship factors.

An excellent example of this methodology, though not in the area of family interaction and psychopathology, is Newcomb's classic study (1961) of the acquaintanceship process. He assessed college students before they met each other and periodically while they lived together. He was able to show that individual attitudes, interests, and values were predictive of later friendship pairings.

Ordinarily, we can not study family members before their becoming a family; certainly, we can not create families by experimental assignment. One important methodology that is possible is to study families before and after a change in composition. For example, the classic study by Raush, Barry, Hertel, and Swain (1974) followed couples through three stages: when they were newlyweds (in the fourth month following marriage), during the first pregnancy (in the seventh month of pregnancy), and during parenthood (in the fourth month after child-birth). With this methodology, we are able to study some members and some relationships in the family (e.g., husband, wife, and marriage) before other members and other relationships exist (e.g., child and parent–child relations).

Studying the family before and after the addition of a new member may be far removed in time from the development of pathology. A prospective study may need to last many years before pathology appears. Furthermore, because any particular pathology is rare, only a small percentage of the population studied will develop the disorder. For these reasons, investigators interested in studying family interaction and pathology by comparisons across time may select a high-risk sample of subjects and follow them during the period in which pathology often occurs. For example, the Goldstein and Rodnick project (Goldstein, Rodnick, Jones, McPherson, & West, 1978; Rodnick, Goldstein, Doane, & Lewis, 1982) selected a sample of disturbed adolescents, measured a variety of family processes, and followed the sample through adolescence and early adulthood, when schizophrenic disorders often occur.

In this section, we have discussed two important comparisons across time: comparisons of functioning before and after family formation and comparisons of functioning before and after the development of pathology. What we have not discussed are the different methodologies for making these comparisons. A later section on developmental research describes these in detail.

Experimental Manipulations

Experimental manipulations are the methodological ideal for sorting out causal factors. If we can experimentally alter the behavior of an individual or a relationship, then we can observe the effects on another individual or relationship. Of course, experimental manipulations that induce pathological reactions are ethically unjustifiable. However, if the manipulations produce only mild and temporary reactions, and if the manipulations mimic processes that occur regularly in the participant's life, then the experiment is usually considered acceptable. For example, through observational analysis, Patterson and his associates (cited in Patterson, 1979) identified certain behaviors by mothers, such as ignoring, that were regularly followed by their child's whining. They then instructed the mothers to manipulate these behaviors with their child during a three-phase experimental period: a period of no ignoring, a period of ignoring, and a period of no ignoring. Measurement of the children's whining during these experimental periods established the causal effects of the mothers' behaviors.

Our ultimate goal in understanding mental disorders is to prevent or ameliorate them. Therefore, most experimental manipulations are designed to be therapeutic, that is, to lessen pathology rather than to exacerbate it. The field has seen literally hundreds of outcome studies on the effectiveness of marital and family therapy (see Gurman & Kniskern, 1978, 1981, for reviews). The methodology of these kind of investigations has been thoroughly discussed (e.g.,

Bergin & Lambert, 1978; Gottman & Markman, 1978), and it is beyond the scope of the present chapter to consider the complexities of conducting good outcome research. However, it is important to note that therapeutic manipulations cannot, by themselves, indicate etiology. If parental training in behavior modification is a successful treatment for certain kinds of child conduct problems, we cannot conclude that the conduct problems were caused by a lack of this training or these skills. In the same manner, we cannot conclude that headaches are caused by lack of aspirin, even though aspirin will eliminate headaches. A successful treatment program can be suggestive of etiology, but other kinds of research, like that just discussed, are necessary to determine that etiology.

DEVELOPMENTAL RESEARCH

Reflection on the methodological requirements of research on family interaction and psychopathology inevitably leads to developmental research designs. The family, its subunits, and the psychopathologies that afflict its members all show developmental changes across time. This feature is perhaps most obvious for individual family members, particularly children. The changes that children go through in their families as they pass from infancy to adulthood and emancipation from their families of origin are as remarkable as they are obvious. Although not nearly so dramatic, developmental changes also appear in parents, as they go from young adulthood, through midlife with its oft-touted crises, and into old age. Not only individual members but subunits of the family, as well as the whole family, show developmental changes over the life span. Most American families consist of couples who have gone through stages of courtship, marriage without children, and marriage with children. Parent–child relations are marked by extreme dependence of the child on the parent in the early years, followed by growing independence from the parent, and then, in many cases, by dependence of the parent on the child. Even sibling relationships, perhaps the most variable of all, go through stages of rivalry, companionship, and independence. All of these individual and subsystem changes contribute to developmental changes in the family as a whole.

Our current understanding also suggests a developmental course for psychopathologies. Common terms such as *premorbid history, prodromal phase, onset, course,* and *residual phase* attest to our view that these disorders develop over time. Therefore, if we are to study psychopathology as it occurs in and is affected by family interaction, we must conduct developmental research.

Longitudinal research designs immediately come to mind as the methodology for studying developmental change. We think of studying individuals over months and years with repeated measurements of their behavior. If we are dismayed by the time and money required by such a study, we perhaps think of cross-sectional research as a more cost-effective, although less valid, approach.

Cross-sectional and longitudinal research are not the only methods of studying development. Other designs and important variations on these two methods can be used to study development. In this section, we will describe these design possibilities, with some comment about their advantages and disadvantages. We will divide the designs into those that use a longitudinal methodology and those that do not. Although both longitudinal and nonlongitudinal designs seek to assess changes over time, only one actually follows subjects over time.

In considering these designs, it is important that we be clear about our central variable: time. We do not necessarily mean chronological time. Sometimes we mean time of life or stage of life. If we are studying the effects of children on distressed marriages, for example, our comparison will *not* be across age groups of married couples, but across groups of couples who are in different stages of childbearing.

Nonlongitudinal Developmental Research

Retrospective Designs. Perhaps the simplest and least costly method of studying changes over time is to ask subjects to report on different time periods in their life. For example, Braiker and Kelley (1979) studied conflict in the development of close relationships by having married couples complete identical questionnaires about four stages of their relationship: casual dating, serious dating, engagement, and marriage.

The flexibility of this design is limited only by the age of the subjects, in that the investigators can presumably ask about any period from the present back to infancy. The major disadvantage is, of course, the reliance on human memory. We don't know how many of the data represent events that actually occurred and how many represent errors of omission and addition. We can not simply assume, as in traditional testing, that errors are randomly distributed around a "true" mean because the subjects actively reconstruct their past with consistent biases (Harvey, Christensen, & McClintock, 1983). Current data on the accuracy of recall over long time periods are extremely discouraging of retrospective research (Mednick & Schaffer, 1963; Robins, 1963; Yarrow, Campbell, & Burton, 1970).

In evaluating retrospective studies, one must, however, consider the nature of the data being gathered and not make blanket judgments about quality. A number of studies of depression (see Orvaschel, Weissman, & Kidd, 1980, for a review) have examined the possible role of parental death in predisposing the child to later depression. Retrospective reports of whether a parental death occurred in childhood are likely to be accurate because of the dramatic nature of the event. However, the exact date or circumstances surrounding the death may be in error.

Follow-Back Designs. In these designs, we start with a set of index subjects, but rather than asking them about early events, we seek earlier data on them, such as childhood records. For example, Barthell and Holmes (1968) identified a sample of hospitalized schizophrenics and psychoneurotics and examined their high-school yearbooks. Data were taken from the index patients and the control subjects, pictured next to the patients. The results supported a social isolation view of schizophrenia in that these patients had fewer social activities listed by their names.

Although the follow-back design represents a major improvement over the retrospective design, two major problems often restrict its use. First, we are limited by what data exist. We may be interested in the nature of the early mother–child relationship in subjects who are now depressed, but early psychotherapy records from these subjects contain only sporadic and unsystematic information on this topic. Second, sampling biases can make the interpretation of results difficult. In our investigation of the childhood antecedents of depression, we may discover that only a portion of the sample saw counselors in their youth and thus have therapist records. It is highly unlikely that this is a random sample. Even when the study examines records that are regularly kept, such as school records, biases may occur. For example, school records may not be complete on children whose families relocated frequently, yet family mobility may be related to the psychiatric outcome of these children.

Follow-Up Designs. These designs are the reverse of the previous ones. Here we start with a sample of childhood records and then assess these subjects currently. For example, Robins (1974) identified people referred for behavior problems in childhood and then assessed these people in adulthood. Like the earlier design, follow-up studies are limited by the data that currently exist. Their biases and incompleteness will affect the results of the study. However, sampling issues are not as much a problem if all the people identified in childhood can be assessed currently. Of course, such a complete assessment may be extremely difficult and expensive.

Under ideal conditions, the follow-up design approximates a longitudinal study. As Achenbach (1982) wrote:

> If (1) all biases affecting the initial pool of records are known; (2) the records provide uniform data on variables important to the research; (3) all subjects are assessed at follow-up; and (4) their histories from the initial records to follow-up are well documented, *then* a follow-up study might approximate the yield of a good real-time longitudinal study. (p. 574; italics in the original)

Of course, as Achenbach noted, these conditions are seldom met.

Cross-Sectional Designs. In these designs, groups of subjects who differ in age or stage are compared at one point in time. Because of its relative lack of expense, compared with longitudinal research, it is perhaps the most common design used for child development. Many studies have examined differences between groups of children at different age or grade levels.

The vulnerabilities of the cross-sectional design are well known but, like the limits of correlational data, are often ignored in the interpretation of data. Cross-sectional research confounds three potential sources of variance: (a) developmental changes, (b) cohort effect, and (c) time of assessment effects (Achenbach, 1982; Schaie, 1965). If families with a younger behavior-problem child were compared with families with an older behavior-problem child, any obtained differences could be due to (a) gradual changes in the family in response to the problems; (b) differences in the two samples of families (perhaps the younger sample represents a more severe population of problems), or (c) a variety of current situational influences, such as a large number of violent television cartoons directed at younger children.

These problems in cross-sectional research are compounded when the investigation is of psychopathology. We do not know enough to predict which families will develop a pathological member, so that comparisons between families who will later develop the disorder and families who currently have the disorder are not possible. The most that can be done is to compare families with individuals at different stages of the disorder. Here again, our lack of knowledge about the course of most disorders is prohibitive. Thus, the difficulty in specifying the independent variable—namely, the stage of the disorder—makes cross-sectional research into psychopathology difficult.

Longitudinal Developmental Research

One-Group Prospective Study. Because of the difficulties inherent in the previous developmental designs, investigators have generally favored longitudinal research that examines behavior repeatedly over time. In the simplest case, one group of subjects is examined prospectively over a period of time. The investigator can definitely establish what changes occur over the repeated measurements but may not know whether the changes are a result of different conditions at the time of testing or whether the changes are generalizable to other cohorts. A more practical problem for psychopathology research is that the incidence of most disorders is so small that investigators would have to conduct longitudinal research on a huge population in order to obtain a subsample that developed the disorder.

Mednick and McNeil (1968) recommended the "high-risk-group method" of studying the development of psychopathology longitudinally. In this method, a sample of children at risk for a disorder are identified, for example, on the basis of a parent's having the disorder or on the basis of current child disturbances. These "high-risk" children are then studied repeatedly over time as some, in fact, develop the disorder. By using this methodology, the researcher obviates the practical problems of studying large populations to obtain a few subjects with the disorder of interest. Furthermore, as Mednick and McNeil (1968) noted, a major advantage of the research method is that it has a built-in control group. Those high-risk subjects who do not develop the disorder are excellent controls for those who do develop the disorder. Of course, the high-risk method is subject to the confounds of one-group prospective studies, namely, cohort and time-of-assessment effects.

In the area of family interaction and psychopathology, the Goldstein and Rodnick studies are perhaps the most well-known example of high-risk research. As mentioned earlier, these investigators identified disturbed adolescents and followed them for a decade to examine family variables associated with the onset of schizophrenia and other disorders.

Longitudinal Sequential Design. This design is a combination of a cross-sectional and a longitudinal design. As illustrated in Figure 1, more than one cohort is studied longitudinally for overlapping periods of time. Cross-sectional comparisons can be made at any point in the study; longitudinal comparisons can be made on more than one cohort, and time lag comparisons can be conducted on different cohorts as they reach a particular age in different years (Achenbach, 1978, 1982). Thus, many more comparisons are possible than in a

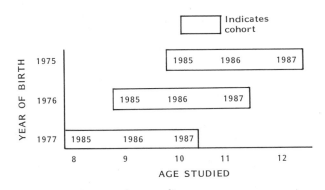

FIGURE 1. Longitudinal sequential design in which three 2-year longitudinal studies are performed simultaneously on samples from three birth cohorts. From "Research Methods in Developmental Psychopathology" by T. M. Achenbach in *Handbook of Research Methods in Clinical Psychology* (p. 577) edited by P. C. Kendall and J. N. Butcher. Copyright 1982 by John Wiley & Sons. Adapted by permission.

simple cross-sectional or longitudinal design. Furthermore, longitudinal changes can be traced over more years than it takes to complete the study. For example, in Figure 1, changes from age 8 to age 12 are studied, even though the investigation follows subjects for only 2 years.

Cross-Sectional Sequential Design. This design is similar to that above, but attempts to control for repeated assessments and increase generalizability by sampling from each cohort on each occasion, rather than measuring the same sample repeatedly (Achenbach, 1978, 1982). As illustrated in Figure 2, the subjects are sampled from the three cohorts in 1985, 1986, and 1987.

These sequential designs do not completely remove all the confounds of age, cohort, and time of assessment (Achenbach, 1982). At most, only two of these factors can be varied at any one time. The choice of a birth cohort and an age of assessment will determine the time of assessment, as any birth cohort will reach a particular age at only one point in time. Similarly, the time of assessment and the age of assessment determine the particular birth cohort, and the choice of the birth cohort and the time of assessment determines the age of assessment. However, these designs do explore more sources of variance than traditional longitudinal and cross-sectional studies.

To the authors' knowledge, these two designs have not been used in the investigation of family interaction and psychopathology, in part, perhaps, because of the newness of these designs and their methodological and practical complexities. However, the use of these designs is limited because of the nature of the phenomenon under investigation: psychopathology. We are not interested so much in the age of the subject, which can be easily specified, as in the stage of the disorder, which is much harder to specify. Nevertheless, one could imagine a study that used these sequential designs in a high-risk study. For example, cohorts of early, middle, and late adolescents with at least one schizophrenic parent might be observed longitudinally as they reached adulthood. Comparisons between cohorts and across time of subjects who did and did not

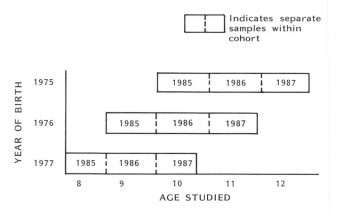

FIGURE 2. Cross-sectional sequential design in which three samples are drawn from each of three cohorts on three occasions from 1985 through 1987. From "Research Methods in Developmental Psychology" by T. M. Achenbach in *Handbook of Research Methods in Clinical Psychology* (p. 577) edited by P. C. Kendall and J. N. Butcher. Copyright 1982 by John Wiley & Sons. Adapted by permission.

develop schizophrenia would provide a more comprehensive picture of schizophrenia than perhaps even Mednick and McNeil (1968) anticipated with their "high-risk method."

EX POST FACTO DESIGNS

Longitudinal designs must clearly be favored as a methodology for assessing family interaction, psychopathology, and the relationship between the two. However, the time and expense of conducting these studies make them prohibitive for many researchers. In addition, practical problems of subject dropout and staff turnover often create methodological difficulties. One could argue that, because of these problems, longitudinal designs should be used only sparingly, when other research strategies have identified promising variables. This argument would suggest that research funding go to simpler, less costly, more practical studies that can generate information that may later warrant longitudinal investigation.

Ex post facto designs, in which subjects are studied "after the fact" or after the development of the characteristic of interest, are able to provide useful information in the face of practical constraints. In such designs, "experimental" groups are defined on the basis of some condition or attribute that the subjects possess independent of contact with the researcher or the research situation. For instance, in the field of family research, a researcher may compare the family communication styles of a group of "nondisturbed" families and a group of families with a depressed parent in an attempt to describe the features differentiating these two types of family systems. The use of *ex post facto* designs allows researchers to address questions about which they might otherwise be able only to speculate. Unfortunately, in sacrificing the control inherent in a longitudinal or in a truly experimental design, a host of other problems arises, some of which the field has yet to address.

Ex post facto designs have essentially two broad limitations, which, although straightforward at base, are far-reaching and complex in their implications. Both of these limitations arise from the fact that the *ex post facto* design is fundamentally correlational in nature. Although the inference of causality between the independent and dependent variables in an experimental design is logically sound, even an introductory statistics student recognizes the problem in extending this practice to correlational data. As cited in every statistics textbook, the problems are two. The first involves directionality. The fact that A and B covary (which is all that can be concluded from an *ex post facto* design, as subjects are not randomly assigned to levels of A) may not necessarily mean that A causes B. Therefore, the simple fact that families with a schizophrenic offspring differ from "normal" families in communication style does not necessarily mean that communication style causes schizophrenia. It is equally plausible that having a schizophrenic offspring causes the family to adopt peculiar communication characteristics. Thus, a clinician falsely concluding the first alternative might treat family communication style in an effort to cure schizophrenia, with no apparent result.

The second problem is more complex: A and B may both be related in some other fashion than the direct causal link discussed above. Commonly noted is the possibility that some third variable causes both A and B and, hence, their observed correlation. In terms of the application of *ex post facto* designs to family research, the observed differences between subject families may be due to some variable other than experimental-group status (e.g., schizophrenic vs. normal). The typical response to this situation is to attempt to control for all variables not of direct relevance that might exert this form of influence on the variables of interest.

A number of methods have been devised to gain control over so-called nuisance variables. The first involves the use of matching, the popular procedure of matching experimental groups on variables that are not of explicit interest, but that may account for any observed differences between groups. More specifically, any variable that might be related to the dependent variables and, additionally, is not equally distributed in the populations represented by the samples in the study is a candidate for matching. Over the years, a number of specific variables have been deemed important factors that are necessary to match the subjects on in family research, such as the age of the target child, the sex of the child, and the social class of the family (Jacob, 1975).

Although this process seems straightforward and logically sound, Meehl (1970, 1971) has pointed out a number of difficulties in the matching procedure as it is used in most research. The first problem involves mismatching or the possibility that matching on one variable may cause mismatching on another. Because family research using *ex post facto* designs often attempts to match groups on a variety of indices, this mismatching is a distinct possibility. Another potential difficulty involves unrepresentative samples. Matching on variables not equally distributed within the various groups often produces samples that are atypical of the population from which they are sampled. For instance, physical child abuse is more common in the lower socioeconomic classes (Gil, 1970), whereas sexual abuse is probably not (Kroth, 1979). A study comparing physically abusive families with sexually abusive ones that attempted to match on the variable of socioeconomic status would more than likely yield a group of unusually wealthy, physically abusive families and a group of unusually poor, sexually abusive families. Neither group would be representative of the population of interest and thus would limit the generalizability of the study's findings.

The last problem with the matching procedure, as noted by Meehl, is conceptually complex but is perhaps the most important. Matching is designed primarily in response to Model A (see Figure 3), the possibility that some "nuisance" variable—for instance, family communication style—has caused both the experimental-group status and the dependent variable. If this is true, then any observed relationship between group status and the dependent variable is due not to a causal relationship between these two factors, but to the influence of the nuisance variable. It is assumed that matching the groups negates the influence of this variable, ensuring that any correlation observed between group status and the dependent variable will be due to some causal relationship. For example, in a study comparing sexually abusive families with normal families on the dependent variable "family enmeshment," matching on the nuisance variable "employment status" would defend against the possibility of a correlation between

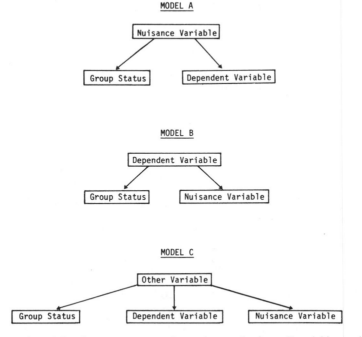

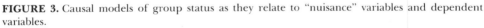

FIGURE 3. Causal models of group status as they relate to "nuisance" variables and dependent variables.

"sexual abuse" and "family enmeshment" simply because both are caused by "employment status."

Unfortunately, Model A is not exhaustive of the ways in which nuisance variables could be related to the variables of interest. For example, the dependent variable could cause both group status and the nuisance variable (Model B). For instance, in the earlier example, family enmeshment could lead to both sexual abuse and unemployment (the family becomes so self-involved that individual family members do not have the energy to devote to extrafamilial pursuits such as effective performance on the job). Or alternatively, some fourth, unspecified variable (such a social isolation) could cause group status, the dependent variable, and the nuisance variable (Model C). If either Model B or Model C were accurate in describing the interrelationship between the relevant variables, then a matching procedure would be unwarranted because it would produce inaccurate results. Thus, matching is appropriate only in cases in which the nuisance variable may act as a causal agent (such as in Model A). However, the causal model relating the variables of interest is often unknown to the experimenter, so the appropriateness or impact of a matching procedure is unclear.

Another way in which "interfering" variables are controlled is through the use of comparison groups. The choice of an appropriate comparison group is, of course, intimately related to the central research question at the focus of the study. Unfortunately, this question is rarely made explicit and must be inferred from the choice of comparison groups. For instance, a study comparing a pathological family group (e.g., physically abusive families) with normal families on some relevant index, such as communication style, is able to distinguish physically abusive families from normal ones but is not capable of definitively delineating the descriptors unique to physical abuse, as the factor of "family distress" has not been controlled for. Thus, any differences observed between the target families and the normal ones may be common to all pathological families.

The addition of carefully considered comparison groups aids in the isolation of the specific variables of interest. For instance, an additional comparison group of another pathological family group would control for the "family distress" factor. Still, one could argue that the observed differences between the physically abusive families and the newly acquired comparison group could be related to the experience of engaging in a socially taboo behavior, not to physical abuse *per se*. Thus, another comparison group of families involved in some other form of taboo behavior—for instance, sexual abuse—could be included to isolate the unique features of physically abusive families even further. Clearly, this procedure could continue *ad infinitum;* the number of factors for which the researcher wishes to control through the use of comparison groups will determine the appropriate extent of this procedure for any given study.

The third method of accounting for interfering variables involves statistical methods of control. Unfortunately, a number of stringent assumptions important to the proper functioning of these tests are often violated when the tests are applied to *ex post facto* designs. For instance, one popular method of achieving the statistical control of nuisance variables involves the use of the analysis of covariance. However, a major problem arises in the process. Analysis of covariance cannot serve as a substitute for random assignment to groups, a procedure that does not (and often cannot) occur in *ex post facto* designs. Thus, statistical forms of control are rarely, if ever, appropriate for *ex post facto* designs.

In sum, it seems clear that there are a variety of problems in the interpretation of findings generated from *ex post facto* designs. Yet, it remains true that, at present, these designs often represent the best source of information practically obtainable about a pathological population or syndrome. What, then, can be done to maximize the validity of the results produced by these designs?

For one thing, researchers should attempt to obtain adequate samples that are truly representative of the population of interest, without regard to matching the samples on nuisance variables. The result would be, at the very least, a descriptive study that would adequately characterize the groups of interest.

Once these representative samples are obtained and relevant data are collected, a number of statistical comparisons can be conducted to account for the variety of causal models that may be operating. For instance, all data from the samples of interest can be analyzed, and additionally, smaller subsamples, matched on relevant nuisance variables, can also be extracted and analyzed. If Model A (see Figure 3) is an accurate representation of the causal relationship among the variables of interest, then the matching procedure will indicate no correlation between group status and the dependent variable. If Model B is accurate, matching would produce one of two results. If the dependent variable is equally causative of group status and the nuisance variable, then no correlation would appear between group status and the dependent variable, and one would conclude (erroneously) that the dependent variable did not cause the group status. However, if the dependent variable is more causative of group status than of the dependent variable, a correlation between the two would persist (although its exact value would be underestimated). Therefore, unless we expect the relationship between the dependent variable and the nuisance variable to be stronger than that between the dependent variable and group status, matching will not disturb the overall accuracy of statistical tests. Because nuisance variables are usually multiply determined (e.g., SES is probably caused by education, intelligence, and a host of other factors), it is unlikely that they would be very strongly determined by the kinds of dependent variables in which family researchers are interested, such as communication style.

To illustrate the above concepts, let us suppose that a researcher interested in the relationship between physical child abuse and parenting attitudes wishes to match experimental and control groups on the nuisance variable of SES. In the case that Model A is accurate (SES causes both physical abuse and parenting attitudes), if a matching procedure were used statistical calculations would reveal no relationship between child abuse and parenting attitudes, an essentially correct finding. If Model B is accurate (parenting attitudes cause SES and child abuse) and matching is used, statistical analyses will reveal (incorrectly) no association between parenting attitudes and child abuse only if parenting attitudes contribute to socioeconomic status to the same degree that they do to child abuse. Such a proposition seems unlikely.

Finally, in the case of Model C, where some fourth variable causes group status, the dependent variable, and the nuisance variable, again the results of a matching procedure will depend on the relative strength of the relationship between this fourth variable and the nuisance variable. In the case of a relationship weaker than the ones between the "other variable" and group status and the dependent variable, statistical tests would accurately indicate a correlation between group status and the dependent variable. However, the researcher must be careful not to infer a causal relationship between these two variables, as they are both caused by another variable.

Thus, analysis of findings from samples representative of populations of interest without the benefit of matching can at least provide descriptive information about the groups of concern. Additionally, analyses using data from matched subsamples will produce accurate findings of a correlational nature except in the unlikely case that the relationship between the causative factor and the nuisance variable is stronger than or equal to that between the causative factor and group status. In these cases, "no effect" will be evident when, in fact, there is one.

Future work in this field should focus on the use of causal modeling strategies to more clearly delineate the models of interest. Although it is true that the validity of models cannot be proved through these procedures, incorrect models can at least be rejected. Of course, the success of a causal modeling procedure is largely dependent on the variables chosen for inclusion. In the case of Model C, where some phantom, "other" variable is an important causative factor, causal modeling would prove inadequate. Nonetheless, it is highly unlikely that important causative factors exist that have not at least been considered by theorists and researchers. Systematic analyses and the development of models that include many of the known possible links to psychopathology have a tremendous chance of specifying the causal relationships among these variables. Last, more sophisticated causal models should be pursued that include not only unidirectional links between variables (which are unlikely) but also more circular and complex interrelationships.

SUMMARY

This chapter has focused on the special, methodological problems of doing research on family interaction and psychopathology. Studying relationships such as couples and families confronts the investigator with complex unitization problems. Dyads, triads, and entire family systems, rather than individuals, are the focus of study. Determining the particular observation, measurement, and analysis procedures appropriate to investigating these relationships requires some difficult choices, often pitting methodological against practical demands. Although important efforts have been made to classify these relationships and the individual tendencies in them, much more theoretical and empirical work remains to be done. Perhaps more complex than these descriptive efforts is the problem of ferreting out causal effects in these larger relationship units. Furthermore, when the major interest is in psychopathology, which is a nonmanipulable, developmental phenomenon, the problems of causal analysis are even more difficult.

Given this complexity, one might ask: Why study family interaction and psychopathology? Why not focus on simpler characteristics that are components of the larger phenomenon? We could study individuals, as all relationships are made up of individuals and as our ultimate interest is in the functioning and welfare of individuals. We could study individual processes such as learning, memory, and emotion, which must certainly make up the phenomenon we call psychopathology.

Such a strategy, however appealing, risks the error made by the proverbial drunk, who lost his keys in a dark area in the park but searched for them by the lamppost because the lighting was better there. Our investigation of family interaction and psychopathology is motivated by a theoretical and personal conviction that relationships are more than the individuals who comprise them; that interaction is a separate phenomenon not currently predictable, perhaps not ever predictable, from knowledge of the interacting individuals; and that psychopathology is something that happens between people as well as within people. Furthermore, this motivation is not founded just on the belief that families, interaction, and psychopathology represent phenomena uniquely different from individual processes, but on the belief that these differences are extremely important—that we will never completely understand either individuals or psychopathology unless we understand relationships and interaction. In short, we brave the complexity and frustration of the darkness because that is where we believe the keys are to be found.

REFERENCES

Achenbach, T. M. (1978). *Research in developmental psychology: Concepts, strategies, methods.* New York: Free Press.

Achenbach, T. M. (1982). Research methods in developmental psychopathology. In P. C. Kendall & J. N. Butcher (Eds.), *Handbook of research methods in clinical psychology.* New York: Wiley.

Barthell, C. N., & Holmes, D. S. (1968). High school yearbooks: A non-reactive measure of social isolation in graduates who later become schizophrenic. *Journal of Abnormal Psychology, 73*, 313–316.

Beavers, W. R., & Voeller, M. N. (1983). Family models: Comparing and contrasting the Olson circumplex model with the Beavers systems model. *Family Process, 22*, 85–98.

Benjamin, L. S. (1974). Structural analysis of social behavior. *Psychological Review, 81*, 392–425.

Benjamin, L. S. (1977). Structural analysis of a family in therapy. *Journal of Consulting and Clinical Psychology, 45*, 391–406.

Benjamin, L. S. (1979). Structural analysis of differentiation failure. *Psychiatry, 42*, 1–23.

Bergin, A. E., & Lambert, M. J. (1978). The evaluation of therapeutic outcomes. In S. L. Garfield & A. E. Bergin (Eds.), *Handbook of psychotherapy and behavior change* (2nd ed.). New York: Wiley.

Birchler, G. R., Weiss, R. L., & Vincent, J. P. (1975). A multi-method analysis of social reinforcement exchange between maritally distressed and non-distressed spouse and stranger dyads. *Journal of Personality and Social Psychology, 31*, 349–360.

Braiker, H. B., & Kelley, H. H. (1979). Conflict in the development of close relationships. In R. L. Burgess & T. L. Huston (Eds.), *Social exchange in developing relationships.* New York: Academic Press.

Cairns, R. B., & Green, J. A. (1979). How to assess personality and social patterns: Observations or ratings? In R. B. Cairns (Ed.), *The analysis of social interactions: Methods, issues, and illustrations.* Hillsdale, NJ: Erlbaum.

Chance, E. (1959). *Families in treatment, from the viewpoint of the patient, the clinician, and the researcher.* New York: Basic Books.

Christensen, A., Sullaway, M., & King, C. E. (1982, November). *Dysfunctional interaction patterns and marital happiness.* Paper presented at the meeting of the Association for Advancement of Behavior Therapy, Los Angeles,.

Christensen, A., Sullaway, M., & King, C. E. (1983). Systematic error in behavioral reports of dyadic interaction: Egocentric bias and content effects. *Behavioral Assessment, 5,* 129–140.

Fiske, D. W. (1978). *Strategies for personality research: The observation versus interpretation of behavior.* San Francisco: Jossey-Bass.

Gil, D. (1970). *Violence against children.* Cambridge: Harvard University Press.

Goldstein, M. J., Rodnick, E. H., Jones, J. E., McPherson, S. R., & West, K. L. (1978). Family precursors of schizophrenic specctrum disorders. In L. C. Wynne, R. L. Cromwell, & S. Matthysse (Eds.), *The nature of schizophrenia.* New York: Wiley.

Gottman, J. M. (1979). *Marital interaction: Experimental investigations.* New York: Academic Press.

Gottman, J. M., & Markman, H. J. (1978). Experimental designs in psychotherapy research. In S. Garfield & A. Bergin (Eds.), *Handbook of psychotherapy and behavior change* (2nd ed.). New York: Wiley.

Gurman, A. S., & Kniskern, D. P. (1978). Research on marital and family therapy: Progress, perspective and prospect. In S. L. Garfield & A. E. Bergin (Eds.), *Handbook of psychotherapy and behavior changes* (2nd ed.). New York: Wiley.

Gurman, A. S., & Kniskern, D. P. (1981). Family therapy outcome research: Knowns and unknowns. In A. S. Gurman & D. P. Kniskern (Eds.), *Handbook of family therapy.* New York: Brunner/Mazel.

Haley, J. (1968). Testing parental instructions to schizophrenic and normal children: A pilot study. *Journal of Abnormal Psychology, 73,* 559–565.

Hartup, W. W. (1979). Levels of analysis in the study of social interaction: An historical perspective. In M. E. Lamb, S. J. Suomi, & G. R. Stephenson (Eds.), *Social interaction analysis: Methodological issues.* Madison: University of Wisconsin Press.

Harvey, J. H., Christensen, A., & McClintock, E. (1983). Research methods. In H. H. Kelley, E. Berscheid, A. Christensen, J. Harvey, T. L. Huston, G. Levinger, E. McClintock, L. A. Peplau, & D. R. Peterson (Eds.), *Close relationships.* San Francisco: W. H. Freeman.

Jacob, T. (1975). Family interaction in disturbed and normal families: A methodological and substantive review. *Psychological Bulletin, 82,* 33–65.

Kelley, H. H., Berscheid, E., Christensen, A., Harvey, J., Huston, T. L., Levinger, G., McClintock, E., Peplau, L. A., & Peterson, D. R. (1983). *Close relationships.* San Francisco: W. H. Freeman.

Kroth, J. I. (1979). *Child sexual abuse: Analysis of a family therapy approach.* Springfield, IL: Charles C Thomas.

Leary, T. (1957). *Interpersonal diagnosis of personality.* New York: Ronald Press.

Liem, J. H. (1974). Effects of verbal communications of parents and children: A comparison of normal and schizophrenic families. *Journal of Consulting and Clinical Psychology, 42,* 438–450.

Lorr, M., & McNair, D. (1963). An interpersonal behavior circle. *Journal of Abnormal and Social Psychology, 67,* 68–75.

Mednick, S. A., & McNeil, T. F. (1968). Current methodology in research on the etiology of schizophrenia: Serious difficulties which suggest the use of the high-risk-group method. *Psychological Bulletin, 70,* 681–693.

Mednick, S. A., & Schaffer, J. (1963). Mothers' retrospective reports in child-rearing research. *American Journal of Orthopsychiatry, 33,* 451–461.

Meehl, P. E. (1970). Nuisance variables and the *ex post facto* design. In M. Radner, & Winokur (Eds.), *Minnesota studies in the philosophy of science: Vol. 4. Analyses of theories and methods of physics and psychology.* Minneapolis: University of Minnesota Press.

Meehl, P. E. (1971). High school yearbooks: A reply to Schwarz. *Journal of Abnormal Psychology, 772,* 143–148.

Moos, R. H., & Moos, B. S. (1976). A typology of family social environments. *Family Process, 15,* 357–371.

Newcomb, T. M. (1961). *The acquaintance process.* New York: Holt, Rinehart & Winston.

Olson, D. H. (1981). Family typologies: Bridging family research and family therapy. In E. E. Filsinger, & R. A. Lewis (Eds.), *Assessing marriage*. Beverly Hills, CA: Sage Publications.

Olson, D. H., Sprenkle, D. H., & Russell C. S. (1979). Circumplex model of marital and family systems: 1. Cohesion and adaptability dimensions, family types, and clinical applications. *Family Process, 18,* 3–28.

Olson, D. H., Russell, C. S., & Sprenkle, D. H. (1980). Circumplex model of marital and family systems: 2. Empirical studies and clinical intervention. In J. P. Vincent (Ed.), *Advances in family intervention, assessment, and theory: An annual compilation on research* (Vol. 1). Greenwich, CT: JAI Press.

Olson, D. H., Russell, C. S., & Sprenkle, D. H. (1983). Circumplex model of marital and family systems: 6. Theoretical update. *Family Process, 22,* 69–83.

Orvaschel, H., Weissman, M. W., & Kidd, K. K. (1980). Children and depression. *Journal of Affective Disorders, 3,* 1–16.

Patterson, G. R. (1976). Some procedures for assessing changes in marital interaction patterns. *Oregon Research Institute Research Bulletin, 16,* (7).

Patterson, G. R. (1979). A performance theory for coercive family interaction. In R. B. Cairns (Ed.), *The analysis of social interactions*. Hillsdale, NJ: Erlbaum.

Patterson, G. R. (1982). *Coercive family process: A social learning approach* (Vol. 3). Eugene, OR: Castalia.

Peterson, D. R. (1979). Assessing interpersonal relationships by means of interaction records. *Behavioral Assessment, 1,* 221–236.

Raush, H. L., Barry, W. A., Hertel, R. K., & Swain, M. A. (1974). *Communication, conflict, and marriage.* San Francisco: Jossey-Bass.

Reiss, D. (1971). Varieties of consensual experience: 1. A theory for relating family interaction to individual thinking. *Family Process, 10,* 1–35.

Reiss, D. (1981). *The family's construction of reality.* Cambridge: Harvard University Press.

Robins, L. (1963). The accuracy of parental recall of aspects of child development and of child-rearing practices. *Journal of Abnormal and Social Psychology, 66,* 261–270.

Robins, L. N. (1974). *Deviant children grown up* (2nd ed.). Huntington, NY: Krieger.

Rodnick, E. H., Goldstein, M. J., Doane, J. A., & Lewis, J. M. (1982). Association between parent–child transactions and risk for schizophrenia: Implications for early intervention. In M. J. Goldstein (Ed.), *Preventive intervention in schizophrenics: Are we ready?* Rockville, MD: National Institute of Mental Health.

Royce, W., & Weiss, R. L. (1975). Behavioral cues in the judgment of marital satisfaction: A linear regression analysis. *Journal of Consulting and Clinical Psychology, 43,* 816–824.

Russell, C. S. (1979). Circumplex model of marital and family systems: 3. Empirical evaluation with families. *Family Process, 18,* 29–45.

Schaie, K. W. (1965). A general model for the study of developmental problems. *Psychological Bulletin, 64,* 92–107.

Skinner, H. A. (1981). Toward the integration of classification theory and methods. *Journal of Abnormal Psychology, 90,* 68–87.

Skinner, H. A., & Blashfield, R. K. (1982). Increasing the impact of cluster analysis research: The case of psychiatric classification. *Journal of Consulting and Clinical Psychology, 50,* 727–735.

Sprenkle, D. H., & Olson, D. H. (1978). Circumplex model of marital systems: An empirical study of clinic and non-clinic couples. *Journal of Marriage and Family Counseling, 4,* 59–74.

Sullaway, M., & Christensen, A. (1983). Couples and families as participant observers of their interaction. In J. Vincent (Ed.), *Advances in family interaction, assessment, and theory: An annual compilation of research* (Vol. 3). Greenwich, CT: JAI Press.

Waxler, N. E. (1974). Parent and child effects on cognitive performance: An experimental approach to the etiological and responsive theories of schizophrenia. *Family Process, 13,* 1–22.

Weiss, R. L., & Margolin, G. (1977). Assessment of marital conflict and accord. In A. R. Ciminero, K. D. Calhoun, & H. E. Adams (Eds.), *Handbook of behavioral assessment*. New York: Wiley.

Wertheim, E. S. (1973). Family unit therapy and the science and typology of family systems. *Family Process, 12,* 361–376.

Wertheim, E. S. (1975). The science and typology of family systems: 2. Further theoretical and practical considerations. *Family Process, 14,* 285–310.

Wiggins, J. S. (1982). Circumplex models of interpersonal behavior in clinical psychology. In P. C. Kendall & J. N. Butcher (Eds.), *Handbook of research methods in clinical psychology.* New York: Wiley.

Yarrow, M. R., Campbell, J. D., & Burton, R. V. (1968). *Child rearing: An inquiry into research and methods.* San Francisco: Jossey-Bass.

Yarrow, M. R., Campbell, J. D., & Burton, R. V. (1970). A study of the retrospective method. *Monographs of the Society for Research in Child Development, 35* (Serial No. 138).

CHAPTER 8

Factors Influencing the Reliability and Validity of Observation Data

THEODORE JACOB, DANIEL L. TENNENBAUM, AND GLORIA KRAHN

INTRODUCTION

During the past 3 decades, researchers and clinicians alike have become increasingly interested in the nature of family interaction in their attempts to understand, modify, and prevent such diverse maladaptations as schizophrenia, depression, alcoholism, and childhood aggression. Overall, such investigations have sought to (a) construct and evaluate theoretical models of marital and parent–child behavior with the aim of understanding the development and functioning of family systems; (b) identify family interactions that reliably differentiate problem from nonproblem families as a first step toward developing more effective methods of treatment and prevention; and (c) assess the influence of various treatment approaches on the nature of intrafamilial interactions.

Increasingly, the preferred information base for these efforts has been the ongoing family-interaction data obtained through the use of laboratory and naturalistic observation procedures. In large part, this move toward observation has been stimulated by dissatisfaction with traditional assessment methods involving questionnaire, interview, and psychological test data. In particular, it has been argued that direct observation methods require fewer assumptions and inferences, are less susceptible to various confounding influences, and reflect

THEODORE JACOB • Division of Family Studies, 210 Family and Consumer Resources Building, University of Arizona, Tuscon, AZ 85721. DANIEL L. TENNENBAUM • Department of Psychiatry, University of Pittsburgh, Pittsburgh, PA 15213. GLORIA KRAHN • Crippled Children's Division, Oregon Health Sciences University, Portland, OR 97202.

greater face validity and generalizability than do the less direct and/or more artificial data-collection strategies (Anthony, 1971; Canter, 1963; Goldfried & Kent, 1972; Jacob, 1975, 1976; Scott & Wertheimer, 1962; Wiggins, 1973).

The value of observational research—providing less inferential methods for developing and testing models of family behavior—depends on the degree to which observed behaviors are generalizable to naturally occurring family behavior. If such applications cannot be made with confidence, the development of compelling family theory and effective treatment programs is surely hindered. Various reliability and validity issues associated with observation procedures must be more clearly understood and ultimately resolved in order for this method's vast potential to be realized. Four issues, which we believe to be most critical in evaluating observation data, will be reviewed in this chapter: observer reliability, context effects, subject reactivity, and cross-measure correspondence.

OBSERVER RELIABILITY

Demonstrated interobserver reliability of family interaction data is essential to the process of drawing valid conclusions from those data. Reviews of the literature, however, suggest that a significant proportion of family researchers who use observational procedures still fail to report any reliability coefficients, and that the majority continue to employ the simple percentage-agreement statistic (Mitchell, 1979; Susman, Peters, & Steward, 1976). This inattention to the reliability characteristics of observer's data is seen to arise not only from a lack of concern, but also from a vague and imprecise conceptualization of reliability and its importance. In the following sections, a definition and context for considering reliability are presented, alternative methods for estimating interobserver reliability are reviewed, and guidelines for selecting reliability estimates is offered.[1]

Definition of Reliability and Its Applications

The concept of *measurement reliability* has been defined variously in the literature. In particular, the concept has been used to describe the "accuracy and stability of measures, as well as the actual conditions under which observations are made" (Hollenbeck, 1978, p. 80); the representativeness and generalizability across coders and conditions (Cronbach, Glesser, Nanda, & Rajaratnam, 1972); and the proportion of true score variance relative to the error score plus true score variance (Nunnally, 1967). Interobserver reliability represents only one aspect of measurement reliability, that having to do with the congruence of measurement between two or more raters observing the same individual at the

---

[1]Distinct from concerns influencing the choice of a reliability index are those factors known to influence the level of interobserver accuracy, regardless of which index is used. Research examining these influences has been reviewed by Johnson and Bolstad (1973), Cone (1977), Kazdin (1977), and Hughes and Haynes (1978).

same time. Thus, interobserver reliability assesses the accuracy of measurement and does not assess temporal stability or difference due to conditions.[2]

Reliability estimation is involved in several phases of family interaction research. A first application occurs during the development of a new coding system or the extension of an established coding system to a new situation or population. Reliability estimates can be used to identify those behavioral codes that are ambiguously defined or those coding procedures that lead to disagreement among coders. These reliability estimates are generally of interest only during initial stages of code development and are rarely reported in the literature.

A second need for reliability estimation occurs during the data collection phase of observation research. Interobserver agreement is typically calculated for individual observation sessions throughout the coding process. This monitoring of agreement can signal when observer retraining may be necessary and, to some extent, can promote coder vigilance (Kent, Kanowitz, O'Leary, & Cheiken, 1977).

A third application occurs in the reporting of research findings. Reliability estimates are presented to indicate the confidence that can be placed in the observational data and their interpretations. Typically, the agreement measures obtained on individual observation sessions during the course of coding are combined into an overall, average percentage agreement figure. Reported less frequently but often of greater relevance to the substantive hypotheses are the reliability estimates calculated for individual codes across sessions. Reliability estimates calculated both within sessions across codes and within codes across sessions are used as demonstrations of the "quality" of the data. A final purpose for determining interobserver reliability is to account for the variance in the observational data. Within a generalizability study framework, observers can be regarded as one facet of a factorial design, which allows for estimating the variance accounted for by coders, and by the interaction of coders with other facets of the design. Interobserver agreement is then reported as a generalizability coefficient. A procedure somewhat similar to this analysis-of-variance approach involves the use of multiple regression. Observers are coded as dummy variables and then entered into the regression equation with other predictors of interest (e.g., Blurton-Jones, & Woodson, 1979).

The implications that the obtained reliability level has for substantive findings differ for the various indices. Within the generalizability framework, a

---

[2]It has been argued that interobserver agreement may not even represent accuracy of measurement unless the observations are compared to some established standard (Herbert & Attridge, 1975), harking back to the well-known measurement maxim that reliability is a necessary but not sufficient condition for validity. Should that note of skepticism not be sufficiently sobering, Yarrow and Waxler (1979) argued that reliability need not represent veridicality. They contended that the coding process itself can obscure the very realities that we wish to study. Adequate interobserver agreement can be obtained and agreement with an established standard demonstrated, but the subtleties and complexities of the ongoing behavior may remain unrecorded. Despite these limitations on the conceptual interpretation of reliability estimates, the need for reliability estimation still remains.

meaningful observer effect (i.e., when observers differ substantially in their codings) need not preclude the interpretation of other main effects (e.g., diagnostic groups differing in their display of specific behaviors), unless they are also evident as interaction effects (e.g., observer by diagnostic group). However, when agreement measures averaged across codes or across sessions serve as the reliability estimate, interpretation of substantive findings is immediately implicated. The lower the values for these agreement measures, the more seriously are the research findings compromised. More specifically, when interobserver agreement is low, neither the presence nor the absence of significant research findings can be presumed meaningful.

Estimates of Reliability

Many reliability indices have been proposed and reviewed in the extant literature. Hollenbeck (1978) presented an excellent review of reliability measures as well as computational illustrations. Hartmann (1977) considered several of the more popular estimates in behavioral analysis and compared their results for several data sets. Four reliability indices are reviewed here, including a discussion of their applicability given the characteristics of one's data, as well as the relative merits and limitations of each estimate. Table 1 (a,b) presents the sample data that will be used to illustrate the computation of several indices.

Percentage Agreement. This is certainly the most commonly used reliability estimate and the easiest to compute. When the data are coded sequentially, a method allowing for a point-by-point comparison between the two raters, this reliability estimate is calculated as the number of points on which the coders agreed (e.g., 6) divided by the number of points in which they agreed plus disagreed (e.g., 8). Percentage agreement can also be calculated when only the aggregates for each code are known. In this calculation, it is assumed that all instances of overlap for the sums of a code recorded by the two observers represent agreement between the observers. Unfortunately, this assumption is not always accurate (e.g., Behavior A in the sample data), and the result is inflated and erroneous estimates. Nevertheless, its use may actually be warranted if subsequent analyses of the data are to be conducted only on frequencies of codes, without considering their sequential order. That is, it may not matter whether observers code behaviors identically at the same time, only that they agree on the relative distribution of codes across the entire observation session, as it is the totals that will be compared.

A major advantage of percentage agreement, in addition to its ease of computation, is its usefulness in providing an immediate estimate of agreement for individual sessions, which facilitates the ongoing assessment of reliability. Variations of the simple percentage-agreement index have been developed. Effective percentage agreement for occurrence is based only on those instances in which one or both observers have coded some behavior. By excluding agreement about nonoccurrence, this index guards against a spuriously high percentage-agreement value when the nonoccurrence of a code is frequent. In similar fashion, an effective percentage agreement for nonoccurrence prevents a mis-

TABLE 1a. Percentage Agreement Calculated on a Point-by-Point Comparison of Sample Data

				Time points				
Observer	1	2	3	4	5	6	7	8
1	A	B	C	D	A	A	B	D
2	A	A	C	D	E	A	B	D
Concurrence	+	−	+	+	−	+	+	+

Percentage agreement (point by point) = 6/8 × 100 = 75%

TABLE 1b. Percentage Agreement Calculated on Aggregate Frequencies of Sample Data

Code	Observer 1	Observer 2	Agree/disagree
A	3	3	3/0
B	2	1	1/1
C	1	1	1/0
D	2	2	2/0
E	0	1	0/1
Total			7/2

Percentage agreement (aggregate) = 7/9 × 100 = 78%

leadingly high agreement index due to a high chance rate of occurrence (Hartmann, 1977). Although these indices prevent the distortions that are evident when high rates of the occurrence or nonoccurrence of a code are present, they still suffer from the same problems as percentage agreement. Most important, the percentage-agreement index fails to take chance agreement into account. The distortion that this leads to is directly related to the differences in base-rate occurrence across the codes. As differences in base rates across codes increase, percentage agreement will increasingly overestimate reliability. (See Jacob, Grounds, & Haley, 1982, for illustrations of how base rates can influence different reliability estimates.) Most coding systems have one or two high-frequency codes (often regarded as the "garbage codes"), which present a serious problem to reliability estimation. Unlike other reliability estimates, the percentage-agreement index has no standardized metric properties and no meaningful lower bound. As a result, it is not suitable for further statistical analysis such as significance testing (Hartmann, 1977). Because of these limitations, percentage agreement is generally regarded as the least desired reliability estimate.

Kappa. Unlike percentage agreement, kappa (Cohen, 1969) does consider the chance occurrence of the behavior codes. Its similarity to a chi-square contingency coefficient is seen in its calculation: the proportion of observed agreements minus the proportion of expected agreements ($PO - PE$), divided by 1 minus the expected agreements ($1 - PE$). The calculation of kappa begins with portraying the observations of the two observers in a matrix in which entries in the diagonals reflect observer agreements, and off-diagonal entries represent disagreements, as depicted in Table 2. The proportion of observed agreements equals the sum of diagonal entries as a proportion of the total number of matrix entries. The proportion of expected agreement is the sum of the marginal products, reflecting the overall frequency of each code for each observer.

Like the percentage-agreement index, kappa can be calculated on data obtained from a single session and can be used immediately and repeatedly during the coding process as a reliability estimate. The matrix display allows for easy identification of those codes that account for the most disagreements. In addition to identifying the sources of confusion, kappa controls for chance agreement and has a known sampling theory and set of statistical properties (Cohen, 1972) that allow for further statistical examination. The use of kappa has been extended to the case of more than two raters (Fleiss, 1971; Fleiss, Nee, & Landis, 1979) and to a weighting procedure that allows for varying degrees of disagreement to be used (Cohen, 1968; Mezzich, Kraemer, Worthington, & Coffman, 1981). The use of kappa has typically been limited to data for which point-by-point comparisons can be made between observers, and where observers agree on the total number of coded units. Procedures are presented in Appendix A for calculating a kappa estimate when only frequency aggregates of codes are known, and when observers differ in the total number of behaviors recorded.

A commonly voiced criticism of kappa is that it is cumbersome to compute. Perhaps of greater concern is that kappa does not allow for estimating the reliability of individual behavior codes. Despite these limitations, kappa is still recommended as one of the most preferred reliability estimates.

Product–Moment Correlation. The interobserver reliability of interval-scaled data is often estimated with a product–moment correlation coefficient. Observational data are most likely to be interval-scaled in one of two situations. In Situation A, the behavior being observed is represented along a single dimension, such as activity level, and gradations of that behavior are recorded (e.g.,

TABLE 2. Calculation of Kappa on Sample Data

		Observer 1					Proportion of total for Observer 2
		A	B	C	D	E	
	A	2	1	0	0	0	3/8 = .375
	B	0	1	0	0	0	1/8 = .125
Observer 2	C	0	0	1	0	0	1/8 = .125
	D	0	0	0	2	0	2/8 = .250
	E	1	0	0	0	0	1/8 = .125
Proportion of total for Observer 2		.375	.250	.125	.250	.000	

$$PO = \text{diagonals/all entries} = 6/8 = .750$$
$$PE = PO1 \times PO2 \text{ for all code entries} = (.375 \times .375) + (.125 \times .250) +$$
$$(.125 \times .125) + (.250 \times .250) + (.125 \times .000) = .219$$
$$\text{Kappa} = PO - PE = (.750 - .219)/(1 - .219) = .680$$

Krahn & Gabriel, 1984; Tronick, Als, & Brazelton, 1977). In Situation B, frequency aggregates of behaviors are compared, such as the total number of negative behaviors.

The product–moment correlation provides an index with a defined distribution and statistical interpretability. It can be applied to the data from a single observation session, and to data in which the total aggregates of frequencies differ between two observers. In addition, it is an index familiar to virtually all audiences. However, a number of problems in applying correlational measures to interobserver reliability estimation warrant attention. First, as has been noted by others (e.g., Hartmann, 1977; Hollenbeck, 1978), the product–moment correlation coefficient is insensitive to differences in level between the two observers. This circumstance might arise in Situation A if one observer consistently recorded a higher level of activity than the other observer at each observation point. In this case, the mean activity levels coded by the observers would differ, but the correlation might still suggest perfect reliability. In Situation B, if Observer 1 consistently recorded more occurrences of each of the behavior codes than Observer 2 (as might occur with event-coded data), these differences in actual numbers of recorded behaviors would not be reflected in the reliability estimate.

A second problem relates to the distribution and range of the variable being examined. Although rarely a problem in Situation A where the behavior codes are interval-scaled, problems of interpretation can arise in Situation B, where frequency aggregates are compared. Recall that a high product–moment correlation between two sets of data requires not that both data sets be normally distributed, but only that the shapes of the distributions be highly similar (Carroll, 1961). That is, variables with highly skewed distributions can correlate perfectly. In Situation B, the variable being correlated is the overall frequency of code occurrence. A high "match" of the observers' distributions is ensured if the base frequency rate differs greatly across the codes. That is, when an observation period contains one or more high-frequency codes as well as several-low frequency codes, the Pearson product–moment correlation between two observers will virtually always be high, even though there may be considerable disagreement about the exact occurrence of the specific codes. Stated in familiar terms, when the product–moment correlation is calculated across all codes, it does not correct for the chance agreement that arises with unequal frequency of usage.

An alternative procedure for calculating a correlation coefficient deals with this difficulty by considering each code separately. That is, correlations are calculated on the frequencies recorded by each of two observers on one code across a number of observation sessions.[3] The magnitude of the correlation is

---

[3]Phi correlation coefficients can be used to examine agreement on individual codes within one observation session. The data then constitute two sets of dichotomous data (occur/nonoccur for Observer 1 and/or Observer 2). When the rate of occurrence of the behavior is equal across the two observers, the value for phi will be almost identical to that for kappa. Factors influencing phi are discussed in Glass and Stanley (1970), and the relationship between phi and kappa is discussed in Hartmann (1977).

influenced by the variability evident in the frequency of the code across the observation sessions. If the sessions represent pretreatment baseline observations or observations of a highly homogeneous group, for example, variance may be restricted and the resulting coefficients will be disappointingly low.

Although the product–moment correlation follows a known sampling distribution and offers statistical advantages, its insensitivity to level differences and its sensitivity to frequency and range distributions can make its interpretation difficult. Reliability, as a reflection of observer agreement, can be highly over- or underestimated, depending on the circumstances. For that reason, the use of this correlation is only cautiously advocated, and only for estimating the reliability of individual codes.

Generalizability Coefficients. The generalizability theory of Cronbach, Gleser, Nanda, and Rajaratnam (1972) provides a means of estimating interobserver reliability within the framework of a factorial design. Observers are regarded as one of several facets (factors) across which results can be generalized. Other facets of interest may be subjects and occasions. Analysis-of-variance procedures provide a method of partitioning the observed variance into the respective components. This partitioning allows for the examination of the main effect of observers, for its interaction with other facets (e.g., observers × occasions), and for temporal stability (i.e., occasions of the main effect). Once the appropriate research design has been determined (e.g., whether the facets are crossed, nested, or some combination is used), a separate analysis of variance is typically conducted separately for each behavioral code. The resulting partitioning of variance can then indicate those codes, if any, that are heavily influenced by observers. A coefficient of generalizability for each code can be calculated from the ANOVA results. This generalizability coefficient is an intraclass correlation and is "completely comparable to the traditional reliability coefficient," (Cronbach *et al.,* 1972, p. 97) except that full attention has to be given to defining the population to which generalization is made and to designing the study on which decisions are based (Cronbach *et al.,* 1972).

Difficulties in application have restricted the use of a generalizability approach in assessments of family interaction data. The data considered in generalizability studies are aggregates of frequencies as coded by the different observers. Point-by-point matching of recorded codes has not been used, although it may be possible to use some form of data that would take temporal sequencing of codes into account (e.g., contingency coefficients as described by Patterson & Moore, 1979).

A second consideration is the substantial number of data required for a generalizability study. The total amount of duplicate coding required for a generalizability study is much more than would be collected for traditional reliability checks. It is also not feasible to make frequent interim reliability checks by the use of generalizability coefficients. Instead, another reliability estimate is needed during the course of coding to ensure reasonable agreement between coders.

A final practical consideration was raised by Mitchell (1979) and illustrated by the data of Jones, Reid, and Patterson (1975). In order to obtain a large reliability coefficient, it is necessary to have a relatively large variance component for subjects. All other things being equal, if one group exhibits a very low frequency of a target behavior (e.g., normal children exhibiting very few non-compliant responses), the generalizability coefficient of this behavior will be lower for this group than for another group that demonstrates a higher frequency of this behavior. This is the same concern about restricted variance that was considered in the discussion of product–moment correlation coefficients.

Notwithstanding these three considerations, generalizability studies offer the opportunity to elegantly and succinctly examine all the defined components of reliability simultaneously: accuracy as measured by interobserver agreement, temporal stability as measured by repeated trials, and context as defined by different tasks.

Additional Considerations in Reliability Estimation

The preceding discussion of reliability indices considered the selection of an index in regard to the nature of the data and the relative advantages and disadvantages of the different indices. In some cases, however, it may be desirable to calculate and report on more than one index. Lytton (1979), for example, reported two percentage-agreement indices, one in which omissions by one coder were regarded as disagreements, and another in which omissions were not included. In other studies, percentage agreement has been calculated during the coding process, and generalizability coefficients have been calculated later (Vincent, Friedman, Nugent, & Messerly, 1979; Wieder & Weiss, 1980). The use of multiple reliability indices is desirable when the indices provide complementary information regarding the nature and the quality of the data.

A second basic consideration in estimating reliability has been expressed in several forms. Briefly, there is general agreement that the estimates of reliability should be calculated on the unit that will be used in subsequent statistical analyses. Departures can lead to either an overly conservative estimate of reliability or an unduly liberal one. When analyses will be conducted on aggregate groupings of codes, the reliability index should be reported on those same groupings. Reliabilities calculated on the more finely discriminating codes will underestimate the reliabilities of code groupings. Conversely, when subsequent analyses will be sequential, the temporal position of the recorded codes must be taken into account. Comparison of frequency aggregates is not adequate, as these estimates will always be greater than or equal to corresponding estimates that take temporal position into account.

The general procedure adopted for estimating the reliability of sequential data has been a point-by-point comparison that is then subjected to percentage agreement or kappa calculation. Gottman (1980) has argued that this strategy is too stringent a criterion and that a more logical approach is to assess reliability on the sequential structures that are evident in the observations made by each observer. This approach requires substantial data collecting by both observers; identifying the sequential structures evident in the coded observations of each coder; and then comparing those sequential structures identified by the observers as occurring significantly more often than chance. Using a related approach,

Patterson and Moore (1979) calculated the conditional probabilities that one behavior would occur given that a specific behavior has just preceded it. The values for these conditional probabilities (or sequential structures) were compared between observers by use of a product–moment correlation. Yarrow and Waxler (1979) described an extension of this approach, in which data from each observer are analyzed and interpreted separately. Comparisons would then be made to show whether the same conclusions would be reached based on each observer's recordings. Although these less traditional approaches to reliability estimation are not without difficulties, they illustrate the importance of relating the reliability estimate to the data and the planned analyses.

Two key questions can serve as guidelines in selecting an estimate of interobserver reliability. First, to what extent can the chance occurrence of codes lead to the overestimation of reliability? Whatever the codes of a system vary in their base rates of occurrence, some capitalization on chance occurrence will operate to overestimate reliability if it is calculated as percentage agreement. When base rates are fairly homogeneous across codes, percentage agreement may be an adequate estimate. However, much more frequently, chance rates will vary considerably, and percentage agreement should be abandoned and replaced with another estimate, such as kappa. Second, is the temporal order of codes important in the subsequent analyses? If sequential analyses are planned, then temporal ordering of codes must be examined in the reliability estimate as well. This examination is done through a point-by-point comparison of the codings. These comparisons are then summarized in a percentage agreement, kappa, or a product–moment correlation, or through the "identified-sequence" procedure advocated by Gottman. On the other hand, when the temporal position of codes will not be of interest in subsequent analyses, kappa based on aggregates or generalizability coefficients may be sufficient.

THE CONTEXT OF OBSERVED INTERACTIONS

In 1974, Bronfenbrenner suggested that much of the extant developmental literature was "ecologically invalid" because of its reliance on laboratory settings and procedures. Because of a similar emphasis on observation within highly controlled laboratory settings, much of the family interaction tradition is vulnerable to this same criticism. Notable exceptions have been the works of Patterson (1982) and his colleagues with delinquent adolescents and their families, as well as the work of Steinglass (1980) and his associates with the families of alcoholics.

To the extent that interactional data are influenced by the context within which they are collected, the generalizability of findings to other, presumably more representative, contexts of family interaction is compromised. At the same time, the high cost of conducting naturalistic observations, the frequent lack of experimental control that characterizes this paradigm, and the increased difficulties surrounding the data quality of at least some naturalistic observation procedures place important limitations on the widespread use of home observations. At the very least, however, the researcher should be aware of the potential impact that contexts can exert on emergent behavior so that appropriate interpretations and qualifications can be considered. In this section, the effects of context are reviewed in terms of the physical setting in which interaction occurs and of the task presented to the interactants.

The Setting as Context

For the most part, studies of family interaction across different settings have involved comparisons between home observations and those made in the laboratory or clinic. Real physical differences existing between these conditions include architecture, furnishings, and noise and lighting levels, all of which may function as cues for different behaviors. In addition, home settings are more familiar, are often less physically constraining for the family members, and are more liable to interruptions by nonparticipating family members and others.

An early study comparing findings across settings was that of O'Rourke (1963). Using Bales's Interaction Process Analysis (1950), he assessed the level of positivity while family members were engaged in decision-making tasks both at home and in the laboratory. Unfortunately, the home observations were always conducted first, so that O'Rourke's findings of greater positivity in the home versus the laboratory may reflect initial reactivity to being observed rather than an effect of the physical setting. Lytton (1974) collected behavioral data in the home and in the laboratory on mothers, fathers, and preschool sons. For these families, ratings based on home observations, interviews, and mother-maintained diaries substantiated theoretical predictions more than ratings based on laboratory observations. Unfortunately, it is not possible to draw strong and unqualified conclusions from this study because (a) the measures taken in the two settings were not completely comparable, and (b) the order of condition was apparently not counterbalanced.

In contrast with the limited literature on families with adolescents and preadolescents, the setting variable has received considerable attention by parent–infant interaction researchers. Belsky (1977), who did control for the order of setting in his observations of mother–infant dyads, observed that, whereas the infants' behavior did not appear to be significantly influenced by the setting, the mothers were more active and more responsive to their infants in the laboratory than in the home. Dyadic interaction also occurred more frequently in the laboratory. Differences between home and laboratory settings have also been observed when infants are separated from their parent; that is, infants have been found to exhibit greater distress when separated from their parents in the laboratory than when separated in the home (Ross, Kagan, Zelazo, & Kotelchuck, 1975). Similarly, Brookhart and Hock (1976) observed infants to exhibit more proximity avoidance of both the mother and a stranger in the home than in the laboratory and more contact maintaining and proximity seeking by the infants when alone with the strangers in the laboratory. On the other hand, no setting differences were observed by Borduin and Henggeler (1981) when infants were exposed to a less stressful situation (i.e., no separation). Taken together, these results indicate that the setting can influence both mother and infant behaviors, but that this context effect depends both on the salience of the task or situation and on the specific behaviors targeted for observation.

Setting effects on marital interaction have received less attention. Gottman (1980) reported on comparisons between home and laboratory observations of distressed and nondistressed couples. In this between-subjects design, the couples who were audiotaped at home were more negative and were more likely to engage in reciprocally negative interactions than were the couples observed in the laboratory. Further, those differences that discriminated the distressed from the nondistressed couples were more evident in the home than in the laboratory. From this study, it seems that the laboratory setting has a moderating and homogenizing influence on marital interactions.

In summary, it appears that physical setting can influence the nature of observed family and marital interactions. A number of general findings can be drawn from this body of research. The first is that the nature of a home–laboratory difference varies with the age of the interactants and the nature of the task. For adults, the laboratory appears to provide more structure and focus than the home. Gottman's distressed couples were seemingly better able to restrain their hostilities in their laboratory discussions than the couples observed at home. He commented that participating couples have often described the laboratory procedures as therapeutic, and he attributes this effect to the laboratory's structured nature and the attendant expectations of cooperation. Belsky's mothers were seen to be more actively involved with their infants and more responsive to the infants' initiations in the laboratory than the home. Mothers at home are seemingly more distracted from their infants. Adults, whether in the role of spouse or parent, appear to be more "on their best behavior" in the laboratory than in the home. Infants, on the other hand, appear to be more immune to differences in physical settings unless they are placed in the stressful situation of being separated from their mothers. Where differences are noted, they are in the direction of increased distress in the laboratory and more competence and independence in the familarity of the home setting. These findings suggest that the effect of the laboratory situation may shift with age, from being distressing for infants to providing facilitative structure for adults. A key question awaiting empirical investigation pertains to the impact of physical setting on the interaction of children and adolescents.

A second general finding, which is most clearly displayed in Gottman's study, is that the results found in one setting generally are not contradictory to those observed in the other. Those behaviors and patterns that discriminate the distressed from the nondistressed couples in the laboratory are generally also evident in the home. What does differ is the magnitude and the number of differences observed in the home relative to a less naturalistic situation.

The Task as Context

An experimental task creates a context within which members relate to one another, imposing an interactional framework within which behavior occurs.

Thus, different task parameters would be expected to exert different demands on the interactants, encouraging certain behavioral relationships and limiting others. From our perspective, two task dimensions are of particular importance in influencing family behavior: (a) the structure that the task imposes on the possible behaviors of the different interactants and (b) the emotional salience of the task for the family members.

The merit in structuring the task for direct observation of parent–child interactions was outlined clearly by Bell in 1964. He cautioned that minimal structuring can result in behaviors' accumulating in an unrepresentative and small number of categories, or of behaviors' being dispersed over a large number of categories, each having only a few, unstable number of observations. Task structure is seen as restricting the behavior of the interactants, both the child and the parent. Behavior can be relatively unrestricted (e.g., free play); can be restricted to a single class, with variation available within the class (e.g., asking family members to solve problems in areas of disagreement); or can be restricted to and within a single class (e.g., providing strict instructions for the parent to follow). Differing degrees of structure can be imposed on different interactants. Bell provided examples from the literature of different combinations of structure for parent and for child. A series of tasks that illustrate these differences in structure are those used by Eyberg and Robinson (1983) in investigating and treating noncompliance in young children. In the first task, the parent is instructed to "follow the child's lead and play along with him." The behavior of both parent and child is relatively unstructured, the only restriction being that the parent not lead the play. In the second task, the parent is instructed to lead the play and have the child follow him or her. The child's behavior is not directly structured, but the parent's behavior is now restricted to the class of "leading the play," although it can vary within the class. In the final task, the parent is asked to instruct the child to clean up the toys. This task represents restricting the parent's behavior to a class (directing the activity) and within the class (cleaning up the toys).

Research on the influence of task structure has been restricted largely to interactions between mothers and their young children. Although relative differences have been noted within tasks, few direct comparisons have been made across tasks. Zegiob and Forehand (1975) compared mothers' behavior as a function of social class, race, and child sex using both a free play situation (Structure Level 1) and a specific task situation (Structure Level 3). Differences that were primarily attributed to social class were noted in maternal cooperation and criticism during free play, and in maternal noncooperation, questions, and use of commands during the task situation. Aragona and Eyberg (1981) compared the verbal behaviors of mothers identified as physically neglecting their children with those of nonproblem mothers and mothers of behavior problem children. The two situations were child-directed interaction (Structure Level 1) and parent-directed interaction (Structure Level 2). Not only were those behaviors that differentiated the groups of mothers in the free play (i.e., type of commands, praise, and criticism) also differentiating in the task situation, but the effects were larger and more clearly evident. In these paradigms where the structure of the task is closely related to the behaviors observed, the general finding is that increased task structure leads to a greater likelihood of observing group differences.

Some insight into the requirements of these two tasks was offered in a study by Mash and Johnston (1982). Middle-class mothers were observed in interaction with their hyperactive school-aged children in a free play and task situation. Analyses were based on aggregate frequencies of maternal behavior, child behavior, and maternal self-ratings on several scales of parental self-esteem and parental stress. During free play, the maternal behaviors were largely predicted by the child behaviors. During the task situation, however, the mothers' behaviors became more predictable by the maternal ratings of parental self-esteem and stress. As the authors indicated, the task situation may be seen as placing additional demands on the mother, demands that lead to observed behaviors that are organized around internal cognitions and affect rather than around her child's immediate behavior. It appears that a strategically structured task can tap into the more stable parenting characteristics, which are hypothesized to determine those parenting behaviors that differ among groups of parents.

Early studies reporting differences in marital interactions as a function of task structure were presented by O'Neill and Alexander (1970). In one study, nondistressed couples ($n = 8$) completed four tasks taken from Watzlawick's structured family interview (1966): (a) Decide on the most troublesome areas in your marriage. (b) Discuss what brought you two together. (c) Decide which partner each of several "blame labels" fits better. (d) Decide on a common story for two cards from the Thematic Apperception Test (TAT). A second sample of 21 couples completed (a) a puzzle task (a block puzzle to be assembled); (b) a discussion of attitudes and opinions on various topics; and (c) a revealed-difference questionnaire. In both studies, ratings of dominance were used and indicated significant task effects. In the first study, the "blame" task elicited more dominance statements from husbands than from wives, whereas the other three tasks showed the exact opposite dominance structure with wives making more dominance statements than husbands. For the second sample, the more structured puzzle task and Revealed Difference Technique (RDT) task yielded greater dominance from husbands than from wives, whereas husband and wife dominance were relatively equal on the less structured topic-discussion task. Based on these findings, the investigators suggested two task dimensions that seemed related to the obtained outcomes: the amount of structure imposed on the family by the task and the amount of stress generated in family members by the task.

When the structure across tasks is held constant but the salience of the tasks varies, few consistent differences have been found. Murrell (1971) observed family triads as they engaged in three written tasks: (a) answering questions about their family; (b) listing adjectives that described their family; and (c) completing an unrevealed-difference questionnaire. The observational measures used were the number of statements exchanged between each of the six pairs of family members (mother to father, father to mother, mother to child, and so on). The stability of each family's rank ordering across the three tasks was determined by Kendall's coefficient of concordance, and significant coefficients for stability were obtained for 22 of 30 families. In an earlier study of family process, Haley (1967) observed American families (40 disturbed and 40 normals) as well as 40 Japanese-American family triads in two discussion tasks: (a) resolving differences of opinion about "neutral items" from a revealed-difference questionnaire and (b) generating a "story" from a set of TAT cards. The measure of interest, a response-deviation score, was based on patterns of speech among the three members, that is, who talked after whom. All correlations on the measure across the two tasks were highly significant: $r = .56$ for American "normals"; $r = .49$ for American "disturbed"; and $r = .77$ for Japanese-Americans. Finally, Jacob and his colleagues (Jacob & Davis, 1973) conducted two studies involving nonproblem adolescent boys and their parents. In the first report, 10 families interacted around three tasks: a plan-something-together task (Watzlawick, 1966), a set of TAT cards, and an unrevealed-difference questionnaire. The families were then rated for talking time, attempted interruptions, and successful interruptions. With few exceptions, family process was not altered as a function of task. In better controlled study with a larger sample, Zuckerman and Jacob (1979) assessed 30 normal family triads across three tasks: (a) composing a story based on TAT cards; (b) discussing and resolving "typical" family problems; and (c) discussing and resolving differences in opinions and attitudes based on an unrevealed-difference technique. All three tasks were similar insofar as they restricted the families to a focus on discussion and consensus, but they differed in the degree to which they were immediately relevant to the family members. The primary measures included the number of speech units, successful interruptions, and attempted interruptions. The only task effect noted was that all family members were more active in the task most salient to them. Comparisons of relative within-family structures, however, showed remarkable consistency across tasks; that is, the same hierarchy (e.g., Father is greater than Mother. Mother is greater than Child.) characterized a family on all measures tasks, regardless of the level differences associated with the particular tasks.

In a study reporting more significant task effects, behavioral measures of dominance and conflict, as well as ratings of activity, dominance, and conflict, were applied to observed interactions of nonproblem mother–father–adolescent triads by Henggeler, Borduin, Rodick, and Tavormina (1979). Comparisons were made between two unrevealed-difference-technique tasks, the first representing "instrumental/external" family issues (e.g., Where should the family go for a vacation?), and the second, "emotional-expressive/internal" issues (e.g., What is the family's biggest problem?). No differences in affect or dominance were noted between tasks, but the instrumental/external task elicited more conflict (in both observed behavior and ratings) than the expressive/internal task. The authors interpreted these findings either as indicating a consensual level of expressivity within a family or as reflecting the safety of expressing disagreement about instrumental but not expressive issues. Alternatively, these tasks may be regarded as representing differences in the salience of the task for the family members. These families, which were selected for their favorable psychosocial adjustment, may have been relatively harmonious in their perception of family and affect (i.e., expressive/internal) but may have had differing preferences about family activities (i.e., instrumental/external). That is, the instrumental/external task may have been more salient to nondisturbed family members in their discussions. Similar findings across tasks might not be obtained for identified problem families.

A study by Floyd and Markman (1983) suggests comparable findings for marital couples. Observations were made of distressed and nondistressed couples on two tasks: (a) discussing their own primary problem and (b) discussing two standard problems taken from Olson and Ryder's Inventory of Marital Conflicts (1970). Although no clear task effect emerged in the multivariate analyses of variance, distressed wives were rated as being significantly less positive than nondistressed wives while discussing their own problem. No such difference was noted in the discussion of the standard problems.

The empirical investigations of task effects on observed family interactions are far from complete or conclusive. Several general conclusions, however, can be extracted. The first is that tasks structured to depict the target areas of concern provide the best opportunity for group differences to emerge. A second general finding is that when tasks are equally structured, those tasks whose context is most immediately salient to family members are again most likely to evidence group differences. And finally, when noninferential process measures are used, intrafamilial structures remain quite similar across tasks, notwithstanding the differences in overall activity that are associated with the various procedures.

REACTIVITY

Reactivity, the impact on emergent behavior of being observed, is rooted in general theoretical issues of the social sciences. Social psychology, for example, has been interested historically in the parameters that affect the process of interpersonal influence. One primary component of these processes, the effect that one person can exert on the performance of another, is the basis of the voluminous literature on social facilitation (Zajonc, 1965). Such areas of study have served to clarify the role of social context in the emergence of individual and interpersonal behaviors. Investigations of observer influence, therefore, can be viewed as another extension of this continued interest in the basic processes that influence social behavior.

Although subject reactivity may affect the interpretation of observational data in many ways, a primary concern is its threat to the external validity of study findings (Campbell & Stanley, 1963). It is a major methodological issue associated with observational procedures in all settings and across all tasks. The same methodological issue has been raised about other data-gathering procedures. Questionnaire research has led to concern about social desirability effects (Crowns & Marlowe, 1960), whereas analyses of face-to-face interviews have described a subject response pattern referred to as *impression management*. Regardless of the manner in which data are collected, then, subjects' reports may be altered by the procedures themselves. Who is affected, in what ways, to what extent, and by what procedures are questions that certainly merit further attention. Efforts to explore these issues will extend the knowledge of individual differences and interpersonal influence, as well as enhance the validity of research findings.

Several recent reviews have discussed much of the literature on reactivity in family research. Most notably, Johnson and Bolstad's early review (1974) of this domain described a number of important factors that must be considered in any analysis of reactivity effects (subject and observer characteristics, the rationale for observation, methods of assessment, and observer salience). More recently, Harris and Lahey (1982), Haynes and Horn (1982), and Kazdin (1982) have reviewed studies of reactivity effects in various settings. All of these authors have concluded that reactivity may occur and that researchers should attempt to minimize such influences as much as possible. In general, however, reviewers have been cautious about drawing more specific or stronger conclusions given the absence of rigorous and programmatic research in this area. Both conceptual and methodological problems—inherent in this research domain—have not been amenable to simple solutions, and thus, the identification of robust and generalizable findings remains to be achieved.

Although reactivity effects have been discussed for many years (Arrington, 1943), systematic research efforts were not undertaken until the 1960s. Since then, the question of reactivity has been addressed in various settings, including the home (Christensen & Hazzard, 1983), the school (Weinrott, Garrett, & Todd, 1978), and the counseling session (Roberts & Renzaglia, 1965). Overall, this literature has been marked by diverse and inconclusive findings, a status that is attributable to the limited number of methodologically sound studies that have been conducted and to the fact that many variables can affect the strength and direction of reactivity effects. Furthermore, theories to guide studies of reactivity effects and to explain the conditions under which they occur have been extremely limited. Primarily, conceptualizations have been borrowed from the experimental literature, where phenomena such as evaluation apprehension (Rosenberg, 1969) have been described and have been found to lead subjects to respond in a more socially desirable manner (Weber & Cook, 1972). Apparently, some subjects are concerned that the experimenter will make a personal evaluation of them based on their performance. To avoid embarrassment, they then act so as to elicit a positive evaluation from the experimenter. In reading the reviews of this literature, however, there appears to be little attempt to go beyond such general models and to develop and test more refined theories of reactivity. Instead, reviewers have focused attention on a more basic, and at this stage necessary, question: What variables appear to be related to the emergence, extent, and direction of reactivity effects? In these critiques, various potentially influential variables have been identified, although only one variable—observer salience—has received any empirical study. Before describing this literature, however, a brief discussion of relevant but understudied variables is offered.

Understudied Variables

Although observational data are gathered for purposes established by the investigator, subjects often develop their own beliefs about the purpose of a study. As a result, family members may be influenced by their understanding of why the observations are taking place. Thus far, the variable of "study rationale" has been evaluated in only one investigation, in which assessments were made of reactivity before and at the completion of therapy (Johnson, Christensen, & Bellamy, 1976). During the week before treatment and for 1 week following treatment, recordings were made during one 15-minute period per day that was designated ("picked") by the parents and during three other randomly chosen 15-minute periods. Although the authors urged caution in interpreting their results, their findings suggested that negative family behaviors changed more during the "picked" time periods, which were more related to the focus of therapy than were the "random" time periods.

Observer characteristics may also influence the emergence of reactivity effects—a contention that draws support from a related literature on interviewer characteristics that has investigated such variables as race, sex, and age (Rosenthal, 1966). In family research, however, only effects due to nonparticipant versus participant (i.e., a family member) observers have been studied (Harris, 1969; Hoover & Rinehart, 1968; Patterson & Reid, 1970). From our vantage point, there appear to be major limitations in using family members as observers of molecular behavior. Most important, such procedures can alter family interaction in unknown ways by imposing the dual role of observer and participant on the family member.

Subject characteristics, including age, social class, adjustment, and personality characteristics, may also affect the extent and the direction of reactivity. As previous research (Christensen & Hazzard, 1983; Tennenbaum, 1980) has suggested that families and family members do differ in their response to observation, greater attention needs to be paid to these variables. At present, three related phenomena—public self-consciousness, guardedness, and social desirability—have been suggested as characteristics that may influence a subject's reactivity. A study by Tennenbaum and Jacob (1985), which found that husbands' level of public self-consciousness predicted their reactivity to spouse observation, offers support for the continued study of these individual-difference variables.

Observer Salience

Two general strategies have been used for assessing reactivity. One approach looks for systematic change in family behavior over time and assumes that such change indicates habituation to observation. In general, little or no habituation has been found in observational studies of families (Christensen & Hazzard, 1983; Patterson & Cobb, 1971). The same is true in reports from quasi-observational studies of marriage, in which spouses keep records of each others' behavior (Margolin & Weiss, 1978; Robinson & Price, 1980; Tennenbaum &

Jacob, 1985; Volkin & Jacob, 1981). To equate minimal change with minimal reactivity, however, is problematic. Most important, absence of change over time could mean either that there is no reactivity effect or that there has been no habituation. Because stronger conclusions are difficult to justify when only this research strategy is used, it is not the method of choice for evaluating reactivity effects.

A second—and in our view, stronger—research strategy for evaluating reactivity effects is to assess subjects' behaviors across conditions that vary along dimensions that are logically and theoretically related to reactivity. This has been the most widely used approach in the empirical literature on reactivity and is therefore reviewed and analyzed here in some detail.

The optimal context against which to evaluate the effects of some obtrusive observational procedure is one in which family members are observed but have no knowledge or awareness that any observation is taking place. Because ethical considerations prohibit this option in its "purest" form, some approximation is usually undertaken. Even in these cases, ethical issues still arise because some deception is often required. An example of such a dilemma and how it can be resolved is found in a study by Christensen and Hazzard (1983). In this effort, the investigators gathered observational data using automatically activated audio-recording equipment installed in families' homes. Although the families gave their consent for such procedures, they were later deceived into believing that an equipment breakdown had occurred and that no recordings were occurring during this "downtime." In actuality, recordings were obtained during this time to approximate observations when the subjects are "unaware" of the observation procedure. To minimize potential harm to the subjects, Christensen and Hazzard did not remove the tapes from the home until the families had been debriefed and had given their consent to the "unaware" procedure. Even with such safeguards, however, these authors decided to conduct this procedure with nondistressed families only, rather than to risk engendering discomfort in families already identified as experiencing significant disturbance. Their cautious approach indicates their sensitivity to the issue as well as the problems inherent in obtaining minimally obtrusive observational data.

As previously noted, observer salience or obtrusiveness has been the variable that has attracted the most attention in the reactivity literature (Bernal, Gibson, Williams, & Pesses, 1971; Christensen & Hazzard, 1983; Conte, 1979; Johnson & Bolstad, 1975; Johnson et al. 1976; Tennenbaum, 1980; Tennenbaum & Jacob, 1985; Vidich, 1956; Volkin & Jacob, 1981; Wells, McMahon, Forehand, & Griest, 1980; White, 1973, 1977; Zegiob & Forehand, 1978; Zegiob, Arnold, & Forehand, 1975). In these various efforts, differences in observer salience have been expected to relate to the quantity or quality of observed behavior.

Laboratory investigations of reactivity during observations of mother–child interactions have led to equivocal results. Studies conducted by Zegiob and her co-workers (Zegiob & Forehand, 1978; Zegiob et al., 1975), for example, compared mother–child interactions during periods when the subjects were informed either that observations were or were not taking place. The findings suggested that mothers altered their behavior so as to maximize the positive behaviors of their child during the informed condition. In a similar study, White (1973) did not find such an effect. Methodological problems present in both studies, however, render the conclusions tentative. Specifically, because all subjects knew (before participating in the study) that they would be observed, their behavior may have been altered even during the unaware condition. At a minimum, the subjects had to believe that no observations were being made during the unaware condition for a valid test of reactivity to be conducted. However, Zegiob and Forehand (1978) found that 39% of the mothers reported being "slightly suspicious" to "certain" of being observed, whereas White (1973) reported that two thirds of his subjects had had at least "some suspicion" of being observed. This lack of a clearly convincing manipulation makes the interpretation of the results problematic.

Another problem that arises in laboratory studies of reactivity is the confounding of "observer" effects with differences in instructional set associated with the various observational conditions. Even though mother–child dyads may remain in the same room with the same toys, for example, being asked "to wait" may lead to different actions on their part than being asked "to interact or play together." In essence, families may be engaging in quite different tasks across the two observation conditions. Given the difficulty in eliminating these confounds in the laboratory setting, assessments of reactivity may be more compelling when conducted in a more natural setting, such as the family's home.

Evaluations of reactivity during naturalistic observations in the home were begun by Bernal in the early 1970s (Bernal *et al.*, 1971). In a clinical case study of a single-parent family, the mother was found to engage in a higher rate of "commands" when an observer was present than in a condition in which an automatically activated tape recorder captured the mother's behavior. Although Bernal developed an innovative method for gathering observational data unobtrusively, the definition of *command* differed across conditions by including nonverbal behavior during the observer-present condition, and as a result, the findings remain difficult to interpret.

An important group study was conducted by Johnson and Bolstad (1975) in which observation was conducted by a tape recorder activated by the families. On alternate days, over a 6-day period, a live observer was also present. Only the tape-recorded interactions—in both observer-present and observer-absent conditions—were used for data analyses. In brief, Johnson and Bolstad found no differences across conditions for the three summary categories of "Child Deviant," "Parent Negative," and "Parent Commands." Although it could be argued that their low salience condition was still too obtrusive to allow for a true test of reactivity to observation, the absence of a significant condition effect certainly suggests that reactivity to direct observation is not a blockbuster phenomenon, able to consistently and dramatically alter all family behaviors of interest.

Subsequent efforts to assess reactivity in families' homes, where even less obtrusive observation procedures were used, also resulted in minimal reactivity effects. Christensen and Hazzard (1983), for example, compared two levels of observer salience using a single-subject ABA design. Using three nondistressed families as subjects, they collected 3 weeks of audio recordings with the families aware of the procedure, followed by one week with the families unaware, and finally a fifth week of recordings with the families once again aware of the observation procedure. The recordings were collected on three tape recorders installed in the home, which were automatically activated at times during which there was a high probability of family interaction. During the unaware week, the families were told that the equipment had broken down and that a needed part would be replaced shortly. In actuality, the machines operated as usual. Two of the three families demonstrated no change on the measured variables. The third family exhibited some changes across conditions, with total interaction and positive interaction being lower during the "unaware" recording week.

Tennenbaum (1980) also used a single-subject (ABA) methodology for evaluating reactivity to home observations. The more salient procedure involved live observation of families during their dinnertime. In addition to taking notes, the observer recorded the interaction on audiotape. Dinnertime was chosen because it minimized the amount of "artificial" structuring of family relationships and patterns of interchange. During a second phase of the study, families had three tape recorders placed in their home; the dining area was always included as one of the settings. Although the subjects were told that these three tape recorders would be randomly activated during the day, only the recorder in the dining area was actually used. Because the equipment remained in the home and, from the families' perspective, was automatically activated at random times in any room, the families were expected to quickly adapt to and become comfortable with the procedure rather than maintaining a high vigilance level for the entire week. The order of phases was balanced across families: two families received the live-random-live order, and two received the random-live-random order. The ratings of the audiotapes on both process measures (talk time, speech rate, and attempted interruptions) and content measures (positivity and negativity) indicated few consistent changes related to observation condition. As in the Christensen and Hazzard study (1983), however, a few changes were observed, suggesting that some family members did react to the observation procedure, although not frequently.

In a related investigation, Wells *et al.* (1980) evaluated the importance of the observer salience dimension during home observations of parent–child interactions. These analyzed data came from the initial assessment phase of a treatment study involving 30 problem children and their families. Home observations were routinely carried out by only one observer, except for planned reliability checks that required the presence of an additional observer in the home. In comparing the interaction generated when one versus two observers were present in the home, the investigators found greater maternal attention to the children when two observers were present. Although one interpretation of this finding is that the mothers were reactive to increased levels of observer salience, an equally reasonable interpretation is that the observers rather than the mothers were reactive. That is, the observers may have seen more examples of actual maternal attention because of the elicitation of increased vigilance on their part by the presence of a reliability checker. These rival hypotheses need to be explored before the meaning of this study can be fully understood.

Two studies (Tennenbaum & Jacob, 1985; Volkin & Jacob, 1981) have now evaluated the reactivity of quasi-observational procedures. Both studies manipulated husband's awareness of whether their wives were observing their behavior via the Spouse Observation Checklist (Weiss & Perry, 1983). Neither study found more than minimal evidence of reactivity effects.

Given the difficulty of eliciting reactivity effects in home observations of families, it is tempting to conclude that observers have only a minimal impact, if any impact at all, on routine family behaviors. Although possibly correct, such a conclusion is as yet unwarranted, given the methodological weaknesses of this extremely limited area of research. Most important, several of the reported studies involved samples ranging from one to four families (Bernal *et al.*, 1971; Christensen & Hazzard, 1983; Tennenbaum, 1980). In addition, reactivity has not been adequately assessed in populations of particular interest to clinical researchers, that is, families in which one or more members are defined as being distressed. Just as distressed families are expected to interact differently from nondistressed families, they may also be differently reactive to observation. Clarification of this more complex concern would certainly aid the interpretation of comparative family-group studies.

Another difficulty to be overcome is that, in order for family behaviors to be comparable across conditions, certain rules need to be followed by the family members. The intrusion, however minimal, of this structuring of family behaviors may lead to unobtrusive conditions' being more salient than would be optimal. For example, Johnson and Bolstad had families follow the same rules during both the observer-present and the observer-absent conditions. Although observer salience is hypothesized to be a dimension, such structuring may lead families to experience the observer-absent condition similarly to how they experienced the observer-present condition. How reactive the observer-absent condition is, therefore, also remains to be determined.

Although initially it is reasonable to evaluate reactivity in its own right, more sophisticated investigations need to consider jointly the relative importance of reactivity effects to other potentially more powerful variables of interest, such as the presence or absence of psychopathology. Even if reactivity effects do exist, they may not be large enough to significantly distort group differences or models of family behavior derived from observational data.

A study currently being conducted by Jacob and his colleagues will begin to address some of these issues (Jacob, Rushe, & Seilhamer, 1986). In this effort, they have incorporated a reactivity study comparing two levels of observer salience into a between-group comparison of families containing fathers who are problem drinkers, social drinkers, or depressives. The minimally salient condition is the same as the "random" condition described in the study by Tennenbaum (1980), in which families were informed that three tape recorders installed in their home would be automatically activated randomly throughout the day. In actuality, only the dining-area tape recorder was activated during dinnertime. As in other minimally obtrusive procedures, a deception was involved, but in this case, families were actually asked to give their consent to a more intrusive procedure than was actually used. During the more salient observation condition, a family member turned on a tape recorder just before dinnertime. Again, choosing dinnertime as the observational period minimized the number of rules that the families were required to follow. The outcome of this study will afford a strong test of the importance of observer salience in a normal family sample as well as indicate whether psychopathology in family members leads to different reactivity effects across the three groups.

At present, the available reactivity literature, as flawed and limited as it is, suggests that family behavior is not dramatically altered by the presence of an observer. Notwithstanding the need for more rigorous and sophisticated research in this area, some consideration should be given to why this may be the case. A major factor may be that family units differ from stranger groupings. One important difference is the lengthy interactional histories of families, which make it more difficult for individual members and the family system to act in novel ways. In order for an observer to affect family behavior, the inertia of maintaining routine interactional patterns needs to be overcome.

Additionally, families are busy environments, with the continual demands of multiple, interrelated tasks. Particularly in home settings, all of these family functions must be accomplished regardless of the presence of an observer. To paraphrase one parent's response when asked about the impact of an observer on his family life, "Taking care of our children takes up much of our time; we were just too busy to be affected by your study."

Finally, most families may have little motivation for altering routine behavior. Researchers are generally unknown to subjects before their involvement, are usually not evaluative in their interactions with the participants, and typically control no important consequences for the families. One population that may be motivated to change and whose behavior may therefore be more reactive to observation is families observed during the course of therapy. Only one study is known to have addressed this issue (Johnson *et al*, 1976), and further work evaluating differences in reactivity across phases of therapy is recommended.

Because so little is currently known concerning reactivity effects, a prudent approach is to design observations so that they are as comfortable as possible for families. Strategies to do so include implementing observational procedures that are as minimally salient as possible. In addition, presenting families with a thorough explanation of the procedures should decrease the apprehensions that may arise. Along with this approach, allowing time for the subjects to become comfortable with the research staff and the observational equipment can facilitate obtaining records of naturally occurring behavior.

Although families may be less reactive to observation than other types of subjects, the notable lack of empirical data suggests a bilevel approach to the issue of reactivity. Investigators should both attempt to minimize potential reactivity effects and begin to address this important methodological concern more systematically.

CROSS-METHOD CORRESPONDENCE

Another major issue related to the interpretation of family studies concerns the degree to which different assessment methods yield similar information regarding a particular family variable or construct. The development of assessment instruments has been based largely on a single methodology (e.g., self-reports, laboratory outcomes, quasi observations, laboratory observations, or naturalistic observations). The gathering of supportive data regarding the instrument's basic psychometric properties has been the researcher's primary task, whereas comparisons with other methods (if undertaken at all) are conducted at a later point in the test development process. Although only a few such cross-method studies have actually been published, the lack of correspondence that has been reported suggests that greater attention should be directed to this issue. If not, it seems likely that family theory will be limited to interpretations unique to particular instruments rather than being generalizable to broader family constructs.

Several authors have begun to describe features of the research context that may help to explain the lack of correspondence that has often been found. Olson (1985), for example, focusing on the structural aspects of family research, suggested that assessment procedures can be categorized by the reporter's frame of reference (insider versus outsider) and by the type of data collected (subjective versus objective). An insider report is one given by a family member, either by answering "subjective" questions on a questionnaire like the Family Adaptability and Cohesion Scales (FACES; Olson & Portner, 1983), or by reporting more "objective" data using self-monitoring or spouse-monitoring procedures. Outsider assessments made by nonfamily members are expected to be inherently different from data gathered by insiders because of the different vantage points used in each of these methodologies. More recently, Reiss and his colleagues (Oliveri & Reiss, 1984; Sigafoos, Reiss, Rich, & Douglas, 1985) have suggested that an analysis of the "pragmatics" of the assessment situation can add further clarity to this issue. Specifically, the relationship between family member and investigator can be quite different depending on the particular assessment method used. The obtained results may therefore be influenced by these different relationships. In reference to his own assessment procedure, Reiss has contended that the subject's uncertainty regarding what is "the appropriate response" on the card-sort procedure gives the investigator more of an insider's view of the family. In contrast, self-report questionnaires, which allow family members to know more easily what responses are expected of them, provide data of more relevance to an outsider's view of the family.

Although theory will help to explain observed differences and to guide research, a more immediate need involves the development of a database that provides empirical descriptions of actual cross-method relationships. Unfortunately, gathering such data is not a simple matter. At the simplest level of analysis, two family members may respond to or perceive the same event in a very different fashion. For example, mothers and fathers may perceive and report their family very differently on the FACES and, as a result, may produce different "scores" on the same variable (e.g., "Cohesion"). To the extent that other evidence is available (e.g., factor analyses of data from different members yielding the same factors), one can also assume that the same concept (trait or construct) is being measured. As more differences are introduced, however, the interpretation of the correspondence becomes more complicated. If one holds constant the general method, for example, a comparison across instruments purporting to measure the same construct (e.g., FACES versus the Family Assessment Measure, or FAM of Skinner, Steinhauer, & Santa-Barbara, 1983) offers another level of complexity. Finally, when instruments based on different methods are compared (e.g., a mother's reports on the FAM versus laboratory observations coded with the Marital Interaction Coding System, or MICS, of Weiss & Summers, 1983), multiple sources of variance are involved in one's assessment and interpretation of correspondence.

In considering this continuum, it is clear that some comparisons are more different from others because of variations in the specific instrument (e.g., FAM versus FACES); the general type of assessment method (report versus observation); the member providing the data (e.g., the mother versus the father or the mother versus ratings of the whole family's participation in a laboratory interaction task); and the concept being assessed (e.g., cohesiveness versus coordination). Stated otherwise, comparisons involving two family assessment procedures can reflect differences between data sources, between instruments, between methods, between concepts, or in any combination of these conditions. Given such complexity, it seems clear that cross-method comparisons can involve much more than differences in general method and that interpretation of low correspondence becomes increasingly difficult as the number of differences between the two assessment procedures increases.

In general, empirical studies of cross-method correspondence among family assessment procedures have been limited and nonsystematic in design. The one exception is the considerable literature on "family power" carried out since the mid-1960s, although even this literature cannot be considered entirely adequate. (For reviews, see Hadley & Jacob, 1973, 1976.) More recently, several investigators have begun to assess correspondence for other family variables. Two studies (Margolin, 1978; Stein, Girodo, & Dotzenroth, 1982) have examined the correspondence between marital assessment procedures based on report (marital satisfaction scales), observational (Marital Interaction Coding System, or MICS), and quasi-observational (Spouse Observation Checklist, or SOC) methods. Margolin (1978) found very low correlations across these measures. Stein *et al.* (1982) reported similar results, although more support was demonstrated for the correspondence between report and quasi-observational procedures. Another investigation (Haynes, Chavez, & Samuel, 1984) used a large sample of 190 couples and compared report (marital satisfaction) and observational (a modified version of the MICS) procedures. Similar to the previous two studies, reported correlations across measures were low, although some were statistically significant because of the large sample size.

In a conceptually related study, Hannum and Mayer (1984) compared Family Environment Scale (FES; Moos & Moos, 1981) scores (family means) with an observational coding system similar to the MICS. In a heterogeneous sample of 22 families, only a few significant correlations across measures were obtained. Focusing on studies of whole families, Reiss and his colleagues have compared the correspondence between the card-sort procedure (a laboratory outcome measure) and two report instruments: the FES (Oliveri & Reiss, 1984) and the FACES (Sigafoos *et al.*, 1985). Again, little, if any, support of cross-method correspondence was found. Although these few studies have been conducted on small, heterogeneous samples, including diverse experimental procedures, their cumulative results suggest that correspondence across methods is quite low, emphasizing the importance of further investigation and thought regarding this issue.

At this point, it seems necessary to begin rigorous and programmatic efforts aimed at determining the degree of correspondence within and across important subsets of family measurement procedures. Concurrently, clarifications of the meaning of observed discrepancies should be attempted. Without such an effort, the integration of family research will be difficult to accomplish. As a first step, instruments with demonstrated psychometric strength should be chosen for comparison. Without such a minimum condition, low correspondence may be attributable to measurement error in one or both instruments, or to the lack of fit between the measures and the constructs that they are reported to assess. A second step would be to determine, where applicable, the relationship between different family members' responses or behaviors within a particular measure. Third, further consideration needs to be given to the derivation of family-level variables from individual members' questionnaire responses or observed behaviors. Such an integration is desired because family researchers have conceptual interests in variables at that level, and because of the practical concern about limiting the number of dependent variables analyzed in any one study. Researchers have taken several approaches to this problem, ranging from retaining individual members' scores for analysis (Oliveri & Reiss, 1984), to using the mean family score (Hannum & Mayer, 1984), to more complicated statistical approaches, for example, first converting raw scores to Z scores and then averaging them to get a family-level score (Sigafoos *et al.*, 1985). However, the advantages of using mean values or more complicated strategies still require empirical demonstration.

Finally, studies in this domain would benefit from including additional instruments in order to help identify variables that may influence subjects' responses. The factors to be considered include the family's social-economic status, its motivation for participation, its level of relationship satisfaction, and its personality characteristics, such as need for approval (Crowne & Marlowe, 1960) and public self-consciousness (Fenigstein, Scheier, & Buss, 1975). Additionally, assessments of family members' desired relationship with the investigator could be developed to further explore the theoretical speculations made by Reiss (Sigafoos *et al.*, 1985). If variance in each measurement procedure could be accounted for more adequately, the resulting tests of cross-method correspondence would be more interpretable, and understanding of this complex issue would be advanced.

APPENDIX

Sample Data Set

This procedure is proposed for calculating kappa when (a) only the frequency *aggregates* for each code are known for each observer, and (b) the observers differ in their *total* number of coded units. The calculation of kappa is demonstrated on the same sample data as presented in text Tables 1 (a,b) and 2.

Kappa Based Only on Frequency Aggregates

Recall that the aggregate data are:

Code	Observer 1	Observer 2
A	3	3
B	2	1
C	1	1
D	2	2
E	0	1

These data are portrayed in a matrix in which all instances of a common code used by both observers are entered in the diagonal, and all mismatches are entered in a new column, X. No other off-diagonal entries are made because none are known. This procedure results in the following matrix and calculations:

		A	B	C	D	E	X	Marg	PO2
	A	3					0	3	.375
	B		1				0	1	.125
Observer 2	C			1			0	1	.125
	D				2		0	2	.250
	E					0	1	1	.125
	X	0	1	0	0	0			
	Marg	3	2	1	2	0			
	PO1	.375	.250	.125	.250	.000			

Header over columns A–E: Observer 1

P Observed = sum of diagonals/sum of all entries = $7/9$ = .778
P Expected = sum of $PO1 \times PO2$ for all codes entries = $(.375 \times .375) + (.125 \times .250) + (.125 \times .125) + (.250 \times .250) + (.125 \times .000)$ = .219
Kappa = $PO - PE/1 - PE$ = $(.778 - .219)/(1 - .219)$ = .716

Note that the total number of entries (i.e., 9) exceeds the number of entries made by either observer alone (i.e., 8). For each code, the number of agreements is considered the smaller of the two aggregate frequencies of the two observers. This method can result in a higher number of "agreements" if this aggregate procedure is used relative to a point-by-point comparison. As one example, the data in Code A demonstrate this phenomenon. In Code A three agreements are noted in the present matrix, and only two in Table 1. For this reason, kappa based on aggregates will always be equal to or higher than kappa based on point-by-point comparisons. It is again asserted that this aggregate-based kappa may be the more appropriate reliability estimate for these data when subsequent analyses will be based on code aggregates. An estimate based on point-by-point matching is unnecessarily conservative unless subsequent analyses will be sequential in nature.

Kappa Based on Aggregates and Unequal Totals

The use of an X entry can be extended to the case where the observers have recorded unequal numbers of behavioral units. Assume the following data set:

Code	Observer 1	Observer 1
A	3	3
B	2	1
C	1	2
D	2	3
E	0	1
TOTAL	8	10

Kappa would then be calculated as:

		A	B	C	D	E	X	Marg	PO2
	A	3					0	3	3/10 = .30
	B		1				0	1	1/10 = .10
Observer 2	C			1			1	2	2/10 = .20
	D				2		1	3	3/10 = .30
	E					0	1	1	1/10 = .10
	X								
	Marg	3	2	1	2	0			
	PO1	3/8	2/8	1/8	2/8	0/8			
	=	.375	.250	.125	.250	.000			

(header: Observer 1)

P Observed = sum of diagonals/sum of all entries = $7/11$ = .636
P Expected = sum of $PO1 \times PO2$ for all code entries = $(.30 \times .375) + (.10 \times .250) + (.20 \times .125) + (.30 \times .250) + (.10 \times .00)$ = .238
Kappa = $PO - PE/1 - PE$ = $(.636 - .238)/(1 - .238)$ = .522

REFERENCES

Anthony, N. (1971). Comparisons of clients' standard, exaggerated, and matching MMPI profiles. *Journal of Consulting and Clinical Psychology, 27,* 253–256.

Aragona, J., & Eyberg, S. (1981). Neglected children: Mother's report of child behavior problems and observed verbal behavior. *Child Development, 52,* 596–602.

Arrington, E. (1943). Time sampling in studies of social behavior: A critical review of technique and results with research suggestions. *Psychological Bulletin, 40,* 81–124.

Bales, R. F. (1950). *Interaction Process Analysis.* New York: Addison-Wesley.

Bell, R. Q. (1964). Structuring parent–child interaction for direct observation. *Child Development, 35,* 1009–1020.

Belsky, J. (1977, March). *Mother–infant interaction at home and in the laboratory: The effect of context.* Paper presented at the Society for Research in Child Development conference, New Orleans.

Bernal, M. F., Gibson, D. M., Williams, D. E., & Pesses, D. I. (1971). A device for automatic audio tape recording. *Journal of Applied Behavior Analysis, 4,* 151–156.

Blurton-Jones, N. G., & Woodson, R. H. (1979). Describing behavior: The ethologists' perspective. In M. E. Lamb, S. J. Suomi, & G. R. Stephenson (Eds.), *Social Interaction Analysis.* Madison: University of Wisconsin Press.

Borduin, C. M., & Henggeler, S. W. (1981). Social class, experimental setting, and task characteristics as determinants of mother–child interaction. *Developmental Psychology, 17,* 209–214.

Bronfenbrenner, U. (1974). Developmental research, public policy, and the ecology of childhood. *Child Development, 45,* 1–5.

Brookhart, J., & Hock, E. (1976). The effects of experimental context and experimental background on infants' behavior toward their mothers and a stranger. *Child Development, 47,* 333–340.

Campbell, D. T., & Stanley, J. C. (1963). Experimental and quasi-experimental designs for research and teaching. In N. L. Gage (Ed.), *Handbook of research on teaching.* Chicago: Rand McNally.

Canter, F. (1963). Simulation of the California Personality Inventory and the adjustment of the simulator. *Journal of Consulting Psychology, 27,* 253–256.

Carroll, J. B. (1961). The nature of the data, or how to choose a correlation coefficient. *Psychometrika, 26,* 347–372.

Christensen, A., & Hazzard, A. (1983). Reactive effects during naturalistic observation of families. *Behavioral Assessment, 5,* 349–362.

Cohen, J. (1968). Weighted kappa: Nominal scale agreement with provision for scaled disagreement or partial credit. *Psychological Bulletin, 70,* 213–220.

Cohen, J. (1969). *Statistical power analysis for the behavioral sciences.* New York: Academic Press.

Cohen, J. (1972). Weighted chi square: An extension of the kappa method. *Educational and Psychological Measurement, 32,* 61–74.

Cone, J. D. (1977). The relevance of reliability and validity for behavioral assessment. *Behavior Therapy, 8,* 411–426.

Conte, J. R. (1979). An experimental investigation of subject reactivity to observation of video camera and human observer (Doctoral dissertation, University of Washington). *Dissertation Abstracts International, 40(6-A),* 3535A.

Cronbach, L. J., Gleser, G. C., Nanda, H., & Rajaratnam, N. (1972). *The dependability of behavioral measurements: Theory of generalizability for scores and profiles.* New York: Wiley.

Crowne, D. D., & Marlowe, D. (1960). A new scale of social desirability independent of psychopathology. *Journal of Consulting and Clinical Psychology, 24,* 349–354.

Eyberg, S., & Robinson, E. (1983). Dyadic Parent Child Interaction Coding System: A manual. *Psychological Documents, 13.* (Ms. No. 2582)

Fenigstein, A., Scheier, M. F., & Buss, A. H. (1975). Public and private self-consciousness: Assessment and theory. *Journal of Consulting and Clinical Psychology, 43,* 522–527.

Fleiss, J. L. (1971). Measuring nominal scale agreement among many raters. *Psychological Bulletin, 76,* 378–382.

Fleiss, J. L., Nee, J. C. M., & Landis, J. R. (1979). The large sample variance of kappa in the case of different sets of raters. *Psychological Bulletin, 86,* 974–977.

Floyd, F. J., & Markman, H. J. (1983). Observational biases in spouse observation: Toward a cognitive/behavioral model of marriage. *Journal of Consulting and Clinical Psychology, 51,* 450–457.

Glass, G. V., & Stanley, J. C. (1970). *Statistical methods in education and psychology* (2nd ed.). Englewood Cliffs, NJ: Prentice-Hall.

Goldfried, M., & Kent, R. (1972). Traditional versus behavioral personality assessment: A comparison of methodological and theoretical assumptions. *Psychological Bulletin, 77,* 409–420.

Gottman, J. M. (1980). Analyzing for sequential connection and assessing interobserver reliability for the sequential analysis of observational data. *Behavioral Assessment, 2,* 361–368.

Hadley, T., & Jacob, T. (1973). Relationship among four measures of family power. *Journal of Personality and Social Psychology, 27,* 6–12.

Hadley, T. R., & Jacob, T. (1976). The measurement of family power: A methodological study. *Sociometry, 39,* 384–395.

Haley, J. (1967). Cross-cultural experimentation: An initial attempt. *Human Organization, 26,* 110–117.

Hannum, J. W., & Mayer, J. M. (1984). Validation of two family assessment approaches. *Journal of Marriage and Family, 46,* 741–748.

Harris, A. (1969). *Observer effect on family interaction.* Unpublished doctoral dissertation, University of Oregon.

Harris, F. C., & Lahey, B. B. (1982). Subject reactivity in direct observational assessment: A review and critical analysis. *Clinical Psychology Review, 2,* 523–538.

Hartmann, D. P. (1977). Considerations in the choice of interobserver reliability estimates. *Journal of Applied Behavior Analysis, 10,* 103–116.

Haynes, S. N., & Horn, W. F. (1982). Reactivity in behavioral observation: A review. *Behavioral Assessment, 4,* 369–385.

Haynes, S. N., Chavez, R. E., & Samuel, V. (1984). Assessment of marital communication distress. *Behavioral Assessment, 6,* 315–321.

Henggeler, S. W., Borduin, C. M., Rodick, J. D., & Tavormina, J. (1979). Importance of task content for family interaction research. *Developmental Psychology, 15,* 660–661.

Herbert, J., & Attridge, C. (1975). A guide for developers and users of observation systems and manuals. *The American Education Research Journal, 12,* 1–20.

Hollenbeck, A. R. (1978). Problems of reliability on observational research. In G. Sackett (Ed.), *Observing behavior: Vol. 2. Data collection and analysis methods.* Baltimore: University Park Press.

Hoover, L. K., & Rinehart, H. H. (1968). *The effect of an outside observer on family interaction.* Unpublished manuscript.

Hughes, H. M., & Haynes, S. N. (1978). Structured laboratory observation in the behavioral assessment of parent–child interactions: A methodological critique. *Behavior Therapy, 9,* 428–447.

Jacob, T. (1975). Family interaction in normal and disturbed families: A methodological and substantive review. *Psychological Bulletin, 82,* 33–65.

Jacob, T. (1976). Behavioral assessment of marital dysfunction. In M. Hersen & A. Bellack (Eds.), *Behavioral assessment: A practical handbook.* New York: Pergamon Press.

Jacob, T., & Davis, J. (1973). Family interaction as a function of experimental task. *Family Process, 12,* 415–427.

Jacob, T., Grounds, L., & Haley, R. (1982). Correspondence between parents' reports on the Behavior Problem Checklist. *Journal of Abnormal Child Psychology, 4,* 593–608.

Jacob, T., Rushe, R. H., & Tennenbaum, D. L. (1986). *Alcoholism and family interaction: An experimental paradigm.* Unpublished manuscript, University of Pittsburgh.

Johnson, S. M., & Bolstad, O. D. (1973). Methodological issues in naturalistic observation: Some problems and solutions for field research. In L. A. Hamerlynck, L. C. Handy, & E. J. Mash (Eds.), *Behavior change: Methodology, concepts and practice.* Champaign, IL: Research Press.

Johnson, S. M., & Bolstad, O. D. (1975). Reactivity to home observation: A comparison of audio recorded behavior with observers present or absent. *Journal of Applied Behavioral Analysis, 8,* 181–185.

Johnson, S. M., Christensen, A., & Bellamy, G. T. (1976). Evaluation of family intervention through unobtrusive audio recordings: Experiences in "bugging" children. *Journal of Applied Behavior Analysis, 9,* 213–219.

Jones, R. R., Reid, J. B., & Patterson, G. R. (1975). Naturalistic observation in clinical assessment. In P. McReynolds (Ed.), *Advances in Psychological Assessment* (Vol. 3). San Francisco: Jossey-Bass.

Kazdin, A. E. (1977). Artifact, bias, and complexity of assessment: The ABC's of reliability. *Journal of Applied Behavior Analysis, 10,* 141–150.

Kazdin, A. E. (1982). Observer effects: Reactivity of direct observation. In D. P. Hartman (Ed.), *Using observers to study behavior.* San Francisco: Jossey-Bass.

Kent, R. N., Kanowitz, J., O'Leary, K. D., & Cheiken, M. (1977). Observer reliability as a function of circumstances of assessment. *Journal of Applied Behavioral Analysis, 10,* 317–324.

Krahn, G. L., & Gabriel, R. M. (1984). Quantifying categorical observations of social interactions through multidimensional scaling. *Developmental Psychology, 20,* 833–843.

Lytton, H. (1974). Comparative yield of three data sources in the study of parent–child interaction. *Merrill-Palmer Quarterly, 20,* 53–64.

Lytton, H. (1979). Disciplinary encounters between young boys and their mothers and fathers: Is there a contingency system? *Developmental Psychology, 15,* 256–268.

Margolin, G. (1978). Relationships among marital assessment procedures: A correlational study. *Journal of Consulting and Clinical Psychology, 46*, 1556–1558.

Margolin, G., & Weiss, R. L. (1978). Comparative evaluation of therapeutic components associated with behavioral marital treatments. *Journal of Consulting and Clinical Psychology, 46*, 1476–1486.

Mash, E. J., & Johnston, C. (1982). A comparison of the mother–child interactions of younger and older hyperactive and normal children. *Child Development, 53*, 1371–1381.

Mezzich, J. E., Kraemer, H. C., Worthington, D. R. L., & Coffman, G. A. (1981). Assessment of agreement among several raters formulating multiple diagnoses. *Journal of Psychiatric Research, 16*, 29–39.

Mitchell, S. K. (1979). Interobserver agreement, reliability and generalizability of data collected in observational studies. *Psychological Bulletin, 86*(2), 376–390.

Moos, R., & Moos, B. S. (1981). *Family Environment Scale: Manual.* Palo Alto: Consulting Psychologists Press.

Murrell, S. A. (1971). Family interaction variables and adjustment of nonclinic boys. *Child Development, 42*, 1485–1494.

Nunnally, J. C. (1967). *Psychometric theory.* New York: McGraw-Hill.

Oliveri, M. E., & Reiss, D. (1984). Family concepts and their measurement: Things are seldom what they seem. *Family Process, 23*, 33–48.

Olson, D. H. (1985). Commentary: Struggling with congruence across theoretical models and methods. *Family Process, 24*, 203–207.

Olson, D. H., & Portner, J. (1983). Family adaptability and cohesion evaluation scales. In E. E. Filsinger (Ed.), *Marriage and family assessment.* Beverly Hills, CA: Sage Publications.

Olson, D. H., & Ryder, R. G. (1970). Inventory of Marital Conflicts (IMC): An experimental interaction procedure. *Journal of Marriage and the Family, 32*, 443–448.

O'Neill, M. S., & Alexander, J. F. (1970, April). *Family interaction as a function of task characteristics.* Paper presented at Rocky Mountain Psychological Association, Salt Lake City, UT.

O'Rourke, V. (1963). Field and laboratory: The decision-making behavior of family groups in two experimental conditions. *Sociometry, 26*, 422–435.

Patterson, G. R. (1982). *A social learning approach: Vol. 3. Coercive family process.* Eugene, OR: Castalia.

Patterson, G. R., & Cobb, J. A. (1971). A dyadic analysis of "aggressive" behavior. In J. P. Hill (Ed.), *Minnesota symposia on child psychology* (Vol. 5). Minneapolis: University of Minnesota Press.

Patterson, G. R., & Moore, D. (1979). Interactive patterns as units of behavior. In M. E. Lamb, S. J. Suomi, & G. R. Stephenson (Ed.), *Social interaction analysis: Methodological issues.* Madison: University of Wisconsin Press.

Patterson, G. R., & Reid, J. B. (1970). Reciprocity and coercion: Two facets of social systems. In C. Neuringer & J. D. Michael (Eds.), *Behavior modification in clinical psychology.* New York: Appleton-Century-Crofts.

Roberts, R., Jr., & Renzaglia, A. (1965). The influence of tape recording on counseling. *Journal of Counseling Psychology, 12*, 10–16.

Robinson, E. A., & Price, M. G. (1980). Pleasurable behavior in marital interaction: An observation study. *Journal of Consulting and Clinical Psychology, 48*, 117–118.

Rosenberg, M. J. (1969). The conditions and consequences of evaluation apprehension. In R. Rosenthal & R. L. Roshow (Eds.), *Artifact in behavioral research.* New York: Academic Press.

Rosenthal, R. (1966). *Experimenter effects in behavioral research.* New York: Appleton-Century.

Ross, G., Kagan, J., Zelazo, P., & Kotelchuck, M. (1975). Separation protest in infants in home and laboratory. *Developmental Psychology, 11*, 256–257.

Scott, W., & Wertheimer, M. (1962). *Introduction to psychological research.* New York: Wiley.

Sigafoos, A., Reiss, D., Rich, J., & Douglas, E. (1985). Pragmatics in the measurement of family functioning: An interpretive framework for methodology. *Family Process, 24*, 189–203.

Skinner, H., Steinhauer, P., & Santa-Barbara, J. (1983). *Family Assessment Measure.* Toronto, Ontario: Addiction Research Foundation.

Skinner, H. A., Steinhauer, P. D., & Santa-Barbara, J. (1983). The Family Assessment Measure. *Canadian Journal of Community Mental Health, 3* (2), 91–104.

Stein, S. J., Girodo, M., & Dotzenroth, S. (1982). The interrelationships and reliability of a multilevel behavior-based assessment package for distressed couples. *Journal of Behavioral Assessment, 4*, 343–360.

Steinglass, P. (1980). Assessing families in their own homes. *American Journal of Psychiatry, 137*, 1523–1529.

Susman, E. J., Peters, D. J., & Steward, R. (1976). *Naturalistic observational child study: A review.* Paper presented at the 4th Biannual Southeastern Conferences on Human Development, Nashville.

Tennenbaum, D. L. (1980). *The effect of observer salience on family interaction in the home.* Unpublished master's thesis, University of Pittsburgh.

Tennenbaum, D. L., & Jacob, T. (1985, November). *An investigation of reactivity effects in spouse observation.* Poster presented at Association for the Advancement of Behavior Therapy (AABT) Convention, Houston.

Tronick, E., Als, H., & Brazelton, T. B. (1977). Mutuality in mother–infant interaction. *Journal of Communication, 7*, 74–79.

Vidich, A. J. (1956). Methodological problems in the observation of husband–wife interactions. *Marriage and Family Living, 18*, 234–239.

Vincent, J. P., Friedman, L. C., Nugent, J., & Messerly, L. (1979). Demand characteristics in observations of marital interaction. *Journal of Consulting and Clinical Psychology, 47*, 557–566.

Volkin, J. I., & Jacob, T. (1981). The impact of spouse monitoring on target behavior and recorder satisfaction. *Journal of Behavioral Assessment, 3*, 99–109.

Watzlawick, P. (1966). A structured family interview. *Family Process, 5*, 256–271.

Weber, S. J., & Cook, T. D. (1972). Subject effects in laboratory research: An examination of subject roles, demand characteristics, and valid interference. *Psychological Bulletin, 77*, 273–295.

Weinrott, M. R., Garrett, B., & Todd, N. (1978). The influence of observer presence on classroom behavior. *Behavior Therapy, 9*, 900–911.

Weiss, R. L., & Perry, B. A. (1983). The Spouse Observation Checklist: Development and clinical application. In E. E. Filsinger (Ed.), *Marriage and family assessment.* Beverly Hills, CA: Sage Publications.

Weiss, R. L., & Summers, K. J. (1983). Marital Interaction Coding System-III. In E. Filsinger (Ed.), *Marriage and family assessment.* Beverly Hills, CA: Sage Publications.

Wells, K. C., McMahon, R. J., Forehand, R., & Griest, D. L. (1980). Effect of a reliability observer on the frequency of positive parent behavior recorded during naturalistic parent–child interactions. *Journal of Behavioral Assessment, 2*, 65–69.

White, G. D. (1973). *Effects of observer presence on mother and child behavior.* Unpublished doctoral dissertation, University of Oregon, Eugene.

White, G. D. (1977). The effects of observer presence on the activity level of families. *Journal of Applied Behavior Analysis, 10*, 734.

Wieder, G. B., & Weiss, R. L. (1980). Generalizability theory and the coding of marital interactions. *Journal of Consulting and Clinical Psychology, 48*, 469–477.

Wiggins, J. S. (1973). Observational techniques: 1. Generalizability and facets of observation. *Personality and prediction principles of personality assessment.* Reading, MA: Addison-Wesley.

Yarrow, M. R., & Waxler, C. Z. (1979). Observing interaction: A confrontation with methodology. In R. B. Cairns, (Ed.), *The analysis of social interaction: Methods, issues, and illustrations.* New York: Erlbaum.

Zajonc, R. B. (1965). Social facilitation. *Science, 149*, 269–274.

Zegiob, L. E., & Forehand, R. (1975). Maternal interactive behavior as a function of socioeconomic status, race and sex of child. *Child Development, 46*, 564–568.

Zegiob, L. E., & Forehand, R. (1978). Parent–child interactions: Observer effects and social class differences. *Behavior Therapy, 9*, 118–123.

Zegiob, L. E., Arnold, S., & Forehand, R. (1975). An examination of observer effects in parent–child interactions. *Child Development, 46*, 507–512.

Zuckerman, E., & Jacob, T. (1979). Task effects in family interaction. *Family Process, 18*, 47–53.

CHAPTER 9

Coding Marital and Family Interaction

Current Status

HOWARD J. MARKMAN
AND
CLIFFORD I. NOTARIUS

You can observe a lot just by watching.

—YOGI BERRA

INTRODUCTION

Despite the truth of Yogi Berra's redundant statement, the study of the family via direct observation is a relatively recent event. The foundations of research on the family were sociological in origin and often employed large-sample self-report questionnaires to uncover relations within the family, as well as between the family and other social institutions. In a rather sweeping judgment, Straus (1964) cast doubt on the validity of research based on self-report measures: "Because of the great importance to both the individual and the society of 'good families' all measurement techniques based on self-report are suspect" (p. 369). Researchers are attracted to self-report measures because they are inexpensive to administer and may appear to be more useful than prudent evaluation would suggest. Many self-report instruments simply do not provide a valid assessment of the family variable(s) of interest to family researchers (e.g., family power).

HOWARD J. MARKMAN • Department of Psychology, University of Denver, Denver, CO 80208.
CLIFFORD I. NOTARIUS • Department of Psychology, Catholic University of America, Washington, DC 20064.

However, some variables, such as marital and family satisfaction, appear to be reliably and validly measured by self-report variables, as are other perceptual variables (e.g., perceived social support received from family relationships).

Although we would support the use of reliable and valid self-report instruments to assess perceptual variables, we would argue, along with Fontana (1966), that observational research may ultimately provide the key to greater understanding of the causes of marital and family distress, as well as to the role of family factors in the development or pathological personality development. In the 20 years or so that have passed since Fontana wrote of the promise of direct observation research, we have reached a reasonable vantage point from which to comment on the state of the field as it exists and on the directions that it appears to be taking. Our focus in this chapter is on the coding systems that comprise the methodological heart of the direct observational study of family interaction. Our goals are to (a) briefly provide a rational for observational research; (b) discuss the major research agendas confronting the observational researcher; (c) describe six interactional dimensions that have guided the development of most coding systems; (d) present a researcher's guide to the prominent coding systems developed for the observational study of marital and family interaction; and (e) provide a commentary on the contemporary state of family interaction research.

WHY OBSERVATION?

Observational research is a costly, labor-intensive endeavor. The truth of this assertion is borne out by the experience of every research team that has engaged in the observational study of human or animal subjects. The best means available to justify the expense of studying the family via observational methods is to consider the rationale for this research strategy and to examine the benefits that derive from observational study of the family.

There is both a conceptual and a methodological rationale for the observational study of the family. From a conceptual point of view, nearly all theories of child development focus on parent–child interaction as the critical determinant of child adjustment. To be sure, the specific content of parent–child interaction that is deemed important tends to be dictated by the different theories. Psychoanalytic models concentrate on the mother–child relationship surrounding the critical developmental stages (e.g., feeding and toilet training). Social learning models focus on parent–child interaction as the mechanism through which modeling and other learning processes determine normal or deviant behavior. The most extreme perspective is taken by the interactional theorists (e.g., Watzlawick, Beavin, & Jackson, 1967), who hypothesize an isomorphism between characteristic dysfunctional family interaction patterns and the development of specific psychological disorders. For example, Watzlawick et al. (1967) consider schizophrenia "the only possible reaction to an absurd or untenable communicational context" (p. 47).

Although every family interaction researcher may not fully endorse the interactional-communications model, most nevertheless share in the belief that (a) family interaction patterns contribute to the etiology and perpetuation of psychopathology and (b) the identification of functional and dysfunctional family interaction patterns is an important step in constructing effective intervention programs for clinically significant problems (cf. Patterson, 1982).

From a methodological point of view, observational research offers investigators the opportunity to collect reliable and valid data unavailable through traditional assessment strategies. Questionnaire assessment of the parent–child relationship has generally failed to yield reliable and generalizable findings (Hetherington & Martin, 1979). Parents are often unwilling or unable to serve as informants about family interaction. Retrospective accounts of family life by parents and children are often unreliable and do not correlate with observational measures. Perhaps the most salient factor mandating observational research is the inability of interactants to describe the ongoing behavioral process, that is, contemporary patterns of interaction. Weick (1968) suggested that this inability stems from our lack of a language system to describe social exchange. The unavailability of a shorthand to describe social interaction is likely to underlie people's failure to conceptualize relationships in process terms (Kelley, 1978). Rotter (1970) suggested the clinical significance of our tendencies to ignore the details of the interaction process:

> It is usually believed that what the patient lacks most is insight into himself, but it is likely that in general what characterizes patients even more consistently is a lack of insight into the reactions and motives of others. (p. 233)

We believe this to be especially true of family relationships.

We have discussed elsewhere the theoretical importance of carefully observing and describing marital interaction (Markman, Notarius, Stephen, & Smith, 1981). The argument is equally pertinent to the study of the family process:

> The important role of description in providing a sound data base for building and testing models and theories has not always been recognized in the behavioral sciences (Hutt & Hutt, 1970). This certainly holds true in the study of marriage, which until recently was characterized by an absence of careful descriptive research. As noted elsewhere, "without careful, detailed description, theorizing about marital interaction is likely to be premature and to generate controversies that produce more heat than light" (Gottman *et al.*, 1977, p. 463).
>
> We believe that a solid data base is a prerequisite to theory development and that the construction of such a data base can best be accomplished by descriptive studies which focus on observable behaviors. We focus on observable behavior to achieve the goals of description because we believe science can only advance knowledge if research results may be replicated by any observer. (p. 236)

Whether or not a particular observational study of the family will expand our knowledge of family process will depend on the quality of the procedures followed. Behavioral observation offers no guarantee that measurements are necessarily reliable or valid (see Markman *et al.*, 1981). Strategic decisions affecting the observational situation, the coding process, and data analysis will all have an effect on the quality of a given study.

OBSERVATIONAL RESEARCH AGENDAS

We turn now to a survey of the issues confronting the family researcher who plans to complete an observational study of the family. Although we are able to identify a number of important decision points, there are no "best" strategies, and we often lack a detailed understanding of how our procedures affect our results. The objective of our presentation is to provide a context for our review of specific coding systems. We will structure our discussion around three primary agendas confronting the family interaction researcher, recognizing that decisions made in one area will have implications for another area. The three agendas are (a) establishing the research situation, (b) coding the interactional data, and (c) extracting meaning from the coded interaction.

Establishing the Research Situation

The initial agenda deals with the research procedure, and decisions made at this point will help to determine how the family experiences the research situation.

Task. First, a decision must be made concerning the task that families will complete. Because observational research is expensive, laboratory situations are usually structured so as to maximize the chance that the family will display behaviors of theoretical interest. Thus, the investigator who believes that family problem-solving is important is most likely to present families with a problem-solving task and to observe how they handle this task, rather than placing families in the laboratory and hoping that the family will naturalistically display problem solving. Problem-solving tasks have been frequently used to generate interactional samples (e.g., Gottman, Markman, & Notarius, 1977; Mishler & Waxler, 1968). Researchers who are more interested in how parents and children control each others' behavior under more naturalistic conditions are likely to observe families with minimal external structure imposed (e.g., Patterson, 1982). Because the task affects the family's interaction (Gottman, Notarius, Markman, Bank, Yoppi, & Rubin, 1976b), these effects must be considered when generalizing beyond the situation studied.

Setting. The setting must also be carefully selected. Shall the family be observed at home, in the laboratory, or in a shopping mall? It will always be reasonable to question the relationship between the interaction observed in the laboratory and the interaction observed at home in terms of the external validity of the interactional record. Some features of the setting will be dictated by how the observational record is preserved and by whether coding of the interaction will be done in real time or will be completed from a permanent record. Thus, passive live observers, participant observers, video or movie cameras, and one-way mirrors are all features of the setting that must be considered.

Recording Interaction. The decision to record the interaction or to use live observation largely depends on the complexity of the coding system. The more complex the system, the greater the need to have a permanent interactional record. The information-processing demands for coders using a complex coding system is simply too great for coders to assess family interaction in real time. Because many coding systems also evolve over time, it is also advantageous to have a permanent interactional record to enable recoding of the data. A permanent interactional record may also be essential for establishing reliability, permitting the coders to go back over segments to make careful judgments and to recode if necessary.

Given current technology, we believe that video recording will be a part of most observational studies and that the awareness of videotaping will be a part of the family's experience of the research setting. Is is not difficult to speculate about significant effects on the family system stemming from recording; yet, it is far more difficult to actually document such effects. The most relevant data come from the marital observation literature, which demonstrates that both distressed and nondistressed couples respond more positively when they are aware of being videotaped (e.g., Vincent, Friedman, Nugent, & Messerly, 1979). The important issue is that the demand characteristics associated with videotaping be *constant* across groups. Because the goal of most interaction studies is to contrast functional and dysfunctional groups rather than to develop normative data about families, we can assert with reasonable confidence that the external validity of observational research is not greatly affected by demand effects associated with the use of videotape procedures.

In addition, we believe that observer effects are much more likely among stranger groups than among families. The family bring with them their own interactional history and context, and this system appears to be relatively robust. Although it is always prudent to question the effects of the situation on the phenomena being observed, it is unwise to automatically suspect the validity of observational data, especially with couples and families.

Family Composition. The final decision in establishing the research paradigm concerns the family composition to be studied. Options include observing dyads (e.g., husband–wife, father–child, and mother–child); triads (e.g., mother–father–child), or larger units (e.g., parents and all children and, perhaps, grandparents). Whatever the conceptual merit of observing whole families, the data-analytic burden becomes exponential as the number of interactants increases. For example, the logistics of keeping track of parallel conversations, of identifying the speaker and the intended receiver, and of tracking the sequence of interactional events can quickly become unmanageable with family groups as small as three or four. For this reason, most researchers have chosen to limit interactional study to couple dyads or parent–child triads. Even in families larger than three, the parents are often observed first with one offspring and then with another (e.g., Mishler & Waxler, 1968).

Coding the Interactional Data

Once the task, the setting, and the family composition have been determined, the research procedures can be established, and the observational record can be obtained. In the following discussion, we will assume that a permanent record of the interaction has been obtained. (Our assumption that the coding task follows the collection of the observational record is for convenience only. In reality, many of the coding issues we will discuss must be decided before data collection begins because they can impact on the research paradigm.)

The Codes and Dimensions. The most important tool necessary for the coding task is the catalog of interactional behaviors that will be judged, rated, or scored, in short, the codebook. The codebook specifies how each behavior in the ongoing interaction stream will be categorized and thus provides the foundation for all substantive conclusions to be drawn from the research. The coding scheme often originates with the researcher's hypotheses about which interactional behaviors are functional and dysfunctional. These hypotheses are then defined as observable behaviors or communication processes, and rules are developed to train observers how to reliably detect the behaviors of interest. For example, a simple hypothesis might be that problem solving in nondistressed marriages is facilitated by a spouse's ability to comment on the ongoing interaction process, that is, to metacommunicate. This global hypothesis is translated into discrete behaviors defining metacommunication, such as (a) comments about the ongoing interaction (e.g., "Why are you yelling at me") and (b) statements directing communication toward problem resolution (e.g., "We have to reach some decision about how to spend money"). The interactional record is then carefully reviewed for examples of metacommunication as defined by the codebook. The hypothesis might then be tested by comparing the recorded frequency of metacommunication observed in "successful" conversations (i.e., conversations in which the interactants arrived at a mutually satisfactory resolution) with the frequency of metacommunication in "unsuccessful" conversations (i.e., conversations in which the interactants did not reach a solution or in which one or both partners were not satisfied with the outcome).

This brief example illustrates the importance of giving careful consideration to the composite codes that are grouped together to define a dimension of interest. Consumers of observational research have an obligation to carefully review the individual codes and their specific behavioral referents in order to assess exactly how each dimension is operationalized. The greater the number and the heterogeneity of the individual codes that are lumped together, and the less the reliance on specific behavioral cues to define each code (i.e., the more inference required in coding), the greater will be the challenge of validly interpreting the results. Another example will help clarify this issue.

Raush, Barry, Hertel, and Swain (1974) developed clear rules for coding the following discrete behaviors: (a) giving information, (b) witholding information, (c) agreeing with the other's statement, and (d) denying the validity of the other's argument with or without the use of counterarguments. Although these individual codes have rather unambiguous behavioral referents, these four codes were grouped together to define the dimension *cognitive*. All analyses then assessed the role of "cognitive" behaviors in the interactional stream, and substantive conclusions were drawn on the basis of this global dimension. Each reader should evaluate for himself or herself the conceptual merit of defining the cognitive dimension in this way and, in general, should not passively accept the investigator's operationalization of any dimension.

In general, readers should be aware of four common approaches to the formation of dimensions. The first represents an empirical approach through which common codes are identified and combined. Factor analysis procedures might be one way of establishing which codes are related (Gottman, 1978). Gottman *et al.* (1977) grouped common codes on the basis of functional similarity, for example, codes that were empirically determined to serve a similar function in the behavior stream were grouped together. A second approach to forming dimensions from individual codes is more conceptual: codes are assumed *a priori* to define a given dimension and are subsequently lumped together. Third, two or more codes may be combined, following the experience that coders are unable to reliably discriminate between codes. Thus, if coders consistently have difficulty discriminating between Codes A and B, these might be combined. Clearly, this third approach should not be used to remedy unclear coding rules. Finally observers can be instructed to code directly a dimension of interest. For example, Mishler and Waxler had coders rate interaction units for the degree of acknowledgment. Often, this last approach requires coders to make global judgments about dimensions and it is not always clear what the exact behavioral referents are that the coders attend to in marking their global ratings (Royce & Weiss, 1975).

Comprehensiveness of the Coding System. An important characteristic of any coding system is the breadth of the dimensions covered. At one extreme, the investigator may consider only one dimension critical for effective family functioning and may therefore structure the coding scheme to tally occurrences of the relevant behaviors. All other behaviors, save the one critical dimension, may be lumped into an "other" category or may simply be ignored. For example, Alexander (1983) has developed a coding system that focuses only on supportive and defensive behaviors. At the other extreme, an investigator may devise a multicode, comprehensive system to assign a specific code to each interactional unit observed. For example, Mishler and Waxler's (1968) coding system has codes for all the major dimensions of family interaction.

Validity of the Coding System. No matter which approach is taken, it is essential to question what we are measuring with our observational codes and what is the relationship between the codes and other behavior. Here we are asking about the validity of the observational coding system. Too often, the decision to study interaction via behavioral observation does not include questioning whether the observational data are valid indexes of what we believe we are measuring.

Following Cronbach and Meehl's classic discussion (1955), it is important to assess the evidence of criterion validity, content validity, and construct validity in any observational coding system. Evidence in support of criterion validity is available when the result of coding interaction can be used to identify membership in a known group (concurrent validity), for example, whether identified interaction patterns differentiate between schizophrenic and nonschizophrenic families. Criterion validity is also established if the interactional codes can predict behaviors measured later in time (predictive validity), for example, if coded family interaction patterns are able to predict a relapse in adolescent schizophrenics after release from the hospital.

When developing and using observational coding systems, it is also important to evaluate content validity. Evidence of content validity is provided when we can demonstrate that our coding system adequately reflects the domain of interest. In evaluating the content validity of any coding system, attention must be paid to the extent to which component codes sufficiently define the domains and concepts of interest. As a practical matter, readers of observational research should examine the content of specific codes to determine the degree to which the code name adequately reflects both the concept to be measured and the actual behaviors that are being measured.

Finally, there is the issue of construct validity: Do the coding categories adequately measure the construct(s) they are intended to measure? Suppose a researcher wished to test the double-bind hypothesis and he or she operationalized this construct as a discrepancy between verbal and nonverbal behavior. We might then assess this construct by comparing families with a known schizophrenic with families with nondisturbed offspring. If we failed to find a difference between these families, we might (a) question whether we had an adequate measure of the construct; (b) question whether our theory was correct; or (c) question whether our observations were adequate enough to observe the double bind. The consumer of observational research should keep these three alternatives in mind as she or he evaluates results from observational coding systems as a convenient way to keep the issue of construct validity in the foreground. (See Markman *et al.*, 1981, for additional discussion of validity issues in observational research.)

The Coding Unit. Whatever approach is taken, the coding task will also require the host of other methodological decisions involved in segmenting or reducing the stream of interactional behavior into analyzable units. Remember that the coding of interactional data is essentially a data reduction procedure. In general, the smaller the coding unit (i.e., the more microanalytic), the less the data reduction; the larger the coding unit (i.e., the more global), the greater the degree of inference required to assign a code and the more heterogeneous the coded behavior. Riskin and Faunce (1972) reviewed several of the common coding units that have been used. The units range from the smallest unit, the "act," defined as a simple grammatical sentence expressing a single idea, to the "speech" or "floor switch," defined as everything spoken until another person starts to talk, to the "idea" defined as all speech that makes up the presentation of a single idea, and finally, to the "theme," defined as a large block of interaction dealing with a global theme. Usually, the larger the coding unit, the more qualitative will be the data analysis. Although the size of the coding unit may have an effect on the substantive conclusions reached, this issue has not been systematically studied. Finally, the size of the coding unit can be an important factor in achieving reliability; large coding units require that coders synthesize the interaction and apply a global judgment involving considerable inference. On the other hand, too small a coding unit may be difficult to code reliably because it provides the coder with an ambiguous context and hence the possibility of multiple meanings.

Data Type. Closely related to the issue of the coding unit is the nature of the boundary that is placed between consecutive coding units. The particular boundary between coding units defines the data type produced by the coding procedure. Two common data types are event data and timed data. Coding units that range from the "act" to the "theme" are all event-based data types. The interaction is encoded as a stream of discrete events, with each event defined as the coding unit. Event data typically yield rate-per-minute proportion scores, the latter defined as Code X divided by the total number of events observed. It is also possible to base a coding unit on a fixed time interval, so that a coding unit occurs, for example, every 10 seconds. Timed data give rise to rates-per-time unit scores, with each code referenced to a particular time unit (e.g., Code V occurs twice per minute). In the analysis of marital interaction, one of the two most popular systems uses timed coding units (Marital Interaction Coding System [MICS]; Weiss, & Summers, 1983), and the other is event-based (Couples Interaction Scoring System [CISS]; Notarius & Markman, 1981). The choice of an event-based system or a time-based system depends largely on the nature of the coding system, the task engaging the interactants, and the purpose of the investigation.

Sampling Strategies. More important than either of the two data types is the decision to sample from the behavior stream or to code continuously. A sample approach has the coder assess at various intervals or has the coder go "on" and "off" periodically. For example, if a coder were instructed to observe the family for 15 seconds, record the code during the next 15 seconds, observe again in the next 15 seconds, and so on, this would be a time-sampling procedure. The disadvantage of a sampling procedure, either timed or event-based, is that it is not possible to obtain accurate frequency estimates of observed behavior, nor is it possible to explore the sequential flow of interaction over time. (See the data analysis discussion below.) We believe that continuous coding is the procedure of choice.

Extracting Meaning from the Coded Interaction (Data Analysis)

Having gathered the observational record and having coded the recorded interactions we must next extract meaning from the strings af codes; in short, the next task is data analysis. We will consider two general data-analytic strategies: nonsequential and sequential. Nonsequential data-analytic procedures will be familiar to most readers. In the simplest case, the code frequencies of two samples may be compared. For example, if one wants to evaluate the hypothesis that functional families, compared to troubled families, have more agreements (AG) than disagreements (DG), a ratio of $AG/(AG + DG)$ may be computed for each family and submitted to a t test to show if the ratio in functional families is significantly different from the ratio observed in dysfunctional families.

Frequency comparisons may also be based on other aspects of the coding system. For example, the coding system may include a measure of intensity, as would be the case in discriminating between "tap," "push," and "shove." Duration measures may also form the basis of nonsequential comparisons. Here, the dimension of interest is how long a respondent engages in a particular behavior or in a particular class of behaviors. A family researcher who is interested in the amount of time that each family member spends talking is most likely to use a duration measure to explore this question. Intensity and duration measures (with the exception of "talk time") have not been commonly used in nonsequential analyses of family interaction.

As researchers compared the frequencies of occurrence scores in distressed and nondistressed families, it became apparent that this data-analytic procedure provided limited information about the observed interaction. Much of the richness of social interaction is lost when analysis is limited to an examination of the frequency or the rate with which each code occurs. For example, it may be more informative to discover that a wife displays negative nonverbal behavior 80% of the time when her husband looks away and becomes quiet, than simply to tally the frequency of the wife's negative nonverbal behavior in general. In the first case, sequence analysis allows the investigator to track ongoing stimulus–response patterns that characterize an interactional system. In the second case, frequency analysis limits the investigator to global characterizations of the behavioral repertoires of individuals. Discussions of sequence analysis can be found in Bakeman (1978, 1979), Gottman (1979), Gottman *et al.* (1977), Hahlweg, Reisner, Kohli, Vollmer, Schindler, and Revenstorf (1984), Margolin and Wampold (1981), and Notarius, Krokoff, and Markman (1981).

Among the interesting questions that can be addressed with sequence analysis are: (a) Does the patterning of family interaction change over the course of a conversation? (b) How does communication skills training change the way in which family members respond to each other? (c) What are the differences in the ways in which parents respond to a symptomatic child and to a normal child? Perhaps more important, sequence analysis is the necessary tool for evaluating important theoretical hypotheses. For example, when reciprocity is conceptualized as the contingent exchange of behaviors, sequence analysis is the proper analytic procedure for evaluating the construct (Gottman *et al.*, 1977).

As noted earlier, the choice of a coding scheme, an interactional setting, and a data-analytic strategy requires the investigator to carefully articulate the research agenda and to planfully coordinate the components of a family interaction study. If the conceptual question necessitates sequence analysis, then the coding record must be continuous (either event or timed). Furthermore, if sequence analysis is planned, the number of dimensions entering data analyses must be kept fairly small; otherwise, the sequential transitions between codes will be too small to provide reliable estimates of observed patterns. The point we wish to stress is a simple one: if careful planning is not carried out at the beginning, it may be impossible to provide answers to the questions most relevant to the research. We emphasize this issue out of respect for the expense (effort and resources) typically involved in completing interactional research and in light of the unfortunate experiences characterizing many beginning projects.

OVERVIEW OF THE FAMILY INTERACTION FIELD

In the preceding section we noted that systems for coding family interaction are essentially data reduction strategies aimed at extracting meaning from the complex stream of behaviors that are exchanged among family members. We have also suggested that coding systems are likely to reflect the originator's theoretical hypotheses about the critical dimensions that define family interaction as well as hunches regarding important interactional behaviors that have yet to be observed adequately. The theoretical underpinnings of most family-interaction coding systems derive from the study of small-group processes, the study of interpersonal behavior, and the study of schizophrenic families. After surveying these literatures and reviewing the major coding systems designed to assess family interaction processes, we identified six primary theoretical dimensions around which most family-interaction coding systems have been constructed. In this section, we briefly review these six dimensions. In our review of the coding schedules, which follows, we organize our presentation, in part, around these six dimensions.

Before describing each of the six dimensions, we wish to emphasize the point that universal relationships between the dimensions and the observational referents that comprise the dimensions do not exist. Often the "same" dimension is operationalized with different behavioral referents by different researchers, a circumstance that perhaps reflects varying theoretical conceptualizations of the dimension of interest. This problem has long been recognized as a source of confusion when one is attempting to synthesize findings across studies (e.g., Riskin & Faunce, 1972). For example, "agreement" and "disagreement" have been described as measures of "conflict" (Jacob, 1975), "positivity" (Gottman, 1979), and "acknowledgment" (Bales, 1950; Mishler & Waxler, 1968). Jacob viewed "affect" as a separate dimension; Gottman considered "affect" a part of the "positivity" dimension. Obviously, interpretation of research findings is critically influenced by the particular way a reviewer or researcher chooses to define each dimension.

In our review of major coding systems, we present the individual codes that define each of the six dimensions. In some cases, our perspective may differ from that of the originators of the coding system. When a reader wishes clarification about the meaning of a particular dimension, it is advisable to examine carefully the composite codes that serve to define the dimension. Below, we briefly orient the reader to the origin of the six primary dimensions hypothesized to discriminate between "normal" and "dysfunctional" families. These dimensions are assumed to be bipolar, with each extreme being characteristic of dysfunction (e.g., high dominance is associated with rigid families, and low dominance is associated with a lack of family structure).

Dominance

There has been a clear convergence among family scholars regarding the belief that dominance is a key process in family interaction (see chapters by Martin and Wahler for a detailed description of this development). In normal development, patterns of parental dominance have been hypothesized as critical determinants of the child's adjustment (Mischler & Waxler, 1968). In psychoanalytic terms, the relative dominance of mother and father is believed to influence the child's resolution of the Oedipal conflict. In social-learning-theory

terms, the power of the caretaker is revealed as an important variable influencing the imitation of critical behaviors, including gender-appropriate roles. Dominance has also been discussed as a critical dimension in small-group theory and
research, most notably in Bales's contention (1950) that certain group members
must take charge of decision making if the group is to function effectively.

Dominance or power has also played a prominent role in theories of schizophrenia and in theories of disturbed family functioning in general. The general
characteristic of these theories is that normal families are assumed to have differential, symmetrical, and clear power structures, whereas disturbed families are
said to be characterized by distorted, asymmetrical, or denied power structures.
For example, in schizophrenic families, theorists have hypothesized that the
mother is significantly more powerful and dominant than the father (Lidz,
Cornelison, Fleck, & Terry, 1957), that the family denies parental power (Haley,
1967), or that the family lacks clear differentiation of power between generations (Minuchin, 1974).

Affect

Next to dominance, affect (both positive and negative) is perhaps the most
widely measured dimension in studies of the family. Social psychologists have
long emphasized the role of affect in group processes in general (Bales, 1950)
and in normal families in particular (Parsons & Bales, 1955). Families characterized by appropriate levels of positive affect are hypothesized to foster the
development of self-esteem and assertion, whereas families characterized by
negative affect are believed to foster low self-esteem and withdrawal from conflict. The affective dimension helps to define the schizophrenogenic mother,
who is described as cold and indifferent (Wynne, Ryckoff, Day, & Hirsch, 1958).
More recently, and with more empirical support, it has been suggested that the
level of criticism expressed by the parents is related to the relapse of hospitalized
schizophrenic offspring (Vaughn & Leff, 1976) and to the onset of the disorder
in high-risk samples (Doane, West, Goldstein, Rodnick, & Jones, 1981). At the
simplest level, positive affect has been said to characterize the nondistressed
family and marriage, and negative affect has been said to characterize the distressed family and marriage. Jacob (1975) found that the affect dimension most
consistently discriminated between functional and dysfunctional families.

Dominance and affect are perhaps the two most salient dimensions of family
interaction. Not surprisingly, these two dimensions also appear in many other
models of group processes and interpersonal behavior. Leary's model (1957) of
interpersonal behavior proposes that all interpersonal behavior is captured by a
two-dimensional space defined by power (dominance–submission) and by interpersonal affiliation (affection–hostility). Schutz (1960) proposed a three-dimen-
sional model with an affective dimension, a dominance dimension (control), and
an inclusion dimension. Similarly, Becker (1964) developed a model of parental
behavior that is reduced to three dimensions: an affective dimension (warmth–
hostility), a control dimension (permissiveness–restrictiveness), and an intensity
dimension (calm detachment–anxious involvement). In addition to dominance

and affect, four other dimensions have received sufficient attention across coding systems and in the theoretical literature to warrant our consideration: communication clarity, information exchange, conflict, and support and validation.

Communication Clarity (Skills)

This dimension derives from family theorists' views on the importance of clear message exchange to effective family functioning. Double-bind messages (Bateson, Jackson, Haley, & Weakland, 1956), incongruence between verbal content and nonverbal cues accompanying message delivery, and speech disruptions or speech fragments (Mishler & Waxler, 1968) are all examples of how communication clarity has been operationalized. Theoretically, the clarity of family communication has been conceptualized both as an etiological factor affecting offspring development, particularly the development of adequate reality testing, and as a concomitant of thought disorder, anxiety, or conflict, which may be a consequence of family psychopathology and not a cause of it. Contemporary social-learning perspectives on marital and family theory and therapy also place a premium on clear, direct communications between family members as a necessary ingredient in effective problem-solving (Gottman, Notarius, Gonso, & Markman, 1976a; Jacobson & Margolin, 1979; Patterson, 1982).

Information Exchange

Observation of family interaction has most frequently taken place when the family have been presented with a problem or issue and they have been asked to come to a decision about the issue. Not surprisingly, the family must exchange facts, state preferences, and share information as they attempt to problem-solve together. Thus, "information exchange" is a dimension that has evolved as researchers developed an exhaustive catalog of interactional behaviors displayed by families as they were observed. Similarly, Bales's work on small groups (1950) also led him to propose information exchange (instrumental behaviors) between group members as an essential component defining the group process. Information exchange is likely to overlap with several other interactional variables, particularly those that relate to the manner in which information is exchanged (e.g., affect).

Conflict

This dimension usually relates to the degree of overt tension that is reflected in a family's interaction. Families characterized by either intense conflict or the complete absence of conflict are believed to be dysfunctional. For example, Lidz *et al.*'s descriptions (1957) of marital schism and skew are global descriptions of families that differ on the level of expressed conflict. Conflict has been operationalized with several process variables, including interruptions, agreements, and disagreements. It is clear that there is substantial conceptual overlap between conflict and affect. High conflict is usually associated with the inappropriate suppression of affect, the inappropriate presence of positive affect, or the expression of negative affect, whereas the absence of conflict is likely to be associated with neutral affect or the genuine expression of positive affect. Similar overlap exists when conflict is operationalized as the relative presence of agreements and disagreements. Ratios of agreements to agreements plus disagreements have been used both as indices of conflict (Jacob, 1975; Riskin & Faunce, 1972) and as an affective index of positivity (Gottman, 1979).

Support and Validation

Support and validation are related concepts that have attracted the attention of various family theorists. For example, Alexander (1973), developing the work of Gibb (1961) on small-group processes, proposed that supportive and defensive communications were the two basic dimensions of family interaction. In general, theorists have suggested that the functional family provides high levels of support and validation to its members, thereby fostering self-esteem, mutual respect, and understanding. On the other hand, the dysfunctional family is marked by indifference to the feelings and thoughts of others and critical evaluation of each other.

REVIEW OF OBSERVATIONAL SYSTEMS

In preparation for writing this chapter, we reviewed the available literature on marital and family coding systems and focused on approximately 20 systems for further study.[1] We will first review Bales's observational system because it has influenced both the codes and dimensions and the coding process used by subsequent observational systems. Next, we will review family observational systems and then marital observational systems. Within the family section, we will order our review by presenting systems with the most breadth first, followed by systems that are focused on a smaller number of dimensions. The systems also vary in terms of the conceptual area to which the system has been applied. Most systems have been developed for and applied to research concerned with the etiology of psychopathology (e.g., schizophrenia and alcoholism). Typically, studies in this tradition have used cross-sectional designs to assess the power of interaction measures to discriminate "abnormal" from "normal" families. Systems have also been used in research evaluating the effects of interventions in families with conduct-disordered children (e.g., aggressive children) as well as to

[1]We wrote letters to the developers of most of these systems requesting up-to-date coding manuals and papers related to their systems. We did not write to the developers of several of the older systems because detailed descriptions of these systems were readily available, and we knew that there had been no recent updates. We received replies to most of our letters, and we are grateful to these researchers for providing us with the information requested. We are sure that other excellent family coding systems are available that we missed in our review, and we apologize to these authors for omitting references to their work.

assess the interaction patterns in these families. Finally, and more recently, developmental psychologists have constructed coding systems to explore the relationship between family interaction processes and child and adolescent development. The influence of a developmental perspective is one of the major recent trends in the family interaction field. Developmental psychologists have long been interested in mother–child interaction; however, only recently have they expanded their focus to the family context of child development (Belsky, 1981; Goldberg & Easterbooks, 1984; Pederson, 1980). In contrast to the first two traditions that focus on dysfunctional family interaction, developmentally oriented family researchers have focused on normal families' interaction.

INTERACTION PROCESS ANALYSIS (IPA)

History and Objectives

The IPA was developed as a method for the "first hand observation of social interaction in small, face-to-face groups" (Bales, 1950, Preface). Bales's overall research objective was to develop a general instrument that would allow for the comparison of interactional phenomena across different types of social groups, including the family. This objective was based on Bales's theoretical assumption that there are formal similarities in face-to-face interaction because of problems of skills and ethics in human relations. Bales's review of observational systems in 1940 led him to three conclusions: (a) most systems tied to the specific purposes of the researchers and thus were not appropriate for discovering general principles concerning social interactions that would span different types of groups; (b) as a result, there were no available norms on rates of theoretical phenomena in various types of small groups; and (c) there was a need for clearly defined categories and coding rules that could be used across time and across different types of social systems. As our review of the various contemporary marital and family interaction systems will indicate, these conclusions remain timely and accurate in the mid-1980s, some 35 years after Bales initiated his research.

With the above objectives in mind, Bales began his research by observing group discussions of Alcoholics Anonymous groups and the Diagnostic Council at the Harvard Psychological Clinic in the 1940s. The observers sat with the group and made observations of the unfolding process—an experience that resulted in the generation of codes to describe the process. Once an initial set of codes was derived, it was applied to a variety of different groups in different settings. These codes were also compared to codes used in existing coding systems at the time of Bales's first publication of the IPA in 1950. Based on this process, the IPA went through 11 or 12 revisions, with the number of categories ranging from 5 to 87. The general guidelines for deciding on a code were twofold: (a) the codes had to be indicators of theoretically relevant group processes, and (b) they had to be amenable to clear definition and reliable observation.

Coding Process

The task coded is a naturally occurring group interaction. The number of group members and the type of group vary, as does the amount of time spent in group discussions. Usually, the typical observation period is about 10 minutes, and the number of participants is usually six or seven adults. Anyone with sufficient training could serve as a coder. The coders are participant observers of the group process and thus sit in with the group and make their ratings live. The perspective of the coder is that of the generalized "other." The coders are instructed to assess the act (defined below) as if it were directed at them in terms of the instrumental value (what it means for the group) as well as the expressive value (what it tells the receiver about the emotional state of the speaker). The observer is explicitly instructed not to take context into account, as well as to ignore prior information about the participants. The basic unit of coding is called the *act* and is a segment of verbal and/or nonverbal behavior that could be coded with one of the 12 IPA codes. The act is usually a single sentence or a complete thought. Thus, the IPA uses an event-sampling procedure. Approximately 15 acts per minute are typically coded. However, coders are also instructed to scan the group every minute (signaled by a light flashing) and to code meaningful nonverbal expressions that might not otherwise be coded. This is an example of time sampling. Each coding unit receives a single code, and a hierarchy is provided to help the coder distinguish between units that might receive more than one code.

Codes and Dimensions

The IPA is seen as the "basic language of social interaction" (Bales, 1951 p. 69). Each coding unit receives one of the twelve IPA codes. In addition, the coder rates who are the speaker and the target of the act. These 12 codes were divided into two major dimensions: instrumental and expressive (socioemotional). The instrumental dimension is further divided into questions and answers, and the expressive dimension is divided into positive and negative. The codes, broken down by dimensions, are listed below:

INSTRUMENTAL		EXPRESSIVE	
Questions	Answers	Positive	Negative
Asks for orientation	Gives orientation	Shows solidarity	Shows antagonism
Asks for opinion	Gives opinion	Show tension release	Shows tension
Asks for suggestion	Gives suggestion	Agrees	Disagrees

Reliability and Validity

Bales (1950) reported that the reliability of the IPA after a great deal of training was very good. Bales (1970) noted that reliability varied with the amount of training and stressed the need for highly trained observers. No doubt, this need was due, in part, to the *in vivo* observation procedures. The validity of the system has been established in numerous studies using the IPA, and readers are referred to Bales (1970) for a review.

Relation to Core Dimension

Dominance or Power (Status). The social relationship between group members, reflected in part by status, is one of the key dimensions of the IPA. Although IPA coders are instructed to ignore the social relationships between the people, it is anticipated that these relationships will emerge when the data are analyzed. Status in the group is assessed by the number of acts and the type of acts received and given to a member relative to the chance distribution of acts.

Three major indices of status are defined: (a) access to resources, defined by the proportion of acts in the three question categories received by a particular individual; (b) degree of control, defined as the proportion of attempted answers and the proportion of positive to negative reactions to attempted answers; and (c) a generalized status index, defined as the sum of the three indices (questions, answers, reactions) divided by 3.

Affect (Socioemotional). One of the IPA's major contributions is the designation of codes into socioemotional (expressive) and instrumental dimensions of interaction. As noted earlier, the expressive dimension is divided into two categories: socioemotional positive codes and socioemotional negative codes. Socioemotional positive codes include "shows solidarity," "shows tension release," and "agrees." Socioemotional negative codes include "disagrees," "shows tension," and "shows antagonism." The expressive codes include ratings of verbal and nonverbal behaviors.

Communication Clarity and Skills (Communication Difficulty). The IPA yields an index of communication difficulty that is the ratio of "asks for orientation" divided by the sum of "asks for orientation" and "gives orientation." The rationale for this index is that "asks for orientation" is viewed as "an index of amount of interaction which the group actually devotes to indicating to each other that problems of perception or communication exist" (Bales, 1950, p. 140). Similarly, "gives orientation" is viewed as an "index of the amount of interaction which the group actually devotes to the solution of problems of perception and communication" (Bales, 1950, p. 140). Thus, difficulty of communication is seen as a increase in "requests for orientation" without an increase in "gives orientation," which provides answers to these requests.

Information Exchange (Instrumental). Along with the expressive dimension, the instrumental dimension is one of the major aspects of the group process assessed by the IPA. The instrumental codes are "asks for orientation," "asks for opinion," "asks for suggestion," "gives opinion," "gives orientation," and "gives suggestion." These codes represent information exchanged in the form of questions and answers.

Conflict (Expressive and Maladaptive Behaviors). The IPA does not assess conflict; however, Bales (1950) proposed an index of expressive and malintegration behavior that can be seen as a measure of conflict. Expressive and malintegrative behavior is defined as a ratio of negative expressive codes ("shows antagonism," "shows tension," and "disagrees") to positive expressive codes ("shows solidarity," "shows tension release," and "agrees"). Bales viewed expressive and malintegrative behaviors as representing pathological group processes because these behaviors serve to reduce tensions in the short run, however, "tend in the long run to set up circular developments which may interfere with the adaptation of the group with the outer situation or with the integration of personalities and activities within the group" (Bales, 1950, p. 139).

Support and Validation (Expressive and Adaptive Behaviors). Although the IPA does not explicitly assess the concept of support or validation, two of the three positive expressive codes ("shows solidarity" and "agrees") represent supportive reactions. These two codes seem to be face-valid measures of the dimension of support.

Commentary

The major strength of the IPA is the separation of interaction into expressive (affect) and instrumental (information exchange) dimensions. These two dimensions are still attracting a great deal of theoretical and empirical attention in understanding marital and family relationships (e.g., Gilligan, 1982). However, although the instrumental dimension remains a very good operationalization of the information exchange dimension, the IPA's measurement of affect is surpassed by more contemporary systems. Although the IPA was ahead of its time in its focus on both verbal and nonverbal behavior, there is no separate coding for an affective dimension of interaction. For example, defining positive affect only as "shows solidarity," "shows tension release," and "agrees" seems to miss a large set of cues for positive affect (e.g., when the subject smiles when asking for an opinion). In other words, instrumental acts can be delivered with positive, negative, or neutral affect.

The IPA's approach to measuring status in terms of the giving and receiving of acts and the response to acts is still the most frequently used operation of this dimension. However, beyond face validity, there is little evidence of the concurrent and predictive validity of this measure for the Bales system and for other systems as well.

The IPA's index of communication clarity is quite different from others that actually assess the content of communication and how clearly it is communicated to other family members. Because the IPA is content-free, it relies on a process definition of communication clarity, assuming that unclear communication will result in an increase in the requests for orientation, information, repetition, and confirmation concerning potentially unclear communication.

Finally, the IPA's conceptualization of conflict is interesting because conflict is seen as pathological only when its rates are increased without a comparable increase in the rate of positive reactions. Although the negative expression codes seem to be a face-valid measure of conflict, there is no evidence to support the validity of this measure. An advantage of using the index of expressive malintegration as a measure of conflict is that it does take into consideration both positive and negative reactions. A disadvantage, however, is that it does confound conflict with support. Similarly, the support codes are confounded with the socioemotional positive codes. Recently, Bales's work has evolved away from act-by-act coding of interaction to a more dimension-oriented approach relying on overall impression after observing a period of interaction (Bales & Cohen, 1979).

FAMILY OBSERVATION SYSTEMS: MISHLER AND WAXLER

History and Objectives

The major aim of Mishler and Waxler's classic research (1968, 1975), was to discover "whether there are distinctive patterns of interactions in families of schizophrenic patients" (1968, p. 1). They noted that their research was stimulated by theories postulating the etiological role of family interaction in the development of schizophrenia. Mishler and Waxler's work was influenced by Bales (1950), and their coding system includes the IPA.

The coding system was designed "to obtain reliable and objective indicators of family interaction related to theory and clinical observation" (Mishler & Waxler, 1968, p. 31). Codes were viewed as "indicators" of specific dimensions of family interaction. The choice of codes and dimensions was guided by research and theory on schizophrenia. The specific dimensions of interest to Mishler and Waxler were expressiveness (affect), power (dominance), speech disruption (communication clarity), and responsiveness (support). The system includes codes that are direct or indirect indicators of these dimensions in order to use "multiple measures of the same concept" and to compare findings in order to assess convergent validity (Mishler & Waxler, 1968, p. 83). Attention to convergent validity illustrates the authors' empirical approach to understanding the association between family interaction and psychopathology.

Codes and Dimensions

Each coding unit receives eight codes, one from each of eight categories described below:

CATEGORIES	CODES
Who spoke to whom	Object, subject
Acknowledgment: Stimulus	Commands, questions, affirmative statements, elliptical affirmative statements
Acknowledgment: Response	Complete acknowledgment, partial acknowledgment, recognition, nonacknowledgment
Affect	Positive affect about relationships, positive states of people, positive qualities of situations, neutral, negative qualities of situations, negative states of people, negative affect about relationships
Focus	Agree, disagree, personal states, personal experience, own opinion, other opinions, item content, task-related statements

Tension	Incomplete sentences, repetitions, incomplete phrase, laughter, number of fragments in one act
IPA	See the section on IPA
Interruption	Interruption, successful interruption
Metacommunication (MC)	MC about communication, MC about procedures, MC about roles (e.g., mother)

Coding Process

Like many early family interaction researchers, Mishler and Waxler used Strodtbeck's (1951) Revealed Difference Task (RDT) as the observational situation. The RDT involves family members separately answering a series of questions (e.g., on child-rearing problems); the researcher then selects situations or vignettes on which the family members disagree. Finally, the family members are asked to reach agreement on the issues in a certain period of time. In Mishler and Waxler's research, the parents and one child discussed nine situations, the average time of discussion was 50 minutes for each family. Families' interactions were audiotaped and then transcribed. Only the transcript was then used for coding purposes. There were two exceptions: as the family interacted, the observer sat behind a two-way mirror and recorded "who speaks to whom," and an audiotape was also used for IPA codes. Similar to the IPA, the basic unit of analysis is called the *act*, which is a simple sentence. Mishler and Waxler's coding procedure requires the use of multiple codes, because each act receives a code from each of eight categories. Each observer rates from three to five categories. A set of acts with the same codes is combined to form the next-larger coding unit, called the *statement*.

Reliability and Validity

The reliability of the system was very good, with coders needing to obtain a minimal level of 85% agreement before starting coding. Percentage agreement did not drop below this level during the course of the study. Evidence of the concurrent validity of the system is reported in Mishler and Waxler (1968). For example, clusters of variables discriminate schizophrenic from normal families in theoretically predicted directions.

Relation to Core Dimensions

Dominance or Power. Mishler and Waxler (1968) acknowledged that there are many different ways to conceptualize power, and they decided to measure "a set of observable behaviors that indicate different strategies" of exercising influence (p. 119). They distinguished between "attention control strategies" that focus attention on the speaker and "person control strategies" that involve attempts to confront and control others in the family. Indicators of attention control include participation rate, talk time (length of statement), and target of speeches. Indicators of person control strategies include attempted and successful interruptions and asking questions. In other words, the speaker is attempting to influence other family members by "forcing that person to stop talking or to respond in a content area limited by the controller" (Mishler & Waxler, 1968, p. 120).

Affect (Expressiveness). Based on theoretical and empirical grounds, Mishler and Waxler asserted that expressiveness was one of the major dimensions of social interaction, in general, and one of the major discriminators between schizophrenic and normal families, in particular. The system enables measurement of both quantity (level of expressiveness) and quality of affective expression (affective quality) in families. The codes hypothesized as direct indicators of expressiveness are derived from the IPA system, and the indirect indicators are derived from the affect category. The IPA codes are assumed to be direct indicators of expressiveness because the IPA takes the voice tone and the context of the speech into account, whereas the affect category classifies "each act according to the literal affective content of the words used" (ignoring voice tone and context) (Mishler & Waxler, 1968, p. 83). In addition, the IPA codes are seen as representing expressiveness toward a member present in the situation, whereas affect categories are viewed as representing the relationship "between two people" (Mishler & Waxler, 1968, p. 96).

Three IPA codes are designated as indicating positive affective quality ("shows solidarity," "tension release," "agreement") and three are designated as representing negative affective quality ("antagonism," "shows tension," "disagreement"). Level of expressiveness is measured by the relative frequency of these six IPA codes, whereas quality of expressiveness is measured by the ratio of positive and negative acts to total expressive acts.

Communication Clarity (Speech Disruptions). As for expressiveness, there are direct and indirect measures of speech disturbance. The direct indicators of speech disturbance include two IPA codes ("tension release" and "shows tension") and two codes from the tension category ("laughter" and pauses"). The indirect measures of speech disturbance include codes from the tension category including "repetitions," "incomplete phrases," and "incomplete sentences." These indicators are summed to create a statistic called "total speech disturbance" as well. Consistent with previous theories of schizophrenia, Mishler and Waxler initially thought that speech disruptions would be indicators of conflict and anxiety and therefore characteristic of schizophrenic families. However, their data indicated that speech disruptions were more likely to characterize the interaction of normals versus schizophrenic families. To explain these findings, speech disturbances were viewed as a sign of "greater adaptability to changing situations" (Mishler & Waxler, 1968 p. 164). In contrast, schizophrenic families were hypothesized to display more "rigid, ordered, almost ritualistic forms of communication" (Mishler & Waxler, 1968, p. 164).

Information Exchange. The information exchange dimension was not one of the primary dimensions of interest to Mishler and Waxler. However, the focus codes (e.g., "item content," "personal experience") and the IPA instrumental codes can be combined to form a dimension of information exchange.

Conflict. Though conflict was not one of the primary dimensions explored in Mishler and Waxler's research, a dimension of conflict can be constructed and would include "simultaneous speech," "agreement," and "disagreement" from both the IPA and focus category, "antagonism," and, most importantly, "interruptions." Interruptions are a key because they have been used in other systems (e.g., Farina, 1960) as a major indicator of family conflict.

   Support and Validation (Responsiveness). Based on theoretical and empirical grounds, Mishler and Waxler asserted that families of schizophrenics are not responsive to the "needs and wishes" of others. Operationally, they focus on the "lack of recognition of the other person's particular qualities, non-acknowledgement of his presence, and indifference to his motives and intentions" (Mishler & Waxler, 1968, p. 192). Thus, there is no validation of the other person nor support for the other person. The use of the term *responsiveness* is almost identical to other researchers' use of the concept of *validation* (e.g., Gottman *et al.*, 1976a), in that Mishler and Waxler (1968) asserted that "to be responsive to or to acknowledge anothers' behavior does not require that one behave as the other wishes but only that one show an understanding of his intention" (p. 192). Similar to the indicators of expressiveness and speech disturbance, there are direct and indirect indicators of responsiveness. The direct indicators of responsiveness are based on the acknowledgment categories, that is, the degree to which the speaker responds to the "nature" of the preceding statement. The indirect indicators are derived from the focus category that identify the reference of the speaker statements (e.g., other family members to experimental procedures). The acknowledgment code requires the observer to make a *global judgment* of the degree of responsiveness or acknowledgment displayed by the speaker.

Commentary

   The major strengths of Mishler and Waxler's system include their use of direct and indirect indicators of dimensions and their measurement of the dimensions of dominance and of support and validation. The major advantage of Mishler and Waxler's approach to measurement of dominance is the division of codes into attention and person control dimensions. Unfortunately, they have not provided validity coefficients to assess the overlap between these two measures of the same construct. However, they have indicated that these dimensions provide different information about family structure and the use of power in families. The use of talk time is consistent with Farina's measure of dominance (1960), which is still popular today. However, talk time is not necessarily a valid measure of dominance, as the most dominant person does not always talk the most (Gottman, 1979). In general, there is very little content validity for the indicators of dominance.

   Compared to other systems available today, Mishler and Waxler's coding of support and validation is better than most, primarily because Mishler and Waxler's system is relatively unique in its coding of this dimension. In addition, rather than relying on global coding of the amount of support or validation perceived, the instructions for coding do take into account the stimulus statement as well as the response. However, there is no evidence for content validity of the global acknowledgment rating. For example, the definition of support and validation used by Misher and Waxler is based strictly on responsiveness to content and does not take into account responsiveness to affect.

The major weaknesses of this system include the measurement of the dimensions of affect and communication clarity. Compared to other available systems, Mishler and Waxler's coding of affect does not clearly distinguish verbal and nonverbal behavior, so that content is confounded with affect (for example, agreement is confounded with positive affect). Further, it is ironic (given the label) that the affect category is based only on content. Thus, the content validity of the affect dimension is clearly questionable.

Compared to other systems available today, Mishler and Waxler's speech disturbance dimension does not provide a comprehensive assessment of the dimension of communication clarity. The advantage of Misher and Waxler's system for this dimension is that it provides a face-valid assessment of fragmentation of speech. However, there are no data to indicate that speech fragmentation is associated with unclear speech. In fact, in the results of their study, normal families had higher rates of speech disturbances than schizophrenic families. Thus, this measure may reflect a dimension of spontaneity in families, rather than communication clarity.

To summarize, Mishler and Waxler's coding system is an excellent example of a comprehensive behavioral observation system that assesses interactional dimensions using both behavioral referents and global judgments. It has reasonable psychometric properties and generates data that help to increase understanding of family interaction.

THE INTERACTION PROCESS CODING SYSTEM (IPCS)

History and Objectives

The IPCS (Bell, Bell, & Cornwell, 1982) was developed to describe the interaction process of normal families with adolescent girls. The original version of the IPCS is based in part on Mishler and Waxler's coding system. Similar to Mishler and Waxler, the IPCS combines both microanalytic codes and global codes. The current version of the IPCS grew out of a large research project that focused on 100 normal families with adolescent girls (see Bell & Bell, 1982a,b, for a description). The overarching goal of this project was to examine the effect of parental power and support on the individuation process of adolescents. The goal of the system is to provide "a large number of narrowly defined codes" that will eventually allow for the "estimation of a wide variety of theoretical variables" and to "facilitate the detection of patterns in verbal interactions" (Bell *et al.*, 1982, p. 1).

Codes and Dimensions

Each coding unit receives seven codes, one from each of the six categories described below:

CATEGORIES	CODES
Who spoke to whom	Subject, object (including entire family)
Topic (function of speech)	Not codable, active task avoidance, metatask, task, non-task, floor control
Orientation (form of speech)	Questions, requests or demands for compliance, assertion of facts with other person as perceiver
Focus (object of speech)	Feelings, ideas, thinking, behavior, condition, possession, location
Support	Level of warmth and acceptance or defensiveness and rejection, assessed by a global rating on a 7-point scale
Acknowledgment (level of validation)	Explicit invalidation, no response, explicit refusal to respond, recognition, response to focus, response to intent, response to focus and intent

Coding Process

A revealed difference task using items from the Moos (1974) Family Environment Scale is used to generate the interaction data. Families have 20 minutes to complete the tasks. Discussions are audiotaped, and because of recording limitations on channels, no more than five people (two parents and three children or one parent and four children) are recorded at one time.

The IPCS requires four separate groups of observers to code the six scales. One group of observers codes "who spoke to whom" and "topic"; "orientation" and "focus" are coded by a separate coder; and "support" and "acknowledgment" are each coded by an individual coder. The basic coding unit is the speech unit, the "shortest sequence of sounds that has independent meaning in interpersonal context" (Bell *et al.*, 1982, p. 2). The coding unit for acknowledgment is the speech: everything said by one speaker before the next speaker speaks. The system is designed to be used by coders working from transcripts made from audiotapes; the coders use both the transcript and the audiotape while coding.

Reliability and Validity

The five major categories of the coding scheme have 77 codes. The intercoder agreement for each of the five major categories ranges from 71% to 92% agreement. The authors do not seem to use Cohen's kappa, the recommended index for assessing agreement (see Chapter 8), nor are they clear on how the individual codes fare vis-à-vis interobserver agreement. Evidence is presented in several papers that summary codes derived from the IPCS discriminate between parents with well-functioning adolescents and parents with poorly functioning adolescents (Bell & Bell, 1982a,b), thus providing some evidence of the discriminative validity of the system for coding *marital* interaction. Unfortunately, no data are available concerning the validity of the system for coding *family* interaction. These data will hopefully be available in the future.

Relation to Core Dimensions

Dominance or Power. Power is one of the major dimensions of interest in the Bells' research program. Power is operationalized by means of the codes from the orientation category, including "requesting or demanding compliance," "asking questions," and "asserting facts." Other indicators of power are the "floor control" code from the topic category, the total number of units used by a particular family member, and successful interruptions. (The latter two statistics have also been conceptualized as indicators of assertiveness.) Thus, dominance is defined as attempts to control the interaction process, as well as attempts to control the behavior of family members.

Affect. Affect is not one of the major dimensions coded by the IPCS. However, there are several codes and categories that can be combined to produce a measure of the affect dimension. The support category of the IPCS loads heavily on the affect dimension. The support category is defined as indicating the quality of the affective relationships between family members, as assessed by voice tone. The coding instructions clearly indicate that the coders are to respond primarily to the affect dimension of speech while coding the support category. In addition, when low levels of support are rated, coders are instructed to rate the level of sadness (another indicator of negative affect). Other indicators of affect in the IPCS include the emotions code of the focus category, which presents the speakers' feelings about a particular object, and codes from the topic (nontask codes) category, including "humor" and "laughter."

Communication Clarity and Skills. The results of several factor analyses of the IPCS codes for marital interaction revealed factors that are labeled as consistent with the communication clarity and skills dimension: "active discussion of differences and disagreement," "turn taking and active listening," and "clear exchange of present opinions and attitudes" (Bell & Bell, 1982). Unfortunately, there is no indication of how the individual codes load on these factors.

Information Exchange. The information exchange dimension is not one of the primary dimensions assessed by the IPCS. However, the focus codes (e.g., presenting information, describing experiences) represent a face-valid measure of the information exchange dimension, and one of the factors mentioned above ("clear exchange of present opinions and attitudes") represents information exchange as well as communication clarity.

Conflict. The dimension of conflict is also not one of the primary dimensions directly coded by the IPCS. An indicator of conflict "active discussion of disagreement" emerged from the results of the factor analysis referred to above.

Support and Validation. The support and validation dimension is one of the primary dimensions coded by the IPCS, and it is measured by both the support category and the acknowledgment category. The codes in the support category reflect the affective quality of the relationships among the family members, and the codes in the acknowledgment category are based on the literal meaning of messages (i.e., content). These two categories are assessed by global coding. The unit of analysis for the support category is the speech unit, and the acknowledgment code is based on an entire speech (a set of statements bounded by a set of statements by other family members).

Commentary

The major strengths of the IPCS system include the measurement of support and validation and of dominance. Because the IPCS system was based, in part, on Mishler and Waxler, it is not surprising that the two systems share the same strengths as well as weaknesses. Unlike the Mishler and Waxler system, the IPCS does not divide the measurement of dominance into attention and person control subdimensions. However, the codes that reflect dominance in the IPCS system are more comprehensive than those of Mishler and Waxler. For example, the IPCS has codes for requesting compliance and thought control (the Mishler and Waxler system does not), while also including the Mishler and Waxler indicators of dominance such as "targets of speeches," "participation rate," "interruptions," and "asking questions." The major weakness of the IPCS coding of the dominance dimension, again similar to that of Mishler and Waxler, is the absence of data to support the validity of the indicators of dominance.

The IPCS measurement of the dimension of support and validation clearly represents both affective and content dimensions of interaction and is another strength of the system. However, no data are available to our knowledge that assess the covariation between these two indicators of support and validation. In this system, support is a higher order dimension that includes affect, enabling support and validation to be assessed by both the content of interaction and the affective qualities present. Distinctions can be made between high and low acknowledgment delivered with negative affect and high and low acknowledgment delivered with positive affect.

The acknowledgment dimension is unique and deserves some commentary. The authors noted, in the beginning of their description of the acknowledgment category for families, that "It can be argued that anyone who would volunteer to learn and use the following coding scheme must be masochistic, crazy, or desperate" (Bell *et al.*, 1982, p. 42). Although we hope that we are in none of these three categories, we agree that the description of the acknowledgment dimension is complicated. The complicated coding instructions may have led to the relatively low reliability for the individual acknowledgment codes and may have necessitated an overall acknowledgment score for establishing an acceptable level of reliability (and we assume for data analysis as well). Although the acknowledgment code requires the observer to make global judgments, these judgments are made before every speech, and therefore, coding inferences are tied more directly to the interactional process. The acknowledgment code is directly based on Mishler and Waxler's acknowledgment code (and responsiveness dimension); however, the IPCS pays special attention to this dimension, and therefore, its treatment is recommended over Mishler and Waxler's. We hope that subsequent versions of this coding system will deal more effectively with the complicated nature of the coding instructions.

There are three major problems with the IPCS. First, the authors have not presented observer agreement data on the majority of the individual codes that are summed to create the dimension of interest. However, this is not a problem if the data analyses are limited to the summary categories. Second, the dimensions are defined on the basis of face-valid criteria with no evidence for the construct validity of these particular arrangements of codes. Third, based on reading the author's studies using the IPCS, it seems that they have not yet presented all of the data they have collected. For example, to this point, only dyadic data (usually on couples) have been presented. This highlights the complexity of family interaction research.

FAMILY INTERACTION CODING SYSTEM (FICS)

History and Objectives

In the early 1960s, the Oregon Social Learning Group, under the leadership of Gerald Patterson, became interested in the study and treatment of aggressive children. Consistent with social learning theory, these researchers were interested in the environmental conditions that were associated with aggressive behaviors and decided to focus on the family home environment, which was hypothesized to foster and to maintain the child's aggressive behavior. Initial attempts to describe these families involved observers in going to homes and writing accounts in longhand of what they observed (Patterson, 1982). In a second early attempt, observers recorded on tape their observations as they watched families. Patterson and associates were not satisfied with these methods and decided that a shorthand was necessary (Patterson, 1982). This decision led to the development of the FICS (Patterson, Ray, Shaw, & Cobb, 1969). The initial version took three years to develop and it underwent six revisions before the researchers felt it was ready to be used for research and clinical purposes. From the outset, this group realized that the FICS would not be adequate for coding low-base-rate behaviors (e.g., fire setting) and hence developed a parent–self-report inventory to assess low-base-rate problem behaviors (Patterson, 1982).

The FICS is probably the most widely used coding system for families with conduct-disordered children, and it has been periodically updated. Moreover, it has served as the basis for some marital-observation coding systems as well as other family-observation systems (e.g., the Dyadic Parent–Child Interaction Coding System; Eyberg & Robinson, 1981; Robinson & Eyberg, 1981). Finally, Patterson and associates have pioneered research on biases in family interaction research, such as observer bias and observer reactivity (see Jones, Reid, & Patterson, 1975, for a review).

The goal of the FICS is to focus on "discrete units of deviant and cohesive behavior" (Patterson, 1982, p. 4) in families during home interaction. Patterson (1982) noted that the FICS was developed to "test hypotheses about limited aspects of behavior" (p. 72) and is not appropriate when other dimensions are of interest. The FICS items were designed to be sensitive to the "process of aggression" and to changes that would occur in family interactions as a function of treatment.

Codes and Dimensions

Currently, 29 codes comprise the FICS, 14 of which reflect aversive behaviors and 15 of which represent prosocial behaviors. The 14 aversive-behavior codes are combined to form a summary index of the level of coerciveness in a family. These codes and dimensions are presented below:

DIMENSION	CODES
Aversive	Command negative, cry, disapproval, dependency, destructiveness, high rate, humiliate, tease, whine, yell, noncompliance, negativism, ignore, physical negative
Prosocial	Approval, attention, command positive, compliance, indulgence, laugh, normative, no response, play, physical positive, receive, self-stimulation, talk, touch, work

Coding Process

As mentioned earlier, the FICS was designed to code family interaction at home. Initially, the researchers tried to obtain samples of free interaction but quickly realized that more structure was needed. Thus, over time, they developed eight rules that families follow for a semistructured interaction task, such as that observations must occur before dinner, that all family members must be present, and that no television or stereo is to be on. The intent here is to maximize the family's providing the information of interest. The coders use a clipboard with a light attached to it that flashes at 30-second intervals.

Individual family members are randomly selected to serve as "targets of the observation." Each family member serves as a target for 5 minutes, and then another family member, randomly selected, becomes the target. For each target, the observer records what the target does (the antecedent behavior) and then codes how other family members respond to the target's behavior (the consequent behavior). The coder uses numbers to record the target, the target's behavior, the respondent, and the respondent's behavior. The basic unit of analysis is called a *frame* and is a 6-second unit of behavior. There are five frames per coding line, equaling 30 seconds; at the flash of the light, the coder switches to a new line. Six-second periods are indicated by an automatic timing device, and coders continuously record what the target is doing and how the various family members are responding to him or her. Thus, the FICS provides for a sequential record of the family's interaction from the target's perspective.

Reliability and Validity

Reliability assessed by interobserver agreement is based on the 30-second coding line. Two observers attend every home visit during a baseline period and every fourth home visit thereafter. This schedule enables evaluation of phenomena such as observer drift and decay. The median percentage agreement for the FICS is .72. thus, the reliability of the FICS as assessed by percentage agreement is very good. In addition, Patterson and associates were pioneers in applying generalizability theory to behavioral observation systems (see Jacob, Chapter 1, for details on generalizability theory). For example, Jones *et al.* (1975) provided evidence of the generalizability to the FICS across facets of observers, settings, and targets.

Patterson (1982) provided an excellent summary of the numerous studies that assess the validity of the FICS. Several studies indicate that families with problem children are more coercive than normal families providing evidence for the concurrent validity of the FICS. In addition, several studies have indicated that FICS codes change in predicted directions after intervention, providing evidence for the construct validity of the systems (Jones, *et al.*, 1975).

Relation to Core Dimensions

Aspects of five of the six dimensions that we have been considering are combined in the FICS's two major dimensions of aversive and prosocial behaviors. In general, aversive codes represent the negative ends of the six dimensions (e.g., "command negative" is high dominance; "cry" and "physical negative" are negative affect; "yell" is high conflict; and "ignore" is low support), whereas the prosocial behaviors represent the positive ends of the six dimensions (e.g., "comply" is low dominance; "laugh," "physical positive," and "touch" are positive affect; "approval" and "attention" are high support). There are no FICS codes that represent the communication clarity and skills dimension. In addition, there are a number of FICS codes that describe what the interactants are doing (e.g., see, talk, work, play) but that do not fall into the six dimensions. Such descriptive codes provide the information about the social ecology of family life and may be of interest to some researchers (Steinglass's HOAM observation system reviewed below has similar characteristics). Thus, the aversive behavior dimension is best described by high dominance, low affect, low support, and high conflict, whereas the prosocial behavior dimension is best described by low dominance, high positive affect, and high support/validation. In addition, the descriptive codes (these might fall into the information exchange dimension) are considered prosocial.

Commentary

The FICS provides one of the best sets of codes to capture negative interaction between parents and school-aged children. The system is designed to be sensitive to chains of negative interaction such as "mother commands → child complies," rather than providing a comprehensive picture of family interaction. Patterson (1982) described two major problems with the FICS. First, the use of a 6 second coding unit is arbitrary and, as noted by Hartup (1979), does not allow for the assessment of the density and duration of behaviors. Timing the length of the event would alleviate this problem. However, to our knowledge, no coding system uses this procedure, although several could with minor modifications. Second, although prosocial codes are included in the system, the FICS focuses on deviant behaviors. Because deviant behaviors are low-base-rate (5%–10%; Patterson, 1982) and the prosocial codes are not well developed, the FICS provides little descriptive information about overall family functioning. To solve this problem, Patterson and his associates have been working on systems that are more comprehensive.

In summary, the FICS focuses on a limited number of dimensions using behavioral referents to clearly define these dimensions. Specifically, the FICS focuses on children's deviant and prosocial behaviors and on parents' response to these behaviors.

DEFENSIVE AND SUPPORTIVE COMMUNICATIONS SCALE

History and Objectives

Alexander and his colleagues at the University of Utah have a long-standing research program with delinquent adolescents and their families. A major tool of their research efforts has been the observational coding of defensive and supportive communication in these families. More recently, Alexander and his associates (e.g., Alexander & Parsons, 1982; Barton & Alexander, 1980) have developed a family therapy program (functional family therapy) that is based, in part, on the empirical research using the defensive and supportive coding system.

Codes and Dimensions

The concept of defensive and supportive communication derives from the work of Gibb (1961), who defined defensive behavior as "that behavior which occurs when an individual perceives threat or anticipated threat in the group" (Alexander, 1983, p. 1). Essentially, defensive behavior produces dysfunctional communication because the speaker is spending energy protecting herself or himself (using projection as a major defense). Supportive behaviors focus on the current task in an empathic manner. Defensive behavior from one family member is hypothesized to increase the probability of defensive behavior in other family members and thus to produce dysfunctional negative interaction patterns in families. Supportive behavior, on the other hand, leads to positive cycles. The four defensive codes are "judgmental dogmatism," "control and strategy," "indifference," and "superiority." The four supportive codes are "genuine information-seeking and -giving," "spontaneous problem-solving," "empathic understanding," and "equality."

Coding Process

Interaction is generated by asking the family to discuss "various topics pertinent to the families situation" (Alexander, 1983, p. 1), and this discussion is videotaped. One coder is assigned to watch and to code each family member. Using a transcript, the coder watches the videotape and records one of four defensive codes or one of four supportive codes every 6 seconds.

Reliability and Validity

The reliability of this coding system is very high, and there is systematic research supporting the concurrent validity of this coding system for families with delinquent adolescents (Alexander, 1973).

Relation to Core Dimensions

Several of the major dimensions are combined in Alexander's dimensions of defensiveness and support of communication. The defensive dimension includes high dominance ("superiority" and "control") and low support ("indifference" and "judgmental"). The supportiveness category includes low dominance ("equality"), high communication skills ("problem solving") and high support ("empathic understanding" and "information seeking"). Thus, defensiveness represents the negative poles of some of the major dimensions, and supportiveness includes the positive poles of some of these dimensions.

Commentary

The strength of Alexander's system is the use of a quantitative strategy to assess dimensions that are usually coded with global ratings. This strength is best seen by comparing Alexander's coding of the dimension of support and validation with Mishler and Waxler's and the Bells'. We can also see how Alexander's two major dimensions incorporate (much like Patterson's FICS) some of the major coding dimensions by combining codes that represent positive or negative ends on the dimensions. Thus, high levels of supportiveness involve high support and validation and low dominance. Alexander's system is a good example of a nonexhaustive coding system that focuses on a small number of theoretically relevant concepts. His research, using the coding system, is an excellent example of linking the results of family observation studies to the development of intervention programs.

SYSTEM FOR THE ASSESSMENT OF FAMILY INDIVIDUATION

History and Objectives

This family-interaction coding system, developed by Condon, Cooper, and Grotevant (1981), grew out of their research focusing on the relationship between family interaction and adolescent social development. The objective of this coding system is to assess three dimensions of individuation: self-assertion (SA), permeability (P), and validation (V). Their theoretical model hypothesizes that these constructs can be assessed through the direct observation of family interaction. The coding system "reflects the fact that some utterances appear to both direct or *move* the conversation while they also *respond* to previous utterances by other participants" (Cooper, Grotevant, & Condon, 1983, pp. 8–9).

Codes and Dimensions

There are two major categories: move and response. In addition, the source and the object of each message are noted. Each coding unit receives a move and a response code. The codes are combined into the three dimensions of individuation that are viewed as important in adaptive adolescent development. The codes and how they load on these dimensions are listed below:

MOVE CODES	RESPONSE CODES
Irrelevant comment (−P)	Initiates compromise (+V)
Suggests action (SA)	Agrees/accepts/incorporates others' ideas (+P)
Suggests location (SA)	Disagrees/challenges others' ideas (−P)
Requests information/validation (+P)	Answers request for information/validation (+P)
Requests action (−P)	Complies with request for action (+P)
No clear move function	Acknowledgment (+V)
	No clear response function

OTHER CODES
Relevant comment
Mind-reads/dictates others' feelings (−V)

Coding Process

The task used is to have the family "plan something together." The authors noted that they chose this task, as opposed to a revealed- or unrevealed-difference task, because these two tasks focused the family too much on conflict. The plan-something-together task involves telling the family that "they have two weeks and unlimited funds to spend on a family vacation. They are asked to plan a day to day itinerary for the vacation and to write down the location and activities planned for each day" (Cooper *et al.*, 1983, p. 51). The families complete the task sitting at home at their kitchen table, and the observers are not present during the discussion. These interactions are audiotaped and then transcribed. The basic coding unit is the utterance, which is sentences or parts of a sentence, and only the first 300 utterances are coded.

Reliability and Validity

The reliability of the system as measured by percentage agreement was 75% or more for each code, with the exception of "acknowledgment" and "incorporates others' ideas." Percentage agreements for these codes were not provided. Evidence of the validity of the system is available in several studies (e.g., Cooper *et al.*, 1983; Grotevant & Cooper, 1983, 1985). For example, Grotevant and Cooper (1983) factor-analyzed the codes, and the dimensions that emerged were consistent with the three dimensions of individuation. The validity of the system is also demonstrated, in part, by correlations in the expected directions between measures of ego development and the behavioral observation data (Grotevant & Cooper, 1983).

Relation to Core Dimensions

Several of the major interactional dimensions are combined in this system's three dimensions. High levels of permeability and validation represent high levels of the support and validation dimension (e.g., "acknowledgment" and "validation"), low levels of dominance ("complies"), low levels of conflict ("agrees"), and high levels of communication clarity and skills ("initiate compromise," "states other feelings," and "suggests actions indirectly"). High levels of separateness indicate high levels of dominance ("requests action") and high levels of conflict ("disagrees"). Although the self-assertion dimension is defined in terms of communication clarity, the codes that represent self-assertion ("suggests action" and "location") seem more consistent with the dominance dimension than with communication clarity and skills. Finally, the "mind-reading" code represents low levels of communication skill.

Commentary

This system was developed for coding a small number of theoretically relevant concepts and therefore is of limited usefulness to researchers with other purposes in mind. However, the strategy of examining the family interaction process for the roots of adolescent individuation illustrates how relatively descriptive, interactionally based strategies can be used to test hypotheses from fields that do not typically use interactional research methods.

The strength of this system (as well as of Alexander's) is the use of an interaction-based strategy to assess the support and validation dimension, whereas this dimension is globally coded by other systems (e.g., the IPCS and Mishler and Waxler's system). This system defines the support and validation dimension in terms of low dominance and high communication skills and has the advantage of also including codes that comprise a more face-valid representative of the validation and support dimension, for example, "acknowledgement," "validation," and "answers requests for information/validation."

The major difference between the present system and Alexander's system is that this system assigns two codes to each unit, a move code and a response code. This dual coding has the advantage of focusing the observer on the sequential nature of the exchange of support and validation in interaction. Another difference between the systems is that Alexander's system was developed to study supportiveness and defensiveness in families that had a delinquent adolescent, whereas the present system was developed to study the process of individuation in families with normal adolescents.

THE FAMILY CONSTRAINING AND ENABLING CODING SYSTEM (CECS)

History and Objectives

This coding system was developed by Hauser and his colleagues (Hauser, Powers, Weiss, Follansbee, & Bernstein, 1983) to study types of family interaction that facilitate or hinder the development of adolescents. The CECS attempts to operationalize Stierlin's theory (1974) concerning how parental interactions affect adolescent maturation. In particular, the CECS focuses on communications that interfere with (constrain) or facilitate (enable) the functioning family members in general and of adolescents in particular.

The CECS is currently being used as part of a large-scale longitudinal research project comparing families with adolescent diabetics, families with psychiatric patients, and normal families with adolescents (Hauser, Jacobson, Noam, & Powers, 1983). Thus, this is one of the few studies that applies observational methods to the study of adolescent families by using a longitudinal design. In addition to the CECS, Powers has developed a companion coding system that focuses on the developmental environments of these families.

Codes and Dimensions

The CECS coding system consists of two major dimensions. The constraining dimension includes codes that function in the interaction sequence to constrain growth, and the enabling dimension includes codes that function in the interaction sequence to facilitate growth. Both the constraining and the enabling dimensions are broken into two subdimensions: cognitive and affective. The CECS codes are presented below:

	COGNITIVE	AFFECTIVE
CONSTRAINING	Distracting	Indifference
	Withholding	Gratifying
	Judgmental	Devaluing
ENABLING	Explaining/Declarative	Acceptance
	Focusing	Active understanding/Empathy
	Problem solving	
	Curiosity	

The coders first decide which of these codes is most applicable to the speech and then rate the degree to which the chosen code is applicable on a 5-point scale ranging from low to high. The coding manual provides a set of rules to help the observer decide which code to use when more than one seems appropriate.

In addition to the constraining and enabling codes, there are two other dimensions that are coded. First, the *discourse change* dimension "focuses upon how a family member changes or resists change following the interventions of other members" (Hauser *et al.*, 1984, p. 197). The unit of analysis is a pair of speeches, and the four discourse change codes are (a) progression (the individual increases his or her contribution); (b) regression (the individual decreases contributions); (c) foreclosure (the individual is repetitive); and (d) topic change (the individual changes the topic). Second, the *adolescent response* dimension "consists of five scales which represent ways in which the adolescent can respond to parental constraining and enabling" (Hauser *et al.*, 1983a, p. 2). The adolescent's response is categorized as either constraining (e.g., submission, opposition) or enabling (e.g., shift, collaboration).

Coding Process

Family members are videotaped discussing a revealed-difference task involving Kohlberg's moral dilemmas (1969). The interactions are transcribed for coding purposes. (It is not clear whether the coders use the tapes for their codings, nor whether the tape is audio or video.) The basic unit of analysis is a speech, which is defined as a statement or a set of statements. The unit of analysis for this coding system is very different from that for the other systems that we have described. The family's interaction is transcribed, and then a person called a *unitizer* goes through the transcript and marks off developmentally important "key events" in the following manner: "(1) all speeches in which the adolescent member takes a position about an outside issue or an event in the family are located by an asterisk; (2) the unitizer proceeds through all following parental speech until he locates the next *adolescent speech* which is then marked with a double asterisk; (3) the unitizer then proceeds through the transcript to locate the next such set of two adolescent speeches with intervening parental speeches" (Hauser *et al.*, 1984, p. 201). Thus, the CECS uses an event sampling and does not provide for a continuous record of family interaction.

Reliability and Validity

The reliability of the CECS was assessed speech by speech for all the codes by the use of both percentage agreement and kappa. The percentage agreement ranged from .81 to .99, and the kappa ranged from .43 to .82. Thus the reliability for the codes is acceptable. However, no reliability data have been presented for the high-level versus the low-level judgments. Substantial data are available on the validity of the system. For example, Hauser *et al.* (1984) found that an adolescent's level of ego development was positively correlated with adolescent enabling behavior and was negatively correlated with adolescent constraining behavior. Further, as predicted, parental constraining and enabling were related in the predicted directions to levels of adolescent ego development.

Relation to Core Dimensions

Several of the major interactional dimensions are included in the CECS codes and dimensions. The constraining affective codes load on the negative end of the affect dimension (i.e., negative affect), and the enabling affective codes load on the positive end of the affect dimension (i.e., positive affect). The enabling affective codes ("acceptance," "active understanding/empathy") also load on the positive end of the support and validation dimension. The constraining cognitive codes include high dominance ("judgmental"), low support ("withholding"), and low communication skills ("distracting"). The enabling cognitive codes all load on the positive end of communication clarity and skills. The adolescent response codes load on low dominance ("submission") and high support and validation ("collaboration"). To summarize, the constraining dimension includes negative affect, high dominance, poor communication, and low support, whereas the enabling dimension includes positive affect, good communication, and high support.

Commentary

The major strength of Hauser's system is the use of an interaction-based strategy to identify interaction processes that may be related to adolescent development. The constraining and enabling dimensions are similar to Alexander's defensive and supportive dimensions, respectively. The major difference is that the CECS adds comprehensiveness of dimensional coverage by including the cognitive and affective dimensions. As with other systems, we can see that the major CECS dimensions incorporate four of the major coding dimensions by combining codes that represent positive or negative poles on these dimensions.

An unique feature of the CECS is that it is used to code *only* key events in the interaction process (e.g., the adolescent's taking a position on an issue). These are events that the researchers believe are the most likely to reveal the developmentally relevant process in which they are interested. This strategy has both advantages and disadvantages. The major advantage is that it is economical because only segments of interaction must be coded rather than the entire interaction sequence. Further, the codes can be "fine-tuned" to reflect the possible theoretically relevant responses to the key event. The major disadvantage is that the CECS does not provide a continuous record of family interaction. It is possible that interactional events relative to constraining and enabling are not sampled.

Another unique feature is the combination of global coding with interaction-based coding. Once the behavioral code is identified, the unit is rated on whether it reflects a low or a high level of that code. The major advantage of this strategy is that it allows for varying degrees of "strength" of code. In contrast, all of the other systems we have reviewed use an all-or-none approach in assigning codes. For example, if a unit meets the minimal standards for a code, it gets the same code. The major disadvantage is that no data are presented on the reliability of these global judgments, and to date, their validity has not been established.

Finally, similar to Grotevant, Cooper, and Condon's research, the work of Hauser and associates illustrates the use of family observation methods to test hypotheses from fields that have not typically used these methods.

AFFECTIVE STYLE (AS)

History and Objectives

One of the most active contemporary research areas in schizophrenia is examining the role of affect in determining relapse. The origins of this recent interest can be traced to the work of George Brown and associates on expressed emotion (e.g., Brown, Burley, & Wing, 1972) and have been elaborated by Vaughn and Leff (1976). For example, Brown *et al.* (1972) divided families into high- or low-expressed-emotion (EE) homes, and the results indicated that there was a 58% relapse rate from high-EE homes compared to a 16% relapse rate in low-EE homes. The expressed-emotion index is comprised of three components: (a) the number of critical comments made by a key relative when talking about the patient and the patient's illness; (b) the amount of hostility and criticism in the remarks; and (c) indications of significant emotional overinvolvement in these interviews. Of the three components of expressed emotion, the one that is considered most important by researchers is the number of critical comments made by the relative in the interview situation. The task typically used is an individual interview with a key relative (e.g., the spouse) who talks about the patient and the patient's illness. Thus, the EE index is not based on a sample of family interaction. The assumption underlying the individual interview seems to be that negativity expressed toward the patient comes out in the family's interactions and that this negativity affects the patient's adjustment to the home after hospitalization.

Doane and associates, as part of the UCLA Schizophrenia Project (Rodnick, Goldstein, Lewis, & Doane, 1984), developed a measure that is similar to the expressed-emotion index, but that was specifically designed to code *interaction*, as opposed to interviews. This measure is called the affective style (AS) interactional system (Doane & Lewis, 1984; Doane *et al.*, 1981). This system has been used, along with Singer and Wynne's (1966) Communication Deviance Index (a noninteraction measure of communication), to predict the onset of psychiatric disorders in an at-risk sample (e.g., Doane *et al.*, 1982)

Codes and Dimensions

The affective style system is composed of eight primary codes that have been variously combined in different studies to form categories. The most up-to-date combinations are presented below:

CATEGORIES	CODES
Benign criticism	Benign criticism
Harsh criticism	Personal criticism, guilt induction, critical intrusiveness
Neutral intrusiveness	Neutral intrusiveness
Support	Primary support, secondary support, indirect support

In previous studies, the categories of benign criticism, harsh criticism, and neutral intrusiveness were combined to form a measure of negative affective tone (Doane *et al.*, 1981).

Coding Process

Two revealed-difference tasks (Strodtbeck, 1954) are used: (a) the adolescent talking to each parent separately and (b) the adolescent talking with both parents. Verbatim transcripts are prepared from videotapes of the interactions and are used for the coding of affective style. An event-sampling procedure is used to generage the coding unit, which is defined as up to six consecutive lines of uninterrupted speech by a speaker. The end of the coding unit is marked when another family member either "significantly interrupts" the speaker or begins a distinct reply of his or her own. Usually, only one code from each category is assigned to each unit, with the more "impactful" code used if more than one code is appropriate.

Reliability and Validity

In initial reports the reliability of the AS system appeared adequate. Cohen's kappa, appropriately calculated without including agreement of nonoccurrences, ranged from .78 to .89 for the four categories (Doane, Goldstein, & Rodnick, 1981). Reliabilities for the individual codes are not available. However, more recently, Doane (personal communication) has indicated that the reliability is hard to achieve without expensive training. The validity of the system is supported by findings that (a) parental affective style was predictive of adolescent psychiatric status (Doane *et al.*, 1981); (b) parental affective style, together with communication deviance, predicted (over a 5-year period) schizophrenic spectrum disorders in young adults (Doane *et al.*, 1981); and (c) parental affective style was found to be associated with expressed emotion assessed during an interview (Valone, Norton, Goldstein, & Doane, 1984).

Relation to Core Dimensions

The affective style system, as the name suggests, reflects the dimension of affect. The theory underlying the system proposes that these three negative affective tone codes should produce negative responses in the patient. The other dimension tapped by the affective style system is support.

Commentary

The AS system focuses on two dimensions of family interaction: affect and support/validation. It is thus not appropriate for a comprehensive description of family interaction. The translation of expressed emotion into the interactional domain is a strength of the AS system. Another strength of the system is its demonstrated utility in predicting the onset of psychiatric disorders in an at-risk population. In current practice, the primary disadvantage of the system is the reshuffling of individual codes to define the categories entering data analysis. It is somewhat unclear how affective-style comparison groups have been formed. In addition, even if affective style predicts psychiatric disturbance, we would like to know more about the interactional patterns that characterize these families, which may help us to understand the precise nature of the risk in these family systems.

Doane and her associate have stimulated other interactional researchers to study the prediction of relapse and/or the development of symptoms using more comprehensive observational systems. For example, the KPI (reviewed below) is being used to predict the relapse of depression (Hooley, 1985).

THE HOME OBSERVATION ASSESSMENT METHOD (HOAM)

History and Objectives

The rationale for this system, developed by Steinglass (1976), was the need for a method of collecting data over long periods of time in the home from a family systems perspective. The goal of the HOAM is to assess the family's regulation of its internal (i.e., home) environment. The HOAM is intended to "capture the unique features of the home, its architecture, the traffic patterns of family members, and interaction in relation to use of space" (Steinglass, 1979, p. 340). Verbal interaction is coded only when necessary. Although the system is applicable to all types of families, Steinglass's research has focused on families with an alcoholic member.

Codes and Dimensions

For each coding unit (2-minute blocks), the four types of codes described below are used:

CATEGORIES	CODES
Contextual	Location, persons in field, alcohol (present/absent, alcohol consumed by other/subject, visible but not consumed, not visible, physical distance
Who to whom	Subject initiates, subject receives, subject initiates and receives
Behavioral characteristics	Physical contact—positive, physical contact—negative, physical contact—neutral, meal activity, working at home, entertainment alone, entertainment with others, conversation with pets, telephone conversation, movement, not observable, sleeping
INTERACTION CATEGORIES	
Type of interaction	Task orientation, problem solving, information exchange, work task

Affective level   Global rating on a 7-point positive-to-negative scale
Outcome from subject's perspective   Resolved, neutral, unresolved

Coding Process

According to the training manual, the family are in charge of the interaction session. They may label, for example, certain areas of the house as being off limits to the coders and can ask the coders to leave if a certain topic comes up or for any other reason. Two-person coding teams come into the home and follow the family members around for periods of up to 4 hours. One coder is assigned to the alcoholic member and the other to another family member (however, it is not clear how this other person is chosen). The coders are instructed to code only "direct interaction between the subject and the other family members." The family are instructed to do whatever they would normally do during the time period when the observer is present. The observers code for 40 minutes, take a break, code again for 40 minutes, break for 15 minutes, and so on. Within the 40 minutes, the basic coding unit is a 2-minute timed block.

Reliability and Validity

Interobserver agreegment for these codes was quite respectable, ranging from .63 for the who-to-whom codes to .96 for the affect codes. The kappa statistic was also used in the calculation of reliability, and once again, the kappa coefficients revealed adequate introbserver agreement. It is interesting that the lowest kappas were for "who to whom" and "number of persons in the field." One reason for this low agreement is that the other observer is sometimes in the field and is sometimes the object of interaction. Evidence for the discriminative validity of the HOAM is presented in Steinglass (1979). For example, HOAM codes and dimensions discriminate between alcoholic and normal families.

Relation to Core Dimensions

Three of the core dimensions are included in the HOAM: information exchange (assessed by the type of interaction codes, e.g., "task orientation," "information exchange," and "work task"); affect (assessed by the affective level rating); and communication skill and clarity (assessed by the problem-solving code and the outcome of interaction, assuming that positive outcome is related to good communication).

Commentary

The HOAM is unique among the systems we have reviewed in its focus on contextual and noninteractional concomitants of family interaction. It provides an excellent description of the "social ecology" of families at home, that is, where families interact and what they do when they interact. This information is particularly important when one's theoretical perspective focuses on the contextual determinants of the outcomes of interest (e.g., drinking behavior). Also the HOAM is the only observational system (to our knowledge) that has been developed for use with alcoholic families.

Obviously, the HOAM is limited in its use for the comprehensive, micro-analytic coding of family interaction. However, the HOAM does provide coverage of three of the core interactional dimensions and thus provides an integration of noninteractional and interactional behavior codes. Of these three dimensions, the HOAM assessment of the information exchange dimension is better than most, and its assessment of communication skill and clarity is weaker than most because it focuses only on problem solving. The assessment of affect relies on a single global code, which may be of questionable utility.

MARITAL OBSERVATION SYSTEMS: COUPLES INTERACTION SCORING SYSTEM (CISS)

History and Objectives

In the early 1970s at Indiana University, the authors of the present chapter (along with John Gottman) started investigating the interaction patterns associated with distressed and nondistressed marriages. The major objective of our research was to identify some of the interactional determinants of marital distress and then, based on these findings, to develop intervention programs to both treat and prevent marital distress. One of the major tools that we have used in our research is the Couples Interaction Scoring System (CISS, pronounced "kiss"). It took over two years to develop the initial version of the CISS. The codes and dimensions that we finally decided to use were guided by

> (1) an assumption concerning the importance of communication processes in marital functioning, (2) our clinical intuitions as we observed distressed and nondistressed couples interacting, and (3) recognition of the importance of nonverbal behavior in determining the meaning of interpersonal messages. (Notarius, Markman, & Gottman, 1983, p. 119)

The CISS codes were derived in part from other available marital observation systems, most importantly the Marital Interaction Coding System (MICS, described later). The CISS has been used to code the interaction data from studies that have used relatively small sample sizes, most of which have compared the problem-solving behavior of distressed and nondistressed couples. A more detailed description of the history of the CISS has been provided by Gottman (1979), Notarius and Markman (1981), and Notarius *et al.*, (1983).

Codes and Dimensions

The unique feature of the CISS is that it is basically two coding systems: a *nonverbal* system that codes nonverbal behaviors and a *content* system that codes verbal behaviors. Two different sets of coders are required to use the CISS. Each coding unit receives *both* a content and a nonverbal code for the speaker and a nonverbal code for the listener. Thus, the CISS is designed to provide a comprehensive interactional record of a couple's problem-solving interaction by means of low-inference behavioral codes.

Content Codes and Dimensions. There were 28 content codes in the original version of the CISS. These codes were combined to form eight summary codes (or dimensions) based on a conceptual analysis of which codes belonged together. (The CISS has been revised several times and has been applied to several different types of couples; the result has been minor modifications of the codes. However, the "summary codes" remain the same.) The eight summary codes and their constituent individual codes are presented below:

SUMMARY CODES	CODES
Problem talk	Generalized problem talk, relationship issue problem talk, nonrelationship issue problem talk, feeling
Mind reading	Mind-reading feelings/attitudes/opinions, mind-reading behavior
Proposing solution	Plan, nonspecific plan, relationship information, nonrelationship information/opinion/feelings
Communication talk	Back on beam—task, back on beam—solution, metacommunication, clarification request
Agreement	Direct agreement, accept responsibility, accept modification, compliance, assent
Disagreement	· Direct disagreement, disagree with rationale, command, noncompliance
Summarizing other	Summarizing other, summarizing both
Summarizing self	Summarizing self

Nonverbal Codes. Three codes—positive, negative, and neutral—are used to assess the nonverbal behaviors of the speaker and the listener. These codes are intended to "identify the effects of a person's nonverbal behavior upon the emotional interpersonal climate that exists between the partners" (Notarius & Markman, 1981, p. 119), not the person's "inner state." To arrive at a nonverbal code, the observer scans facial expression, voice tone, and body position or movement and provides a summary impression based on the combination of these three nonverbal channels. (Early versions of the CISS used a hierarchy rule that instructed the coders to first scan the face. If a code could be applied, this would be the affect code. If facial expression was neutral, they would proceed to the voice tone and so on.) Examples of cues used for CISS affect codes are presented below:

	POSITIVE	NEGATIVE
Face	Smile	Frown
	Head nod	Sneer
Voice	Caring	Cold
	Warm	Tense
Body	Touching	Rude gestures
	Open arms	Hand tension

Coding Process

We use three types of tasks to generate interaction: discussion of the couple's top problem areas; discussion of problems not directly related to the couple (e.g., an Inventory of Marital Conflict task, Olson & Ryder, 1970); and more recently, a discussion of how the couple's day went (Levinson & Gottman, 1983). The couples usually talk for about 10 to 15 minutes, and their discussion is videotaped. The videotapes are transcribed verbatim, and the coders use the transcript and the videotape while coding.

The basic coding unit is called the *thought unit* and represents the smallest unit of speech that is intelligible. The transcripts are "slashed" into thought units, and the units are numbered before coding starts. As mentioned earlier, each thought unit receives three separate codes (speaker content, speaker nonverbal, and listener nonverbal).

Reliability and Validity

The reliability of the CISS, assessed by Cohen's kappa and by generalizability studies, has been established in several investigations. For example, Gottman (1979) reported that Cohen's kappas for content codes averaged .909 and for nonverbal codes averaged .715. The validity of the CISS has been established in several studies, the results of which were summarized by Notarius, *et al.*, 1983). Specifically, distressed couples tend to engage in relatively long negative-affect sequences, whereas nondistressed couples are able to exit from these sequences.

Relation to Core Dimensions

Dominance. The CISS has no codes to directly assess dominance because of our view that dominance is best assessed by examining the *consequences* of several codes in the interaction stream, rather than by examining *rates* of behavior (Gottman, 1979). For example, Gottman (1979) presented a statistical procedure for assessing dominance defined as assymmetry in predictability of behavior.

Affect. The CISS nonverbal codes directly assess positive, negative, and neutral affect. Affect is therefore defined as strictly based on nonverbal cues and is rated for the listener as well as the speaker.

Communication Clarity and Skills. Several of the CISS summary codes directly assess communication skills and deficits: "mind reading," "problem solving," "summarizing other," and "summarizing self." These codes can be combined with the nonverbal codes to form more sensitive indicators of the quality of communication (Gottman *et al.*, 1977). As for dominance, research has indicated that the most sensitive indications of the quality of a couple's communication can be obtained from sequential analysis that identifies patterns of functional and dysfunctional communication. For example, summarizing oneself repeatedly is a sign of distressed marriages (Gottman *et al.*, 1977).

Information Exchange. The "problem talk" summary code and the "relationship and nonrelationship information" codes that comprise the "proposing solution" summary code provide an assessment of the information exchange dimension.

Conflict. The ratio of the "agreement" summary code to "agreement" and "disagreement" is one indicator of conflict available from the CISS. However, research has indicated that sequential analyses of CISS verbal and nonverbal codes provides the most sensitive indication of the conflict dimension. For example, strings of problem talk with negative affect are a sign of conflict in a distressed marriage, whereas in nondistressed marriages, a person (usually the wife) responds to a negative message with a *neutral* message, thus breaking the powerful negative affect cycle during a problem discussion (Notarius *et al.,* 1983).

Support and Validation. The "summarizing other" summary code provides an assessment of this dimension. However, once again, the best assessment of the support and validation dimension is through the antecedents and contingencies of several verbal and nonverbal behaviors (e.g., agreement, summarizing other, and head nods), rather than through examining the rates of one behavior designed to assess the level of support and validation.

Commentary

We are obviously biased when it comes to the CISS and our research using this system, and the reader should keep this in mind when evaluating our comments. The major strengths of the CISS include the separate coding of verbal and nonverbal behaviors and the use of sequential analyses of CISS codes to assess some of the core interactional dimensions. In addition, we feel that our research strategy of conducting comprehensive studies with small numbers of subjects has been productive in advancing our understanding of marital interaction. Other marital-interaction researchers have followed the same strategy (e.g., Billings, 1979; Birchler, Weiss, & Vincent, 1977; Hahlweg, Revenstorf, & Schindler, 1984). Further, because the major marital-observation systems have been developed and modified to reflect the best features of each, a comparable database has emerged that has enabled a rapid growth of our knowledge concerning the development, maintenance, treatment, and prevention of marital distress.

In contrast to the family interaction field, which has generally examined family interaction in relation to psychopathology, the marital interaction field has generally focused on marital distress as the outcome variable of interest (or response to marital intervention programs). The marital field is now turning to examining the role of marital interaction in the development and treatment of psychopathology, particularly the affective disorders (Coyne, present volume, Chapter 14; Hooley, 1985; Notarius & Pellegrini, 1986).

One major weakness of the CISS is the conceptual formation of summary codes. Although there is some eivdence that the individual codes function similarly in the stream of interaction and hence support their being combined in the same summary code (Gottman, 1979), factor analysis studies with similar results would add confidence in the content validity of the summary codes.

MARITAL INTERACTION CODING SYSTEM (MICS)

History and Objectives

The MICS is probably the most widely used and most frequently evaluated marital observation system (see Jacobson, Elwood, & Dallas, 1981; Markman *et al.*, 1981; Weider & Weiss, 1980; Weiss & Margolin, 1977; Weiss, Hops, & Patterson, 1973). The original version of the MICS (Hops, Wills, Patterson, & Weiss, 1972) was basically a marital version of the Family Interaction Scoring System (described earlier). There have been three revisions of the MICS, the most recent of which is presented in Weiss and Summers (1983). The MICS has been used to compare the interaction of distressed and nondistressed couples and to evaluate marital therapy programs, and it has influenced the development of other marital observation systems. A more detailed description of the history and objectives of the MICS, as well as a review of the research conducted with the MICS, has been provided by Weiss and Summers (1983).

Codes and Dimensions

The current version of the MICS contains 32 behavioral codes. In the past, the codes have been combined into summary dimensions ranging from two dimensions (positive and negative) to six dimensions (verbal positive, verbal negative, nonverbal positive, nonverbal negative, problem description, and problem solving). However, in the most recent version, 28 of the codes have been combined into eight dimensions (Weiss & Summers, 1983). These codes and dimensions are presented below:

DIMENSIONS	CODES
Problem description	Problem description—internal, problem description—external
Blame	Complain, criticize, mind-read—negative, putdown
Proposal for change	Positive solution, compromise, negative solution
Validation	Agree, approve, accept responsibility, compliance
Invalidation	Disagree, deny responsibility, excuse, interrupt, no response, non-compliance, turn off
Facilitation	Paraphrase/reflection, mind-reading—positive, humor, positive physical contact, smile/laugh, assent
Irrelevant	Talk, normative
Nonverbal affect	Positive physical contact, smile/laugh, normative nonverbal behavior, turnoff, assent

There are also codes that describe listener attention ("attention" and "not tracking") and speech style ("questions and "commands").

Coding Process

The task used is a problem discussion of an issue that is relevant to the couple. Discussions should last for 10 minutes and are audio- or videotaped. The basic coding unit is a behavioral unit "defined as behavior of homogeneous content, irrespective of duration or formal grammatical accuracy, emitted by a single partner" (Weiss & Summers, 1983, p. 89). Two coders rate every tape, recording codes in 30-second blocks (signaled by a tone) for the purposes of reliability checks. Disagreements between coders are resolved by discussions, and the final set of codes is entered into a computer program (available from Robert Weiss, Psychology Department, University of Oregon, Eugene, Oregon).

Reliability and Validity

The reliability of the MICS, assessed by interobserver agreement has been demonstrated in numerous investigations (e.g., Birchler, Weiss, & Vincent, 1975; Wieder & Weiss, 1980). Further, a generalizability study has indicated that variance in MICS codes is attributable to couple differences and interactions between couples and occasions (Wieder & Weiss, 1980).

Evidence for construct and discriminative validity of the MICS codes (not necessarily the dimensions, see "Commentary" section) has been summarized by Weiss and Summers (1983). For example, MICS codes reliably discriminate between distressed and nondistressed couples (e.g., Birchler *et al.,* 1975) and reflect changes in marital therapy programs (e.g., Jacobson, 1977).

Relation to Core Dimensions

The MICS dimensions of "blame," "proposal for change," and "facilitation" all reflect the communication clarity and skill dimension. The MICS dimensions of "validation" and "invalidation" reflect the support and validation dimension; "nonverbal affect" reflects the affect dimension; "command" and "compliance" codes reflect the dominance dimension; and "problem description" and "irrelevant talk" codes reflect the information exchange dimension. The MICS "agreement" and "disagreement" codes, as well as exchanges of positive and negative behaviors, represent the conflict dimension. It should be noted that several MICS codes (e.g., "agree" and "positive physical contact") can be incorporated into different dimensions. Therefore, the dimensions are not independent of each other.

Commentary

The MICS is an excellent example of an observational system that has slowly changed, based on other coding systems, the results of observational studies, and the increased sophistication of data-analytic techniques. For example, Weiss and his associates have increased the sensitivity of the MICS to nonverbal behavior, have modified the coding process to facilitate sequential analyses, and have revised the dimensions of the MICS in response to criticisms (early versions of the MICS were criticized for collapsing codes into only two major categories: positive and negative). The major strengths of the current version of the MICS include its comprehensive coverage of communication and problem solving in couples' interaction, its suitability for sequential analyses, numerous observational studies that provide the beginnings of a normative baseline of marital interaction in problem-solving situations (Weiss & Summers, 1983, reported that there have been 45 studies using the MICS), the possibility of using the MICS with audiotaped interaction data, and the fact that Weiss will code and analyze interaction data with the MICS for researchers.

The major difference between the MICS and the CISS is that the CISS codes each unit with a separate content and nonverbal code, whereas the MICS codes each unit with either a verbal or a nonverbal code (although some verbal codes, such as "blame," are defined based on verbal and nonverbal cues). Otherwise, despite some differences in the summary dimensions, the MICS and CISS codes are very similar. This is not surprising because the CISS was based in part on the MICS and the MICS has added CISS codes (e.g., mind reading).

Consistent with our critique of other systems, a major problem with the MICS is the lack of construct validity for the dimensions. That is, do all the codes that comprise a dimension function in the interactional stream in the same way? And do the constructs measure what they claim to measure? This problem is exacerbated by the inconsistent lumping of schemes across studies.

Finally, the work of Weiss and his associates with the MICS provides an excellent example of how observational systems can be used in a systematic research program linking research, clinical practice, and the evaluation of intervention programs.

KATEGORIENSYSTEM FÜR PARTNER-SCHAFTLICHE INTERACTIONS (KPI)

History and Objectives

The KPI (Hahlweg et al., 1984a) was developed in Munich, West Germany, and represents one of the few observational systems developed outside the United States. The KPI was designed to evaluate the effects of behavioral marital therapy (BMT) on the interaction of a sample of distressed and nondistressed German couples (see Hahlweg et al., 1984b). The KPI was based on the CISS, the MICS, and an earlier German version of the KPI (Wegener, Revenstorf, Hahlweg, & Schindler, 1979). The major objective of the KPI is to measure the communication and problem-solving skills taught in BMT and similar marital therapy programs. Hahlweg et al. (1984b) argued that the CISS and the MICS have limited validity when it comes to directly assessing communication skills. A more detailed description of the KPI is provided by Hahlweg et al. (1984a).

Codes and Dimensions

The KPI contains 26 behavioral content codes and 3 nonverbal codes (positive, neutral, and negative). Following from the CISS, each coding unit receives both a content and a nonverbal code. The nonverbal codes and coding procedures are identical to those of the CISS.

The content codes are divided into 10 dimensions. For the purposes of data reduction (e.g., for sequential analyses), these 10 dimensions can be further divided into 5 and then 3 higher order dimensions. In addition to the codes that form these dimensions, there are codes for inaudible statements and statements that do not fit into the other codes. Moreover, the listener receives a content code called "listening" and a nonverbal code whenever the speaker receives more than one code for a unit. This procedure enables alternative coding of speaker and listener. The content codes and dimensions are presented below:

DIMENSIONS	CODES
Self-disclosure	Expression of feelings, expression of wishes
Positive solution	Constructive proposal, compromise
Acceptance of other	Paraphrase, open question, positive feedback
Agreement	Direct agreement, accept responsibility, assent
Metacommunication	Metacommunication, clarification request
Problem description	Problem description, neutral questions
Criticism	Global negative, specific negative
Negative solution	Negative solution
Justification	Excuse, deny responsibility
Disagreement	Direct disagreement, yes-but, disagreeing statements, blocking

HIGHER ORDER DIMENSIONS	LOWER ORDER DIMENSIONS AND CODES
Direct expression	Self-disclosure, positive solution
Acceptance and agreement	Acceptance of partner, agreement, positive listening, neutral listening
Critique	Criticism, negative solution
Refusal	Disagreement, justification, negative listening
Neutral information	Problem description, megacommunication

HIGHEST ORDER DIMENSIONS	LOWER ORDER DIMENSIONS
Positive communication	Direct acceptance, acceptance and agreement
Negative communication	Criticism, refusal
Neutral information	Neutral information

Coding Process

The task used is a 10-minute discussion of a problem of moderate intensity selected from a problem list or from an interview. The discussion is videotaped and is then coded by two observers without the use of a transcript. The basic unit of analysis is a "verbal response that is homogenous in content without regard to its duration or syntactical structure" (Hahlweg *et al.*, 1984a, p. 186). To facilitate reliability analyses, observers code in 30-second blocks.

Reliability and Validity

The reliability of the KPI, assessed by interobserver agreement and generalizability coefficients, has been demonstrated in several studies (Hahlweg *et al.*, 1984a, b). Evidence for the discriminative and construct validity of KPI codes is presented in Hahlweg *et al.* (1984a,b). For example, KPI codes discriminate between distressed and nondistressed couples in the expected direction, and sequences of KPI dimensions are sensitive to changes in the expected directions as a function of marital therapy.

Relation to Core Dimensions

Consistent with the KPI's objective of assessing communication skills, the majority of the KPI dimensions reflect the communication clarity and skills dimension. These include "self-disclosure," "positive solution," "negative solution," "justification," "direct expression," "criticism," "critique," "positive communication," and "negative communication." The KPI dimensions of "agreement," and "disagreement," as well as sequences of positive and negative communication, reflect conflict. The KPI dimensions of "acceptance of other," and "criticism" and the "positive and negative listening" codes reflect the support and validation dimension. The KPI dimensions of "metacommunication," "problem description," and "neutral information" reflect the information exchange dimension. Finally, the nonverbal codes reflect the affect dimension.

Commentary

The KPI is a relatively new addition to the available set of marital observation systems. Its developers have incorporated the best features from older systems and have added codes and dimensions that have the potential to provide a more detailed assessment of communication skills. The results from observational studies in West Germany using the KPI have replicated and extended the findings from the United States (see Markman *et al.*, 1981, for a review). The history of the KPI illustrates how the marital observation field has grown, based on the cross-fertilization of codes, coding procedures, and data analyses.

The major strengths of the KPI are (a) its comprehensive coverage of communication and problem-solving skills; (b) its codes that discriminate between distressed and nondistressed couples; (c) its suitability for sequential analyses (in the case of the KPI, K-gramm analyses [Hahlweg *et al.*, 1984b] are used); (d) its reasonable comparability to the MICS and the CISS; and (e) the lack of the need to transcribe the interaction, which enables great time savings.

The major weakness of the KPI is that speaker nonverbal behavior is coded only when there are multiple speaker codes. This code provides only a sporadic sampling of listener nonverbal behavior. Yet, the authors believe that the code is important enough to be included in their higher order dimensions (e.g., "acceptance and agreement," "refusal," and "positive communication"). If researchers are interested in listener behaviors, then the CISS procedures should be followed. It should be noted that the major reason that the KPI includes listener codes is to guarantee an ongoing speaker–listener exchange, which is important in sequential analyses. A second problem is that there is no evidence that the codes that comprise a dimension function in the same way and that the dimensions really measure what they claim to measure.

Finally, similar to the MICS and CISS, the work of Hahlweg, Revensdorf, Schindler, and associates nicely illustrates the integration of basic and applied research as well as the systematic development of the marital interaction and intervention fields.

CONCLUSIONS AND RECOMMENDATIONS

Having reviewed and commented on the major coding systems available for the study of marital and family interaction, we urge readers not to lose sight of the most salient principles guiding interaction research. Simply stated, the key assumption underlying interactional research is that interaction among family members is the most salient *proximal* causal agent determining psychological (and often physical) well-being among family members (Notarius & Pellegrini, 1984). Because the interactants are not able to report validly on the interaction process, observational research strategies are the necessary analytical tool to uncover these proximal interactional factors. We believe that the developers of the system we have presented would be in nearly unanimous agreement with the above premise.

Less agreement among researchers will be found about the implementation of specific research protocols. Our review amply demonstrates this point: There is wide-ranging diversity in the interactional situations studied, the coding procedures constructed, and the data-analytic strategies used to extract meaning from the ongoing behavior stream. Out of this diversity, we believe that there are procedures to be recommended as well as some to be discouraged. Thus we offer our recommendations; however, readers must realize that any set of recommendations is influenced strongly by the overall objectives of the research plan. Thus, in order to provide a context for our recommendations, we will briefly summarize the approach we advocate for advancing interactional research in the next decade.

Researchers have taken two basic approaches to identify the proximal (interactional) determinants of psychopathology in family members. The two approaches actually represent extreme ends of a continuum, and most contemporary research falls somewhere between these extremes. The first approach is to hypothesize a critical role for one or two dimensions and to assess just these dimensions; in some cases using *global* coding of the interaction (e.g., affective style, and CECS). The utility of this approach will depend on the theoretical merits of the particular dimensions or on serendipity in uncovering a salient interactional dimension. The second approach directs attention to a comprehensive microanalytical study of the interactional stream to reveal the salient behaviors associated with good and poor family functioning (e.g., IPCS, MICS, and CISS). An important outcome of this approach is the generation of *specific* interactional hypotheses to account for dysfunctional family systems.

A focus on one approach over the other is best decided on according to how well the research problem is understood: If the phenomenon being investigated is poorly understood, then we would argue for microanalytical descriptive studies to extend our knowledge base and to generate meaningful interactional hypotheses for continued study. If the research problem is better understood, then the existing knowledge base should enable the researcher to focus on a more limited range of behaviors, on more thematic, global codes, or on both. An example will help clarify this point.

In the early 1970s, the state of knowledge concerning interactional differences between distressed and nondistressed couples was quite limited. Distressed and nondistressed couples had rarely been observed, and when they were observed, the measures used (e.g., talk time) provided little information about how spouses actually communicated with each other (e.g., Raush, Marshall, & Featherman, 1970). Because of the lack of knowledge of the interactional differences between distressed and nondistressed couples, there was a need for descriptive microanalytical study of functional and dysfunctional couples. As the field went in this direction, we have gained greater understanding of the interaction correlates of marital distress and success. The findings have stimulated interaction-based models of marital functioning (e.g., Gottman, 1979; Weiss, 1980), and they have influenced the current practice of marital therapy from a social learning perspective (e.g., Gottman et al., 1976a; Jacobson & Margolin, 1979; Stuart, 1980).

Specific research questions may continue to support the use of the comprehensive descriptive systems; however, we are beginning to see the next generation of marital interaction coding systems. Incorporating previous research findings, these new systems code larger units of interaction. For example, where the CISS found the microanalytical "problem-feeling"–"agreement" sequence to discriminate between distressed and nondistressed couples and labeled this *validation*, the next-generation codebook looks for more global "problem-feeling"–"agreement" transactions and codes them directly as support/validation (e.g., Gottman, 1983; Julien, Markman, Johnson, & Widenfelt, 1986). Part of the reason for favoring an evolution from microanalytical codes to more global codes is that precise microanalytical coding can reveal patterns that are beyond the capabilities of human judges to discover. A coder may be able to tally the single reciprocal exchange of negative behaviors but would be hard-pressed to track the persistence of these exchanges over six or more floor switches, as was revealed by sequence analysis on the microanalytical codes (Gottman et al., 1977). However, once revealed, these larger patterns or themes may be amenable to more global coding procedures.

There are four important caveats that we must add to this framework. First, the progression from microanalytical codes to more global codes does not eliminate the need to establish the reliability and validity of the emergent global codes. Second, there is a dangerous pitfall for beginning a research program with "a descriptive mission." The danger is captured succinctly in the phrase "mindless description." Thus, the researcher who lacks a guiding theoretical framework and decides to code "everything" is likely to get swamped by the data and is unlikely to learn a great deal about family interaction. Third, global coding systems do have the potential to generate interactional hypotheses that can serve as the basis for more detailed microanalytical systems. In essence, one could argue for the very opposite research progression from the one we have advanced. In fact, if sound research and appropriate data analysis procedures are used, then a progression from global-hypothesis-generating coding to micro-analytical descriptive coding is certainly a defensible strategy. Although our reading of the literature supports the utility of the approach we have advocated, we encourage readers to come to their own conclusions on the issue of global versus microanalytical coding strategies.

Finally, it is important to consider what interactional processes are implicated in the origins, the maintenance, and the remediation of underlying specific disorders. Many of the early family interaction systems have been developed to study the family origins of schizophrenia, and thus, it is not surprising to see an emphasis on dominance, affect, and communication clarity. The relevance of these coding systems to the study of other disorders—for example, affective disturbance—is questionable. Other interactional processes are likely to be of interest in families of affective disorders, such as negative self-evaluation and other evaluations. At this time, there is a paucity of specific coding systems that explore the role of family interaction and affective disorders, psychophysiological disorders, subclasses of schizophrenia, and personality disorders. As we turn to our recommendations for future coding systems, it is worth remembering that we are offering suggestions only for the current dimensions being assessed. We do not intend to imply that these are the only dimensions of importance, and in fact, we would argue that other dimensions will become salient as the field broadens its focus to study other forms of psychopathology besides schizophrenia. We have seen the beginnings already in the contributions of the coding systems developed by researchers investigating normal families and their impact on adolescent development.

Below, we conclude with a series of recommendations for interactional research on the family. Because there are interdependencies between the research situation, the coding process, and the data analysis, we have chosen to present recommendations in each of these areas.

Research Situation

Task. We have seen that numerous family interaction tasks have been used to generate meaningful interactional records. To the extent that different tasks are used, a comparison of results across studies becomes difficult or impossible. In order to facilitate comparison across studies, all future studies should include one common task. While there are few data to guide us, tasks that reflect typical problem-solving situations (e.g., a discussion of one of the family's top problems) are preferable to less salient tasks (e.g., various types of revealed-difference tasks), because we believe that a family's ability to solve *real-life* problems is critical to adaptive functioning. Most observation systems do assess family problem-solving by using a revealed-difference task. However, these tasks vary in relevance to the family's functioning (e.g., child-rearing issues, family-environment scale items, planning a family vacation, and Kohlberg's moral dilemmas).

Family Composition. There are very few data to support a recommendation for the ideal family group to be studied. There is currently a strong emphasis on system processes and on studying the family as a whole. Some family therapists might even argue for the importance of studying the extended family. However, the technical problems presented by family groups even as small as four may currently be insurmountable. The general trend has been: the greater the number of interactants, the simpler the coding system and the data analysis plan. Our preference is to keep the family unit small and the coding and the data analysis "complex."

Accordingly, we recommend that family researchers focus on the marital dyad and/or on the parents and one offspring. At this time, we are not convinced that the study of family groups larger than three will be profitable. We do not intend to imply that family interaction is constant across different family compositions or that the interactional study of larger family groups is unimportant. Instead, until there is further development of tools to facilitate the study of larger family groups, the outcomes are not likely to be commensurate with the effort.

Sample Size. There is necessarily an inverse relationship between sample size and the complexity of coding and data analysis. Although it is possible to survey a large random sample with a questionnaire, it is often difficult to study 20 to 30 couples or families in an interactional paradigm. Consistent with the approach we have argued, we believe it most advantageous to work with a relatively small number of subjects without sacrificing depth of study. In place of a large number of subjects, we would argue for replication of findings with independent samples. The study of marital interaction amply illustrates the strength of this approach, with replication appearing in independent laboratories in the United States, West Germany, and the Netherlands (see Hahlweg, Baucom, & Markman in press, for a review).

Interactional studies with small numbers can also be justified through a comparison of typical effect sizes that derive from large-sample questionnaire techniques with those from small-sample interactional paradigms. In general, interactional studies have accounted for a far greater share of the variance in discriminating between functional and dysfunctional families than have interview or questionnaire studies (Gottman, 1979).

Coding Interactional Data

Regardless of the approach followed (microanalytical vs. global coding), it is important for interactional researchers to recognize that six primary dimensions have guided theoretical efforts to date. Accordingly, we would recommend that interactional coding schedules be constructed around the six primary dimensions. Our review of current coding systems suggests the following, concerning how these dimensions should be defined.

Dominance. We have seen that dominance has usually been operationalized with verbal frequency measures, including (a) who speaks first, (b) who speaks last, (c) who speaks the most, (d) percentage of total speaking time, and (e) passive acceptance of the solution (Farina, 1960). Dominance has also been operationalized with several noninteractional measures, such as the number of "wins" on a revealed-difference task. However, verbal frequency measures have not discriminated between functional and dysfunctional families (Jacob, 1975). Assuming that dominance is, in fact, an important dimension of family interaction, we must question the adequacy of verbal frequency measures to assess dominance. Gottman (1979) offered a cogent critique of the verbal frequency measures of dominance. First, Gottman questioned the usual assumption that high or low frequency of certain verbal behaviors is related to dominance. For example, the family member who speaks the most is usually assumed to be the most dominant. However, Gottman suggested that the "dominant member may be a person who does not speak very often, who rarely interrupts, but who is highly influential" (p. 69) and can therefore be considered dominant. Second, dominance may not be related to any one variable; rather, it may be reflected in the pattern across several variables. For example, the well-timed interruption, the carefully placed agreement, and the strategic display of negative affect may all serve to define the dominant person. Gottman concluded that dominance must therefore be operationalized in terms of the consequences of behavior and not in terms of the rates of behavior. Therefore, we recommend that investigators replace verbal frequency measures with procedures that assess the consequences of behavior through coding rules or data analysis.

Affect. Affect has been operationalized with codes ranging from "humor" and "laughter" to "support." The most critical facet of the operationalization of this dimension is the degree to which coders attend to verbal and nonverbal behaviors. Some investigators have chosen to rely solely on the "literal affective content of the words used" (Mishler & Waxler, 1968, p. 83) and thus to ignore nonverbal cues, whereas other researchers have tended to emphasize nonverbal cues as the primary affective dimension (Gottman, 1979). We regard the coding of affect without attention to nonverbal cues as raising problems. For example, the coding of a transcript entry "Oh, nice job" as positive affect when the message delivery was laced with sarcasm cannot yield readily interpretable results.

When coding affect, it is also important to consider the level of specificity that will be assessed. When affect has been attended to, it has usually been catagorized as positive, negative, or neutral. It may be important to recognize differences, for example, between fear, sadness, disgust, contempt, and anger rather than coding all of these as negative. Recent advances in the precise coding of facial expression now enable these finer discriminations (see Ekman & Friesen, 1977). The optimal level of specificity coded ultimately depends on the conceptual questions under study. A researcher who wishes to understand parents' feelings toward their offspring may want to make inferences based on specific affects observed, and detailed coding may be very useful. Another researcher, who wishes to focus exclusively on the behavior exchange process may reason that, as the family members themselves are not likely to discriminate among specific affects, a global coding of positive, negative, and neutral (with attention given to nonverbal behavior) may be sufficient.

In summary, we recommend that, at a minimum, nonverbal behaviors be used to code positive, negative, and neutral affect.

Communication Clarity and Skills. Family observation systems have not focused much attention on this dimension despite its importance in several major theories of schizophrenia. When communication clarity and skills have been assessed, codes are used that represent conflict (e.g., "interruptions") or support and validation dimensions. Given the paucity of attention in contemporary systems, it is not surprising that the most popular measure of this dimension is still Singer and Wynne's Communication Deviance Index (CDI) (1966). The CDI "reflects an inability of the parent or parents to establish or maintain the shared focus of attention during transactions with another person" (Doane *et al.*, 1981, p. 679). Although this definition focuses on interaction, the 41 CD codes are used to code Rorschach or Thematic Appreception Test protocols from individuals. Thus, the CDI does not directly assess family interaction. Doane *et al.* (1982) questioned whether a high level of communication deviance assessed in this manner "has any real relation to communication problems across interpersonal contexts within the family" (p. 220). Wynne (1984) reached the same conclusions about the use of nonobservational methods to assess interaction: "Preliminary data . . . suggest that studies of the communication of family members meeting directly with one another provide better predictors of offspring adjustment than do individual parental measures" (p. 553).

Marital systems, on the other hand, have placed great emphasis on assessing communication and problem-solving skills based on the couple's interaction generated by realistic tasks. For family researchers interested in assessing communication skills, we recommend using the communication and problem-solving codes from the KPI because (a) it has incorporated the MICS and CISS codes, and (b) the relative frequency of KPI codes discriminates between distressed and nondistressed couples (Hahlweg *et al.*, 1984b). For researchers interested in communication clarity, we recommend modifying the CD codes and using them to code family interaction generated by realistic problem-solving tasks.

Information Exchange. Most systems either treat this dimension as a reservoir for codes that do not reflect other dimensions of interest (e.g., CISS) or do not code it at all (e.g., CECS). Yet, most interaction falls into this dimension (e.g., Gottman *et al.*, 1977). This state of affairs is ironic because most comprehensive, microanalytical systems have high content validity for this dimension (e.g., expressing feelings and opinions). One reason for the paucity of attention to the information exchange dimension is that codes that reflect information exchange do not generally discriminate between functional and dysfunctional couples and families (Mishler & Waxler, 1968). However, when these codes also receive nonverbal (affect) codes, and when interaction sequences are examined, patterns of information exchange emerge that do discriminate between functional and dysfunctional groups (Gottman *et al.*, 1977; Hahlweg *et al.*, 1984b). Thus, most systems are losing a great deal of information about family interaction by ignoring this dimension. We therefore, recommend that information exchange be assessed and that nonverbal cues accompanying these messages also be assessed.

Conflict. Conflict has been operationalized with codes initially suggested by Farina (1960), including "simultaneous speech," "disagreement" (or agreement–disagreement ratios), "interruptions," and "failure to reach agreement." These codes clearly do not cover the full range of conflict behaviors, and in fact, two of these codes ("interruptions" and "simultaneous speech") seem to represent flexible communication in a family, rather than conflict (Mishler & Waxler, 1968). Moreover, the concept of conflict implies a sequence of negative interaction and is therefore difficult to assess by means of frequency analyses or outcome measures (e.g., failure to reach agreement). For example, both distressed and nondistressed married couples display conflict behaviors, and although some studies have revealed that the frequency of these behaviors discriminates between these two groups, chains of these behaviors have been found to have significantly more discriminatory power (Gottman *et al.,* 1977; Hahlweg *et al.,* 1984b; Margolin & Wampold, 1981). Therefore, we recommend that, for assessing conflict, investigators (a) devote attention to improving the content validity of codes that reflect the conflict dimension and (b) replace verbal frequency measures with procedures and codes that allow the assessment of chains of interaction that reflect conflict.

Support and Validation. Systems have assessed this dimension by using both global ratings and specific behavioral codes. As noted earlier, several systems (e.g., Alexander, 1973) have developed specific behavioral codes, as opposed to only global impressions, that provide information about the process of the exchange of support and validation in families. We have also seen that these codes ("genuine information-seeking," "spontaneous problem-solving," and "empathic understanding") reflect other dimensions (e.g., communication clarity and skills). Thus, support and validation comprise a higher order dimension defined as a composite of some of the other core dimensions. We recommend that investigators continue to rely on specific codes to assess this dimension as well as focus on the antecedents and consequences of support and validation in families using sequential analyses.

Data Analysis

The most important recommendation concerning data analysis is for researchers to explore their data with measures other than frequency measures. It is intuitively obvious that the sequential patterning of behavior between family members is likely to be of critical importance in discriminating between functional and dysfunctional family systems. Yet, as intuitively appealing as this assumption may be, it is procedurally appealing (i.e., it is easy) to compare families on simple frequency measures. For example, do schizophrenic parents utter more unclear statements than do normal parents? Do fathers of aggressive children receive less validation from their mates than fathers of depressed children? It is not that these questions are uninteresting; it is only that they do not go far enough and that they should not be the exclusive focus of data analysis.

Thus, we urge researchers to consider the sequential patterning of interaction in their analysis of observational data. In the study of marital interaction, verbal frequency measures proved to be far less potent in discriminating between distressed and nondistressed couples than did sequential patterns (Gottman *et al.,* 1977; Margolin & Wampold, 1981). Furthermore, sequential patterns appear to be more stable across situations than do frequency measures (Gottman, 1980). The study of family interaction sequences is just beginning; we believe that these techniques will greatly increase our understanding of family interaction in the coming years.

As noted earlier, the use of sequence analysis demands that researchers follow the law of parsimony to keep the number of interactional dimensions studied relatively small. A balance must be struck between combining individual codes to define a small number of dimensions that are each coherent (i.e., each has content validity) and keeping individual codes separate to yield unambiguous interactional units. As a practical suggestion, we believe that 8 to 10 summary dimensions should be the maximum number used to enter data analysis. As the number of interactants gets larger, this maximum number of summary codes may have to be reduced because the number of transitions will increase rapidly. The number of cells with frequencies too low to analyze meaningfully can quickly become a problem if there are too many codes and/or too many interactants for the number of data collected.

All of the data analysis procedures commonly used today are structured to uncover replicable patterns or to reveal relatively high-frequency behaviors that discriminate between the groups under study. It is worth noting that current techniques are not sensitive to detecting infrequent behaviors that may strongly affect family sentiment and behavior because of both the data-analytic procedures and the difficulty of observing low-frequency events. One way of exploring infrequent events might be to punctuate the behavior stream at theoretically meaningful moments (e.g., as in the CECS) or at moments that appear important after observing the family. A comparison might then be made between the interaction patterns that characterized the family system before and after the "critical event." The observed differences might then be attributed to the significant, though infrequent, event. Our point is a simple one: Infrequent but salient events present a special data-analytic challenge.

Coda

The careful and precise analysis of family interaction still holds tremendous potential for unraveling the role of the family in psychopathology. We remain convinced that the *proximal* source of family distress and well-being lies in the microlevel of exchange between family members. The family's communication patterns that emerge each day, over time, define the family and shape the daily sentiments of each family member, and they exist, awaiting our discovery.

REFERENCES

Alexander, J. (1973). Defensive and supportive communications in family systems. *Journal of Marriage and Family, 35,* 613–617.

Alexander, J. (1983). *Defensive and supportive interaction manual.* Unpublished manuscript, University of Utah, Salt Lake City.

Alexander, J., & Parsons, B. V. (1982). *Functional family therapy.* Monterey, CA: Brooks/Cole.

Bakeman, R. (1978). Untangling streams of interaction. In G. Sackett (Ed.), *Observing behavior: Vol. 2. Data collection and analysis methods.* Baltimore: University Park Press.

Bakeman, R. (1979). *Analyzing event sequence data computer programs ESEQ and ELAG.* Unpublished manuscript, Georgia State University, Atlanta.

Bales, R. (1950) *Interaction process analysis.* Cambridge, MA: Addison-Wesley.

Bales, R. (1970). *Personality and interpersonal behavior.* New York: Holt, Rinehart & Winston.

Bales, R., & Cohen, S. (1979). *SYMLOG.* New York: Free Press.

Barton, C., & Alexander, J.F. (1980). Functional family therapy. In A. S. Gurman & D. P. Kniskern (Eds.), *Handbook of marital therapy.* New York: Brunner/Mazel.

Bateson, G., Jackson, D. D., Haley, J., & Weakland, J. (1956). Toward a theory of schizophrenia. *Behavioral Science, 1,* 251–264.

Becker, W. C. (1964). Consequences of different kinds of parental discipline. In M. L. Hoffman & L. W. Hoffman (Eds.), *Review of child development research* (Vol. 1). New York: Russell Sage Foundation.

Bell, D. C., & Bell, L. G. (1982a). Family process and child development in unlabeled (normal) families. *The Australian Journal of Family Therapy, 3,* 205–210.

Bell, L. G., & Bell, D. C. (1982b). Family climate and the role of the female adolescent: Determinants of adolescent functioning. *Family Relations, 31,* 519–527.

Bell, L. G., & Bell, D. C. (1982c, August). *Parental validation as a mediator in adolescent development.* Paper presented at meetings of the American Psychological Association, Washington, DC.

Bell, D. C., Bell, L. G., & Cornwell, C. S. (1982). *Interaction process coding scheme.* Unpublished manuscript, University of Houston.

Belsky, J. (1981). Early human experience: A family perspective. *Developmental Psychology, 17,* 3–23.

Billings, A. (1979). Conflict resolution in distressed and nondistressed married couples. *Journal of Consulting and Clinical Psychology, 47,* 368–376.

Birchler, G. R., Weiss, R. L., & Vincent, J. P. (1975). Multimethod analysis of social reinforcement exchange between maritally distressed and nondistressed spouse and stranger dyads. *Journal of Personality and Social Psychology, 31,* 349–360.

Brown, G. W., Birley, J. L. T., & Wing, J. F. (1972). Influence of family life on the course of schizophrenic disorders: A replication. *British Journal of Psychiatry, 121,* 241–258.

Condon, S. L., Cooper, C. R., & Grotevant, H. D. (1981). *Manual for the analysis of family discourse.* Austin: University of Texas.

Cooper, C. R., Grotevant, H. D., & Condon, S. M. (1983). Individuality and connectedness: Both foster adolescent identity formation and role-taking skill. In H. D. Grotevant & C. R. Cooper (Eds.), *Adolescent development in the family: New directions for child development.* San Francisco: Jossey-Bass.

Cronbach, L. J., & Meehl, P. (1955). Construct validity in psychological tests. *Psychological Bulletin, 52,* 281–302.

Doane, J. A., & Lewis, J. M. (1984). Measurement strategies in family interaction research: A profile approach. In N. Watt, E. J. Anthony, L. Wynne, & J. Rolf (Eds.), *Children at risk for schizophrenia: A longitudinal perspective.* New York: Cambridge University Press.

Doane, J. A., West, K. L., Goldstein, M. J., Rodnick, E. H., & Jones, J. E. (1981). Parental communication deviance and affective style as predictors of subsequent schizophrenia spectrum disorders in vulnerable adolescents. *Archives of General Psychiatry, 38,* 679–685.

Doane, J. A., Jones, J., Fisher, L., Ritzler, B., Singer, M., & Wynne, L. (1982). Parental Communication Deviance as a predictor of competence in children at risk for adult psychiatric disorder. *Family Process, 21,* 211–223.

Ekman, T., & Friesen, W. V. (1977). Manual for the facial action coding system. Palo Alto, CA: Consulting Psychologist Press.

Eyberg, S. M., & Robinson, E. A. (1981). *Dyadic parent–child interaction coding system: A Manual.* Available from S. M. Eyberg, Department of Medical Psychology, Oregon Health Sciences University, Portland, OR 97201.

Farina, A. (1960). Patterns of role dominance and conflict in parents of schizophrenic patients. *Journal of Abnormal Social Psychology, 61,* 31–38.

Ferreira, A. (1963). Decision making in normal and pathologic families. *Archives of General Psychiatry, 8,* 68–73.

Ferreira, A., & Winter, W. (1965). Family interaction and decision making. *Archives of General Psychiatry, 13,* 214–223.

Fontana, A. (1966). Familial etiology of schizophrenia: Is a scientific methodology possible? *Psychological Bulletin, 66(3),* 214–227.

Framo, J. L. (1979). Family theory and therapy. *American Psychologist, 34,* 988–992.

Gibb, J. (1961). Defensive communications. *Journal of Communication, 3,* 141–148.

Gilligan, C., (1982). *In a different voice.* Cambridge, Harvard University Press.

Goldberg, W., & Easterbrooks, A. (1984). The role of marital quality in toddler development. *Developmental Psychology, 20,* 504–515.

Gottman, J. M. (1978). Nonsequential data analysis techniques and observational research. In G. P. Sackett (Ed.), *Observing behavior: Vol. 2. Data collection and analysis methods.* Baltimore: University Park Press.

Gottman, J. M. (1979). *Marital interaction: Empirical investigations.* New York: Academic Press.

Gottman, J. M. (1980). Consistency of nonverbal affect reciprocity in marital interaction. *Journal of Consulting and Clinical Psychology, 48,* 711–717.

Gottman, J. M. (1983). *Rapid couples interaction scoring system.* Unpublished manuscript, University of Illinois, Champaign.

Gottman, J. M., Notarius, C. I., Gonso, J., & Markman, H. J. (1976a). *A couple's guide to communication.* Champaign, IL: Research Press.

Gottman, J. M., Notarius, C. I., Markman, H. J., Bank, S., Yoppi, B., & Rubin, M. (1976b). Behavior exchange theory and marital decision-making. *Journal of Personality and Social Psychology, 34,* 14–23.

Gottman, J. M., Markman, H. J., & Notarius, C.I. (1977). The topography of marital conflict: A sequential analysis of verbal and nonverbal behavior. *Journal of Marriage and the Family, 39,* 361–377.

Grotevant, H., & Cooper, C. (1983, April). *The role of family communication patterns in adolescent identity and role taking.* Paper presented at the Meeting of the Society for Research in Child Development, Detroit.

Grotevant, H., & Cooper, C. (1985). Patterns of interaction in family relationships and the development of identity exploration in adolescence. *Child Development, 56,* 415–428.

Hahlweg, K., Reisner, L., Kohli, G., Vollmer, M., Schindler, L., & Revenstorf, D. (1984a). Development and validity of a new system to analyze interpersonal communication (KPI). In K. Hahlweg & N. S. Jacobson (Eds.), *Marital interaction: Analysis and modification.* New York: Guilford Press.

Hahlweg, K. Revenstorf, D., & Schindler, L. (1984b). Effects of behavioral marital therapy on couples' communication and problem-solving skills. *Journal of Consulting and Clinical Psychology, 52(4),* 553–566.

Hahlweg, K., Baucom, D., & Markman, H. J. (In press). Recent advances in behavioral marital therapy and in preventing marital distress. In J. R. H. Fallon (Ed.), *Handbook of behavioral family therapy,* NY: Guilford Press.

Haley, J. (1967). Speech sequences of normal and abnormal families with two children present. *Family Process, 6,* 81–97.

Hartup, W. (1979). Levels of analysis in the study of interaction: An historical perspective. In M. Lamb, S. Summit, & G. Stephenson (Eds.), *Social interaction analysis: Methodological issues.* Madison: University of Wisconsin Press.

Hauser, S., Powers, S., Weiss, B., Follansbee, D., & Bernstein, E. (1983a). *Family constraining and enabling coding system (CECS) manual.* Unpublished manuscript, Boston.

Hauser, S. T., Jacobson, A., Noam, G., & Powers, S. (1983b). Ego development and self-image complexity. *Archieves of General Psychiatry, 44,* 325–332.

Hauser, S., Powers, S., Noam, G., Jacobson, A., Weiss, B., & Follansbee, D. (1984). Familial contexts of adolescent ego development. *Child Development,* pp. 195–213.

Heatherington, E. M., & Martin, B. (1979). Family interaction. In H. Quay & J. Werry (Eds.), *Psychological disorders of childhood.* New York: Wiley.

Hooley, J. (1985, September). *Familial factors predictive of relapse in depression.* Paper presented at

International Conference on the Impact of Family Research on our Understanding of Psychopathology, Tegensee, West Germany.

Hops, H., Wills, T. A., Patterson, G. R., & Weiss, R. L. (1972). *Marital interaction coding system.* Eugene: University of Oregon Research Institute.

Hutt, S. J., & Hutt, C. (1970). *Direct observation and measurement of behavior.* Springfield, IL: Charles C Thomas.

Jacob, T. (1975). Family interaction in disturbed and normal families: A methodological and substantive review. *Psychological Bulletin, 82,* 33–65.

Jacobson, N. S. (1977). Problem solving and contingency contracting in the treatment of marital discord. *Journal of Consulting and Clinical Psychology, 45,* 442–452.

Jacobson, N. S., & Margolin, G. (1979). *Marital therapy: Strategies based on social learning and behavior exchange principles.* New York: Brunner/Mazel.

Jacobson, N. S., Elwood, R., & Dallas, M. (1981). The behavioral assessment of marital dysfunction. In D. Barlow (Ed.), *Behavioral assessment of adult dysfunction.* New York: Guilford Press.

Jones, R. R., Reid, J. B., & Patterson, G. R. (1975). Naturalistic observations in clinical assessment. In P. McReynolds (Ed.), *Advances in psychology assessment* (Vol 3.). San Francisco: Jossey-Bass.

Julien, D., Markman, H. J., Johnson, H., & VanWidenfelt, B. (1986). *Interaction Dimensions Scoring System (IDS).* Unpublished manuscript, University of Denver, Denver.

Kelley, H. (1978). *Personal relationships: Their structure and processes.* Hillsdale, NJ: Erlbaum.

Kohlberg, L. (1969). Stage and sequence: The cognitive-developmental approach to socialization. In D. A. Goslin (Ed.), *Handbook of socialization theory and research.* Chicago: Rand McNally.

Leary, T. (1957). *Interpersonal diagnosis of personality.* New York: Ronald Press.

Levenson, R., & Gottman, J. (1985). Physiological and affective predictors of changes in relationship satisfaction. *Journal of Personality and Social Psychology, 49,* 85–94.

Lidz, T., Cornelison, A., Fleck, S., & Terry, D. (1957). The intrafamilial environment of schizophrenic patients: 2. Martial schism and marital skew. *American Journal of Psychiatry, 114,* 241–248.

Margolin, G., & Wampold, B. (1981). Sequential analysis of conflict and accord in distressed and nondistressed marital partners. *Journal of Consulting and Clinical Psychology, 49,* 554–567.

Markman, H. J., Notarius, C. I., Stephen, T., & Smith, T. (1981). Behavioral observation systems for couples: The current status. In E. Filsinger & R. Lewis (Eds.), *Assessing marrage: New behavioral approaches.* Beverly Hills, CA: Sage Publications.

Minuchin, S. (1974). *Families and family therapy.* Cambridge: Harvard University Press.

Mishler, E. G., & Waxler, N. W. (1968). *Interaction in Families: An experimental study of family processes and schizophrenia.* New York: Wiley.

Mishler, E., & Waxler, N. W. (1975). The sequential patterning of interaction in normal and schizophrenic families. *Family Process, 14,* 17–50.

Moos, R. (1974). *The social climate scales: An overview.* Palo Alto, CA: Consulting Psychologists Press.

Notarius, C.I., & Markman, H. J. (1981). The couples interaction scoring system. In E. Filsinger & R. Lewis (Eds.), *Assessing marriage: New behavioral approaches.* Beverly Hills, CA: Sage Publications.

Notarius, C. I., & Pellegrini, D. (1984). Marital processes as stressors and stress mediators: Implications for marital repair. In S. Duck (Ed.), *Personal relationships: Vol. 5. Repairing personal relationships.* London: Academic Press.

Notarius, C. I., & Pellegrini, D. (1986). Family adaption to parental dysfunction: A pilot study. Unpublished manuscript, Catholic University of America, Washington, DC.

Notarius, C. I., Krokoff, L., & Markman, H. (1981). Analysis of observational data. In E. Filsinger & R. Lewis (Eds.), *Assessing marriage: New behavioral approaches.* Beverly Hills, CA: Sage Publications.

Notarius, C. I., Markman, H., & Gottman, J. (1983). Advances in the couples interaction scoring system. In E. Filsinger (Ed.), *Handbook of marital and family assessment.* Beverly Hills, CA: Sage Publications.

Olson, D.H., & Ryder, R. G. (1970). Inventory of marital conflicts (IMC): An experimental interaction procedure. *Journal of Marriage and the Family, 32,* 443–448.

Parsons, T., & Bales, R. F. (1955). *Family, socialization, and interaction process.* Glencoe, IL: Free Press.

Patterson, G. R. (1982). *Coercive family process*. Eugene, OR: Castilia.

Patterson, G. R., Ray, R. S., Shaw, D. A., & Cobb, J. A. (1969). *Manual for coding of family interactions* (rev. ed.). New York: Microfiche Publications.

Pederson, F. (1980). Research issues related to fathers and infants. In F. Pederson (Ed.), *The father–infant relationship*. New York: Praeger.

Raush, H., Marshall, K., & Featherman, J. (1970). Relations at three early stages of marriage as reflected by the use of personal pronouns. *Family Process, 9*, 69–82.

Raush, H. L., Barry, W. A., Hertel, R. K., & Swain, M. A. (1974). *Communication, conflict, and marriage*. San Francisco: Jossey-Bass.

Riskin, J., & Faunce, E. E. (1972). An evaluative review of family interaction research. *Family Process, 11*, 365–455.

Robinson, E. A., & Eyberg, S. M. (1981). The dyadic parent–child interaction coding system: Standardization and validation. *Journal of Consulting and Clinical Psychology, 49*, 245–250.

Rodnick, E. H., Goldstein, M. J., Lewis, J. M., & Doane, J. A. (1984). Parental communication style, affect and role as precursors of offspring schizophrenia-spectrum disorders. In N. F. Watt, J. Anthony, L. Wynne, & J. E. Rolf (Eds.), *Children at risk for schizophrenia: A longitudinal perspective*. Cambridge: Cambridge University Press.

Rotter, J. B. (1970). Some implications of a social learning theory for the practice of psychotherapy. In D. J. Levis (Ed.), *Learning approaches to therapeutic behavior change*. Chicago: Aldine.

Royce, K., & Weiss, R. (1975). Behavioral cues in the judgment of marital satisfaction: A linear regression analysis. *Journal of Consulting and Clinical Psychology, 43*, 816–824.

Schultz, W. C. (1960). *The interpersonal underworld: FIRO-B*. Palo Alto, CA: Science and Behavior Books.

Singer, M., & Wynne, L. (1966). Principles for scoring communication defects and deviances in parents of schizophrenics: Rorschach and TAT scoring manuals. *Psychiatry, 29*, 260–288.

Steinglass, P. (1976). *Home observation assessment method*. Unpublished manuscript, Center for Family Research, Washington, DC.

Steinglass, P. (1979). The home observation assessment method (HOAM): Real-time observations of families in their homes. *Family Process, 18*, 337–354.

Steirlin, H. (1974). *Separating parents and adolescents*. NY: Quadrangle.

Straus, M. (1964). Measuring families. In H. T. Christensen (Ed.), *Handbook of marriage and the family*. Chicago: Rand McNally.

Strodtbeck, F. (1951). Husband and wife interaction over revealed differences. *American Sociological Review, 16*, 468–473.

Strodtbeck, F. (1954). The family as a three-person group. *American Sociological Review, 19*, 23–29.

Stuart, R. (1980). *Helping couples change: A social learning approach to marital therapy*. New York: Guilford.

Valone, K., Norton, J., Goldstein, M., & Doane, J. (1984). Parental expressed emotion and affective style in an adolescent sample at risk for schizophrenia spectrum disorder. *Journal of Abnormal Psychology, 93*, 448–457.

Vaughn, C. E., & Leff, J. P. (1976). The influence of family and social factors on the course of psychiatric illness. *British Journal of Psychiatry, 129*, 125–137.

Vincent, J., Friedman, L., Nugent, J., & Messerly, L. (1979). Demand characteristics in observations of marital interaction. *Journal of Consulting and Clinical Psychology, 47*, 557–566.

Watzlawick, P., Beavin, J., & Jackson, D. (1967). *Pragmatics of human communication*. New York: Norton.

Wegener, C. Revenstorf, D., Hahlweg, K., & Schindler, L. (1979). Empirical analysis of communication in distressed couples. *Behavior Analysis and Modification, 3*, 178–188.

Weick, K. E. (1968). Systematic observational methods. In G. Lindzey & E. Aronson (Eds.), *Handbook of social psychology* (rev. ed., Vol. 2). Reading, MA: Addison-Wesley.

Weiss, R. L. (1980). Strategic behavioral marital therapy: Toward a model for assessment and intervention. In J. P. Vincent (Ed.), *Advances in family intervention, assessment, and theory* (Vol. 1). Greenwich, NY: JAI Press.

Weiss, R. L. & Margolin, G. (1977). Assessment of marital conflict and accord. In A. R. Ciminero, K. S. Calhoun, & H. E. Adams (Eds.), *Handbook of behavioral assessment*. New York: Wiley.

Weiss, R. L., & Summers, K. (1983). Marital interaction coding system: 3. In E. Filsinger (Ed.), *Marriage and family assessment.* Beverly Hills, CA: Sage Publications.

Weiss, R. L., Hops, H., & Patterson, G. R.(1973). A framework for conceptualizing marital conflict: A technology for altering it, some data for evaluating it. In F. W. Clark & L. A. Hamerlynck (Eds.), *Critical issues in research and practice: Proceedings of the Fourth Banff International Conference on Behavior Modification.* Champaign, IL: Research Press.

Wieder, G. B., & Weiss, R. L. (1980). Generalizability theory and the coding of marital interaction. *Journal of Consulting and Clinical Psychology, 48,* 469–477.

Wynne, L. C. (1984). Communication patterns and family relations of children at risk for schizophrenia. In N. F. Watt, E. J. Anthony, L. C. Wynne, & J. E. Rolf (Eds.), *Children at risk for schizophrenia: A longitudinal perspective.* Cambridge: Cambridge University Press.

Wynne, L. C., Ryckoff, I., Day, J., & Hirsh, S. (1958). Pseudomutuality in the family relations of schizophrenics. *Psychiatry, 21,* 205–220.

CHAPTER 10

Participant Observation Procedures in Marital and Family Assessment

GAYLA MARGOLIN

The term *participant observation*, in its general usage, refers to assessment procedures in which the observer is clearly visible to the person being observed (Wiggins, 1973). The observer may maintain a passive, noninteractive role or may directly interact with the person being observed. In the marital and family literature, that definition covers three types of observation procedures. First, there have been direct observations by noninteractive and uninvolved trained coders, that is, objective observations by a "blend-into-the-woodwork" type of observer (e.g., Patterson, 1982). Second, there are observations that family members make of one another during the natural course of daily interactions. Techniques that record these observations also have been referred to as *quasi-observational* or *quasi-behavioral* (Weiss & Margolin, 1986), because the observer's objectivity is affected by the extensive and intensive interaction that has occurred and continues to occur between himself or herself and the person being observed. Third are observations in which the person doing the reporting is also the target of the observation (or is one of several targets). This type of observation is an example of self-monitoring.

This chapter focuses on the latter two assessment procedures: observations of oneself or of another family member. When distinctions are made between these two formats, they will be referred to, respectively, as *self-monitoring* and *other monitoring*, or *observations by significant others*. *Participant observation*, as used in this chapter, refers to both formats.

As noted by Sullaway and Christensen (1983), participant observation falls

GAYLA MARGOLIN • Department of Psychology, University Park, University of Southern California, Los Angeles, CA 90089-1061.

under the more general rubric of verbal report procedures, as opposed to objective observations. However, because participant observation is a monitoring procedure, as contrasted to a one-time reporting task, it embodies several important distinctions from most other forms of self-reporting. First and foremost, the data are prospective rather than retrospective. In most self-report procedures, the reporter is required to think back and then mentally summarize all that has happened up to the point of inquiry. Unbeknownst to the examiner, the data may be primarily a function of recent experiences, such as the couple's fight on the way to the examiner's office, or more distant experiences, such as the partner's affair that occurred five years ago. The difficulty with retrospective information is the high degree of selectivity that goes into the data. In contrast, in participant observation, data are collected immediately or within a relatively brief time interval. Moreover, the format of observations is predetermined and preplanned before the observation ever begins. The reporter is instructed regarding what aspects of his or her own behavior or what aspects of his or her interactions with someone else are to be observed. The observation period begins only *after* the reporter has received and perhaps even practiced these instructions. With these respective procedures, previous experiences function in a circumscribed fashion as a backdrop for current observations, rather than as the sole basis for the reporter's judgment.

A second important distinguishing feature of participant observation is that each observation refers to a limited time interval, perhaps several seconds, several hours, or an entire day. Whatever the length of this interval, observations are repeated at the same interval across time, thereby giving a sequential dimension to the data. With such repeated observations, we can explore how the events at one point in time are related to events at a later time, for example, how a couple's argument in the morning affects their interactions that evening or the following day. The reason for looking at data from a sequential perspective is that important relationship dimensions vary across time. More important than knowing an overall or summary level of marital satisfaction, it is essential to understand how and why satisfaction varies from day to day or from week to week.

The third identifying feature is the structure of participant observation, which relates to the prospective and time-limited nature of the data. Formats for collecting the data must be carefully constructed so that they expressly fit the nature and the timing of the observations. Observations are made onto written records so that the recorder does not need to remember his or her observations for more than one time interval. These records serve as a prompt regarding what exactly is to be observed as well as a reminder to repeat the observation at the prespecified intervals. There are, of course, countless possibilities for formating participant observations. The essential component, however, is that observations are made systematically, so that one observation can be compared with another.

Just from the brief description thus far, it should be obvious that participant observation (either self-monitoring or the monitoring of a significant other) is an educational process for the client. With other types of self-report, the reporter simply states what already is clear to him or her. Alternatively, with direct observation by nonparticipants, the family members perform prespecified tasks or act in a certain fashion while the therapist (or research assistant) faces the task of collecting, analyzing, and interpreting the data; the results of the assessment then are presented to the clients as a *fait accompli*. With participant observation, however, the search for information is an open-ended process, and client and therapist are active collaborators in exploring the relationship in a new manner. The database available through participant observation will bring to light important relationship dynamics for the family members just as it does for the therapist. Thus, participant observation is an active therapeutic component. Close attention to targeted aspects of the relationship, followed by greater awareness of interaction processes is likely to set the stage for change in the family system (Paquin, 1981).

This chapter has been written to describe how participant observation has been used in marital and family research and therapy. The rationale for participant observation from the theoretical and practical perspectives is presented. Options for participant observation are discussed, followed by a presentation of specific procedures currently in use. The psychometric features of these procedures are considered, and finally, areas for the further development of participant observation are identified.

RATIONALE FOR PARTICIPANT OBSERVATION

The Stimulus–Organism–Response Paradigm

Despite the lip service paid to stimulus–organism–response paradigms of assessment, very few of our assessment procedures do this model justice. In most assessment situations, stimuli are presented in the form of questionnaires, tests, or interviews and responses are obtained in the form of open-ended statements, forced choices, or true–false answers. These assessment formats elicit associations between one response (a psychological test) to another response (a significant nontest characteristic). Errors occur in the interpretation of these data when we forget that the test stimuli represent a highly restricted stimulus situation. A stimulus–response (S–R) analysis, in contrast, seeks to examine the relationship between environmental conditions (antecedents and consequences) and samples of the criterion response. Empirical data on these S–R relationships have typically been obtained through functional analyses that uncover aspects of the environmental conditions that are relevant to the criterion response.

Although traditional functional analysis tends to be impractical or too costly for most clinicians, participant observation can be used to estimate relationships between criterion variables and environmental conditions. With data collection repeated across time, participant observation allows us to examine the specific situations in which problem behaviors are likely to occur, as well as those situations in which they are unlikely to occur. Once the target response has been defined, participant observation can be used to monitor stimulus and/or consequence events; this analysis leads to a set of hypotheses about which antecedent stimuli and which consequences are controlling the target behavior.

In many stimulus–response assessments, very little information is obtained about organismic variables that may, indeed, hold the key to understanding how specific interventions affect specific individuals. Often, it is presumed that psychological assessment procedures measure organismic traits when, in fact, they are simply measuring responses (Tyron, 1979). Knowing what individual variables interact with what stimulus conditions to produce particular response patterns is a different matter. The same organismic variables that are of interest in individual psychotherapy are also of interest in relationship therapy, for example, competencies, constructs, expectancies, subjective values, and rules (Mischel, 1973). In relationship therapy, however, attention tends to be focused on person variables that mediate interactional events, such as communication skill levels, relationship expectations, and the range and intensity of spouses' affective experience and expression (Margolin, 1983a). Although a few of these organismic variables are evident to outside observers, most reflect internal states of experience. These states are communicable, however, when participant observations on oneself monitor the association between internal states and changes in relationship conditions.

Cognitive and Affective Explanations of Marital Distress

The question can be raised why it is important to assess cognitive or affective events. Why risk the accuracy and reactivity inherent in these subjective indices when there is an incredible amount to be learned simply through direct observation of the interaction? Although still unproven, it is assumed that the etiology and maintenance of marital and family distress rest on a combination of behavioral, cognitive, and affective factors. Despite the plethora of findings regarding behavioral differences between distressed and nondistressed relationships, theoretical explanations always include cognitive factors as important mediators of observable interactions. There are the short-term momentary cognitions related to the way that participants process information. Spouses are not simply passive receptors of environmental stimuli; they actively evaluate and interpret such stimuli based on their idiosyncratic sets and schemata (Jacobson, 1984). The communication deficit explanation of marital distress, for example, suggests that distressed spouses intend their messages to be received far more positively than they are, in fact, received (Gottman & Porterfield, 1981; Gottman, Notarius, Markman, Bank, Yoppi, & Rubin, 1976). This hypothesis, of course, cannot be tested through the observations of an outsider. Yet, through participant observations, a comparison can be made between the sender's and the receiver's perceptions of each communication.

Because of the continuous nature of the relationships, participants formulate general ideas and conclusions about one another, themselves, and the relationship (Huston & Robins, 1982). The long-standing cognitions, in the form of attributions, expectations, and attitudes, have been central to concepts of relationship distress. Overall experiences of "satisfaction" have long been the fundamental goal of marital therapy. In addition, it is assumed that relationship distress may be a function of unrealistic or irrational relationship beliefs (Epstein, 1982; Jacobson & Margolin, 1979; Sager, 1976) regarding the nature of relationships. A third focus has been on spouses' attributions about who or what is causing the problem, as well as efficacy expectations about whether or not the problem can be solved (Doherty, 1981a,b; Weiss, 1980).

It is, in some ways, ironic that affective dimensions should have received less attention than either behaviors or cognitions in the understanding of marital and family problems. Emotional responses, in terms of both the overall emotional tone of a marriage and the momentary emotional flashes, are very important components of close relationships. As Bersheid (1983) noted:

> The very phrase "close relationship" carries the implication of passions spent or antici-
> pated, of feelings of every size, shape, and description, of, at the very least, some
> experience of "affect"—an antiseptic term, but one that encompasses without prejudice
> the entire range of quality and intensity of human emotion and feeling, from mild
> irritation to raging hatred to blinding joy to placid contentment. (p. 110)

Certainly, different types of affective experiences accompany relationship distress versus satisfaction. Yet, it is not sufficient to view emotional reactions simply as the outcome of the general state of a couple's marriage. Emotional responsiveness may actually be part of the problem. Margolin and Weinstein (1983) suggested that affective responsiveness involves the related but separate dimensions of affective experience and affective expression. Relationships suffer when there is either a deficit in emotional experience (e.g., spouses experience one another as emotionally distant or indifferent) or an excess of emotional experience (e.g., a spouse is overwhelmed by one persistent emotion that seems to crowd out all other emotions). Vastly different levels of emotional experience between the two spouses also can be a problem. Excesses or deficits in the expression of emotions are the second dimension of affective problems. Examples include (a) when spouses fail to recognize and describe their own emotional experiences; (b) when all emotional experiences are automatically subsumed under one general class of emotions, such as anger without recognition of fear or hurt; or (c) when the expression of emotions is ill timed or insensitive to the partner's reaction.

To a certain degree, affect can be assessed by outsiders. One of the major coding systems for describing couples' interaction, the Couples' Interactional Scoring System (CISS; Gottman, 1979), examines each behavioral unit for positive, negative, or neutral affect based on a hierarchical scanning of vocal tone, facial cues, and body posture. Because of the considerable difficulty in reading affective cues, however, several investigators have turned to the spouses themselves to rate their affective reactions as they participate in an interaction. Through participant observation procedures, affect has been assessed on a moment-to-moment basis as well as on more molar daily levels of interaction.

Behavioral-Affective-Cognitive Sequences

The study of relationships, even at its most basic level, translates into the study of interpersonal events that, it turns out, are relatively complicated units.

Interpersonal events are comprised of the ongoing exchange of overt observable behaviors, as well as the subjective reactions such as the momentary thoughts and emotions that accompany those behaviors. These events take place against a backdrop of relatively stable attitudes, attributions, and beliefs. Adding to this already complex picture is the fact that each of these components affects and is affected by the other. Within a given individual, overt behaviors affect and are affected by covert reactions. Looking across individuals, we find that one person's overt behavior affects the other person's covert and overt responses. Huston and Robins (1982) concluded that

> the fundamental characteristic of a relationship is *behavioral interdependence;* that is, each person's overt behavior affects the overt behavior and subjective events of the other. In addition, any relationship that endures long enough to allow both partners to form attitudes and beliefs about each other and the relationship (subjective conditions) can be viewed as exhibiting *psychological interdependences.* By "psychological interdependence" we mean that these attitudes and beliefs are the result, at least in part, of the interaction. (p. 903)

How do we study these aspects of relationships? A primary feature of these behavioral-cognitive-affective cycles is the rapidity with which they occur. According to Peterson (1977), all three components may all happen at once; certainly, there is not a given temporal order of events. There is, furthermore, the problem of segmenting interaction into meaningful units. Without an obvious beginning or ending to any one interaction, we must make rather arbitrary decisions about what constitutes a meaningful unit. Finally, attention must be paid to the sequential dimension of these data.

Within the ongoing stream of behavior, the recurring patterns are those that tend to be of most interest. By carefully examining recurring patterns, we can identify molecular chains of behavior and the accompanying subjective reactions that feed into these problem cycles.

The assessment of interactional events, as just defined, depends, to a large extent, on self-monitoring. Outside observers can evaluate only the overt behavioral dimensions of these sequences and can only estimate the affective dimensions. In contrast, by having family members report on their own interaction processes, we can gain access to subjective reactions and also come to appreciate the meaning and value placed on the overt behaviors.

Practical Considerations

The rationale for participant observation also takes into account practical considerations, namely, the limitations of observations by outsiders or nonparticipants. As previously stated, outside observers do not have access to the important subjective reactions that are of interest to the study of close relationships. In addition, even many of the overt behaviors of intimacy cannot be observed by an outsider because of their low frequency or their private nature. Finally, using any type of formal schema for observations by trained outsiders (as discussed in Chapter 8) requires tremendous resources, and such schemata are thus rarely used other than by a select group of marital and family researchers. Participant observation, in contrast, could bring formal assessment into the realm of most clinicians and could expand the options of researchers who rely exclusively on one-time verbal reports.

OPTIONS IN DECIDING ON PARTICIPANT OBSERVATION INSTRUMENTS

Participant observation is not a unitary set of procedures. On the contrary, the exact format of participant observation is limited only by the creativity of the therapist or the experimenter working in conjunction with the family members. Although the section below describes specific procedures for participant observation, which have been standardized and, in a few cases normed, participant observation procedures can also be individualized to meet the unique requirements of each evaluation situation. Following is a set of the factors to be considered when deciding on a participant observation procedure.

Observation of Self or Other

One of the major benefits of studying close relationships, as opposed to individuals, is the fact that we are not dependent on the report of one person. The number of persons involved in the assessment process determines the number of available perceptions. In participant observation, a choice is to be made about whether individuals observe themselves, in which case they can assess behavioral, cognitive, and affective reactions, or they observe each other, in which case they are limited to behavioral observations and behavioral manifestations of affective reactions. Participant observation, at least from a social learning perspective, has focused predominantly on observing another family member, for example, parents keeping records on a child's behavior or spouses keeping records of one another's behavior. The advantage of this external focus is that family members become more aware of exactly how much of a positive nature the other person is doing. When tracking negative behaviors, however, the external focus often has the unfortunate effect of creating an atmosphere of fault-finding and blaming, unless the observer is surprised by the *low* frequency of these behaviors.

As argued elsewhere (Margolin, 1983a), relationship satisfaction is not based solely on being a recipient of interactions; it also takes into account perceptions of oneself as a spouse or as a parent. For this reason, a focus on oneself through self-monitoring is as important as the focus on someone else. Self-observations can help someone become more aware of his or her reactions to the interaction, and this awareness may be the first step toward changing oneself. Self-observation can also provide a basis for teaching other family members about oneself.

One of the best uses of participant observation is the comparison between "how I view myself" and "how you view me." Having two persons monitor themselves *and* one another provides data on the degree of overlap versus discrepancy in their perceptions. Examining the source of those discrepancies may illuminate why certain conflicts typically arise in the relationship.

Immediate versus Delayed Observation

Immediate observation requires the reporter to engage in two tasks simultaneously, that is, to participate in an interaction and to observe that interaction. The more individuals are asked to report on processes that they do not normally attend to, the more difficult the task is. As spouses engage in a conversation, for example, they may be asked to simultaneously rate their reactions to what is being said. Introducing this rating procedure into the the conversation means that the evaluations that might have occurred in an offhand fashion now are to be formalized and regularized. Spouses may also be asked to observe and report on their own internal processes, a procedure that requires tremendous awareness of covert reactions that spouses may or may not typically attend to.

An alternate form of participant observation is to assess family members' reactions after they have completed a specific phase of interaction, for example, after they have completed a structured discussion, or after there is a natural break in the interaction. Because these procedures ask the reporter about overt and covert events that occurred at an earlier time, they are considered retrospective verbalizations (Ericsson & Simon, 1980). Although less intrusive than assessments that are simultaneous to the event, these procedures are likely to entail some sacrifice in accuracy. It is difficult, if not impossible, actually to retrieve an internal state that occurred at a particular moment during task performance. Nonetheless, it is possible, on completing the task, to describe general reactions. It is also possible, with detailed probing procedures, to recall events or critical incidents from larger time frames, such as the course of the entire day. The specificity of these events, however, cannot be as great as with more immediate recall.

Another alternative is to return to the task, through the use of videotape or role play, and to use the respondents' reactions to a "relived" experience as an indication of their reactions to the original event. The reenactment presents the respondents with the same cues as occurred during the original task and allows the respondents to speculate and theorize on what internal and interactional processes were occurring. Furthermore, the original task has occurred with little disruption or interference. Unfortunately, however, there are no guarantees that the responses in the replayed task will replicate the original task. Observers of videotape playback, for example, often attend to details on the videotape (how overweight they look) that were unimportant during the original interaction.

Structured versus Open-Ended Inquiry

Another dimension to consider in participant observation is the format for the observation, which typically ranges from highly structured to entirely open-ended. Structured formats involve rating tasks in which the respondent decides whether a predetermined behavior has occurred or to what degree a reaction was experienced. These data result in a comprehensive picture of dimensions deemed important by the experimenter or the therapist. Because this task involves recognition more than recollection, it is not overly demanding on the respondent. There is a drawback, however, in using these same procedures over repeated trials. Respondents' awareness of what they will be asked may change the course of the actual interaction.

The alternative is to use an open-ended procedure that simply asks the respondents to verbalize, or to recollect and then verbalize, what they were doing, thinking, or feeling, or what was significant about the event. With this ambiguous instruction, the respondent does not know what to attend to on the next trial. Persons who are unaccustomed to introspection or to verbal accounts of their internal states may have some difficulty with this task. On the positive side, however, this procedure brings forth dimensions that are important to the participant, rather than the predetermined dimensions of the experimenter. Even the variability among participants in the selection of important dimensions may be an important source of data.

Micro- versus Macrobehavior

A factor related to degree of specificity is the molarity of the unit of observation. Peterson (1977) aptly pointed out that the choice of unit is important theoretically and clinically. Those who study moment-to-moment reactions are likely to intervene on this level, whereas those who study more major sequences are likely to intervene at that level. The molecular types of analysis often define behavior in terms of the individual, for example, "husband smiles," "wife feels happy," or "wife complements husband." Molar analyses involve larger units of behavior (e.g., "When wife calls husband to see how he is doing at work, she catches him at a busy moment and he snaps at her; she hangs up feeling irritated and vowing never again to call him"). McClintock (1983) described 10 levels of molarity, illustrating how analyses move from molecular to molar, and from individual to dyadic. Interaction units can be even larger, involving an individual and a family subsystem or multiple family subsystems (Margolin, 1981b). The wife who became irritated after calling her husband, for example, might express her irritation at one of the children, and then, even later, the husband and wife might have an argument regarding the children while failing to mention the original source of their tensions. This example combines several interactional units, which can be examined separately or as an aggregate.

There is the risk, at either end of the continuum of molarity, that family members will not be able to provide the types of data that are being sought because they are either too general or too specific. Thus, a match must be sought in terms of units that are understandable and meaningful for the respondent so that she or he can classify and store relevant information while still providing data that are useful to the therapist.

Consideration of the molarity issue brings us back to the stimulus–organism–response model. Rarely is it useful in marital and family therapy simply to count discrete behaviors. What is more important is to identify the context surrounding problem behaviors. When a spouse complains of feeling distanced from the mate, for example, it may be important to get an open-ended description of what stimulus brought on that feeling of distance, what response was made to that feeling (e.g., withdrawal or seeking attention), and finally, what was the consequence for the mate. Through such procedures, problem sequences can be identified. Such procedures also lead to hypotheses about what part of the sequence might be the focus of an intervention, for example, the dysfunctional response to feeling distant, the cognition that contributes to that feeling in the first place, or the mate's eventual reaction.

As will be illustrated below in the description of specific procedures, the dimension of molarity has been dichotomized according to setting. Participant observation at home has consisted of molar behaviors, whereas observation in the therapist's or researcher's office has focused on molecular types of analyses. Practical considerations rather than theoretical issues have been the source of this dichotomy. The types of interactions that occur during a therapy session are briefer and can be subjected to highly detailed scrutiny, particularly if audiotape or videotape procedures are available. It is more difficult to apply the same degree of scrutiny to a couple's interactions at home. Also, because there is a much wider and richer range of behaviors from which to sample at home, molar interactional behaviors have been the target of home assessment.

PARTICIPANT OBSERVATION PROCEDURES

Nonstandardized Procedures

Monitoring of behaviors in the home setting initially began with parent training procedures. As part of the treatment of acting-out, difficult-to-control youngsters, parents were helped to identify specific problem behaviors. The parents were then presented with a structured format for assessing how frequently that behavior occurred and/or how frequently a more desirable alternative behavior occurred. At this early stage, the procedures were highly individualized, depending on the specific behavior to be observed and the estimated base rate of that behavior. Fighting with siblings, for example, could be assessed through a simple frequency count across the entire day. Or if fighting was particularly frequent directly before dinner, the parents' monitoring of fighting could be limited to that one high-risk period. Certain problem behaviors, such as noncompliance, lend themselves to a percentage-of-occurrence strategy. That is, the number of times the child complies or does not comply is assessed relative to the number of commands that were issued. The parent making such observations is to keep track of his or her own behavior (e.g., commands), as well as of the types of responses by the child.

A number of reasons were given for these monitoring procedures (Patterson, 1975). First, the data collected before therapy served as a baseline index of exactly how frequently the target behavior occurred. Second, the charting identified under what circumstances problem behaviors occurred or did not occur. Third, because problem behaviors change slowly, these procedures could be a useful index of slow but perceptible change and thus could be a helpful reminder to keep working on the problem behavior. Fourth, sometimes the mere act of monitoring the occurrence of problem behaviors led to a reduction in those behaviors.

The focus on discrete behaviors that initially characterized family therapy was also adopted in marital therapy. The focus was generally on counting someone else's behavior rather than one's own behavior. Rappoport and Harrell (1972) suggested that the husband and wife independently prepare lists of three specific undesirable behaviors. Then, the spouses prepared another list indicating how they usually responded to the undesirable behaviors. Spouses were then to observe what happened before and after the target behaviors occurred. From such procedures, spouses learned to identify the cues that set the occasion for undesirable behaviors and the consequences that maintained those behavior.

Jacobson (1979) elaborated on spouse tracking by using a multiple-baseline design. Each spouse simultaneously monitored three problem behaviors. Problem solving was then introduced in one conflict area at a time. The results, which were confirmed by nonparticipant observation measures as well, indicated that all six of the couples studied improved significantly. In five of the six cases, the multiple-baseline analysis of the participant observation data confirmed that behavioral intervention rather than nonspecific therapeutic procedures was responsible for the improvement.

Recent trends in participant observation procedures have focused on the association between overt transactions and the internal reactions of individual family members. As Margolin and Weinstein (1983) described, spouses' subjective reactions of feeling distant from one another, feeling unappreciated, or feeling angry and irritated with one another can be better understood through monitoring procedures that are structured to study fluctuations in those feelings. A couple that complains of feeling emotionally distant, for example, can be asked to regularly appraise those feelings. In one such case, the couple was instructed to rate emotional closeness versus distance three times a day along a 5-point scale ("extremely close" to "extremely distant"), and to indicate what factors contributed to each rating. These records gave the couple and the therapist the opportunity to examine the variability of ratings (Did the ratings fluctuate, or did one feeling pervade?), to compare and contrast the two separate records (Did the spouses feel close at the same time, or did one feel close when the other felt distant?), and to analyze what situations altered each partner's feelings.

Macrolevel Observation in the Home

In contrast to the individualized approach to participant observation just described, other procedures have been designed with a set format that permits comparison across couples. These procedures typically are more comprehensive than the individualized approach because they must apply to more than one couple. Each of these procedures makes some effort to integrate specific behaviors with more global, subjective reactions.

Spouse Observation Checklist (SOC). As perhaps the most well-known participant observation procedure in the marital literature, the SOC (Weiss & Perry, 1979) truly captures the behavioral marital therapist's commitment to ferreting out the details of spouses' lives together. The SOC is an eight-page listing of pleasing and displeasing relationship behaviors. The most recent revision of the SOC contains approximately 400 items that span 12 relationship dimensions: Companionship, Affection, Consideration, Sex, Communication Process, Coupling Activities, Household Management, Financial Decision-Making, Education–Employment, Childrearing, Personal Habits, and Self and Spouse Independence. "Spouse called me just to say hello" is an example of a Consideration Please, and "Spouse refused to make a decision on a significant issue" is an example of a Communication Displease. As is evidenced in these examples, spouses report on one another rather than on themselves. There are, in addition, some "we" items, for example, "We discussed the children." Although items were categorized *a priori* as pleases and displeases, Christensen and Niles (1980) reported that virtually all the items categorized as pleasing are indeed rated as pleasing by a majority of individuals. For items classified *a priori* as displeasing, however, there is more variability in how spouses actually rate them.

The SOC was designed to obtain repeated recordings of a couple's daily interactions. It is formatted into one recording package for an entire week. Spouses are to complete the SOC before retiring each night, reading through the entire inventory and placing a checkmark to indicate what items occurred during the previous 24 hours. Spouses then tally their subtotals for each of the 12 categories to get an overall profile of the areas in which pleasing versus displeasing behaviors are likely to occur. The final tally page also contains a section for spouses to rate (on a 1–9-point scale) their overall satisfaction with the marriage for that day. Comparing fluctuations in the satisfaction ratings with fluctuations in the behavioral rates offers valuable information about the relative significance of these behavioral categories in the marital satisfaction of a given individual.

The SOC, which has been used in a number of research studies, has provided support for a behavioral exchange explanation of marital distress. According to expectation, distressed compared to nondistressed couples report fewer pleasing behaviors and more displeasing behaviors. Please–Displease ratios are approximately 4 : 1 for distressed and 12 : 1 to 30 : 1 for nondistressed couples (Birchler, Weiss, & Vincent, 1975; Margolin, 1981a). Although overall Please and Displease scores discriminate distressed and nondistressed couples, not all of the content categories discriminate between these groups. The frequency of Instrumental Displeases, weighted by valence, was a powerful discriminator in the Barnett and Nietzel (1979) sample, but Instrumental Pleases, Affectional Pleases, and Affectional Displeases were not. Margolin (1981a) also found significant differences between distressed and nondistressed couples on Instrumental Displeases as well as on Affectional Pleases, Communication Pleases, and Communication Displeases. The SOC has also been used as a therapy outcome measure and has been shown to be a sensitive index of pretherapy to posttherapy change (Margolin & Weiss, 1978b; Patterson, Hops, & Weiss, 1974; Weiss, Hops, & Patterson, 1973).

Interactional Records (IR). As contrasted with the frequency count approach of the SOC, Peterson's IR (1977, 1979) is based on a critical events format. Spouses independently identify the most important interaction that occurs each day. They then discuss between themselves which interaction to record so that both are writing about the same incident. Independent accounts of the incident are constructed according to the following open-ended instructions:

> Please use this form to describe the most important interaction you two had today. In your own words, from your own viewpoint, tell:
> 1. The conditions under which the exchange took place. Where and when did it happen? How were you both feeling as the interaction began?
> 2. How the interaction started. Who made the first move? What did that person say or do?
> 3. What happened then. Please write a fairly detailed description of the exchange from start to finish. Who did and said what to whom? What were you thinking and feeling as the action went on? What ideas and emotions did your partner seem to have? How did it all come out? (Peterson, 1979, p. 224)

The underlying purpose of these procedures is to identify interaction sequences, which Peterson has defined as interactions in which a reciprocal contingency prevails.

Casual inspection of the records obtained by Peterson showed that they offer rich accounts of significant events in the daily lives of participants. The problem, however, was how to interpret and code these data. To take both covert and overt experience into account, the records were coded in terms of affect (e.g., "I hate you"), construal ("I think it is your fault that our bank account is overdrawn"), and the expectations that each partner held in regard to the subsequent response of the other. Eighteen categories of affect were grouped into four major categories. Affection–Affiliation, Calm–Neutrality, Aggression–Disapproval, and Distress–Dysphoria. Twenty-two categories of construal also were grouped into four general categories: Positive Relationship, Sense of Control, Negative Relationship, and Loss of Control. Finally, the 10 expectation categories were clustered into overall categories of Compliance, Positive Affect, Withdrawal, and Negative Affect.

The IR has been examined for basic frequencies of identified categories as well as for interaction sequences. The frequency data show expected differences among disturbed, average, and satisfied couples. Affectionate expressions and construals of positive relationship are most common among satisfied couples. Aggression, negative relationship, and expectations of negative affect are most common among couples in treatment. For the sequential analyses, action–reaction units were categorized, with the eight most frequent patterns being Mutual Enjoyment, Support, Aggression–Injury, Mutual Affection, Cooperation, Noncooperation, Aggression–Retaliation, and Conciliation. As anticipated, Mutual

Enjoyment, Mutual Affection, and Conciliation appeared to occur frequently among the nondistressed couples, and Aggression—Injury was frequently found among distressed couples.

Protzner, King, and Christensen (1981) elaborated on Peterson's method of data collection but used somewhat different coding procedures. They adopted patterns similar to those used by Peterson but also categorized incidents in terms of contextual features (e.g., a recreational event, a household task, and exchange of ideas). Not surprisingly, household tasks were the most frequent setting for negative interactions, and recreational events were the most frequent setting for positive interactions. The most frequently occurring patterns were Mutual Enjoyment, Collaboration—Cooperation, Support, Aggression—Retaliation, Lack of Support, and Mutual Affection.

Marital Satisfaction Time Lines (MSTL). The MSTL, developed by Williams (1979), is similar to Peterson's procedure in that spouses are to report on behaviors that influence their satisfaction ratings. To use the MSTL, spouses independently rate each 15-minute segment during the day as positive, neutral, or unpleasant. They then report the most and the least pleasant behavior that occurred during the morning, afternoon, and evening and also indicate what could have been done to improve the interaction during any neutral times. Compared to the SOC and the IR, which call for global ratings over an entire day, the MSTL focuses on a smaller unit of analysis, namely, satisfaction ratings every 15 minutes and behavioral records for each third of the day. Similar to the IR, the MSTL is an open-ended approach in which spouses report on what they believe to be the most important events, rather than reporting the occurrence versus the nonoccurrence of a predetermined list of behaviors.

A comparison on the MSTL between happy and distressed couples showed that total time together and positive time together were higher for the happy couples, and that negative time was higher for the distressed couples (Williams, 1979). There was, however, a subgroup of negative couples that spent an inordinate amount of time together. The content of the interaction intervals was markedly different for the happy couples and for the distressed couples. The ratings of happy couples were usually associated with the commission or omission of positive behavior, in contrast to the ratings of unhappy couples, which were associated with the omission or commission of negative behaviors.

Interview Procedures. There are, in addition, participant observation procedures that have been designed to collect data through brief interviews, either through face-to-face or telephone contact. Wahler (1980; Dumas & Wahler, 1983), for one, developed an insularity measure to assess the quantity and quality of mothers' daily contact with people in the neighborhood. On a quantitative basis, this interview assesses the mean number of daily contacts, the percentage of daily contact with friends, the percentage with kinfolk, and/or the percentage with helping-agency representatives. On a qualitative basis, the interview assesses the topic of the interaction (e.g., the children and finances), as well as the valence of the interaction (good, neutral, or bad). Based on these data, Wahler defined an "insular" parent as one who reports at least twice as many of her daily contacts with kinfolk and/or helping-agency representatives as with friends, or one who reports at least one third of all her daily contact as neutral or negative. Although more an individual than a family measure, the assessment of insularity, Wahler found, significantly improves the prediction of treatment outcome in parent training programs. He suggested that mothers who themselves experience high levels of aversive stimuli from the environment fare poorly in treatment programs that require them to provide consistent social contingencies to their children. These results "point to the indirect, though powerful, impact of ecological variables upon mother–child behavior change and, consequently, to the danger of ignoring such variables in parent-training" (Dumas & Wahler, 1983, p. 31).

In contrast to procedures that focus on only one set of dyadic relationships (e.g., husband–wife, parent–child, or parent–outsider), Christensen and Margolin (1981) developed the Daily Behavior Report (DBR), a procedure used to examine the interrelationship between marital and child problems. Telephone interviews are used to collect reports of "family tensions" and to target problem behaviors. Tension events are operationally defined by each family to identify the specific ways in which each member of the family communicates her or his dissatisfactions with the other members. Typical examples of tension events include yelling, blaming, withdrawing, and crying. The telephone interview examines who actually participated in the conflict and who were uninvolved observers, for example, children who heard their parents arguing in another room. Having events coded in this fashion permits examination of temporal patterns (e.g., Do marital tensions tend to precede parent–child or sibling tensions?). After collecting information on the tension events for the morning, afternoon, and evening, the telephone interviewer then obtains daily frequencies of problem behaviors for the child and for the marital relationship. Each family identifies at least three target behaviors for the child (e.g., tantrums, refusing to go to bed, and not completing chores) and three target behaviors for the marriage (e.g., arguments about the children, sexual intimacies, and talking about the day's events). Last, the reporter indicates general satisfaction with the marital relationship and the parent–child relationship.

Comparisons between distressed and nondistressed families on the DBR revealed twice as many tension events per day for distressed as for nondistressed families (Christensen & Margolin, 1981). Tension incidents involving one partner and at least one child were more frequent in both groups than parent–parent tensions or sibling tensions. The data for both groups also indicated that the conditional probability that any type of tension event would occur, given its previous occurrence, was higher than the base-rate probability of that event. Finally, analyses of the satisfaction ratings looked at correlations between daily satisfaction with the spouse and the children. To examine whether the one target child did indeed play a unique role in the marriage, correlations between spouse satisfaction and satisfaction with the most deviant child were compared to correlations between spouse satisfaction and satisfaction with the other children. The expected pattern was found in distressed families, in that correlations for the target child were significantly greater than for the other children.

Margolin (1983b) incorporated several of the procedures presented thus far into a new telephone procedure that includes four separate sections and is administered on a daily basis to both husband and wife. The first part evaluates overall satisfaction with each family member and assesses the types of activities that the spouses or the whole family engage in (e.g., how many meals were eaten together, television watching time, and time in recreational, social, and work activities). Part 2 borrows Wahler's format to assess each spouse's individual contact with nonfamily members and the quality of the spouses day in non-family-oriented activities. Part 3 expands on the DBR to assess marital and family tensions. Similar to the DBR, this telephone interview assesses how many tensions occurred and who was involved. The questionnaire additionally examines (a) what caused the tension (e.g., conflict of ideas, values, or opinions; negative characteristics of self or other; psychological state of self or other; or physical state of self or other); (b) how long the tension lasted; (c) how the tension was demonstrated (e.g., direct discussion, arguing, indirect action, or withdrawal); (d) what was the outcome of this event; and (e) whether there was any kind of physical contact. The final section of the interview employs Peterson's IR to assess the most important marital event of the day. These telephone procedures, taken as whole, provide a comprehensive analysis of spouses' lives as individuals, as marital partners, and as family members.

This overview of participant observation in the home points up two types of procedures: daily written records and daily interviews. Because compliance is sometimes an issue with participant observation procedures, the daily telephone call offers several advantages. First, the phone call both guarantees that data will be collected every 24 hours and serves as a prompt for the respondent to pay attention to the target responses. It thus circumvents the problem of "forgetting" to record data and attempting to fill in the gaps at the end of the week. On the other hand, the telephone interviews are a more costly procedure that, depending on the amount of information to be obtained, requires 15 to 30 minutes of staff time per call. A compromise strategy adopted by some is to make one or two data-collection telephone calls during the week to prompt the respondents and to encourage them to record data on a daily basis.

Microlevel Observation in the Laboratory

Participant observation in the laboratory, which has focused primarily on couples rather than families, elicits spouses' evaluations of and their reactions to their own communication process. Interest in obtaining spouses' subjective impressions of moment-to-moment interactions stems from the communication deficit hypothesis and cognitive theories of marital distress. The communications deficit explanation of marital distress predicts a discrepancy in the way spouses intend their messages to be received and the way messages are sent (Gottman *et al.*, 1976). This theory is complicated by the fact that there are at least two levels of interpersonal interaction: a content level, which conveys information directly through the meaning of words, and a relationship or affect level, which indicates to the recipient how the sender intends the message to be received (Knudson, Sommers, & Golding, 1980). Cognitive explanations of marital distress suggest that attributions about the spouse's behavior or conclusions drawn from the partner's behavior, rather than the behavior *per se*, constitute the primary problem (Doherty, 1981a,b; Epstein, 1982).

Procedures for testing these hypotheses involve obtaining spouses' reactions to their own brief discussions. These procedures vary according to whether reactions are obtained during the discussion or retrospectively, once the discussion is complete. The procedures also vary in terms of structure and format. In some studies, spouses have been required simply to rate their reactions along a general positive–negative dimension, whereas in others they rate a greater number of specific dimensions (e.g., the degree to which they experienced a wide range of emotions). Still other procedures require open-ended impressions of thoughts and feelings at various points in the discussion.

Spouse-monitoring procedures in the laboratory typically involve the same type of problem-solving discussion as are coded by outside observers. After selecting a topic that represents a true-life disagreement, the couple proceeds to discuss that topic for 10 to 15 minutes. They may be instructed simply to discuss the topic or to attempt to resolve the topic. The discussions are typically audiotaped or videotaped and proceed without any direct interference or intervention on the part of the therapist or researcher.

Thomas, Carter, and Gambrill (1971) developed the first electromechanical device for spousal recording of discrete behaviors (e.g., agree, question asking, and opinion giving). This system was designed both for private recording of spouse observations during an assessment phase and for public coding, by the transmission of light signals during an intervention phase. This system, referred to as *SAM* after its acronym *SSAMB* (Signal System for the Assessment and Modification of Behavior), was tremendously flexible in terms of who received and registered signals. The therapist could signal along with a marital pair, or with parents and one or more children, or family members could signal without the therapist. The major drawback of this system, however, was that it applied only to verbal responses.

Tremendous advances in laboratory-based participant observation came from Gottman and his colleagues (1976), who built a "talk table" that allows spouses to code ongoing communications along a 5-point Likert scale from supernegative to superpositive. As each spouse finished speaking the listener rated the *impact* of the message received, and the speaker rated the *intent* of the message sent. Initial results from these procedures showed that impact, but not intent, ratings differentiated distressed and nondistressed couples. In a further study involving analogue procedures rather than naturalistic communication, Gottman and Porterfield (1981) conducted a specific test of sender versus receiver deficits. Each message that was sent was received by both the sender's spouse and an opposite-sexed, married stranger. The results suggested that wives in dissatisfied marriages have trouble communicating nonverbally to their husbands but not to a married stranger. The inferential data suggested that the husband's receptive difficulties are confined to interactions with the wife.

Using the talk table approach, Notarius, Vanzetti, and Smith (1981) explored another variable: spouses' expectations about the interactional consequences of communication messages. A spouse's prediction of the impact of his or her message was believed to be an indirect measure of beliefs about how the partner would respond. The prediction ratings, along with intent and impact ratings, all discriminated distressed from nondistressed couples. Distressed husbands, in particular, predicted that their wives would receive their messages negatively nearly three times as often as did nondistressed husbands. The distressed wives, in fact, did not receive the messages as negatively as predicted. In nondistressed couples, the husbands overpredicted positive reactions compared to the number of positive messages the wives actually received.

Markman (1979, 1981; Floyd & Markman, 1981; Markman & Poltrock, 1982) has provided still other important contributions based on the talk table procedure. Markman (1979, 1981) found that impact ratings by premarital couples on the "talk table" were significantly predictive of global marital satisfaction at 2½- and 5-year follow-ups. These data suggest that the perceptions of non-rewarding or negative communication from the spouse actually preceded the development of marital dissatisfaction. In his more recent work, Markman (1982) has developed a procedure called the *communication box,* which is similar to the talk table, but that records data directly onto a stereo cassette tape. This procedure currently is being tested with a variety of clinical and nonclinical populations (Floyd & Markman, 1984).

Ratings of communication positiveness have also been used by Margolin (1978; Margolin & Weiss, 1978a), but through somewhat different procedures. Rather than rate every floor switch, as in the talk table procedure, Margolin (1978) used a frequency measure of communication helpfulness. That is, every time either spouse observed an instance of communication helpfulness, she or he recorded this observation through a hand-held electromechanical system. Because of the difficulties in maintaining conversational continuity while observing and coding, spousal observations were collected while watching videotaped playbacks of problem-solving sessions, rather than during the discussions. Low correlations between distressed spouses on this measure indicate that partners hold quite different ideas of what constitutes communication helpfulness.

In a more recent study, Margolin, Hattem, John, and Yost (1985) asked spouses to make 10-second ratings of themselves and of one another along a positive–negative dimension. Couples coded themselves through videotaped playback and also coded a standardized videotaped interaction of two actors portraying a married couple in a problem-solving discussion about the wife's new job. The spouses showed more agreement when coding the standardized tape than when coding their own tapes, a finding indicating greater agreement in spouses' perceptions when coding a neutral rather than a personally relevant stimulus. Furthermore, the women were coded more positively as a group than were the men. The women rated themselves more positively than they rated the husbands. Interestingly, the men characterized by high and moderate marital adjustment also rated the women more positively than they rated themselves. Only men with low marital adjustment showed the opposite pattern of rating themselves as more positive and less negative than the women. Finally, the agreement between spouses was compared to agreements between a spouse and a trained observer. On both the standard tape and the couples' own tapes, the spouses agreed more with one another than they did with the trained coders. These data provide partial support for Gottman's hypothesis (1979) of a "private communication system" in couples. However, the absence of differences according to level of marital adjustment contradicts Gottman's findings that this private communication system exists in the communication of nondistressed couples more than of distressed couples.

Weiss and his associates (Weiss, 1984; Weiss, Wasserman, Wieder, & Summers, 1981) also examined how spouses evaluated their own interaction. According to Weiss, such evaluations combine two sources of information: spouses' previous history with one another and the immediate experience provided by the interaction itself:

> Their history is the *context* of variables preexisting to their interaction. It includes cognitive and affective influences as well as actual competencies and resources available to the couple. In a word, context includes everything that the couple brings with them to the interaction. (p. 2)

The behavioral data generated by the interaction itself are the *process* of the interaction.

The participant observation measures used by Weiss included measures before the discussion, during the discussion, and after the discussion. First, the spouses completed three global self-report measures that served as context variables. Before the discussion, the spouses also completed a 34-item expectancy scale that asked about likely acts and feelings during the discussion. The process measure was a Video Rating Scale (VRS), in which spouses made 15-second ratings of perceived helpfulness from the partner. Third, the outcome measure was the Interaction Rating Scale, which assessed the degree of the spouses' satisfaction with the interaction and the amount of progress they felt had been made. These multiple measures were used to sort out what degree of the couples' process ratings were associated with context, expectancy, and outcome.

The Weiss *et al.* results indicate that context (i.e., global measures of satisfaction and stability) and expectancy measures accounted for more than one third of the variance in the couples' impact ratings. Context measures accounted for substantially more of the negative impact variance than of the positive impact variance, and expectancy variables accounted for more positive than negative impact variance. Looking from process to outcome, Weiss found that impact ratings accounted for one third of the variance in the spouses' rating of discussion outcomes. What the Weiss study points out is the overlap between different types of self-report measures. The 15-second ratings correlated with the global ratings made immediately after the discussion. The ongoing ratings also correlated with the expectancy ratings and the global self-report measures taken before the conversation. Weiss's study, as well as the Margolin *et al.* study, also examined the relationship between self-report variables and ratings by outsiders, which will be addressed below under "Validity."

The approaches to microlevel participant observation discussed thus far all involve ratings, that is, either a rating for each "floor switch," regular ratings at 10- or 15-second intervals, or satisfaction ratings made after the discussion has been completed. An alternative, less structured approach is to conduct a detailed inquiry into spouses' perceptions of their communication process. This approach, which certainly is familiar in the therapy session, involves periodically interrupting the couple and inquiring into thoughts and feelings associated with the previous statement or interaction.

An inquiry process developed by Knudson *et al.* (1980) consisted of a semistructured interview organized around certain standard questions. A videotaped playback of the couple's discussion was interrupted at three predetermined points to allow the experimenter to inquire into the participants' interpersonal perceptions. Questions during the inquiry were designed to elicit the spouses' direct perceptions of themselves and one another, metaperspectives (i.e., the respondent's perception of the other's direct perspective views), and metametaperspectives (i.e., the respondents' perceptions of how the other saw the respondent seeing the other). Each of these perspectives for each spouse was rated according to Leary's circumplex model. Knudson *et al.* acknowledged that the inquiry interview, although appearing to be a useful method, can also be a tedious and frustrating procedure. Obtaining spouses' metametaviews was particularly difficult and raised questions about whether the inquiry assessed perceptions that had actually occurred in the original interaction or whether spouses generated perceptions as a response to the experimenter's request. The authors hypothesized that there were large individual differences in the extent to which spouses' reactions reflected previous perceptions.

Knudson *et al.*'s results focus on perceptual differences between spouses as reflected in the participant observation of couples who engage in conflict discussions versus those who avoid conflict discussion. In general, differences in perceptions increased across time for the conflict-avoidant group and decreased across time for the conflict-engagement group. Furthermore, conflict-avoidant spouses actually felt that there was more agreement when agreement, in fact, had decreased.

In general, participant observations in the laboratory require spouses to become "commenters" on their own communication. Although there are numerous ways to obtain this information and numerous bits of information that are of interest, attention thus far has focused primarily on the general impact of various segments of interaction. It is likely that impact ratings during the discussion may be quite different from impact ratings to videotape playback. Spouses' attention in these two tasks appears to be focused on quite different dimensions. Informal clinical experience with these procedures, particularly the videotape playback, suggests that they are quite powerful and may serve important intervention functions as well.

UTILITY OF PARTICIPANT OBSERVATION

Reliability

As in any assessment procedure, there are two levels of reliability to consider: reliability of data collection and reliability of data interpretation. *Reliability of data collection* refers to the repeatability and precision of measurement. *Reliability of interpretation* refers to the degree of uniformity in the conclusions drawn about the test data. In other words, what degree of match exists for two independent interpretations of identical data sets? This second type of reliability is particularly a problem for participant observation. Because very few of the measures described here have norms or "cutoff" scores, there is very little with which the scores or data from a given individual can be compared. For the most part, participant observation conforms to a "person-oriented" focus of assessment, or as Mischel (1977) wrote, "The interest here is not in how people compare to others, but in how they can move close to their own goals and ideals if they change their behavior in specific ways as they interact with the significant people in their lives" (p. 248).

The reliability related to consistency of measurement also raises some problems. In standardized as opposed to individualized participant-observation procedures, the assessment stimuli and the instructions to the respondents may be held constant. Still, there are obvious problems for test–retest or interrater reliability. Inherent in the definition of participant observation is the idea that behavior will fluctuate across different environmental situations. Rather than seeking temporal stability, participant observation searches out the variability in behavior as related to environmental changes. Similarly, inherent in the definition of participant observation is the fact that the major instrument for observing and for recording data is the individual. Obviously, there is tremendous variability in how two or more individuals perceive and label events. In fact, one of the purposes of participant observation is to understand the cognitive and perceptual distortions that differentiate how two family members observe the same event.

Despite these basic problems for reliability, there are reliability data on participant observation procedures to be examined. As may be anticipated by its behavioral foundations, interobserver reliability is the main consideration in participant observation. This consideration has been explored by examining husband–wife agreement on marital events and parental agreement on child and family behaviors. Overall, interobserver agreement tends to be low. Agreement levels generally are greater than chance but usually fall below the levels deemed acceptable for observational research with nonparticipants. As seen in the studies described below, level of agreement, furthermore, seems to be a function of relationship adjustment, with low agreement exhibited by persons in distressed, compared to nondistressed, relationships.

A series of interobserver reliability studies have been conducted on the SOC. Using a modified version of the SOC, which had "I" items as well as "Spouse" items, Christensen and Nies (1980) found that only 18% of the items had agreement levels greater than 70%. Interestingly, the highest agreement items all were Pleases, whereas 15 of the 20 lowest agreement items were Displeases. Correlations between husbands and wives on Please and Displease totals were higher than on individual items. The correlations on total Pleases were .49 and .41, respectively, for wives and husbands, and the correlations for Displeases were .22 and .36 for wives and husbands.

Christensen, Sullaway, and King (1983) examined the same data for systematic sources of bias. All items on the modified SOC were rated for egocentric bias (i.e., greater endorsement of "I" items than for "Spouse" items), social desirability, objectivity (i.e., the amount of inference required of the observer), molarity (i.e., the size of the behavioral unit), observability, and importance. This study showed greater agreement in happy couples than in unhappy couples. These authors concluded that "Perhaps happy couples are less biased or more attentive observers or simply more similar in the way they view interaction events" (p. 137). Spouses exhibited greater agreement on more objective and more molar items. These types of items, however, received low ratings on importance. The study also presents support for the egocentric bias hypothesis, in that spouses tended to overreport their own behavior and underreport their partners' behavior. Interestingly, as the length of the relationship increased, egocentric bias on negative behavior shifted, indicating more blame and/or denial of responsibility for negative behaviors.

Jacobson and Moore (1981) also explored interspouse reliability on the SOC but based their results on 12 days rather than only 1 day. For the first 6 days, both spouses monitored the behavior of one person. The tasks then were reversed for the final 6 days. The mean agreement between spouses was 47.8%, with a range of 31.0% to 78.6%. The mean percentage agreement of 52% for nondistressed couples was significantly higher than the 42% agreement for distressed couples. It also was noted that agreement was significantly higher for the second 6 days (50%) than for the first 6 days (46%). Consensus between spouses was affected by the degree of inference needed to rate different behaviors. Consensus was higher for categories such as companionship, affection, and sex, which required little inference regarding the intent or the feeling state of the perpetrator. Elwood and Jacobson (1982) considered the possibility that spousal consensus may be higher in couples seeking therapy. These couples, compared to volunteer couples, may be more motivated to observe accurately if they presume that accurate observation will facilitate successful treatment. Elwood and Jacobson's results, however, did not support this hypothesis. Overall agreement was 38.6%, and 53.1% was the highest consensus rate for a single couple.

Spousal agreement also was examined on the MSTL (Williams, 1979). With respect to the amount of time together, happy couples agreed on 92.6% of the recording intervals, and therapy couples agreed on 89.6%; these percentages are not significantly different. However, happy couples showed more agreement (76.8%) than unhappy couples (67.0%) on the quality of their time together. Williams noted that, although distressed couples may be in agreement about the general state of their relationship, they showed marked discrepancies in their ratings of ongoing interaction.

Parental agreement on child behavior presents a more demanding situation because both parents do not necessarily have to the same database or observe the same interactions. Christensen and Margolin (1981) examined the agreement between mothers' and fathers' DBR reports of tension events in the family. One parent, usually the mother, was the standard reporter. The father then provided reliability checks at least one day per week. The highest agreement (.69) occurred for marital tensions, which, by definition, include both spouses. In contrast, the correlation for total family tensions was .42, and that for parent–child tensions was .46. Several factors may have contributed to these significant but still low correlations. First, even though reliability checks were directed to the time period that both parents were together, they may not have been in exactly the same location and may not have observed the same events. Thus, one parent may not have known about an incident of tension unless it was brought to his or her attention by the other. Second, as the range of tension events in a single day was low, the size of the correlation coefficient was limited. Third, the secondary observer, who was usually the father, provided only one report per week and thus was not a familiar with nor as invested in the procedures as the primary reporter. Finally, the decision that there is tension is a very subjective evaluation. Parents often have different tolerance points for family disruption and different definitions of deviant behavior. Distressed families, in particular, tend to argue about what falls into the "normal" range for children. For these reasons, there can be considerable disagreement between spouses on whether a child has exhibited a deviant or disruptive behavior.

Bernal, Klinnert, Russell, Schultz, Bolstad, Rosen, North, and Chao (1978) were faced with a similar reliability problem on parent telephone interviews that assessed whether a child had engaged in 32 specific behaviors during the previous 24 hours. These authors also experienced disappointments in parental agreement even when the parents were asked to monitor only when they both were in the home. Bernal *et al.* concluded "that in the normal course of events, the two parents spent their time in different parts of the home or community, doing different things, and varying in their degree of vigilance over their children" (p. 14). As a creative solution, reliability checks also were attempted between the mother and the child. Here, too, however, the interpretative and experiential discrepancies proved to be a problem; for example, a mother might say that her son hit his brother, whereas the son might argue that it was a playful punch. Once intent is entered into the definition of behavior, errors in measurement are inevitable. Bernal, Klinnert, and Schultz (1980) explored the reliability of the telephone interviewer as another potential source of error. When two interviewers recorded data from the same phone call, Bernal *et al.* found 100% agreement. Thus, with relatively straightforward telephone interview procedures, the error resides more in data collection than in data recording.

These reports on interobserver reliability highlight the difficulties of observing behavior, particularly one's own behavior or that of another family member. Taking a rather pessimistic view of reliability in participant observation, particularly with respect to reports of covert processes, Nisbett and Wilson (1977) identified several factors that affect participant observation but that tend to go unnoticed or unreported. First, removal in time, or the length of separation between the report and the actual occurrence of the event, is a factor that decreases accuracy. Second, there are mechanisms of judgment to consider, such as serial order effects, positioning effects, contrasting effects, and other "anchoring" effects. It is easy to imagine, for example, how a judgment regarding a partner's behavior is affected by that person's previous behavior, but this connection may not be reported. Contextual cues (e.g., disagreeing with a spouse *in front of others*) are highly plausible causes for emotional reactions but are not necessarily spontaneously salient. Fourth, we sometimes fail to monitor the non-occurrence of expected events (e.g., the absence of a friendly inquiry about one's day) and focus instead on outright manifestations of hostility or lack of consideration. Fifth, when reactions to others are determined by nonverbal cues, the verbal labels for those cues are often lacking. Sixth, it often is assumed that a parity exists between the magnitude of a cause and an effect. For example, because it often is difficult to comprehend how a small, relatively irrelevant detail can cause a huge argument, there is a tendency to attribute a larger cause to the event.

Taking a more positive view, Ericsson and Simon (1980) argued that there are factors that mediate the reliability of verbal reports. They reiterated the point that it is important to minimize the time lag between the task and the probe so that relevant information is still in the short-term memory. Second, they emphasized the importance of requesting information that depends on one's memory rather than information that can be obtained without consulting one's memory (e.g., "How did you feel *when* . . ." versus "How would you feel *if* . . ."). Other factors to consider include the degree of practice with the observing and reporting task, anticipation of what the recall task involves, and the specificity of the cues used to access the memory.

Although not specifically addressing participant observation, Boice (1983) similarly emphasized the importance of training people to be good observers. He pointed to biological links that are related to being a good observer (e.g., sex and age) but interpreted these simply as biological substrates *on which experience can be built.* He also suggested that personality traits thought to be associated with being a good observer (e.g., introversion, self-awareness, and the ability to view others and/or oneself dispassionately) need to undergo empirical investigation.

Taken as a whole, these reviews of observational ability point out a myriad of factors that detract from the reliability of participant observation and define directions that may improve on its accuracy. The practical application of these suggestions translates into (a) structuring the observation task so that the respondents know what to expect; (b) training the respondents in the specific procedures; (c) providing time to practice the recording procedures; and (d) reviewing and giving feedback on the respondent's performance.

Reactivity and Stability

Reactivity concerns the question of whether the assessment processes *per se* lead to changes in the target behavior (e.g., Ciminero, Nelson, & Lipinski, 1977). With both participants and nonparticipant observation, social desirability factors, or the value judgments made about the target behavior, tend to influence the subject's behavior (Lipinski & Nelson, 1974). With participant observation, there is the additional impact of the respondents' receiving immediate and direct feedback on their behavior. They know exactly what is being observed. They also know how they performed from one trial or one interval to the next. Furthermore, because the respondents are generally not highly trained in the assessment task, nor are they generally supervised while performing the task, there is the possibility that they will redefine the task over time. That is, the respondent may alter the initial definition of the target response or may refine the original description of how the task is to be carried out. Although observer drift may have the inadvertent benefit of increasing the relevance of the task for that particular respondent, it decreases the comparability of data across subjects.

As Margolin and Jacobson (1981) noted, there are several ways in which the SOC or other daily tracking forms may be reactive:

> First, simply reading items on the form alerts spouses to a variety of activities to which they have not paid much attention. Awareness of these items might encourage spouses to engage in new behaviors or take notice of behaviors that, in fact, already are occurring but have not received attention. On the other hand, this awareness may cause discouragement over the vast number of possibilities overlooked in the couple's current relationship. Second, knowledge that the partner will be using the same list may foster various forms of impression management, i.e., emitting new behaviors to receive credit for more pleases. Third, repeated exposure to SOC data provides spouses with feedback regarding the relative frequencies of pleases and displeases, the frequency with which specific behaviors occur, and relative frequencies between the two spouses. This type of data might provide couples with a new perspective on their relationship. (pp. 408–409)

Unfortunately, it is impossible to assess the SOC's immediate reactivity because there is no suitable baseline against which to compare these data (Jacobson, Elwood, & Dallas, 1981). Thus, the best that can be done is to examine the difference between early and later weeks of data collection. Although comparisons across a two-week period of data collection did not reveal changes (Robinson & Price, 1980; Wills, Weiss, & Patterson, 1974), comparisons across four weeks of SOC data collection did show declines in Pleases for nondistressed couples (Margolin, 1981a) and declines in Displeases for distressed couples (Margolin & Weiss, 1978b).

Williams (1979) examined reactivity on the MSTL through the congruence of husbands' and wives' adjustment scores on the MAS. She hypothesized that the correlation between husband and wife MAS scores would increase as a function of behavioral recording in the home. Although high at pretest ($r = .85$), the MAS correlations increased significantly at posttest ($r = .91$), suggesting greater agreement after a home-based recording procedure. Williams also considered the possibility that adjustment scores, in general, would be affected by the recording procedures. Contrary to expectation, the MAS scores did not change; the husbands' scores on the Marital Conventionalization Scale (Edmonds, 1967), however, were significantly affected.

Volkin and Jacob (1981) systematically addressed the question of whether positive behaviors emitted by the monitoring spouse can lead to changes in observed behavior or changes in the recorder's overall evaluation of the marriage. These authors compared the impact of wives' monitoring under two conditions: where the husbands were aware and where the husbands were unaware of the monitoring procedure. One type of reactive effect would be that the husbands actually change the rate at which they emit positive behaviors. The comparison of aware and unaware husbands, however, revealed no such differences. The other reactivity manipulation examined the effects of drawing the wife's attention to her husband's positive behavior by measuring changes in her daily satisfaction, but, this manipulation also showed no reactivity.

Reactivity is also an issue in participant observation procedures in the laboratory. Here, however, we have to contend with the additional reactive effects concomitant with the laboratory situation (e.g., videotaping and having observers behind a one-way mirror). Thus far, there have been no direct tests of the reactivity of participant observation in the laboratory. In a study on observational bias, however, Vincent, Friedman, Nugent, and Messerly (1979) found that both distressed and nondistressed couples could "fake good" or "fake bad" in response to verbal instructions. Yet, in discussions more focused on the couple's actual problems, Cohen and Christensen (1980) found that nondistressed couples did not change their behavior when asked to act at their best and their worst. These results address only one aspect of the reactivity question for participant observation, that is, how couples present themselves in the interaction. How they may alter their ratings of themselves or how these alterations may be a function of the level of marital distress remains to be tested.

Validity

The validity of participant observation has been explored in several ways in the marital and family literature. First, as reported previously, construct validity has been evaluated by comparing distressed and nondistressed couples and families. Considerable evidence exists that distressed and nondistressed samples differ both on macrolevel measures, such as the SOC, the IR, the DBR, and the MSTL, and on more microlevel measures, such as Gottman's "talk table" and the Knudson *et al.* critical events inquiry. Concurrent validity, which has received an equal amount of attention, is determined by examining the correspondence between participant observation measurements and other measurement of marital adjustment, namely, nonparticipant observations or global self-reports.

Comparisons with Nonparticipant Observers. Data from nonparticipant observers has been used primarily to assess the validity of microlevel observation in the laboratory rather than macrolevel reports from the home setting. Robinson and Price (1980) provided one exception, however, in that they compared spouses' monitoring of themselves and one another on an abbreviated version of the SOC (positive behaviors only) with trained coders' monitoring of nine positive behaviors selected for home observation. The accuracy with which the couples recorded pleasurable behaviors varied according to their level of adjustment. Despite the small sample size, the couples high on marital adjustment were significantly more accurate than were the couples that were low on adjustment. Low-adjustment couples consistently underestimated the rate of pleasurable behavior by approximately 50%.

In the laboratory setting, increasing attention has been directed to exploring the correspondence between participant and nonparticipant observers when coding the same interaction samples. These comparisons examine the degree of overlap between the subjective, untrained participant observations of spouses and the objective, detailed observations of trained coders. Because untrained, emotionally involved couples are certainly not directly comparable to outside coders, the comparisons are best conceptualized as a measure of convergent validity rather than of interobserver reliability.

Gottman (1979) provided one such comparison between couples' perceptions on the talk table and coders' data on the affect portion of the CISS. According to Gottman, couples with higher marital satisfaction are likely to develop their own private message system and thus to agree less with outside observers. Although there was no statistical comparison, the percentage agreement scores between the nonclinical couples and the affect coders (.509) was somewhat lower than between the clinical couples and the same coders (.671). Floyd and Markman (1983) continued this line of inquiry with talk table ratings by comparing the mean levels of insider and outsider ratings. They reported that spouses' ratings of their partners' behavior were not consistent with observers' ratings of the partners' behaviors but observers' ratings were consistent with spouses' ratings of their own behavior. Moreover, as trained coders observed, distressed wives behaved the most negatively and produced the most negative ratings of their partners' behavior.

Weiss's 1 to 5 rating system (1984) for participant observation was compared to the Marital Interaction Coding System (MICS; Wieder & Weiss, 1980). Positive MICS behaviors correlated with couples' ratings of positive intervals ($r = .57$) and negative intervals ($r = -.42$). Negative MICS behaviors, however, did not correspond with couples' positive or negative ratings. Weiss's viewpoint that "couples and coders may be in agreement about positive behavior, yet hold different views about what is truly negative" (p. 17), was further borne out by the association between sequential patterns on the MICS and the couples' ratings. The MICS pattern of one proposal, followed by another proposal, was not viewed as a particularly helpful sequence by the couple. As part of this same study, Weiss et al. (1981) had couples rate separate positive and negative interactions involving other couples. Couples' median correlation with outside coders on the positive tape (.59) was higher than on their own tapes, but agreement on the negative tape ($-.01$) was exceptionally low.

To shed more light on these issues, Margolin et al. (1983) used kappa as the index of agreement on event-by-event comparisons between participant and nonparticipant observers. The major finding of this analysis is that agreement between couples and outside coders was higher on a standard tape (made by actors) than on the couples' own tape. In other words, the spouses perceived the interaction more similarly to outside coders when they themselves were not the target of the observation. In participant observation, however, when they were the target of observation, agreement with objective coders was quite low. Further inspection shows these data to be in accord with the Weiss et al. (1981) finding that differences between insider and outsider coders primarily surround negative behaviors. On the standard tape, when outside coders rated behavior as negative, the most likely response by the couple was a negative rating. Yet, on the couples' own tapes, when negative behavior was coded by outsiders, a positive rating was the most likely response by the couple. Either couples distort in a positive direction when viewing themselves, or their perceptions and recollections of the recent interaction simply are not as negative as the observations of an outsider.

Patterson (1982) reviewed the literature on the parallel question for parent–child relationships: What degree of correspondence exists between parents' observations of parent–child interaction and an outsider's observations of the same interaction? Describing a preliminary study by Peine (1970), Patterson reported that mothers, compared to outside observers dramatically underestimated the level of deviancy. In a replication of that study, Patterson found, similarly, that mothers underestimated the frequency of most behavioral events when observing their own parent–child interaction. Yet, similar to the marital couples' observations of a neutral stimulus rather than their own interaction, mothers' observations of other mother–child dyads was much closer to the rates recorded by observers. Lorber, Reid, Felton, and Caesar (1982) explored how mothers' errors in tracking behavior may be related to their own behavior. They found that abusive mothers' behavioral tracking skills, as assessed by an analogue task, was significantly related to mothers' actual rates of emitted aversive behaviors *in vivo*, the rate of the abused child's emission of aversive behavior, the mothers' reaction to the child's behavior, and the mothers' self-reports of tension while viewing the stimulus child. These findings lend support to Patterson's prediction (1982) that future studies will demonstrate that parents of problem children may be highly selective in their errors of tracking and labeling behavior as deviant.

Comparisons with Global Measures of Marital Satisfaction. The other commonly cited validity evidence is the correspondence between participant observation measures and global measures of satisfaction. Because the same respondent is the source of data for both these measures, the question being examined is the degree to which long-standing relationship reactions, as measured by global indices of satisfaction and stability, relate to participant observation.

Weiss (1984) presented the most detailed analysis of microlevel participant observation and global satisfaction. He found, for example, that the Dyadic Adjustment Scale (a well-researched measurement of satisfaction), the Marital Status Inventory (a measurement of marital stability), and the Love–Liking Scale (another measure of overall relationship sentiment) all correlated with impact ratings. Weiss also explored how positive and negative impact ratings on a particular discussion correlated with spouses' one-time rating of that same discussion. As anticipated, the 15-second ratings were closely associated with the one-time ratings of satisfaction with the discussion and with an evaluation of progress in that discussion. Weiss's work strongly suggests that participant observation measurements of communication impact are associated with overall marital satisfaction as well as with satisfaction with the particular conversation.

The concurrent validity between molar participant-observation measures and global satisfaction ratings has been computed in two ways: through correlations with one-time measures of satisfaction and through correlations with daily measures of satisfaction. The association is stronger in the second type of correlation than in the first because of the similarity in the size of the behavioral unit. Christensen and Nies (1980), for example, found no significant correlations between the modified SOC and the MAS but did find significant correlations between the SOC and daily happiness ratings.

My own data on this question have been somewhat mixed. On a sample of disturbed couples only (Margolin, 1978), Pleases but not Displeases correlated with MAS scores. Yet, on a sample of both distressed and nondistressed couples, Margolin and Wampold (1981) found the MAS to correlate positively with SOC Pleases and negatively with SOC Displeases. A more recent study by Margolin, Talovic, and Weinstein (1983) correlated the SOC with the Areas of Change Questionnaire (AC), another one-time measure of satisfaction. For women, SOC total Displeases correlated significantly with AC measure of Desired Change and Perceived Change. No significant correlations were found, however, for men.

Data holding more relevance for clinical interventions come from the exploration of SOC data and daily satisfactions ratings. To what extent do daily reports of pleasing and displeasing behaviors account for fluctuations in daily ratings of marital satisfaction? Wills *et al.* (1974), the first to explore this question, conducted regression analyses on 12 consecutive days of data from seven nondistressed couples. Five predictor variables from the SOC (Affectionate Pleases and Displeases, Instrumental Pleases and Displeases, and Quality of Outside Interaction) collectively accounted for 25% of the variance in the spouses' daily satisfaction. Jacobson, Waldron, and Moore (1980) found negative behaviors, particularly negative verbal interactions, to be strongly associated with fluctuations in daily satisfaction for distressed spouses. In contrast, positive behaviors, particularly shared recreational events for husbands and positive communication for wives, were most predictive of daily satisfaction ratings for nondistressed couples. Margolin (1981a) also found that distressed, compared to nondistressed, couples were influenced by the occurrence of Displeases. These findings, however, revealed no differences in the effect of pleasing behaviors on satisfaction. Finally, in the most recent study on this topic, Jacobson and his colleagues (Jacobson, Follette, & McDonald, 1982) found that distressed spouses were significantly more reactive than nondistressed spouses to their partners' positive behaviors as well as to their negative behaviors. Taken as a whole, these data lend considerable support to the impact of negative behaviors on daily satisfaction ratings for distressed couples. Whether distressed and nondistressed couples differ in the extent to which positive behaviors affect their overall satisfaction still remains an open question.

Overall, there is strong evidence of the discriminant validity of most participant observation measures as seen in comparisons between distressed and nondistressed samples. Data are more sparse and less consistent on the question of concurrent validity. Correlations with global measures of marital satisfaction, although often significant, are not particularly strong. Indices of agreement with nonparticipant observers are even less convincing, particularly with respect to the coding of negative behaviors.

Before leaving validity considerations, a brief comment is in order about predictive validity. The only data regarding predictive validity are found in Markman's work (1979, 1981) on the talk table. As stated previously, he found impact ratings to be predictive of overall satisfaction at 2½- and 5-year follow-ups. Overall, however, predictive validity, which holds the most important key to understanding marital and family distress, has been neglected. It is important to determine whether the patterns that we observe through participant observation measures are simply descriptive of marital distress or are related to the etiology of distress. Thus far, the data point to concomitants of marital distress. Variables associated with a change in status from nondistressed to distressed are still to be identified.

FUTURE DIRECTIONS

The procedures that have been reviewed in this chapter represent only the tip of the iceberg of what can be assessed through participant observation. Because these procedures have been designed to answer specific research questions, their general applicability and clinical utility are yet to be determined. For the most part, specific methodologies within the participant observation framework have been paired with specific questions; for example, moment-to-moment ratings have been adopted as the principal way of examining communication process. It is important to emphasize, however, that these pairings are not the only nor necessarily even the best options for addressing important questions in marital and family assessment. This final section suggests how participant observation can further advance our knowledge of marital and family therapy processes and integrate with our treatment efforts.

Macrolevel Assessment in the Laboratory and Microlevel Assessment at Home

There are a number of practical reasons that microlevel observation has been relegated to the laboratory setting and macrolevel observation has been relegated to the home (e.g., laboratories, and not homes, are equipped with videotape; sessions in the laboratory are time-limited, thereby restricting the molarity of the patterns that occur; and couples may not be able to engage in the evaluation of microlevel patterns without the constant supervision of a therapist or an experimenter). Yet, despite the practicalities, much can be learned by generalizing methodologies across settings.

The laboratory procedures currently in use focus attention on relatively minute behaviors. Procedures such as the moment-to-moment ratings provide a standard measure that can be repeated over time and that can be used to compare couples. These ratings, however, should be augmented by having couples interpret the ratings by describing the larger context. More important than knowing that a certain segment is a "5" or a "1" is knowing why the interval was rated that way. Having spouses specify the cues that lead to the rating (e.g., "She stopped looking at me" or "He changed the topic") is a start toward understanding what is important in a couple's communication. Having spouses aggregate data even further—that is, looking for the connections that pair one person's action with the other person's reaction—is the next step. Probing questions can be asked that direct the participants' attention to the impact of their behavior on one another or to the connections between behaviors, thoughts, and feelings. The basic unit of analysis, although still relatively detailed, would represent an interaction sequence rather than an isolated behavior or reaction.

Currently, in my own laboratory, spouses are asked to take the "spectator" role when watching themselves on videotape and to teach the examiner what is important in their communications: What are the important turning points? What patterns do they see that are either typical or atypical? We are finding, of course, that individuals vary in their abilities to categorize, label, and articulate patterns that are important to them. Some persons reflect on patterns that they were aware of during the original conversation, whereas others see the interaction from an entirely new stance as they watch themselves on tape. What has been surprising is how often what the spouses report differs from the observations of the nonparticipant observers, in this case, the impressions of trained clinicians. In one such case, the husband had just started to mimic the wife's gestures and tone of voice. The clinician figured that the husband's actions probably infuriated the wife. As the wife and the clinician watched the replay of the tape, the wife spontaneously commented on that particular incident: "I just love it when he does that. Sometimes I get so carried away on a point and then he does something that helps me see how ridiculous it's become. This really loosens me up." This comment, which in this case came from a nondistressed wife, illustrated the important point that behaviors can have very different meanings across relationships. My colleagues and I are still figuring out how to code these open-ended responses. It is evident, however, that they are a rich source of data and point out important patterns that are not obvious to an outside observer.

Alternatively, microlevel observations may be important in the home setting. The rapid escalation of arguments is a phenomenon familiar to all marital and family therapists. Home data that capture only the molar units (e.g., "We had an argument") do not provide a sufficiently detailed analysis of these events. There are at least two possibilities for a more in-depth exploration of such events. A critical events approach offers one possibility. After each argument, for example, spouses could write down or dictate into a tape recorder their answers to a prearranged series of questions. A second possibility is to tape-record the actual arguments so that there is a record that the spouses can examine in detail later. Based on Gottman's data (1980) comparing communication samples made at home to samples made in the laboratory, there is substantially more negativity in the home setting, where spouses are surrounded with familiar cues. These data underscore the importance of submitting home data to the fine-grained analysis typically done in the laboratory.

Greater Focus on Family Interaction

Participant observation has been used predominantly to assess marital, as opposed to family, interaction. When it is used in a family context, there has been a tendency for the mother to be the primary, if not the sole, reporter.

These tendencies maintain two unfortunate biases: (a) that children cannot be relied on for data collection and (b) that fathers' contribution to the data collection process is less important than mothers'. It is suggested, instead, that children aged 8 and older can, indeed, be taught how to monitor their own behaviors or parent–child interactions. Children, just as adults, vary in the extent to which they can reflect on their own actions and in the extent to which they may distort data in a face-saving direction. Obviously, the recording procedures for children must take into account their developmental level and are likely to be more specific and concrete than those for some adults. Having the child collect data, however, offers an alternative perspective to the family members as well as to the therapist. Making use of those data in the therapy session communicates to the child that his or her observations and opinions play an important role in therapeutic decisions.

Likewise, including fathers in participant observation communicates that the father's involvement is important. One of the frequent characteristics of stressed families is that the parents have different ideas about parenting roles, different perceptions of what actually occurs in the family, or different values about what is appropriate child behavior. Having parents monitor the interactional patterns makes it possible to sort out and discuss these differences on the basis of actual data. The data may demonstrate, for example, that the child is actually more noncompliant with one parent than with the other, and that, furthermore, the parents respond differently to the noncompliance. Relying solely on the reports of one parent subtly conveys that that parent is more responsible for the family problems and more responsible for making therapy work.

The Identification of Different Types of Family Problems

The contrasted-groups approach of comparing distressed with nondistressed couples and families gives, at best, limited evidence for the utility of participant observation. This approach, although common across all forms of marital and family assessment, does not do justice to the different types of family pathology. Because the same interaction patterns would not be expected from an enmeshed versus a distancing family, we lose information when all dysfunctional families are collapsed into one group. Williams's data (1979) nicely illustrated this point when two distressed couples sent inordinate amounts of time together, compared with other distressed couples that rarely saw each other. She happened upon two very different types of marital distress.

Unfortunately, an adequate system for categorizing family pathology is still lacking. Nonetheless, as the clinical literature makes frequent reference to distinctions between different types of family dysfunction, these distinctions should not be ignored in our attempts to validate participant observation measures. Although participant observation measures are designed to measure more refined constructs than simply whether a couple is distressed, validity studies have not progressed beyond the stage of examining to what degree the participant observation measure is associated with overall adjustment. It is recommended that more attention be paid to different subtypes of family problems, and that participant observation be used to compare and contrast the interaction patterns that characterize these different subgroups.

SUMMARY

This chapter reviews the theoretical basis for participant observation, describes the procedures currently in use, and examines the supporting data for these procedures. There is substantial evidence that these procedures accurately discriminate well-adjusted from disturbed family systems. There is, however, less evidence for the general applicability or the clinical utility of these measures. The range of procedures that fall under the rubric of *participant observation* varies considerably, from moment-to-moment observation in the laboratory to once-per-day charting of behaviors and events at home. The range of possibilities for participant observations is limited only by the creativity of the investigator and the client or subject. As indicated by the procedures reviewed here, the core ingredient of participant observation is viewing our research subjects and clients as also being experts, and colleagues. Rather than relying strictly on outsiders' impressions of overt family transactions, we enlist the assistance of family members to help us understand their particular brand of marital or family disturbance. Mischel (1977) wisely advised, "if we don't stop them by asking the wrong questions, and if we provide appropriate structure, they often can tell us much about themselves and, indeed, about psychology itself" (p. 249).

REFERENCES

Barnett, L. R., & Nietzel, M. T. (1979). Relationship of instrumental and affectional behaviors and self-esteem to marital satisfaction in distressed and nondistressed couples. *Journal of Consulting and Clinical Psychology, 47*, 946–957.

Bernal, M. E., Klinnert, M. D., Russell, M. B., Schultz, L. A., Bolstad, C., Rosen, P. M., North, J. A., & Chao, C. (1978). *Parent telephone interviews: Normative data on an economical procedure for assessment of conduct problem children.* Unpublished manuscript.

Bernal, M. E., Klinnert, M. D., & Schultz, L. A. (1980). Outcome evaluation of behavioral parent training and client-centered parent counseling for children with conduct problems. *Journal of Applied Behavior Analysis, 13*, 677–691.

Berscheid, E. (1983). Emotion. In H. H. Kelley, E. Berscheid, A. Christensen, J. H. Harvey, T. L. Huston, G. Levinger, E. McClintock, L. A. Peplau, & D. R. Peterson (Eds.), *The psychology of close relationships.* San Francisco: W. H. Freeman.

Birchler, G. R., Weiss, R. L., & Vincent, J. P. (1975). Multimethod analysis of social reinforcement exchange between maritally distressed and nondistressed spouse and stranger dyads. *Journal of Personality and Social Psychology, 31*, 349–360.

Boice, R. (1983). Observational skills. *Psychological Bulletin, 93*, 3–29.

Christensen, A., & Margolin, G. (1981, August). *Correlational and sequential analysis of marital and child problems.* Paper presented at the American Psychological Association Convention, Los Angeles.

Christensen, A., & Nies, D. C. (1980). The Spouse Observation Checklist: Empirical analysis and critique. *American Journal of Family Therapy, 8*, 69–79.

Christensen, A., Sullaway, M., & King, C. E. (1983). Systematic error in behavioral reports of dyadic interaction: Egocentric bias and content effects. *Behavioral Assessment, 5,* 131–142.

Ciminero, A. R., Nelson, R. O., & Lipinski, D. P. (1977). Self-monitoring procedures in behavioral assessment. In A. R. Ciminero, K. S. Calhoun, & H. E. Adams (Eds.), *Handbook of behavioral assessment.* New York: Wiley.

Cohen, R. S., & Christensen, A. (1980). Further examination of demand characteristics in marital interaction. *Journal of Consulting and Clinical Psychology, 48,* 121–123.

Doherty, W. (1981a). Cognitive processes in intimate conflict: 1. Extending attribution theory. *American Journal of Family Therapy, 9(1),* 3–12.

Doherty, W. (1981b). Cognitive processes in intimate conflict: 2. Efficacy and learned helplessness. *American Journal of Family Therapy, 9(2),* 35–44.

Dumas, J. E., & Whaler, R. G. (1983). Predictors of treatment outcome in parent training: Mother insularity and socioeconomic disadvantage. *Behavioral Assessment, 5,* 301–314.

Edmonds, V. H. (1967). Marital conventionalization: Definition and measurement. *Journal of Marriage and the Family, 29,* 681–688.

Elwood, R. W., & Jacobson, N. S. (1982). Spouses' agreement in reporting their behavioral interactions: A clinical replication. *Journal of Consulting and Clinical Psychology, 50,* 783–784.

Epstein, N. (1982). Cognitive therapy with couples. *American Journal of Family Therapy, 10,* 5–16.

Ericsson, F. A., & Simon, H. A. (1980). Verbal reports as data. *Psychological Review, 87,* 215–251.

Floyd, F. J., & Markman, H. J. (1981). *Insiders and outsiders assessment of distressed and nondistressed marital interaction.* Paper presented at the meeting of the Association for the Advancement of Behavior Therapy, Toronto.

Floyd, F. J., & Markman, H. J. (1983). Observational biases in spouse observation: Toward a cognitive/behavioral model of marriage. *Journal of Consulting and Clinical Psychology, 51,* 450–457.

Floyd, F. J., & Markman, H. J. (1984). An economical observational measure of couples communication skill. *Journal of Consulting and Clinical Psychology, 52,* 97–103.

Gottman, J. M. (1979). *Marital interaction: Experimental investigations.* New York: Academic Press.

Gottman, J. M. (1980). Consistency of nonverbal affect and affect reciprocity in marital interaction. *Journal of Consulting and Clinical Psychology, 48,* 711–717.

Gottman, J. M., & Porterfield, A. L. (1981). Communicative competence in the nonverbal behavior of married couples. *Journal of Marriage and the Family, 43,* 817–824.

Gottman, J., Notarius, C., Markman, H., Banks, S., Yoppi, B., & Rubin, M. E. (1976). Behavior exchange theory and marital decision making. *Journal of Personality and Social Psychology, 34,* 14–23.

Huston, T. L., & Robins, E. (1982). Conceptual and methodological issues in studying close relationships. *Journal of Marriage and the Family, 44,* 901–925.

Jacobson, N. S. (1979). Increasing positive behavior in severely distressed marital relationships: The effects of problem-solving training. *Behavior Therapy, 10,* 311–326.

Jacobson, N. S. (1984). The modification of cognitive processes in behavioral marital therapy: Integrating cognitive and behavioral intervention strategies. In N. S. Jacobson & K. Hahlweg (Eds.), *Marital interaction: Analysis and modification.* New York: Guilford Press.

Jacobson, N. S., & Margolin, G. (1979). *Marital therapy: Strategies based on social learning and behavior exchange principles.* New York: Bruner/Mazel.

Jacobson, N. S., & Moore, D. (1981). Spouses as observers of the events in their relationship. *Journal of Consulting and Clinical Psychology, 49,* 269–277.

Jacobson, N. S., Waldron, H., & Moore, D. (1980). Toward a behavioral profile of marital distress. *Journal of Consulting and Clinical Psychology, 48,* 696–703.

Jacobson, N. S., Elwood, R., & Dallas, M. (1981). The behavioral assessment of marital dysfunction. In D. H. Barlow (Ed.), *Behavioral assessment of adult disorders.* New York: Guilford Press.

Jacobson, N. S., Follette, W. C., & McDonald, D. W. (1982). Reactivity to positive and negative behavior in distressed and nondistressed married couples. *Journal of Consulting and Clinical Psychology, 50,* 706–714.

Knudson, R. M., Sommers, A. A., & Golding, S. L. (1980). Interpersonal perception and mode of resolution in marital conflict. *Journal of Personality and Social Psychology, 38,* 751–763.

Lipinski, D., & Nelson, R. (1974). The reactivity and unreliability of self-recording. *Journal of Consulting and Clinical Psychology, 42,* 118–123.

Lorber, R., Reid, J. B., Felton, D., & Caesar, R. (1982, November). *Behavioral tracking skills of child abuse parents and their relationships to family violence.* Paper presented at the meeting of the Association for the Advancement of Behavior Therapy, Los Angeles.

Margolin, G. (1978). A multilevel approach to the assessment of communication positiveness in distressed marital couples. *International Journal of Family Counseling, 6,* 81–89.

Margolin, G. (1981a). Behavior exchange in distressed and nondistressed marriages: A family cycle perspective. *Behavior Therapy, 12,* 329–343.

Margolin, G. (1981b). The reciprocal relationship between marital and child problems. In J. P. Vincent (Ed.), *Advances in family intervention assessment and theory: An annual compilation of research* (Vol. 2). Greenwich, CT: JAI Press.

Margolin, G. (1983a). An interactional model for the assessment of marital relationships. *Behavioral Assessment, 5,* 103–127.

Margolin, G. (1983b). *Marital conflict: Interpersonal and intrapersonal factors* (Continuation report on NIMH Grant 1RO1 36595).

Margolin, G., & Jacobson, N. S. (1981). The assessment of marital dysfunction. In M. Hersen & A. S. Bellack (Eds.), *Behavioral assessment: A practical handbook.* New York: Pergamon Press.

Margolin, G., & Wampold, B. E. (1981). A sequential analysis of conflict and accord in distressed and nondistressed marital partners. *Journal of Consulting and Clinical Psychology, 49,* 554–567.

Margolin, G., & Weinstein, C. D. (1983). The role of affect in behavioral marital therapy. In M. L. Aronson & L. R. Wolberg (Eds.), *Group and family therapy 1982: An overview.* New York: Brunner/Mazel.

Margolin, G., & Weiss, R. L. (1978a). Communication training and assessment: a case of behavioral marital enrichment. *Behavior Therapy, 9,* 508–520.

Margolin, G., & Weiss, R. L. (1978b). Comparative evaluation of therapeutic components associated with behavioral marital treatment. *Journal of Consulting and Clinical Psychology, 46,* 1467–1486.

Margolin, G., Talovic, S., & Weinstein, C. D. (1983). Areas of Change Questionnaire: A practical approach to marital assessment. *Journal of Consulting and Clinical Psychology, 51,* 920–931.

Margolin, G., Hattem, D., John, R. S., & Yost, K. (1985). Perceptual agreement between spouses and outside observers when coding themselves and a stranger dyad. *Behavioral Assessment, 7,* 235–247.

Markman, H. J. (1979). Application of a behavioral model of marriage in predicting relationship satisfaction of couples planning marriage. *Journal of Consulting and Clinical Psychology, 47,* 743–749.

Markman, H. J. (1981). Prediction of marital distress: A 5-year follow-up. *Journal of Consulting and Clinical Psychology, 49,* 760–762.

Markman, H. J. (1982, November). *Couples' observation of their own communication: Implications for prevention and treatment of marital distress.* Paper presented at the meeting of the Association for the Advancement of Behavior Therapy, Los Angeles.

Markman, H. J., & Poltrock, S. (1982). A computerized system for recording and analysis of self-observations of couples' interaction. *Behavior Research Methods and Instrumentation, 14,* 186–190.

McClintock, E. (1983). Interaction. In H. H. Kelley, E. Berscheid, A. Christensen, J. H. Harvey, T. L. Huston, G. Levinger, E. McClintock, L. A. Peplau, D. R. Petersen (Eds.), *The psychology of close relationships.* San Francisco: W. H. Freeman.

Mischel, W. (1973). Toward a cognitive social learning reconceptualization of personality. *Psychological Review, 80,* 252–283.

Mischel, W. (1977). On the future of personality assessment. *American Psychologist, 32,* 246–254.

Nisbett, R. E., & Wilson, T. D. (1977). Telling more than we can know: Verbal reports on mental process. *Psychological Review, 84,* 231–259.

Notarius, C. I., Vanzetti, N. A., & Smith, R. J. (1981, November). *Assessing expectations and outcomes in marital interaction.* Paper presented at the meeting of the Association for the Advancement of Behavior Therapy, Toronto.

Paquin, M. J. R. (1981). Self-monitoring of marital communication in family therapy. *Social Casework: The Journal of Contemporary Social Work,* pp. 267–272.

Patterson, G. R. (1982). *Coercive family processes.* Eugene, OR: Castalia.

Patterson, G. R., Hops, H., & Weiss, R. L. (1974). A social learning approach to reducing rates of marital conflict. In R. Stuart, R. Liberman, & S. Wilder (Eds.), *Advances in behavior therapy*. New York: Academic Press.

Patterson, G. R., Reid, J. B., Jones, R. R., & Conger, R. E. (1975). *A social learning approach to family intervention: Vol. 1. Families with aggressive children*. Eugene, OR: Castalia.

Peine, H. (1970). *Behavioral recording by parents and its resultant consequences*. Unpublished master's thesis, University of Utah, Salt Lake City.

Peterson, D. R. (1977). A plan for studying interpersonal behavior. In D. Magnusson & N. Endler (Eds.), *Personality at the crossroads: Current issues in interactional psychology*. New York: Wiley.

Peterson, D. R. (1979). Assessing interpersonal relationships by means of interaction records. *Behavioral Assessment, 1,* 221–236.

Protzner, M., King, C., & Christensen, A. (1981). *Naturalistic interaction of married couples: A descriptive analysis*. Paper presented at the Western Psychological Association meeting, Los Angeles.

Rappoport, A. F., & Harrell, J. (1972). A behavioral exchange model for marital counseling. *Family Coordinator, 22,* 203–212.

Robinson, E. A., & Price, M. G. (1980). Pleasurable behavior in marital intervention: An observational study. *Journal of Consulting and Clinical Psychology, 48,* 117–118.

Sager, C. (1976). *Marriage contracts and couple therapy: Hidden forces in intimate relationships*. New York: Brunner/Mazel.

Sullaway, M., & Christensen, A. (1983). Couples and families as participant observers of their interaction. In J. P. Vincent (Ed.), *Advances in family intervention assessment and theory*. Greenwich, CT: JAI Press.

Thomas, E. J., Carter, R. D., & Gambrill, E. D. (1971). Some possibilities of behavior modification with marital problems using "SAM" (signal system for the assessment and modification of behavior). In R. D. Rubin, H. Fensterheim, A. Lazarus, & C. M. Franks (Eds.), *Advances in behavior therapy*. New York: Academic Press.

Tyron, W. W. (1979). The test-trait fallacy. *American Psychologist, 34,* 402–406.

Vincent, J. P., Friedman, L. C. Nugent, J., & Messerly, L. (1979). Demand characteristics in observations of marital interaction. *Journal of Consulting and Clinical Psychology, 47,* 557–566.

Volkin, J. I., & Jacob, T. (1981). The impact of spouse monitoring on target behavior and recorder satisfaction. *Journal of Behavioral Assessment, 3,* 99–109.

Wahler, R. G. (1980). The insular mother: Her problems in parent–child treatment. *Journal of Applied Behavior Analysis, 13,* 207–219.

Weiss, R. L. (1980). Strategic behavioral marital therapy: Toward a model for assessment and intervention. In J. P. Vincent (Ed.), *Advances in family intervention, assessment, and theory: An annual compilation of research* (Vol. 1). Greenwich, CT: JAI Press.

Weiss, R. L. (1984). Cognitive and behavioral measures of marital interaction. In N. S. Jacobson & K. Hahlweg (Eds.), *Marital interaction: Analysis and modification*. New York: Guilford Press.

Weiss, R. L., & Margolin, G. (in press). Assessment of conflict and accord: A second look. In A. Ciminero (Ed.), *Handbook of behavioral assessment* (Vol. 2). New York: Wiley.

Weiss, R. L., & Perry, B. A. (1979). *Assessment and treatment of marital dysfunction*. Eugene, OR: University of Oregon and Oregon Marital Studies Program.

Weiss, R. L., Hops, H., & Patterson, G. R. (1973). A framework for conceptualizing marital conflict, a technology for altering it, some data for evaluating it. In L. A. Hamerlynck, L. C. Handy, & E. J. Mash (Eds.), *Behavior change: Methodology, concepts, and practice*. Champaign, IL: Research Press.

Weiss, R. L., Wasserman, D. A., Wieder, G. R., & Summers, K. (1981, November). *Subjective and objective evaluation of marital conflict: Couples vs. the establishment*. Paper presented at the 15th Annual Convention of the Association for the Advancement of Behavior Therapy, Toronto.

Wieder, G. B., & Weiss, R. L. (1980). Generalizability theory and the coding of marital interactions. *Journal of Consulting Psychology, 48,* 469–477.

Wiggins, J. S. (1973). *Personality and prediction: Principles of personality assessment*. Reading, MA: Addison-Wesley.

Williams, A. M. (1979). The quantity and quality of marital interaction related to marital satisfaction: A behavioral analysis. *Journal of Applied Behavior Analysis, 12,* 665–678.

Wills, T. A., Weiss, R. L., & Patterson, G. R. (1974). A behavioral analysis of the determinants of marital satisfaction. *Journal of Consulting and Clinical Psychology, 42,* 802–811.

CHAPTER 11

Self-Report Instruments for Family Assessment

HARVEY A. SKINNER

There are many approaches to the assessment of family functioning. Popular techniques include the unstructured clinical interview (Fitzgerald, 1973); focused or structured interviews (Watzlawick, 1966); projective tests (Elbert, Rosman, Minuchin, & Guerney, 1964); self-report instruments (Moos & Moos, 1981); and performance on experimental tasks such as the revealed-difference technique (Jacob, 1975). The various methods differ with respect to their focus on past events versus the assessment of ongoing behavior. Also, there is considerable debate regarding how much emphasis should be placed on examining the characteristics of individual family members, their various interactions, or the family system as a whole (Bodin, 1968; Gurman & Kniskern, 1981; Lebow, 1981). Because each perspective may provide unique as well as corroborating information on areas of health or pathology in the family, there are obvious advantages in attempts to integrate these viewpoints. However, practical constraints and different theoretical orientations of staff often result in the use of a more circumscribed approach to family assessments in a given setting.

This diversity reflects both the presence of a number of competing theories and the multidisciplinary nature of family therapy and research. Adherents to a given theoretical persuasion tend to emphasize a selected scope of variables. This emphasis can cause difficulties in communication among the various "schools" of clinicians and researchers who are actively engaged in family work. According to Fox (1976), "it is often difficult to compare the kinds of families and family problems being treated by different types of family therapists, much less develop a uniform system of classification" (p. 461). In addition, problems have been noted in the links between family theory and measurement. Several recent articles have underscored the need for a better integration of theories of family

---

HARVEY A. SKINNER • Addiction Research Foundation, 33 Russell Street, Toronto, Ontario, Canada M5S 2S1.

functioning and corresponding assessment techniques (Cromwell & Peterson, 1983; Fisher, 1982; Reiss, 1983; Schumm, 1982).

The aims of this chapter are twofold. First, a general framework for test development is described. Based on the principles of construct validation, the framework emphasizes an active interplay between theory formulation and test construction. Second, the framework is used as a basis for evaluating three popular self-report assessment techniques, including the Family Environment Scale (Moos & Moos, 1981), the Family Adaptability and Cohesion Scales (Olson, Portner, & Lavee, 1985), and the Family Assessment Measure (Skinner, Steinhauer, & Santa-Barbara, 1983).

TEST DEVELOPMENT FRAMEWORK

The history of structured assessment has witnessed a progression from (a) a rational approach with little or no empirical analyses to (b) an empirical strategy that largely set aside theoretical considerations until after the test was constructed, and finally to (c) the construct validation viewpoint that integrates theory formulation with test construction (Wiggins, 1973). This progression is exemplified by the Personal Data Sheet (Woodworth, 1917), the Minnesota Multiphasic Personality Inventory (Hathaway & McKinley, 1951), and the Personality Research Form (Jackson, 1974), respectively. The principles of construct validation provide a powerful methodology for the development and evaluation of theory-based assessment tools (Campbell & Fiske, 1959; Cronbach & Meehl, 1955; Embretson, 1983; Jackson, 1971; Loevinger, 1957; Messick, 1981; Skinner, 1981, 1984).

A synopsis of the construct validation approach is given in Table 1. Basically, the *theoretical component* involves an explicit definition of each construct as well as specification of functional links among constructs in the model of family functioning (nomological network). Given these construct definitions, the next step is to generate a large pool of items that are rated according to their clarity, their content saturation, and their clinical relevance. The *structural component* entails the development and the empirical evaluation of a preliminary version of the instrument. The test should be administered to relevant samples, and various statistical analyses should be conducted in order to evaluate item properties, scale reliabilities, and intercorrelations. The outcome of these analyses should be a revised and possibly much briefer version of the instrument. The *external validation* component involves a series of studies aimed at establishing the validity properties of the instrument. These studies should establish the degree of convergence among alternative methods of assessing the theoretical constructs, should evaluate the predictive power of the instrument with respect to family therapy outcome, should compare the instrument with other family assessment measures, and should explore the clinical relevance of profiles derived from the instrument.

TABLE 1. Construct Validation Strategy for Test Development

1.   Theoretical Component
     (a) Prepare a precise definition of each construct
     (b) Specify structural relationships among constructs in the theory (nomological network)
     (c) Generate a large pool of items
     (d) Choose items for preliminary scales

2.   Structural Component
     (a) Administer preliminary scales to relevant samples
     (b) Conduct statistical analyses to evaluate item and scale measurement properties
     (c) Select "best" items for each scale

3.   External Validation Component
     (a) Compare scales with expert clinical ratings and behavioral observations (*construct validity*)
     (b) Evaluate prognostic value of scales with respect to treatment outcome (*predictive validity*)
     (c) Examine correlation of scales with other family-assessment instruments (*concurrent validity*)
     (d) Determine the perceived relevance of profiles to family therapists (*clinical validity*)

Theoretical Component

What constitutes a scientific theory, and why should a theory of family functioning be developed in the first place? A model may be thought of as a set of constructs with hypothesized connections among them (a nomological network). Based on the model, certain inferences may be drawn and predictions made. When enough constructs are linked to empirical data through rules of correspondence or operational definitions, then the model becomes a *scientific theory* with elements that are open to empirical evaluation. In his doctrine of falsifiability, Popper (1972) argued that the essential aspect of a "scientific" theory is that it suggests refutation rather than proof. Empirical evidence is valuable for its power to falsify hypotheses. Theoretical conjectures and auxiliaries are corroborated to the extent that they have survived increasingly risky tests (Meehl, 1978).

According to Harre (1972), models serve both logical and epistemological functions. As a heuristic, a model helps to simplify phenomena, to make the problem more readily handled, and to stimulate new research directions. During the formative stages of scientific enquiry, models are useful primarily for their descriptive power in organizing a set of nonrandom observations. As scientific disciplines mature, emphasis shifts from the description of events to the establishment of explanatory theories (Hempel, 1965). Here, models are used as an explanation or representation of the real causal mechanism that underlies the phenomena. Perhaps the best example of this process is the periodic system of elements, which began with preliminary groupings, such as potassium and sodium, because of observations about their common characteristics; was then systematized by Mendeleev in his formulation of the periodic table; and was subsequently refined through understanding of atomic structure and chemical valency.

The first section of this book provides a description of various theoretical orientations to family studies of psychopathology. Earlier reviews of family theory have pointed out that either the structural-functional or interactional models have tended to be most popular, followed by the developmental framework (Cerny, Dahl, Kamiko, & Aldous, 1974; Klein, Calvert, Garland, & Poloma, 1969). A more recent review has indicated that the field is beginning to develop integrative conceptual models that expand on and refine existing theories (Olson, Russell, & Sprenkle, 1980). For instance, there would appear to be increasing support for the three constructs of cohesion, adaptability, and communication. Similarly, Fisher (1976) identified five common dimensions in his review of family assessment: (a) structural descriptors (e.g., roles, boundaries); (b) controls and sanctions (e.g., flexibility); (c) emotions and needs (e.g., affective expression); (d) cultural aspects (e.g., social position); and (e) developmental aspects (e.g., life stage). Thus, there would appear to be increasing consensus about important constructs to be assessed in family functioning, even though there may be wide disagreement among various "schools" about the developmental processes involved and the interrelationships among these concepts.

Another trend is the increased focus on integrating the presenting symptoms of psychopathology (e.g., alcoholism) with family system dynamics. Russell, Olson, Sprenkle, and Atilano (1983) proposed the concept of *functional consequences* as a means of linking presenting symptoms to family interaction. For example, excessive drinking may function to facilitate the expression of warmth and caring between spouses (Steinglass, Davis, & Berenson, 1977). Gurman and Kniskern (1981) discussed the levels of inference involved in assessment when moving from the individual to system properties. Similarly, Cromwell and Peterson (1983) described a multisystem—multimethod framework for conceptualizing and assessing different levels of the family system. This framework (Table 2) proposes a hierarchy of relationships (individual, dyadic, and family system) and their assessment by alternative methods (e.g., self-report, therapist ratings, and

TABLE 2. Multisystem—Multimethod Framework[a]

Assessment method	Family level		
	Individual	Dyad	Family system
Self-report			
Therapist ratings			
Behavior observations			

[a]Adapted from Cromwell and Peterson (1983).

behavioral observations). However, Reiss (1983) criticized the framework on several counts and called for more specific theory and instruments linking family processes and individual behaviors. In a subsequent clarification, Peterson and Cromwell (1983) defended their logic for integrating family assessment, systems thinking, and clinical interventions.

To provide a concrete illustration of the construct validation approach to test construction, a series of practical steps is outlined in the appendix to this chapter. These guidelines have evolved from work on the development of the Family Assessment Measure (Skinner *et al.*, 1983). The guidelines are useful as a "cookbook" for guiding the construction of new instruments, as well as for evaluating the merits and limitations of existing instruments for family assessments.

Structural Component

This component addresses internal properties of the instrument (e.g., item–scale correlations and scale reliabilities and intercorrelations), as well as the extent to which the item properties conform to a particular structural model. The *cumulative* measurement model is the most widely used method of combining items into a single-scale score (Wiggins, 1973). A central assumption is that the number of items endorsed provides an index of the degree of the underlying construct that is present. For example, with the hypothetical construct of affective expression, one might order individuals along a continuum (low–high affective expression) according to the number of items endorsed that reflected the range, timing, and intensity of their feelings and emotions. Items are generally selected to optimize scale homogeneity (inter-item correlation), and to form a predominantly undimensional scale.

Various steps involved in the structural component are outlined in the appendix. Jackson (1970, 1971) and Nunnally (1978) provided details regarding the statistical analyses. Basically, one wants to select a subset of "good" items from the preliminary item pool. A good item should correlate highly with its own scale and should correlate minimally with other content scales and measures of response-style biases. The field of personality assessment has expended considerable research on the influences of response styles, such as social desirability, defensiveness, acquiescence, and carelessness (Wiggins, 1973). Unless these response styles are minimized in an instrument, one will have difficulty in supporting a content interpretation of a given scale. Response-style issues have also received attention in family therapy research and practice, for example, pseudomutuality and denial (Gurman & Kniskern, 1981). However, there has been a notable absence to date of response-style research in the development of family assessment instruments.

External Validation

This component involved a series of studies that explicate what a particular scale does measure (convergent validity), as well as what it does not measure (discriminant validity). The basic design is to assess two or more constructs by two or more measurement methods. Campbell and Fiske (1959) termed this design a "multitrait–multimethod matrix." Evidence for *convergent validity* is provided when a particular scale correlates highly with other independent measures (e.g., therapist rating and behavioral observations) of the same construct. That is, a self-report scale that indicates problems in the area of role performance should be corroborated by independent (nontest) assessment of that construct.

Discriminant validity is evidenced by demonstrating the scale's lack of correlation with irrelevant constructs assessed by the same (self-report) or different methods. Thus, to establish the construct validity of a scale, one must demonstrate that most of the scale score variance may be attributed to the underlying construct, rather than to irrelevant constructs (scale overlap), response style (e.g., social desirability), or measurement error.

Other important aspects of external validation include predictive validity, concurrent validity, and clinical validity (see Appendix). Of most immediate relevance to therapists is the predictive validity of the instrument with respect to therapy planning and outcome. In brief, can the instrument aid in making treatment decisions? Another aspect is the comparison of the instrument with existing measures for family assessments (concurrent validity). Finally, if a new instrument is to gain clinical acceptance this measure must provide information that is consistent with the clinical experience and background of therapists.

FAMILY ASSESSMENT INSTRUMENTS

Self-report techniques for family assessments are of fairly recent origin. This section describes three instruments that have evolved from systematic programs of research. Each instrument represents a distinct conceptual approach and is evaluated by means of the construct validation framework (Table 3). The reader is also directed to reviews by Forman and Hagan (1983, 1984) of 10 family assessment instruments, and to a comprehensive review by Cromwell, Olson, and Fournier (1976) of earlier instruments.

Family Environment Scale

The Family Environment Scale was one of the first instruments developed specifically for family assessments, and is the only instrument to date that has been formally published (Moos, 1974; Moos & Moos, 1981). The Family Environment Scale is one of a series of social climate scales developed by Rudolf Moos. This instrument is composed of 10 subscales that assess three broad domains:

1. *Relationship Dimensions:* Cohesion, Expressiveness, and Conflict
2. *Personal Growth Dimensions:* Independence, Achievement Orientation, Intellectual-Cultural Orientation, Active-Recreational Orientation, and Moral-Religious Emphasis
3. *System Maintenance Dimensions:* Organization and Control

TABLE 3. Comparison of Three Family Assessment Instruments

Component	Family Environment Scale[a]	Family Adaptability and Cohesion Scales[b]	Family Assessment Measure[c]
1. *Theoretical*			
Orientation	Social climate (interactionist)	Family systems (circumplex model)	Family systems (process model)
Construct definitions	Well defined	Well defined	Well defined
Nomological network	Specified	Well specified	Well specified
2. *Structural*			
Measurement model	Cumulative	Cumulative	Cumulative
Family level	Whole	Whole	3 levels (whole, dyads, individual)
Item analyses	Extensive	Extensive	Extensive
Scale reliability	Very good	Very good	Very good
Scale correlations	Low to moderate	Low	Moderate to high
Response styles	Not studied	Examined social desirability	Examined denial and social desirability
Normative data	Extensive	Extensive	Moderate
3. *External*			
Construct validity	Limited	Limited	Limited
Predictive validity	Broad evidence	Limited	Limited
Concurrent validity	Limited	Limited	Limited
Clinical validity	Limited	Limited	Limited

[a]Moos and Moos (1981).
[b]Olson, Portner, and Lavee (1985).
[c]Skinner, Steinhauer, and Santa-Barbara (1983).

The Family Environment Scale has three forms: the Real Form (Form R), which assesses individuals' perceptions of their family environments; the Ideal Form (Form I), which taps people's conception of ideal family environments; and the Expectations Form (Form E), which focuses on people's expectations about family settings. Moos and Spinrad (1984) prepared an annotated bibliography for 1979 through 1983 that gives abstracts of over 200 studies that have used the Family Environment Scale.

Theoretically, the Family Environment Scale has evolved from an interactionist perspective that purports that behavior is a joint function of the person and the environment (Bowers, 1973; Endler & Magnusson, 1976; Mischel, 1973). Traditionally, personality assessment has tended to focus on the person with the measurement of personality traits. However, a growing body of evidence has shown that a substantial proportion of variance in behavior can be accounted for by situational and environmental factors. The measurement of social climate is one of the main ways in which human environments may be characterized (Moos, 1973). This perspective assumes that environments have unique "personalities" just as individuals have. Thus, the Family Environment Scale was developed to measure the social climate of the family according to relationship, personal development, and system maintenance dimensions.

Construct definitions are well defined for the 10 subscales on the Family Environment Scale. Links among the constructs (nomological network) are discussed within a general conceptual framework for linking stressful life circumstances and adaptation (Moos, 1984). General relationships between family environment constructs and person variables have been evaluated in path analysis models, for example, on the functioning of married persons with impaired partners (Finney, Moos, Cronkite, & Gamble, 1983).

The revised manual (Moos & Moos, 1981) describes the development and applications of the Family Environment Scale. The instrument is based on a cumulative measurement model and assesses whole family functioning. The 90 true–false items were drawn from an original pool of 200 items. Items were selected according to five psychometric criteria: even split in item response frequency, higher correlation with its own subscale than with another subscale, equal number of true- and false-keyed items on each scale, low to moderate scale intercorrelations, and maximum discrimination among families. The average item–scale correlations ranged from .27 for Independence to .44 for the Cohesion and Intellectual-Cultural Orientation subscales. Detailed results from the item analyses are not given in the manual, nor is specific information provided regarding characteristics of the families used in the analyses. Both test–retest and internal consistency reliability estimates are reported. For instance, the internal consistency (coefficient alpha) estimates ranged from .61 for Independence to .78 for the Cohesion, Intellectual-Cultural Orientation, and Moral-Religious Emphasis subscales. These reliability estimates are quite good given the small number of items (9) comprising each subscale. Intercorrelations among subscales are in the low to moderate range and are reported separately for adults ($N = 1,468$) and adolescents ($N = 621$). The influence of response style (e.g., social desirability) was not investigated.

The manual presents detailed normative data for each subscale based on a normal family sample ($N = 1,125$). Subscale means and standard deviations are also given for distressed families ($N = 500$), as well as for families of different sizes, families with one member over age 60, black and Mexican-American families, and single-parent families. Moos and Moos (1981) also described the computation of a family Incongruence Score for quantifying the extent of disagreement among family members about their family climate. Normative data are given for normal and distressed families.

Relationships among subscales on the Family Environment Scale have been evaluated in several studies. Fowler (1981) factor-analyzed the subscale intercorrelations and identified two factors: (a) cohesion versus conflict and (b) organization and control activities. Fowler (1981) noted that these two factors have been found previously in small-group research. Fowler (1982a) replicated this factor structure in a subsequent study that also controlled for the effects of social desirability. Subscale correlations with a social desirability index ranged from .02 for Moral-Religious Emphasis to .44 for Cohesion. A third study (Fowler, 1982b) compared the two factors from the Family Environment Scale with personality characteristics assessed by the Personality Research Form.

Using cluster analysis procedures, several studies have attempted to derive family typologies using the Family Environment Scale. Moos and Moos (1976) applied cluster analysis to 100 family profiles and identified six types of family environments: three were oriented toward personal growth (independence, achievement, and moral-religious emphasis), two toward interpersonal relationships (conflict and expressiveness), and one toward system maintenance (structure). This typology was used in a subsequent study as a basis for classification rules for seven family types (Billings & Moos, 1982). Differences in environmental stressors and coping responses were examined as mediators between family types and family members' levels of functioning.

With respect to external validation, the Family Environment Scale manual (Moos & Moos, 1981) provides a synopsis of research that supports the predictive validity of this instrument. The Family Environment Scale has been used to compare normal with distressed families (families with one or more "dysfunctional" members), to study changes in therapy, to predict treatment outcome, and to compare family environment with other aspects of family life (e.g., adult career and occupational patterns). For example, Karoly and Rosenthal (1977) found that parents receiving a behaviorally oriented training program perceived more family cohesion and support than did parents in a control group, who did not perceive changes in their families. Druckman (1979) reported that families who completed a treatment program for juvenile offenders had higher pretest scores on the Intellectual-Cultural Orientation subscale than did families who dropped out of treatment.

Moos and colleagues have used the Family Envrionment Scale in a systematic program of research evaluating the outcome of treatment for alcoholism (e.g., Finney, Moos, & Newborn, 1980; Finney *et al.,* 1983; Moos, Bromet, Tsu, & Moos, 1979; Moos, Finney, & Chan, 1981; Moos, Finney, & Gamble, 1982; Moos & Moos, 1984). For instance, Finney *et al.* (1980) found that alcoholic patients in families with greater perceived cohesion were functioning better on a variety of outcome measures both 6 months and 2 years after treatment. A family emphasis on intellectual and cultural matters and an active recreational orientation were linked to less alcohol consumption and less depression at follow-up. In general, a more cohesive and supportive family environment resulted in a better prognosis for an individual who had been treated for alcoholism.

The clinical utility of the Family Environment Scale has been explored in several case studies. Fuhr, Moos, and Dishotsky (1981) compared each family member's real (Form R) and ideal (Form I) family environments, and identified key areas of agreement and disagreement about aspects of family functioning. Feedback of this information was integrated with the therapeutic process. Similarly, Moos and Fuhr (1982) illustrated how the Family Environment Scale can be used in conceptualizing environmental factors, enhancing clinical case descriptions, and formulating intervention strategies.

Little research has been published to date that compares the Family Environment Scale with other measures of family functioning (concurrent validity).

One major study, conducted by Bloom (1985), examined commonalities among items from the Family Environment Scale (Moos & Moos, 1981), the Family Adaptability and Cohesion Scales (Olson, Portner, & Bell, 1982), the Family Assessment Measure (Skinner *et al.*, 1983), and The Family Concept Q Sort (van der Veen, 1969). The results of this study will be described in the "Discussion" section below.

Limited data are available regarding the construct validity of the Family Environment Scale. Oliveri and Reiss (1984) compared the Family Environment Scale with a card-sort procedure, which is a family problem-solving task from which direct measures of family behavior are obtained and scored according to configuration, coordination, and closure dimensions. Although the construct definitions for each instrument suggested a good deal of similarity, Oliveri and Reiss (1984) found no empirical associations between the self-report and the direct observational procedures. The authors concluded that the instruments tap essentially unrelated domains of family functioning. That is, the Family Environment Scale assesses how individual family members perceive the family and describe it to an investigator, whereas the card-sort procedure examines family behavior in a situation with unclear external demands.

In an earlier study, Russell (1980) conducted a modified multitrait–multi-method analysis of four different methods of assessing family cohesion and adaptability. Evidence for convergent validity was weak. The Cohesion subscale from the Family Environment Scale did not correlate with other measures of family cohesion. This finding prompted Russell (1980) to question the validity of the Moos and Moos (1981) subscale as a measure of family cohesion.

Family Adaptability and Cohesion Evaluation Scales

The Family Adaptability and Cohesion Evaluation Scales (FACES) were developed by David Olson and colleagues to provide an operational measure of the two primary dimensions in their circumplex model (Olson, Russell, & Sprenkle, 1979, 1983; Olson, Sprenkle, & Russell, 1979; Russell, 1979). They argued that cohesion and adaptability represent two significant clusters of concepts from the family therapy literature. Family *cohesion* is defined as the emotional bonding that family members have with one another. Family *adaptability* concerns the ability of a marital or family system to change its power structure, role relationships, and relationship rules in response to situational and developmental stress. Family *communication* is a third dimension in the circumplex model that is hypothesized to facilitate movement on the two central axes. Each dimension in the circumplex model is differentiated into four levels (Figure 1). Family cohesion ranges from extremely low (disengaged), through moderate or balanced levels (separated, connected), to extremely high cohesion (enmeshed). Similarly, family adaptability ranges from extremely low (rigid), through moderate levels (flexible, structured), to extremely high adaptability (chaotic). In composite, the two basic dimensions form 16 potential types of family systems as depicted in Figure 1.

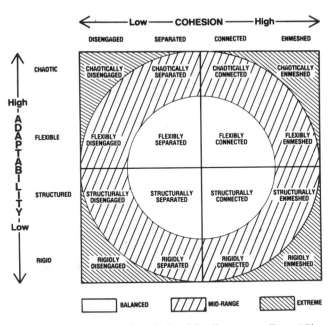

FIGURE 1. Circumplex model: 16 types of marital and family systems. From "Circumplex Model of Marital and Family Systems: 1. Cohesion and Adaptability Dimensions, Family Types, and Clinical Applications" by D. H. Olson, D. H. Sprenkle, and C. S. Russell, 1979, *Family Process, 18,* 17. Copyright 1979 by D. H. Olson. Reprinted by permission.

The circumplex model hypothesizes a curvilinear relationship with effective family functioning (Figure 1). That is, families with balanced levels of cohesion and adaptability function more adequately than those at the extremes of these dimensions. However, in a theoretical update, Olson, Russell, & Sprenkle (1983) acknowledged the importance of family *satisfaction*, which hypothesizes that families extreme on both dimensions will function well *if all* family members like it that way. The circumplex model is dynamic because it assumes that individuals and family systems will change throughout the family life cycle, and that a different family type (level of adaptability and cohesion) may be more effective during one life cycle than during another.

Although FACES was developed to provide a self-report measure of family cohesion and adaptability, empirical research (e.g., Sprenkle & Olson, 1978) on the circumplex model has also been conducted by means of the Simulated Family Activity Measure (SIMFAM) by Straus and Tallman (1971). The original FACES started with 204 statements: 104 for family cohesion and 100 for family adaptability. The clinical relevance of items was rated by 35 marriage and family counselors, and the instrument was administered to 410 young adults. Items were selected that had (a) high content saturation indicated by the counselor ratings and (b) a high factor loading on a designated factor from the young adult data. From these analyses, the first version of FACES was formed, which consist-ed of 54 cohesion items, 42 adaptability items, and 15 social desirability items. Internal consistency reliability estimates were .83 for family cohesion and .75 for family adaptability. In two validation studies, Portner (1981) and Bell (1982) found that nonproblem families were more likely than clinical families to fall into the balanced areas of the circumplex model.

A second version of this instrument, FACES II, was developed to provide a briefer measure with simple sentences and a revised 5-point response scale. The 50 items of FACES II were included as part of a national sample of 1,140 couples and 412 adolescents surveyed across different stages of the family life cycle (Olson, McCubbin, Barnes, *et al.*, 1982, 1983). On the basis of item factor analy-ses and reliability estimates, the 50-item scale was reduced to 30 items, which now comprise the final version of FACES II. The internal consistency reliability estimates for Cohesion (16 items) was .87, and for Adaptability (14 items), it was .78. Item–scale correlations are not presented, which would be helpful in determining the content saturation for each item. The authors did report an item factor analysis restricted to two factors (Varimax rotated?), in which the family cohesion items had a median loading of .49 on Factor I (range from .35 to .61), and the Adaptability items had a median loading of .41 on Factor II (range from .10 to .55). Although the item factor analysis is reported under the heading of "Construct Validity," this analysis pertains only to the internal struc-ture of the instrument. Construct validity, as generally defined (Wiggins, 1973), involves relating a given measure of a concept (e.g., adaptability) to data from other methods of assessing this same construct.

FACES II is administered in two formats: "How would you describe your family now?" (*perceived* family), and "How would you like your family to be?" (*ideal* family). Then, an individual's level of *satisfaction* with the current family system is computed by examining the magnitude of the perceived-ideal discrep-ancy score. Differences between family members' perceptions and ideals are useful clinically for identifying problem areas (Olson & Portner, 1983). Norms on FACES II are given separately for parents and adolescents who participated in the Olson, McCubbin, Barnes, Larsen, Muxen, & Wilson (1983) national survey (2,083 parents and 416 adolescents). Significant differences were found between stages of the family life cycle. For example, wives tended to rate cohe-sion and adaptability higher across all stages than did husbands. Also, there was a trend for both husbands and wives to rate cohesion and adaptability as greater in the early and later stages of the life cycle (they reached a low point during the adolescent stage). Thus, one of the strengths of FACES II is the availability of normative data for families at different stages in the life cycle.

Olson *et al.* (1983) also reported a lack of agreement between family mem-bers in their FACES II scores. With respect to Cohesion, the correlation between husbands and wives was .46; between husbands and adolescents, .46; and be-tween wives and adolescents, .39. Similarly, on Adaptability, the husband–wife correlation was .32; the husband–adolescents correlation, .31; and the wife–adolescent correlation, .21. This general lack of agreement indicates that family members may have quite different perspectives on the family system.

The correlation between Cohesion and Adaptability on FACES II was not reported by Olson, Portner, & Bell (1983). This correlation is important for establishing the extent to which empirical data from FACES II correspond to the hypothesized circumplex structure. The term *circumplex* was proposed by Guttman (1954) to describe a condition in which variation among individuals appears to be continuous in the form of a closed circle. In practice, the structure need not be exactly circular but should approximate a circle or a hyperspheroid in shape. Circumplex structures have been popular in the study of interpersonal variables (e.g., Wiggins, 1979) and in the examination of the social behavior of parents and children (e.g., Benjamin, 1974). The circumplex model (Figure 1) proposed by Olson and colleagues would assume that Cohesion and Adaptability on FACES II have a low correlation. Otherwise, if the two measures are highly correlated, there would be very few examples of extreme family types. Table 5 from Olson, Portner, & Bell (1982) gives the distribution of parents and adolescents according to the 16 possible family types in the circumplex mode. Given these distributions, I estimated the correlation between Adaptability and Cohesion for parents to be .57. No cases were found in two of the extreme types (chaotic-disengaged and rigid-enmeshed).

This issue was addressed in a recent revision of the instrument, designated FACES III (Olson *et al.*, 1985). Following further item-analysis work on the 50-item pool of FACES II, Olson *et al.* (1985) selected 10 items for Adaptability and 10 items for Cohesion to form the *20-item* FACES III scale. In this third version, the correlation between Adaptability and Cohesion is virtually zero ($r = .03$), and a good distribution of scores was noted on the 16 types of the circumplex model. Moreover, items in FACES III were selected to suppress a social desirability response style. The new Adaptability subscale is uncorrelated with social desirability ($r = .00$), whereas Cohesion correlates moderately with social desirability ($r = .35$). Internal consistency reliability estimates based on 2,412 individuals are .77 for Cohesion and .62 for Adaptability, is slightly lower than the data reported for FACES II. This drop in reliability is due, in part, to the smaller number of items (10) in each subscale in FACES III.

These improvements in FACES III should greatly enhance the structural fidelity of the instrument with respect to the underlying circumplex model. New normative data are being collected with families at different stages in the life cycle. Finally, FACES III and all other instruments reported in Olson, McCubbin, Barnes, Larsen, Muxen, & Wilson (1982) have been programmed for use on the IBM-PC microcomputer. (Further details regarding FACES III may be obtained by writing directly to David Olson, Family Social Science Department, 290 McNeal Hall, University of Minnesota, St. Paul, Minnesota, U.S.A. 55108.)

With respect to external validation (Table 3), Olson *et al.* (1983) reported that FACES II distinguished between balanced and extreme families at different stages of the family life cycle. Also, this study found that different types of family systems are perceived as functional at varied stages of the life cycle. Couples perceived greater cohesiveness early in their marriages, whereas families with adolescents tended to exert greater independence and less cohesion. Olson (personal communication) reported that a construct validation study is in progress that is comparing family self-reports using FACES III with therapist's observations of the family collected by means of the Clinical Rating Scale (Olson & Killorin, 1985). Other studies in progress are addressing various aspects of the external validation component.

In review, this instrument is closely linked with a comprehensive model of family and marital systems (the circumplex model), and Olson and his colleagues have taken FACES through several generations in order to improve its psychometric properties. Although FACES is still evolving, the care taken in revising both the instrument and the underlying circumplex model should lead to significant advances in this approach to family assessment.

Family Assessment Measure

The Family Assessment Measure was developed to provide quantitative indices of family strengths and weaknesses (Skinner *et al.*, 1983). The current version of this instrument (FAM III) consists of three components: (a) a General Scale, which focuses on the family as a system; (b) a Dyadic Relationships Scale, which measures relationships between specific pairs in the family; and (c) a Self-Rating Scale, which taps the individual's perception of his or her functioning in the family. Each scale provides a different perspective on the family functioning.

Theoretically, the Family Assessment Measure is based on a process model of family functioning that integrates different approaches to family therapy and research (Steinhauer, Santa-Barbara, & Skinner, 1984). A schematic representation of the process model is given in Figure 2. The overriding goal of the family is the successful achievement of a variety of basic, developmental, and crisis tasks (Task Accomplishment). Successful task accomplishment involves the differentiation and performance of various roles (Role Performance); communication of essential information (Communication), including the expression of affect (Affective Expression); the degree and quality of family members' interest in one another (Involvement); and the process by which the family members influence and manage each other (Control). From a more general perspective, how tasks are defined and how the family proceeds to accomplish them may be greatly influenced by the specific culture and family background (Values and Norms).

The process model of family functioning emphasizes family dynamics. Although it is important to identify dimensions that are relevant to family health or pathology, the process model also attempts to define the processes by which families operate. Thus, the model emphasizes *how* basic dimensions of family functioning interrelate. Moreover, the model encourages formulation at both the total-family-system and the individual-intrapsychic levels (Steinhauer, 1984; Steinhauer & Tisdall, 1984).

The Family Assessment Measure was developed according to the construct validation paradigm outlined in Table 1 and described in the appendix. The first step involved an explicit definition of each construct in the process model. Then, a large pool of over 800 items was generated, and these items were rated according to clarity, content saturation, and clinical relevance. The best 30 items for each subscale of the seven constructs in the process model were retained for a

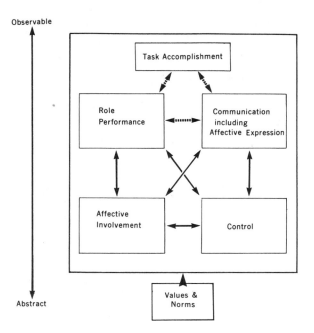

FIGURE 2. Family functioning model.

preliminary version of the FAM. Within each subscale, the items were balanced to give an equal number of healthy and pathological keyed responses (5-point rating). The individual was asked to answer each item for his or her family *as a whole*. In addition to the seven construct subscales, three subscales were included as marker variables for response style biases (Social Desirability, Defensiveness, and Family Conventionalization).

The FAM was administered to 433 individuals who represented 182 clinical and nonclinical families. Statistical analyses were conducted that examined the discriminatory power of each item, scale reliability, intercorrelations among scales, and the influence of response-style biases (Skinner, Santa-Barbara, & Steinhauer, 1981). The median internal consistency reliability was substantial at .93 for the 30-item subscales, and at .87 for the best 10 items selected for each subscale. Intercorrelations among the content subscales ranged from .55 to .79. This degree of correlation suggests that a general factor of family health or pathology underlies the content subscales. Correlations between the FAM constructs and response styles indicated only a marginal tendency to deny or minimize problems (Defensiveness); a moderately positive correlation with Social Desirability (mean $r = .44$); and a substantial correlation with Family Conventionalization (mean $r = .61$). The FAM significantly differentiated between clinical and nonclinical families. Mothers provided the most critical information in that mothers of nonclinical families rated their family functioning as most healthy, whereas mothers of clinical families gave the most pathological FAM profiles.

From these analyses, a briefer 15-item instrument, designated FAM II, was developed. This version has been used in several research projects. For example, Garfinkel, Garner, Rose, Darby, Brandes, O'Hanlon, and Walsh (1983) compared the characteristics of families of patients with anorexia nervosa and normal controls. Mothers and daughters in the anorexic group reported significantly increased difficulties in Task Accomplishment, Role Performance, Communication, and Affective Expression in their families, in comparison with controls. However, the fathers did not report any familial problems. This finding suggests either that the fathers had marked differences in their perception of family problems, or that they were less willing to acknowledge family problems.

Feedback from users of FAM II combined with statistical analyses of its measurement properties indicated a need to provide more differentiated information about areas of family functioning. Accordingly, a third revision of the instrument (FAM III) was devised that assesses the family from three different levels:

1. *General Scale* (50 items) focuses on the level of health or pathology in the family from a systems perspective. This scale provides an overall rating of family functioning, seven measures (subscales) relating to constructs in the process model (Figure 2), plus two response style subscales (Social Desirability and Defensiveness).
2. *Dyadic Relationship Scale* (42 items) focuses on relationships among specific pairs (dyads) in the family. For each dyad, an overall rating of family functioning is provided along with seven indices (subscales) relating to constructs in the process model.
3. *Self-Rating Scale* (42 items) focuses on the individual's perception of his or her functioning in the family. An overall index is provided along with seven measures relating to the process model.

FAM III generally takes around 30 to 45 minutes to administer, and it may be completed by family members who are at least 10 to 12 years old. A hand-scorable version is available that may be quickly scored and graphed on profile sheets. Also, a prototype version of FAM III has been developed for administration using an IBM-PC microcomputer. The FAM III Administration and Interpretation Guide provides normative data separately for adults ($n = 247$) and adolescents ($n = 65$) from *normal* families. Also, normative data from various clinical families (over 2,000 individuals) are available by writing to H. Skinner. These groups include families in which one member has a major physical disorder (e.g., cystic fibrosis), families involved in therapy, families with gifted and disturbed children, and families in which one member has a major psychiatric disorder (e.g., depression).

Skinner *et al.* (1983) described statistical analyses on FAM III using 475 families (933 adults and 502 children). Internal consistency reliability estimates (coefficient alpha) for the overall ratings were substantial: General Scale (.93), Dyadic Relationships Scale (.95), and Self-Rating Scale (.89). With respect to the briefer subscales (5–6 items), the median reliability was .73 for the 9 subscales from the General Scale, .72 for the 6 subscales from the Dyadic Relationships

Scale, and .53 for the 6 subscales from the Self-Rating Scale. Intercorrelations among the subscales were moderate to high in a sample ($n = 277$) of clinical families: General Scale (.39–.70), Dyadic Relationships Scale (.63–.82), and Self-Rating Scale (.25–.63). The median correlation of subscales with social desirability was −.53 (General Scale), −.35 (Dyadic Relationships), and −.35 (Self-Rating). Similarly, the median correlation with defensiveness was −.48 (General Scale), −.28 (Dyadic Relationships), and −.28 (Self-Rating).

The correspondence between the FAM General Scale profiles of husbands and wives in the same family was examined. In 74 normal couples, the mean correlation between husband and wife profiles was .36 (standard deviation = .43). Thus, overall, there was only a moderate level of agreement between spouses in rating family functioning, and wide variability in congruence between couple's profiles was noted. With 43 clinical couples, a somewhat higher level of correspondence was in evidence between husband and wife profiles ($r = .51$; standard deviation = .41). These findings parallel results reported by Olson and Portner (1983) for congruence between spouses on FACES II.

The discriminating power of FAM III in differentiating problem from non-problem families was examined by Skinner et al. (1983). "Problem" families were defined as currently having one or more family members receiving professional help for psychiatric or emotional problems, alcohol or drug problems, school-related problems, or major legal problems. Of the 475 families examined, 28% were designated as problem families. A multiple discriminant analyses was conducted to identify linear combinations of subscales from the General Scale that significantly differentiated among (a) problem versus nonproblem families and (b) family position (father, mother, and child). Two dimensions were major discriminators among these groups. The first dimension was defined by problems in the area of control, values and norms, and affective expression and served mainly to differentiate children from adults. That is, children were more likely than adults to report problems on these subscales. The second dimension, on the other hand, clearly distinguished problem from nonproblem families. Specifically, problem families tended to report more dysfunction in the areas of Role Performance and Involvement.

Currently, FAM III is being used in a number of research studies that address external validity (Table 4). Both FAM and the underlying process model are involved in an active program of refinement.

DISCUSSION

The construct validation paradigm provides a comprehensive framework for the development of family assessment instruments that are closely linked with theoretical models of family functioning. Indeed, the test construction process usually results in an active interplay of refinements to both the instrument and the underlying theory. The status of the three family assessment instruments reviewed in this chapter is summarized in Table 3. With respect to the theoretical component, both FACES and FAM offer advantages in that these

TABLE 4. Synopsis of Projects Using FAM-III

Investigator	Location	Project description
H. Skinner T. Jacob	University of Toronto University of Pittsburgh	Compare FAM-III with behavioral indices from laboratory interactions and home observations; three family types: (1) alcoholic father, (2) depressed father, (3) normal father.
S. Markovich	Hospital for Sick Children, Toronto	FAM-III used as a measure of factors contributing to maternal stress and mother–child interaction with the developmentally delayed preschool child.
D. Jansen	Blue Hills Academy, Aurora, Ontario	FAM-III used for clinical purposes and in an outcome study of a 5-day residential treatment center and home-care program.
N. Cohen	Thistletown Regional Centre, Rexdale, Ontario	Using FAM-III as part of a battery of tests looking at change in disturbed and developmentally delayed preschoolers and their families in an intensive treatment program. Results will be compared to those of similar children receiving unintensive treatment and to normal controls.
P. Martin	Hinks Treatment Centre, Toronto	Using FAM-III in a longitudinal study to examine the characteristics and developmental course of personality functioning during early adolescence aiming at delineating precise criteria for the reliable identification of the young adolescent who is "at risk" for future serious personality disturbance and psychiatric disorder.
R. Simmons	Hospital for Sick Children, Toronto	FAM-III used in the psychosocial assessment of individuals with cystic fibrosis and their families, using clinical groups. The general scale of FAM-III is also used as part of a battery of tests in a longitudinal study of the parent–infant interaction of infants with cystic fibrosis.
J. Duggan	Mental Health Center, Kansas City, Missouri	FAM-III used to study the interrelationship of six patient self-report measures of family functioning, including Family Concept Test, Family Environment Scale, Family Adaptability and Cohesion Evaluation Scales, Family APGAR, and FAM-III.

(continued)

TABLE 4. (*Continued*)

Investigator	Location	Project description
B. Toner	Toronto General Hospital, Department of Psychiatry, Toronto	FAM-III used in a long-term follow-up of diagnoses made 6–14 years ago of bulimic anorexia nervosa and dietary-restricting anorexia nervosa. The study also has a normal control group.
E. Gelcer	Clarke Institute of Psychiatry, Toronto	FAM-III used in a study to compare families with a child in one of four classifications: (1) gifted–disturbed, (2) disturbed–not gifted, (3) gifted–not disturbed, and (4) normal.
L. de Groot	Alberta Children's Hospital, Edmonton	Is evaluating the computerized version of FAM-III developed for the IBM-PC microcomputer.
A. Westhues	University of Toronto, Toronto	FAM-III will be used in four Children's Aid Societies to test the effectiveness of a training program in a systems-based approach to practice that is hoped to result in more effective placement of children in adoptive and foster homes. Two branches will receive training; two will not; and one will act as a control group.

instruments are based on models that emphasize critical dimensions and family dyadics. The Family Environment Scale has evolved from a more general theory of social climates and interactionism. With respect to the structural component, the three instruments have undergone fairly extensive empirical analyses and subsequent refinements. More attention needs to be given to the influences of response-style biases (e.g., social desirability) on scale scores. Further empirical work is needed in order to demonstrate how well FACES corresponds to the hypothesized circumplex structure. FAM requires additional normative data, as well as attempts to reduce the high correlation among subscales. Finally, all three instruments require much further work with respect to external validation. To be fair, one must appreciate that well-designed validity studies are expensive and time-consuming.

Although the three assessment instruments are based on different theoretical models, these models share a number of common elements (see Forman & Hagan, 1983, 1984). In a recent study, Bloom (1985) factor-analyzed the item pool from these instruments and derived a 75-item scale comprising 15 dimensions of family functioning. These findings would suggest that the three instruments tap similar dimensions. Unfortunately, Bloom (1985) did not present intercorrelations among subscales across the three instruments, which would provide evidence regarding their concurrent validity. Further work is clearly needed that would study relationships among these instruments.

The assessment of family functioning presents many challenges. Indeed, the complexities involved in family assessments are certainly at a "postgraduate" level compared with the assessment of individuals. Although the three instruments reviewed in this chapter require additional refinement and validation, there is reason to be optimistic that self-report family assessments will offer important roads to understanding and treating families. At the same time, there are clear limits on any single method. A fundamental mechanism of science is convergence across different assessment methods aimed at different levels in the family (e.g., Table 2). Self-report instruments are not a substitute for a good clinical assessment of a family, or for behavioral observations recorded in real-life or experimental situations. The different assessment methods complement each other by providing different perspectives or "windows" on family functioning. A skillful integration of different assessment methods will yield the greatest insights into understanding family functioning.

ACKNOWLEDGMENTS

The author thanks Sheila Henderson, Bonnie Levine, and Wen-Jenn Sheu for their assistance in the preparation of this chapter. Also, I want to acknowledge my colleagues, Paul Steinhauer and Jack Santa-Barbara, for their vital contributions to the development of the Family Assessment Measure. David Olson and Rudolf Moos provided valuable material on their instruments.

APPENDIX: GUIDELINES FOR DEVELOPING A SELF-REPORT INSTRUMENT FOR FAMILY ASSESSMENT

I. Theoretical Component

Step 1. Define Constructs

The crucial point is to have a precise definition of the construct. This should include a description of the domain that this construct covers (e.g., communication), as well as a clear idea of the boundaries between related concepts (e.g., roles). A thorough mastery of the construct definition is essential.

Step 2. Generate Items

Pick one construct definition. Think of various behaviors, situations, and emotions that exemplify the construct. These exemplars should span the full domain from healthy (well-adjusted) through maladjusted families. Try composing several items that reflect on each exemplar. Approximately half of the items should be keyed (scored) in an "agree" direction, and the other half should be keyed in a "disagree" orientation with respect to one's family. Assume that a high score indicates maladjustment. Once you feel that the item possibilities for a particular construct have been exhausted, move on to a new construct definition.

Step 3. Edit Items

When a large pool of items has been generated for each construct, a panel of editors should be set up to scrutinize each item. In order for an item to be considered for the preliminary form of the test, this item must pass the following editorial hurdles:

A. *Content Saturation*
   (1) Is the item clearly related to the construct definition?
   (2) Does the item have clinical relevance?
   (3) Are there adequate positive and negative instances (exemplars) of the construct?
   (4) Does the item demand knowledge that the respondent does not have or inferences that he or she is unable to make?
   (5) Is the behavior manifestation of sufficient frequency?
B. *Convergent and Discriminant Properties*
   (1) Does the item overlap excessively with a different construct?
   (2) Can the judges correctly sort the items into groups according to the construct definitions?
C. *Item Wording*
   (1) Is the wording clear and unambiguous?
   (2) Is the item in any way misleading?
   (3) Will a respondent with a specified level of education understand the item?
   (4) Is the item concise and simple?
D. *Response Styles*
   (1) Is the item worded so that most respondents will not give the same answer?
   (2) Is the item judged to be free from extreme levels of social desirability bias?
   (3) Does the item require very sensitive information that the respondent may deny or resist giving?
   (4) Is there a balanced number of agree-keyed and disagree-keyed items in the pool?

Where possible, the board of editors should be composed of individuals other than those who wrote the items. If consensus cannot be reached, the rule should be to revise or discard the item. The process of writing and judging items is frequently quite illuminating in uncovering "fuzzy" thinking with respect to the construct definition and the boundaries between concepts. Hence, the constructs may need further clarification and revision.

II. Structural Component

Once a preliminary version of the test has been administered to relevant samples, an item analysis should be conducted (see Jackson, 1970; Nunnally, 1978) that asks "statistically" most of the questions raised in Step 3.

Step 4. Item-Level Analyses

A. *Item Mean, Standard Deviation, and Distribution Characteristics (Skewness and Kurtosis).* The item should be endorsed by a reasonable proportion of the sample and should have good variability.

B. *Item–Scale Correlations.* The item should correlate highly with its own scale (content saturation) and should correlate minimally with other scales (discriminant validity).

C. *Item–Response-Style Correlation.* The item should correlate minimally with response-style measures such as denial or social desirability.

Step 5. Scale-Level Analyses

A. *Scale Mean, Standard Deviation, Skewness, and Kurtosis.* The scale scores should demonstrate good variability and should conform to a normal distribution.

B. *Reliability Estimates.* The scale should demonstrate good internal-consistency reliability (e.g., coefficient alpha) and temporal stability (test–retest).

C. *Correlations among Scales.* A particular scale should provide sufficient unique information and should not be too highly correlated with other scales on the instrument.

D. *Correlations with Response Styles.* The scale should be minimally influenced by response styles (e.g., social desirability and defensiveness).

This phase in the test development program may require several iterations between generating (revising) items and analyzing their psychometric properties before an acceptable version of the instrument is achieved. In an extreme case, one may need to go back to the original model, substantially revise the constructs, and begin the test development program again.

Step 6. Normative Data

The interpretation of an instrument is usually facilitated by comparing an individual's (or family's) responses with a reference population (a normative group). For instance, one might compare how a given family rates on cohesion relative to a representative sample of "normal" families. In a clinical setting, the level of pathology in a particular family may be compared to that of a sample of typical families seen at the clinic. Thus, depending on the intended uses of the instrument, normative data (mean, standard deviation, and distribution of scale scores) should be collected for representative samples of clinical and nonclinical families.

III. External Validation

This component involves a series of validation studies that may take a number of years to complete.

Step 7. Construct Validity

These studies are aimed at establishing that a given scale actually assesses the construct that it is purported to measure. Generally, this research involves assessing two or more constructs (e.g., adaptability, cohesion, and communication) by two or more methods (e.g., self-report, therapist ratings, and behavioral observations). Then, the degree of convergent and discriminant validity (Campbell & Fiske, 1959) may be evaluated, often by the use of factor analysis methods (Joreskog, 1978).

Step 8. Predictive Validity

This research is usually of most direct interest to therapists, who want to know whether the instrument is predictive of important criteria (e.g., differential response to therapy, long-term prognosis, or compliance with treatment). Hence, the instrument must be used in treatment evaluation studies.

Step 9. Concurrent Validity

A new instrument should generally be compared with existing instruments for family assessment, such as the Family Environment Scale (Moos & Moos, 1981). These studies would establish commonalities among instruments, as well as the unique components measured by each.

Step 10. Clinical Validity

This research focuses on the extent to which the assessment instrument provides information about family functioning that is seen to be of immediate relevance to family therapists (Skinner & Blashfield, 1982). It is unlikely that an instrument will be widely used if therapists do not find the concepts meaningful and the assessment data concordant with their clinical experience.

REFERENCES

Bell, R. Q. (1982). *Parent/adolescent relationships in families with runaways: Interaction types and the circumplex model.* Unpublished doctoral dissertation, Family Social Service, University of Minnesota.

Benjamin, L. S. (1974). Structural analysis of social behavior. *Psychological Review, 81,* 392–425.

Billings, A. G., & Moos, R. H. (1982). Family environments and adaptation: A clinically applicable typology. *American Journal of Family Therapy, 10,* 26–38.

Bloom, B. L. (1985). A factor analysis of self-report measures of family functioning. *Family Process, 24,* 225–239.

Bodin, A. M. (1968). Conjoint family assessment. In P. McReynolds (Ed.), *Advances in psychological assessment.* Palo Alto, CA: Science and Behavior Books.

Bowers, K. S. (1973). Situationism in psychology: An analysis and a critique. *Psychological Review, 80,* 307–336.

Campbell, D. T., & Fiske, D. W. (1959). Convergent and discriminate validation by the multitrait–multimethod matrix. *Psychological Bulletin, 56,* 81–105.

Cerny, V., Dahl, N., Kamiko, T., & Aldous, J. (1974). International developments in family theory: A continuation of the "Pilgrim's Progress." *Journal of Marriage and the Family, 36,* 169–173.

Cromwell, R. E., & Peterson, G. W. (1983). Multisystem–multimethod family assessment in clinical context. *Family Process, 22,* 147–163.

Cromwell, R. E., Olson, D. H., & Fournier, D. G. (1976). Tools and techniques for diagnosis and evaluation in marital and family therapy. *Family Process, 15,* 1–49.

Cronbach, L. J., & Meehl, P. E. (1955). Construct validity in psychological tests. *Psychological Bulletin, 52,* 282–302.

Druckman, J. (1979). A family oriented policy and treatment program for juvenile status offenders. *Journal of Marriage and the Family, 41,* 627–636.

Elbert, S., Rosman, B., Minuchin, S., & Guerney, B. (1964). *A method for the clinical study of family interaction.* Paper presented at the American Orthopsychiatric Association, Chicago.

Embretson, S. (1983). Construct validity: Construct representation versus nomothetic span. *Psychological Bulletin, 93*, 179–197.

Endler, N. S., & Magnusson, D. (1976). Toward an interactional psychology of personality. *Psychological Bulletin, 83*, 956–974.

Finney, J. W., Moos, R. H., & Newborn, C. R. (1980). Posttreatment experiences and treatment outcome of alcoholic patients six months and two years after hospitalization. *Journal of Consulting and Clinical Psychology, 48*, 17–29.

Finney, J. W., Moos, R. H., Cronkite, R. C., & Gamble, W. (1983). A conceptual model of the functioning of married persons with impaired partners: Spouses of alcoholic patients. *Journal of Marriage and the Family, 45*, 23–34.

Fisher, L. (1976). Dimensions of family assessment. *Journal of Marriage and Family Counselling, 2*, 367–382.

Fisher, L. (1982). Transactional theories but individual assessment: A frequent discrepancy in family research. *Family Process, 21*, 313–320.

Fitzgerald, R. V. (1973). *Conjoint family therapy.* New York: Jason Aronson.

Forman, B. D., & Hagan, B. J. (1983). A comparative review of total family functioning measures. *American Journal of Family Therapy, 11*, 25–40.

Forman, B. D., & Hagan, B. J. (1984). Measures for evaluating total family functioning. *Family Therapy, 11*, 1–36.

Fowler, P. C. (1981). Maximum likelihood factor structure of the Family Environment Scale. *Journal of Clinical Psychology, 37*, 160–164.

Fowler, P. C. (1982a). Factor structure of the Family Environment Scale: Effects of social desirability. *Journal of Clinical Psychology, 38*, 285–292.

Fowler, P. C. (1982b). Relationship of family environment and personality characteristics: Canonical analyses of self-attributions. *Journal of Clinical Psychology, 38*, 804–810.

Fox, R. E. (1976). Family therapy. In I. B. Weiner (Ed.), *Clinical methods in psychology.* New York: Wiley.

Fuhr, R. A., Moos, R. H., & Dishotsky, N. (1981). The use of family assessment and feedback in ongoing family therapy. *American Journal of Family Therapy, 9*, 24–36.

Garfinkel, P. E., Garner, D. M., Rose, J., Darby, P. L., Brandes, J. S., O'Hanlon, J., & Walsh, N. (1983). A comparison of characteristics in the families of patients with anorexia nervosa and normal controls. *Psychological Medicine, 13*, 821–828.

Gurman, A. S., & Kniskern, D. P. (1981). *Handbook of family therapy.* New York: Brunner/Mazel.

Guttman, L. (1954). A new approach to factor analysis: The radex. In P. F. Lazarsfeld (Ed.), *Mathematical thinking in the social sciences.* Glencoe, IL: Free Press.

Harre, R. (1972). *The philosophies of science.* London: Oxford University Press.

Hathaway, S. R., & McKinley, J. C. (1951). *The Minnesota Multiphasic Personality Inventory* (rev.). New York: Psychological Corporation.

Hempel, C. G. (1965). *Aspects of scientific explanation.* New York: Free Press.

Jackson, D. N. (1970). A sequential system for personality scale development. In C. D. Spielberger (Ed.), *Current topics in clinical and community psychology* (Vol. 2). New York: Academic Press.

Jackson, D. N. (1971). The dynamics of structured personality tests: 1971. *Psychological Review, 78*, 229–248.

Jackson, D. N. (1974). *Personality research form.* Port Huron, MI: Research Psychologists Press.

Jacob, T. (1975). Family interaction in disturbed and normal families: A methodological and substantive review. *Psychological Bulletin, 82*, 33–65.

Karoly, P., & Rosenthal, M. (1977). Training parents in behavior modification: Effects on perceptions of family interaction and deviant child behavior. *Behavior Therapy, 8*, 406–410.

Klein, J. G., Calvert, G. P., Garland, T. N., & Poloma, M. M. (1969). Pilgrim's Progress: 1. Recent developments in family theory. *Journal of Marriage and the Family, 31*, 677–687.

Lebow, J. (1981). Issues in the assessment of outcome in family therapy. *Family Process, 20*, 167–188.

Loevinger, J. (1957). Objective tests as instruments of psychological theory. *Psychological Reports, 3*, 635–694.

Meehl, P. E. (1978). Theoretical risks and tabular asterisks: Sir Karl, Sir Ronald and the slow progress of soft psychology. *Journal of Consulting and Clinical Psychology, 46*, 806–834.

Messick, S. (1981). Constructs and their vicissitudes in educational and psychological measurement. *Psychological Bulletin, 89,* 575–588.

Mischel, W. (1973). Toward a cognitive social learning reconceptualization of personality. *Psychological Review, 80,* 252–283.

Moos, R. (1973). Conceptualization of human environments: An overview. *American Psychologists, 28,* 652–665.

Moos, R. (1974). *Combined preliminary manual for the family, work and group environment scales.* Palo Alto, CA: Consulting Psychologists Press.

Moos, R. (1984). Context and coping: Toward a unifying conceptual framework. *American Journal of Community Psychology, 12,* 5–25.

Moos, R., & Fuhr, R. (1982). The clinical use of social-ecological concepts: The case of an adolescent girl. *American Journal of Orthopsychiatry, 52,* 111–122.

Moos, R., & Moos, B. (1976). A typology of family social environments. *Family Process, 15,* 357–372.

Moos, R., & Moos, B. (1981). *Family Environment Scale manual.* Palo Alto, CA: Consulting Psychologists Press.

Moos, R., & Moos, B. (1984). The process of recovery from alcoholism: 3. Comparing functioning in families of alcoholics and matched control families. *Journal of Studies on Alcohol, 45,* 111–118.

Moos, R., & Spinrad, S. (1984). *The Social Climate Scales: An annotated bibliography, 1979–1983.* Palo Alto, CA: Consulting Psychologists Press.

Moos, R., Bromet, E., Tsu, V., & Moos, B. (1979). Family characteristics and the outcome of treatment for alcoholism. *Journal of Studies on Alcohol, 40,* 78–88.

Moos, R., Finney, J., & Chan, D. A. (1981). The process of recovery from alcoholism: 1. Comparing alcoholic patients and matched community controls. *Journal of Studies on Alcohol, 42,* 383–402.

Moos, R., Finney, J., & Gamble, W. (1982). The process of recovery from alcoholism: 2. Comparing spouses of alcoholic patients and matched community controls. *Journal of Studies on Alcohol, 43,* 888–909.

Nunnally, J. C. (1978). *Psychometric theory* (2nd ed.). New York: McGraw-Hill.

Oliveri, M. E., & Reiss, D. (1984). Family concepts and their measurement: Things are seldom what they seem. *Family Process, 23,* 33–48.

Olson, D. H., & Killorin, E. (1985). *Clinical rating scale for the Circumplex Model.* St. Paul: Family Social Science, University of Minnesota.

Olson, D. H., & Portner, J. (1983). Family adaptability and cohesion evaluation scales. In E. E. Filsinger (Ed.), *Marriage and family assessment.* Beverly Hills, CA: Sage Publications.

Olson, D. H., Russell, C. S., & Sprenkle, D. H. (1979). Circumplex model of marital and family systems: 2. Empirical studies and clinical intervention. In J. Vincent (Ed.), *Advances in family interaction, assessment and theory.* Greenwich, CT: JAI.

Olson, D. H., Sprenkle, D. H., & Russell, C. S. (1979). Circumplex model of marital and family systems: 1. Cohesion and adaptability dimensions, family types, and clinical applications. *Family Process, 18,* 3–28.

Olson, D. H., Russell, C. S., & Sprenkle, D. H. (1980). Marital and family therapy: A decade review. *Journal of Marriage and the Family, 42,* 973–993.

Olson, D. H., McCubbin, H. I., Barnes, H., Larsen, A., Muxen, M., & Wilson, M. (1982). *Family inventories: Inventories used in a national survey of families across the family life cycle.* St. Paul: Family Social Science, University of Minnesota.

Olson, D. H., Portner, J., & Bell, R. (1982). *FACES II: Family Adaptability and Cohesion Evaluation Scales.* St. Paul: Family Social Science, University of Minnesota.

Olson, D. H., McCubbin, H. I., Barnes, H., Larsen A., Muxen, M., & Wilson, M. (1983). *Families: What makes them work.* Beverly Hills, CA: Sage.

Olson, D. H., Russell, C. S., & Sprenkle, D. H. (1983). Circumplex model of marital and family systems: 4. Theoretical update. *Family Process, 22,* 69–83.

Olson, D. H., Portner, J., & Lavee, Y. (1985). *FACES III.* St. Paul: Family Social Science, University of Minnesota.

Peterson, G. W., & Cromwell, R. E. (1983). A clarification of multisystem–multimethod assessment: Reductionism versus wholism. *Family Process, 22,* 173–177.

Popper, K. R. (1972). *The logic of scientific discovery.* London: Hutchison.

Portner, J. (1981). *Parent/adolescent relationships: Interaction types and the circumplex model.* Unpublished doctoral dissertation, Family Social Science, University of Minnesota.

Reiss, D. (1983). Sensory extenders versus meters and predictors: Clarifying strategies for the use of objective tests in family therapy. *Family Process, 22,* 165–171.

Russell, C. S. (1979). Circumplex model of marital and family systems: 3. Empirical evaluation with families. *Family Process, 18,* 29–45.

Russell, C. S. (1980). A methodological study of family cohesion and adaptability. *Journal of Marital and Family Therapy, 6,* 459–470.

Russell, C. S., Olson, D. H., Sprenkle, D. H., & Atilano, R. B. (1983). From family symptom to family system: Review of family therapy research. *American Journal of Family Therapy, 11,* 3–14.

Schumm, W. R. (1982). Integrating theory, measurement and data analysis in family studies survey research. *Journal of Marriage and the Family, 8,* 983–998.

Skinner, H. A. (1981). Toward the integration of classification theory and methods. *Journal of Abnormal Psychology, 90,* 68–87.

Skinner, H. A. (1984). Models for the description of abnormal behavior. In H. E. Adams & P. B. Sutker (Eds.), *Comprehensive handbook of psychopathology.* New York: Plenum Press.

Skinner, H. A., Santa-Barbara, J., & Steinhauer, P. D. (1981, June 3–5). *The Family Assessment Measure: Development of a self-report instrument.* Symposium presented at the Canadian Psychological Association Annual Meeting, Toronto.

Skinner, H. A., Steinhauer, P. D., & Santa-Barbara, J. (1983). The Family Assessment Measure. *Canadian Journal of Community Mental Health, 2,* 91–105.

Sprenkle, D. H., & Olson, D. H. (1978). Circumplex model of marital and family systems: 4. Empirical study of clinic and non-clinic couples. *Journal of Marital and Family Therapy, 4,* 59–74.

Steinhauer, P. D. (1984). Clinical applications of the process model of family functioning. *Canadian Journal of Psychiatry, 29,* 98–111.

Steinhauer, P. D., & Tisdall, G. W. (1984). The integrated use of individual and family psychotherapy. *Canadian Journal of Psychiatry, 29,* 89–97.

Steinglass, P. D., Davis, D. I., & Berenson, D. (1977). Observations of conjointly hospitalized "alcoholic couples" during sobriety and intoxication. *Family Process, 16,* 1–16.

Steinhauer, P. D., Santa-Barbara, J., & Skinner, H. A. (1984). The process model of family functioning. *Canadian Journal of Psychiatry, 29,* 77–88.

Straus, M. A., & Tallman, I. (1971). SIMFAM: A technique for observational measurement and experimental study of families. In J. Aldous (Ed.), *Family problem solving.* Hinsdale, IL: Dryden Press.

van der Veen, F. (1969). *Family concept inventory.* Unpublished manuscript, Institute for Juvenile Research, Chicago.

Watzlawick, P. (1966). A structured family interview. *Family Process, 5,* 256–271.

Wiggins, J. S. (1973). *Personality and prediction: Principles of personality assessment.* Reading, MA: Addison-Wesley.

Wiggins, J. S. (1979). A psychological taxonomy of trait-descriptive terms: The interpersonal domain. *Journal of Personality and Social Psychology, 37,* 395–412.

Woodworth, R. S. (1917). *Personal data sheet.* Chicago: Stoelting.

CHAPTER 12

The Sequential Analysis of Family Interaction

John M. Gottman

This chapter is essentially an advertisement for the sequential and time-series analysis of observational data. It is currently reasonable to make the following statement: *Anyone who has collected data over time and ignores time is missing an opportunity.* It will be helpful to back up this statement with several examples and with a discussion of conceptual issues.

I would like to begin with a few examples from my own work. First, let us discuss the concept *metacommunication*. This concept was introduced in the original double-bind paper on schizophrenia (Bateson, Jackson, Haley, & Weakland, 1956) that was so seminal for the family interaction field. A metacommunication qualifies or comments on communication. It can be a nonverbal act that says "All that follows is really play," or it can be a statement that comments on the process of communication, such as, "You're interrupting me," or "That's not what we were discussing." The concept had arisen from Bateson's observations of otters at the zoo in San Francisco when he was unemployed. In fact, most social scientists who refer to metacommunication cite Bateson for this application of the term rather than the family interaction application. In the double-bind paper, Bateson and his colleagues proposed that the schizophrenic has a deficit in precisely this domain, that is, an inability to metacommunicate, which is the way out of the classic double-bind message. Thus, in 1957, metacommunication was catapulted to a prominent position in the study of social interaction in families. The hypothesis never achieved comparable visibility in the study of marriages.

I studied how satisfied and dissatisfied couples differ in the way they go about resolving an important current issue about which they disagree. What I discovered was that there was no significant difference in the *relative frequency* with which satisfied and dissatisfied couples used metacommunication. However, the sequential analysis performed on these data (Gottman, 1979) showed

JOHN M. GOTTMAN • Department of Psychology, University of Washington, Seattle, WA 98195.

dramatic differences in the way metacommunication was used by the two groups of couples. Satisfied couples frequently used short chains of metacommunication that seemed to function as a repair mechanism for the interaction. The metacommunication was usually followed by an agreement by the partner. For example,

A: You're interrupting me
B: Sorry, what were you saying?

Then the conversation would continue. The metacommunication was usually delivered with neutral affect even if the conversation itself had become negative. For dissatisfied couples, metacommunications were to be delivered with negative affect, followed by a "countermetacommunication" that had the same affect, rather than by an agreement. For example,

A: You're interrupting me.
B: I wouldn't have to, if I could get in a word edgewise.
A: Oh, now I talk too much, is that it?
B: You could say that you do rattle on and on about nothing.

And so on, almost indefinitely. Metacommunication between dissatisfied couples was what is called an *absorbing state*, to use the language of Markov chains; it was difficult to exit once entered. Furthermore, the affect from the conversation tended to transfer (sequentially) to the metacommunicative chain, so it could not function as a repair mechanism.

I want to make several points about the preceding set of results. First, the sequential analyses revealed differences between the two groups of couples that were not revealed by the analysis that ignored sequence. This alone ought to be enough reason to employ sequential analysis.

Second, the sequential analysis revealed patterns that were not even dreamed of by the original double-bind paper that drew attention to metacommunication. What is the implication of this latter fact? The implication is that sequential analysis is an important tool for *generating* theory with good description, as well as for testing theory.

The example I gave showed no base-rate or unconditional-probability differences in metacommunication between couples. Let me now give an example in which base-rate differences do exist and imply a host of differences in social processes, which can be revealed only by sequential analysis. In a monograph on how young children become friends, Gottman (1983) found that there were large differences between unacquainted children who did and did not "hit it off" in terms of the amount of agreement displayed by the quest child. (*Hitting it off* was indexed by a questionnaire completed by the mothers regarding the children's progress toward friendship after the experiment.) A low level of agreement indexes a stacatto rhythm in the play of children who do not hit it off—a pattern that indicates that children will play for relatively few number of turns before they escalate by making the play more demanding. Furthermore, these children are less likely to engage in extended fantasy play and more likely to engage in conflict than are children who do become friends. Here, base-rate differences between groups do exist and these differences can be *understood* by sequential analyses that illuminate a set of social processes that the base-rate differences entail.

A third example will be useful for an additional reason. Many married couples who attempt to resolve an issue go through a middle phase in a discussion in which they disagree a great deal. This disagreement seems to pave the way for later compromise on the issue because they discover the areas of agreement and disagreement between them in this middle phase. Couples who *avoid* conflict during this middle phase of the discussion often have greater difficulty with compromise, which usually occurs in the last third of the conversation.

Notice how natural this latter description was, and how rich it is theoretically. It is also consistent with other literature on decision making in areas other than marital interaction (Fisher & Ury, 1981). Also, notice that this discussion is not even possible without the conceptual tools provided by sequential analysis. Furthermore, the sequential analysis needs to be of a certain character, called *nonstationary*, which means that the second third of the discussion (in which the couples argue or avoid conflict) is *intrinsically different* from the last third of the discussion, for which the goal is compromise.

Finally, in this advertisement, I want to discuss the great *conceptual* clarity that is provided just by thinking about social interaction in terms of sequences. Just about all of the interesting hypotheses we have about how social systems function imply at their base an imagined scenario of interaction. What is really interesting is that this scenario is invariably sequential in character. In short, we tend to think sequentially anyway, so why not give free rein to this thinking with analytic tools that supplement it?

To illuminate this idea of the conceptual clarity to be gained by sequential analysis, let us consider one example from the literature on nonverbal behavior in family interaction, namely, the notion of *channel inconsistency*. This notion was also inspired by the double-bind hypothesis. The idea is that one channel communicates a message such as "Come hither" while the other channel communicates a message such as "Get away from me." The result is supposedly a double bind for the receiver of the inconsistent message. If this hypothesis were true, the *consequences* of the inconsistent message would be predictable. The receiver would act like someone who has been placed in a double bind. On the other hand, let me suggest the rival hypothesis that, whenever one channel contains negative affect (e.g., "Go away"), this is the channel that is listened to, and the overall message is not at all inconsistent. The hypothesis is that negative affect predominates wherever it occurs. If anything, the overall message may be interpreted as "This person is negative but is trying to qualify, constrain, or temper the negativity." In my opinion, although I think she would not agree, the continuing work of Daphne Bugental in this area supports this latter interpretation. A direct test of the hypothesis would be provided by a sequential analysis. Simply examine the consequences of naturally occurring double-bind messages. This test has yet to be performed. This is an example in which theoretical clarity about the anatomy of messages would be gained by thinking in sequential terms.

Another example of the conceptual clarity provided by thinking in sequential terms concerns reciprocity. The reciprocity of self-disclosure has been implicated as the *sine qua non* of acquaintanceship and close friendship by researchers on self-disclosure (Dindia, 1983). If research on this reciprocity hypothesis took a temporal form, a self-disclosure by one person would make a subsequent self-disclosure by the other more likely, and in fact, the intimacy of the self-disclosures would match in more satisfying relationships, or ones in which attraction was high. Despite the temporal nature of this hypothesis, it had never been tested sequentially until Dindia's work (1983) that used Sackett's lag-sequential technique. Instead, in previous research, the amounts of self-disclosure by both people were correlated across dyads. This is not a logical test of the reciprocity hypothesis, which, by its very nature, argues for *contingency* and hence must examine sequences. The correlation that collapses data across time examines only rates of the disclosures. Dindia found that there was no evidence for the reciprocity of self-disclosure using the sequential analysis.

Ginsberg and Gottman (1986) studied the importance of the reciprocity of self-disclosure in accounting for variance in the closeness of college roommates. There was no evidence that reciprocity was important.

Why should this be the case? The answer is that so many other things happen in a natural conversation other than reciprocal self-disclosure, such as laughing, disagreeing, and giving advice and support, that reciprocal self-disclosure is unusual. In fact, it is difficult to write a script of purely reciprocal self-disclosure that does not seem absurd. No doubt, most good friends do find out about one another, but it may, in fact, be important that this mutual discovery be *noncontingent* in many friendships. Self-disclosure in children past middle childhood, for example, usually entails support, understanding, and problem solving. Even in adolescents' conversations with their friends in which mutual self-exploration is important, only one problem at a time tends to be discussed (Gottman & Mettetal, 1986). The methodological point that I am really trying to make here is that we need to learn how to think theoretically about social processes unfolding in time. To do that, we will require the quantitative ideas of sequential analysis.

At times, specific interaction sequences have been posited by family therapists, and these have not been found in subsequent research. The importance of the not finding specific sequential structure in specific interaction situations ought to be noted, and it ought to influence the nature of therapeutic intervention. Unfortunately, it rarely does. Consider Lederer and Jackson's *quid pro quo* hypothesis of marital functioning (1968), which proposed that satisfying marriages were characterized by a reciprocal exchange of positive events or actions. Their hypothesis led to a new form of marital therapy called *reciprocal contracting* (e.g., Stuart, 1969).

However, there was never any empirical evidence supporting the *quid pro quo* hypothesis, and there was some evidence (Murstein, Cerretto, & McDonald, 1977) that the extent to which people held such a philosophy of marriage predicted marital *dissatisfaction*. A series of studies reported in Gottman (1979) found no evidence *within one problem-solving interaction* that positive reciprocity is a variable that discriminates satisfied from dissatisfied couples. Negative reciprocity, on the other hand, did discriminate couples; that is, dissatisfied couples were more likely than satisfied couples to reciprocate negative affect. There was even some evidence for the contention that dissatisfied couples were *more* likely to reciprocate positive affect than satisfied couples. Gottman proposed the hypothesis that temporal linkage among married couples itself was an index of distress.

To understand this result, think of the early stages of acquaintanceship. When one is invited for dinner, one wishes to reciprocate because it demonstrates responsiveness. Temporal structure in the early stages of relationship formation is indicative of responsiveness. This is what Gottman (1983) found for the acquaintanceship of young children. Similarly, in a distressed marriage, if after a fight one's spouse is positive, one wishes to reciprocate because it implies one is also being responsive. *Not* to reciprocate positive affect in the context of prior negative affect communicates a great deal. So a positive *quid pro quo* may make much more sense in the context of unhappy marriages than in happy ones. In a satisfied marriage, people tend to be positive fairly independent of their partner's prior actions and more based on their own prior behavior; to use sequential language, *autocontingency* will probably be more predictive here than *cross-contingency*.

Note that the sweeping nature of the original Lederer and Jackson hypothesis has, of course, never received an adequate test. Only short time spans have been considered, and primarily problem-solving conversations. The role of positive affective experiences in marriages has never been fully explored; work is under way in our laboratory on this issue. It is possible that some form of the hypothesis is true. My only point is that conceptual clarity is added to the hypothesis by thinking sequentially.

I hope I have convinced you that it would be useful to learn about sequential techniques. As the Talmud says, "We are given life. The only question is how to live it." What I am saying is that we are endowed with sequential thinking, the only question is how best to conduct these analyses.

DATA, DATA, DATA

Several technological innovations that have occurred since 1970 make it possible to describe social interaction in considerably more detail than was previously possible. One of these innovations is the widespread availability of videotape equipment. Over the past decade, it became possible for researchers with budgets between $10,000 and $15,000 to construct video laboratories or portable field equipment that (a) merges picture and sound from two or more cameras; (b) puts a visible time code on the picture; (c) can operate in natural or low-light settings; and (d) permits playback at various slow and fast speeds. Recently, it has become possible to read a time code by computer, which now makes it feasible to code directly from the videotape into a microcomputer and also for the computer to control the videotape recorder. To equip such a laboratory, however, will currently cost the researcher about $30,000. About $15,000 to $18,000 is for hardware, and the rest is for the development of the necessary specialized software. Budgets must include new kinds of technical support personnel.

The importance of video and computer technology is obvious. As opposed to live observation, coding can take place at leisure; multiple passes at the data are possible, which make it possible to code observational data in more detail, with multiple coding systems at several levels of analysis (micro to macro; behavioral to symbolic). We can now detect events that we never noticed before—not that they were not there, only that they were too subtle to detect. Along with these *technological* advances have come a new set of "conceptual" technologies with which researchers have had to become familiar.

The 1970s saw the emergence of sophisticated observational techniques for the study of emotional expression and nonverbal behavior in general (see, for example, Harper, Wiens, & Matarazzo, 1978; Scherer & Ekman, 1982). These include the Facial Action Coding System (Ekman & Friesen, 1978) for the description of facial movement using an anatomically based system rather than adjectives. We also have witnessed the emergence of an unfortunately largely qualitative field of sociolinguistics. Nonetheless, this field has called our attention to the detailed study of *conversation*. We have a long way to go before this area will be systematic and rigorous. For an introductory reference, see Coulthard (1977).

Also in the 1970s, there were breakthroughs in our conceptualizations of interobserver reliability, mostly through generalizability theory (Cronbach, Gleser, Nanda, & Rajaratnam, 1972) and corrections for agreement by chance (Fleiss, 1971). Most of the innovations in observational methods are due to two laboratories, those of Gerald Patterson and of Gene Sackett. The recent innovations in reliability assessment are not yet reflected by editorial standards even in our best journals; it is most likely that reliability between observers will still be reported as agreement-to-agreement-plus-disagreement proportions for some time to come. This is unfortunate.

It is important to mention that we have been overwhelmed by detail and by the cost of observational research. We are struggling with the problem at several junctures in our research. First, in the design of coding systems, researchers are now turning toward the employment of *several* coding systems to describe different aspects of the data; coding units vary from micro to macro, and categories vary from specific to global. Currently, we need to have the motto "Let 100 flowers bloom" because we need the detailed systems *and* we need systems that are integrative. Second, we are struggling with the problem at the data analysis juncture. Many researchers use detailed observational systems and struggle mightily with reliability problems only to drastically collapse the many codes into a few summary codes for analysis. This is an unfortunate waste of information. One problem that researchers face is this: Many analyses on few subjects capitalize on chance and increase Type I error rates. The solution is this: *Replicate.* I would argue that, at this juncture, all proposals include a study and a replication and extension study. We need a process of sifting and winnowing *within* each laboratory. For an introduction to the most recent techniques of observational research, the reader is directed to Bakeman and Gottman (1986).

DATA COLLECTION

Not all data sets collected over time are candidates for sequential analysis. In fact, Bakeman (personal communication) has pointed out that the recording strategy is critical in determining if the data can be analyzed sequentially at all. For example, a common method of gathering data is to do something like this: Have a click go off in the observer's ear every 6 seconds, and then the observer records one thing that has occurred within that interval. If two events have occurred within the interval, one is ignored, as is the time order of the events. These data are difficult to interpret sequentially. The same is true of time-sampled data. If sequential analysis is to be performed on the data, it is important to consider this at the outset, in planning the data collection phase of the research.

Bakeman and Gottman (1986) discussed three types of data that are amenable to sequential analyses. One data type is timed-event-sequential, in which a code can follow itself and is detected as often as its duration, relative to some way of using a record. Another is event-sequential, in which a code cannot follow itself. In this case, only episodes and episode transitions are noted. For example, if the timed-event-sequential data for three codes, A, B, and C, were AAACCB-BABACCCCCCBBAACCB, the event-sequential data would be ACBABAC-BACB. Because no code follows itself in the event-sequential case, there are zeros on the diagonal of an antecedent-code × consequent-code matrix; these are called *logical zeros*. A third data type is called *cross-classified events*. In this case, an observer scans for a particular kind of event (e.g., object struggles among preschool children) and then notes temporal information for each of the events of interest (antecedent and consequent behaviors, for example). The cross-classification of each event becomes a count in a particular cell of a contingency matrix.

DATA REDUCTION

Often, we collect observational data in more detail than we plan to analyze. Sometimes, we do this because we are not sure which subcategories of a coding system we plan to combine into a summary code. This has been called the *lumping problem,* as opposed to the *splitting problem,* which involves leaving distinctions between codes intact. Sequential techniques can be used to make these lumping and splitting decisions. For example, I found (Gottman, 1979) that two codes—"disagree" (e.g., "No that's wrong. I think we can't afford that yet") and "yes but" (e.g., "Yes, that's true, but I don't really think we can afford it yet")—had the same consequence: they both led to disagreement by the partner. So I combined yes-but and disagreement. Thus, codes can be combined if they have the same or similar consequences. Parkhurst and Gottman (1986) combined types of demands made by children on the basis of the likelihood that they would elicit either compliance or noncompliance from a peer.

Patterson and Moore (1979) explored the idea of expanding their coding system from a micro to a more macro level by changing the unit of interaction. They were trying to use sequential analysis to discover "repetitive interactive patterns" that they could then call "games." They analyzed the interactions of one child, Tina, with her family. First, they noticed that "Tina's aversive behaviors fluctuated in an orderly fashion, i.e., they seemed to recur every 25 minutes." They determined this from visual inspection of a graph of the frequency of Tina's aversive responses for 50 consecutive one-minute intervals.[1]

They also noticed that Tina's aversive behavior tended to be displayed in bursts, that Tina's "complaining" was the most common initiator of one coercive chain, and that Tina's "arguing" was the next most frequent event for initiating extended coercive interchanges. They then used lag-sequential analysis (Sackett, 1979) and found that the mother tended to reward Tina's complaining. They wrote:

> Mother's reaction to Tina's individual "Complain" behaviors (97 isolated events) suggested strongly that Tina's complaining significantly increased the probability that the mother would subsequently react positively towards her. Forty-five percent of the reactions by others to these "Complaints" were prosocial. . . . If Tina ran off two "Complaints" in a row, the mother reacted by providing positive consequences 67% of the time. . . . The data strongly suggest that Tina's first "Complain" was often not effective in removing the mother's aversive intrusion, but produced another aversive intrusion which finally produced a positive response from the mother, i.e., an exemplar of negative reinforcement for complain patterns. . . . It seemed likely that if Tina had stopped after her first complain (CP) she should have received an aversive antecedent plus an aversive consequence. However, going on to a third or fourth CP appeared to produce a more favorable outcome. (pp 88–90)

In this way, Patterson and Moore built up two- and three-event chains.

Gottman (1983) did a similar analysis of unacquainted children's conversations. He identified a set of sequences that indexed social processes of interest and then designed a macrocoding system that *coded* for these longer chains using a larger interaction unit. This is a very different strategy from relying on statistics to find the sequences. Experience has proved that relying on statistics in sequential analysis is very dangerous. There are simply too many sequences to examine once we have three- or four-event chains. To give an example, suppose that we have a 20-category coding system that we use with triads (e.g., mother, father, and child). Then there are 60 codes at Time 1, 60 possible at Time 2, and so on; if we are interested in three-event chains, there will be $60 \times 60 \times 60 = 216,000$ cells in the sequential matrix! Four-event chains have 12,960,000 cells! The Type I error problem is enormous here. The solution is to be really familiar with one's data. It simply will not do to have research assistants do the observation; of course, coding cannot be done by the investigator who knows the hypotheses, but invesigators must watch their tapes and know how to code. There is no substitute for intimate familiarity with one's data set. Only then can one know what to look for.

---

[1]They could have tested this observation by using a spectral analysis of Tina's data. See Gottman (1981) for examples, and see Williams and Gottman (1981) for a description of a computer program written to conduct the analysis.

It is important to note that the sequential method I have used for lumping data into summary codes makes much more sense than multivariate techniques such as factor analysis. The multivariate techniques cluster on the basis of between-subject correlation between the frequency or the probability of codes. If people who do a lot of Code A also do a lot of Code B and people who do little of Code A do little of Code B, then the advice would be to lump A with B. However, this could be a mistake. For example, some children rejected by peers are high in both aggressive and prosocial behavior. This is so because they interact a great deal, and their behavior has a lot of variety in it. It does not make sense to lump two codes on the basis of multivariate techniques applied to data collapsed over time. To clarify this point, assume that we have two codes, "Husband Fear" and "Wife Whining." Suppose we had two alternative sources of information about a lumping decision for these codes: (a) the relative frequencies of these codes load on the same factor; or (b) both the husband's fear and the wife's whining predict subsequent anger by the partner, in a sequential sense. In most cases, a lumping decision is equivalent to saying that codes are equivalent or substitutable for one another. Which source of information makes most sense if we are going to speak of such an equivalence and are still interested in the time course of an interaction? I would argue that the factor-analytic method is misleading.

TIME SERIES FROM CATEGORICAL DATA

I would like to suggest that investigators who collect categorical data over time also think of creating time-series data. There are several good reasons for doing this.

First, one can obtain an overall visual picture of an interaction. This can be useful in two ways. One is for creating taxonomies of interactions. For example, Gottman (1979) created a time series from data obtained from marital interaction. The variable was the total positive minus the total negative interactions up to that point in time. In some couples, both the husband's and the wife's graphs were quite negative. These couples tended to be high in reciprocating negative affect. In some couples, one partner's graph was negative and the other's was positive. These couples tended to have one partner who gave in most of the time in response to the partner's complaints. Couples whose graphs were flat at the start of an interaction tended to have social skill deficits in listening, whereas couples whose graphs were flat at the end of an interaction tended to have social skill deficits in negotiation. Thus, the time-series graphs led to a classification of interactional styles that related to response deficits. The time-series graph then became a useful diagnostic tool in itself for studying individual couples. There was a trick inherent in this application of time-series analysis. With one summary variable, it was possible to obtain dyad-by-dyad plots of the interaction. Often, there were not enough data for dyad-by-dyad sequential analysis of the categorical data. It turned out that the shapes of the graphs were related to group profiles of interaction sequences in a regular way. In other words, even though a particular couple did not have enough data for detailed sequential analysis, just by the time-series plot it was possible to be confident about the kinds of predictions one could make about the sequences in this couple's interaction. Recently, I have developed a rapid version of the Couples Interaction Scoring System that cuts by one tenth the coding time necessary to generate the point graphs.

A second use of a time-series graph is that it makes it possible to discover the limitations of a coding system. This is a remarkable result that may seem almost magical on first hearing. It is possible to use a coding system to identify critical moments for more detailed coding with another system. How can this be done? First, one needs to create a time-series variable that indexes something important about the interaction. I used cumulative positive minus negative affect; Brazelton, Koslowski, and Main (1974) used a total positive-engagement score in mother–infant face-to-face interaction. One can then use the graphs to scan for shifts in slope or level. These moments may be rare critical events that the coding system itself does not know about. An example comes from a videotape that Ted Jacob had that was coded by a version of the Marital Interaction Coding System (MICS). The interaction began in a very negative way but changed dramatically in the middle and became quite positive. The event that triggered the change seemed to be the husband's summarizing what he thought was the wife's complaint and then accepting responsibility for the problem. The MICS has no code for summarizing the other (which is a very rare event, but quite powerful), although it does have a code for accepting responsibility, but this code was not included in Jacob's version of the MICS. I refer to this use of time series as *Godeling* because, like Kurt Godel's work, it is concerned with using a system to view itself and to discover its own limitations (Godel, 1932).

In addition to these reasons for creating time-series data from categorical data, time-series analysis has some powerful analytic options that I will briefly discuss in a moment. First, I would like to mention three options for creating time-series data from categorical data. One option, used by psychophysiologists, is the *interevent interval*. This involves graphing the time between events of a certain type over time. Cardiovascular psychophysiologists, for example, plot the average time between the R waves of the EKG within a time block of sufficient size. The reader will be amazed at how nicely this works even for very crude diary data; for example, it can be used to create a time series from daily records of cigarettes smoked.

A second option is the *moving probability window*. Here we compute the proportion of times an event was observed with a particular time block of observations, and then we slide the window forward in time. This option *smoothes* the data as we use a larger and larger time unit, a useful procedure for graphic display, but not necessary for many time-series procedures (particularly those in the frequency domain).

A third option is the *univariate scaling* of codes. For two different approaches, see Brazelton *et al.* (1974) and Gottman (1979).

Each option produces a set of time series for each variable created, for each person in the interacting unit. Analysis proceeds within each interacting unit ("subject"), and statistics of sequential connection are then extracted for standard analysis of variance or regression. I discussed a detailed example of the analysis of this kind of data obtained from mother–infant interaction in Gottman, Rose, and Mettetal (1982). A review of time-series techniques is available in Gottman's (1981) book, together with 10 computer programs (Williams & Gottman, 1981). In this chapter, I will restrict myself to the discussion of three analytic procedures and a suggestion of how to use them together.

There are two types of bivariate analyses: frequency domain and time domain. In the frequency domain, we can obtain (using Williams and Gottman's 1981 program CRSPEC) two statistics: (a) the coherence, which assesses how strongly correlated the two time series are (see Porges, Bohrer, Cheung, Drasgow, McCabe, & Keren, 1980), and (b) the phase, which assesses the lead–lag relationship between the two time series. The time-domain analyses improve to some degree on the frequency domain by controlling for autocorrelation in each series to infer cross-correlation between the series (see Gottman & Ringland, 1981). A detailed introduction to time-series methods is available in Gottman (1981).

Many options exist for multivariate time-series analysis, such as two-stage least squares (Williams and Gottman's TSREG), that relate one "dependent-variable" time series to a set of "independent-variable" time series. The phase information from the cross-spectral bivariate analyses can be used to add lagged variables into the multivariate model.

Multivariate cross-spectral procedures are also available (Brillinger, 1975; Koopmans, 1974), but they are extremely complicated to use at present, and until we have more examples of their successful use, I would advise against relying on them.

Figure 1 is a summary of these recommendations.

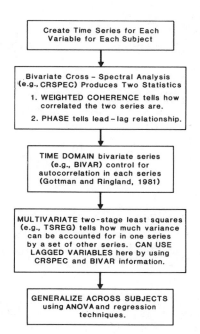

FIGURE 1. Flowchart of proposed time/series analyses.

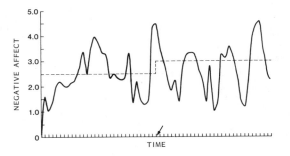

FIGURE 2. Time-series example.

Time-series methods are considerably more powerful than techniques of categorical analysis, which will be discussed in the next section. The balance to be struck is to find a set of time-series variables that have sufficient precision to be clearly interpretable; this is sometimes difficult when adding codes or using a moving probability window or an interevent procedure.

Interrupted time-series analyses are also useful for assessing the effects of extremely rare events. An "indicator" time-series variable can be used, and the data record can be considered an interrupted time-series quasi experiment. Figure 2 illustrates this data-analytic option. The rare event occurred at time = 30 (see arrow). The Gottman–Williams program ITSE used a sixth-order autoregressive model to fit the data. The t test for change in slope was not significant ($t = -.13$, $df = 44$), but the t test for change in level was significant ($t = 2.15$, $df = 44$).

SEQUENTIAL ANALYSIS OF CATEGORICAL DATA

There are many ways of thinking about a sequence of observations if they come from several interacting people. I recommend the following. If there are two codes, A and B, and two people, 1 and 2, this arrangement creates four codes: A1, A2, B1, B2. In my discussion, I will assume that the data from each "subject" (dyad, family, or group) consists of a stream of continuous observations, or of several streams of continuous observations. For purposes of discussion, I will often refer to a sample data set in which there are only two codes, A and B, obtained from one subject:

ABABABAAABBABABABAABBABABABAABBABABABABBBAAA

This will be our raw data record. I will now discuss sequential analysis. I purposely made this data set short so that the reader could follow along and do the simple computations with me. In practice, much longer data sets are required to give confidence in the stability of a sequential analysis. In a sequential analysis, it is important to realize that what we detect are repetitive patterns. This means that a sequence has to happen over and over again to be detected. We cannot do a sequential analysis on one pair of events, no matter how interesting. The statistics, which can be used within a couple or a family, need lots of observations, and the conclusions we arrive at are only statistical, not deterministic. We will be concluding that these patterns occur on a probabilistic basis, not always in deterministic, invariable fashion.

This chapter is, as I mentioned previously, an advertisement. It is not a complete guide to how to do sequential (or time-series) analysis. I refer the reader to forthcoming books by Bakeman and Gottman and by Gottman and Roy on sequential analysis that discuss the subject in some detail. What I would like to do in this section is to offer an overview.

You will have to know only one theorem and to learn only one formula to do sequential analysis. The formula you need to learn is the likelihood ratio chi-square, $LR\chi^2$, defined as

$$LR\chi^2 = 2 \sum_i O_i \log (O_i/E_i) \tag{1}$$

The O represents the observed values, and the E represents the expected values. This equation is something like the familiar Pearson chi-square statistic:

$$\text{Pearson } \chi^2 = \sum_i \frac{(O_i - E_i)^2}{E_i} \tag{2}$$

The $LR\chi^2$ is nice because it has some special mathematical properties. The $LR\chi^2$ is also called G^2. The G stands for Goodman, who was a pioneer in the field now known as *qualitative data analysis*.

The theorem you need to know about is a remarkable result that has to do with what are called *nested* or *hierarchical models* in statistics. This theorem involves a big model and a little model, the latter being a special case of the former. For example, in analysis of variance, the big model may have interaction terms, and the little model may not have these terms in it. Usually, in statistics, the little model is the mathematical representation of the null hypothesis. The little model will be the big model with some terms set to zero (which will usually mean different parameters for the little model). The theorem is that if we compute the likelihood function of the big model (call it Model A), L_A, and the likelihood function of the little model (call it Model B), L_B, then twice the log of the ratio of the two likelihood functions, $2 \log_e (L_A/L_B)$ will be distributed asymptotically as a chi-square with degrees of freedom equal to the difference in the number of parameters in the two models. Now, I realize that that is a mouthful and seems very complex at first hearing, but it is actually a really amazing result and worth studying for some time.

It is possible to heuristically derive from this relation (if one assumes a multinomial distribution) the usual Goodman likelihood ratio formula (see Gottman & Roy, in press).

The thing that is critical in applying Equation (1) is to recognize what a "model" is. I suggest that

A MODEL IS *ANY* SET OF ASSUMPTIONS THAT PRODUCE
ESTIMATES OF THE EXPECTED VALUES, THE E_i

The word *any* is emphasized in the above definition of a model because any reasonable way of getting the expected values will do. (A caution needs to be added: Only maximum likelihood methods for obtaining the *E*s will produce asymptotic chi-square statistics.) There are profound implications of this definition that ought to free up researchers.

We will need two additional concepts to proceed with our discussion. The first concept is the *timetable*. The timetable is a contingencylike table that summarizes antecedent–consequent relationships. This summary is done by means of a moving time window. The moving time window is a way of counting. For example, if we have two codes, A and B, and our data are ABBAB, our first pair is AB, our second pair is BB, our third pair is BA, and our fourth is AB. We are sliding a two-unit window along the data and counting. Note that the data are dependent because the last element of one pair is the first element of the next. Similarly, the antecedent can be a pair of events, in which case we would have a three-unit window. For the data just presented, the first triple would be ABB, and the second would be BAB. The table we fill would consist of counts of specific antecedents followed by specific consequents. For example, Table 1 is a summary of the two-way table obtained with a two-unit time window to the longer data set previously presented. The timetable can be a cube if we go back two time lags into the past. The determination of the size of the timetable is called finding the *order of the Markov chain*. We want to know how far back into the past we can go and keep gaining new information.

The second concept we need is what I call the *contextual design*. In any study, we will probably have a timetable for each cell of our experimental design. For example, our design may be a 2 × 2 factorial design with one factor the social class of married couples (blue collar/white collar) and the other factor marital satisfaction (high/low). Each cell of the design contains a timetable for each couple. As does the text of Table 1, Table 2 illustrates a full 2 × 2 factorial contextual design. There are two factors: (a) blue or white collar and (b) happy or unhappy marriage. In each cell, there is a 6 × 6 timetable (husband positive, H+; husband neutral, Ho; husband negative, H−; wife positive, W+; wife neutral, Wo; and wife negative, W−).

We can now discuss sequential analysis in terms of two steps: issues involved in forming the timetable and issues involved in analyzing the contextual design.

TABLE 1. A Contingency-like Two-Way "Timetable"

Antecedent code (Time *t*)	Consequent code (Time *t* + 1)	
	A	B
A	6	16
B	16	5

TABLE 2. Example of a Contextual Design with Varying Timetables

Group	Antecedent affect	Consequent affect					
		H+	Ho	H−	W+	Wo	W−
White collar	H+	0	12	0	8	11	12
	Ho	8	0	29	33	509	168
	H−	2	30	0	3	87	54
Unhappy	W+	7	32	5	0	15	2
	Wo	15	506	75	17	0	70
	W−	11	162	67	1	64	0
	H+	0	24	2	34	49	15
	Ho	23	0	31	96	873	133
Happy	H−	5	36	0	4	43	16
	W+	27	79	13	0	41	5
	Wo	57	894	40	28	0	24
	W−	11	121	18	4	39	0
Blue collar	H+	0	19	1	11	17	5
	Ho	15	0	46	53	520	93
	H−	1	41	0	23	142	97
Unhappy	W+	13	43	22	0	26	5
	Wo	21	524	134	19	0	62
	W−	3	99	100	4	54	0
	H+	0	17	13	30	58	25
	Ho	27	0	40	72	729	108
Happy	H−	8	50	0	24	123	54
	W+	31	70	16	0	48	6
	Wo	54	725	146	40	0	61
	W−	24	117	44	7	62	0

THE THREE ISSUES IN FORMING THE TIMETABLE

In forming the timetable, we need to decide three things: (a) the *order* of the timetable (i.e., how far back in the past to go); (b) the *stationarity* of the timetable (e.g., whether the first part of the data stream is like the second part); and (c) the *homogeneity* of the data (i.e., whether to pool the data across subjects).

In each case, we use Equation (1). For example, suppose we have had couples discuss two topics, and we are not sure whether to analyze the discussions separately; to determine if the data should be broken into two parts, we have a big model that says the data *should* be broken into two parts and a little model that says the data should not (the little model is usually less interesting than the big model). The little model computes a timetable for all the data and gives us our E_i. The big model breaks the data into two parts and gives us our O_i. For further detail on how to perform these computations, see Gottman and Roy. Ting-Toomey (1982) computed the likelihood ratio test for homogeneity across two topics that married couples discussed. Her likelihood ratio was 86.79 with

210 degrees of freedom, not significant. Because she found no significant difference, this means that the two conversations could be pooled and analyzed as one kind of interaction.

Ting-Toomey also used the likelihood-ratio chi-square test to determine for the appropriate order of the model. In comparing a zero-order model (no sequential structure) to a first order model, she found that the likelihood-ratio chi-square was 566.46 for satisfied couples and 709.51 for dissatisfied couples, with 196 degrees of freedom. Thus, the first-order model cannot be rejected, that is, there is sequential structure in the data for both of these groups. She then examined the first-order compared to the second-order model. This comparison assesses whether there is any payoff in going back one additional time unit into the past, that is, to consider triads of events. She found a likelihood-ratio chi-square of 931.50 for satisfied couples and a likelihood ratio of 1598.06 for dissatisfied couples, with 2940 degrees of freedom, both not significant. Hence, she decided to stop with the first-order model.

The reader may be interested in referring to another example of the application of these tests. Hawes and Foley (1976) applied the Anderson and Goodman (1957) tests in a study of group decision-making. They used a nine-category coding system: (a) chairperson assert; (b) chairperson request; (c) chairperson propose; (d) faculty assert; (e) faculty request; (f) faculty propose; (g) student assert; (h) student request; and (i) student propose. Seven meetings, each lasting about two hours, of three academic committees were videotaped. Hawes and Foley used the likelihood ratio statistic for testing stationarity; the data were divided into fourths. Lack of stationarity was found for two meetings of one of the committees. The order of the Markov chains was also tested by means of the Attneave test, which can be shown to be mathematically equivalent to the Anderson and Goodman tests (see Gottman & Roy, in preparation, for a proof). First-order analyses provided a better fit to the data than zero-order (no sequential dependency). Homogeneity was also tested; Hawes and Foley concluded that the committees needed to be separately analyzed. The paper is useful because it shows that the computations are practical.

All of these tests are what might be called *omnibus tests*. For example, they do not assess stationarity for specific sequences. They are crude tests, and various other options exist that are much more specific and potentially more interesting. These options are discussed in detail in Gottman and Roy (in preparation).

The point I want to make about these three issues in forming the timetable is that each issue is an opportunity for learning about your data. The issue of *order* tells you, in general, how long your interaction chains are. The issue of *stationarity* tells you whether different parts of the interaction are different. The issue of *homogeneity* tells you how to classify the subjects in your sample. Each issue is an opportunity for discovery, rather than a prohibition. Unfortunately, these issues have been viewed in the latter restrictive sense in much of the literature. I am recommending an approach here that is similar in spirit to Cronbach *et al.*'s reconceptualization (1972) of reliability and validity.

The implication of this view is that the data should not be considered absolutely stationary or not stationary, but that it depends on the purposes of the research which decision is reached. For further details see Gottman and Roy (1986).

ISSUES IN THE CONTEXTUAL DESIGN

I want to briefly describe how the contextual design can be analyzed if, of course, the decision has been made to pool data across subjects. Much of this discussion is available in any good text on log-linear models, such as Bishop, Fienberg, and Holland (1975).

As I previously noted, it's not very interesting to state the order of the sequential structure. Usually, our hypotheses are that some particular sequence varies with contextual variables in our experimental design, such as age and sex. Procedures have become available in the last decade (Bishop *et al.*, 1975) that mimic analysis of variance. We can now estimate the result of specific effects (such as age) and their interactions on frequency counts using log-linear models.

We begin with the data. This is called the *saturated table*, not really a model, as a model is any reasonable way of obtaining expected counts. The counts of this table are denoted O_i. Any other representation of the data is a simplification, called a *model*, and it involves dropping terms from the saturated table model. For example, in a two-way table, the counts $n_{i,j}$ are represented by the independence model in the familiar way of multiplying column, $Q(i)$, and row probabilities, $R(j)$, by the total, N:

$$n_{i,j} = NQ(i)R(j)$$

which can be written in log form as

$$\log n_{i,j} = \log N_2 + \log Q(i) + \log (R_j)$$
$$= \mu + \mu_A + \mu_B$$

In its last form, this equation represents the independence model in an additive form; much as in the analysis of variance, there is no nonadditive interaction term.

We test a model such as the independence model (or any other model) by computing

$$G^2 = 2 \sum_i O_i \log (O_i/E_i)$$

With appropriate degrees of freedom. As I noted earlier, a "model" for a table is simply a logical way of obtaining the E_i terms (i.e., the expected counts). There are algorithms for obtaining the E_i once we specify the model. The most commonly used algorithm is iterative proportional fitting (IPF), also called the Deming–Stephan algorithm. In general, this algorithm works by putting ones in each cell of the design and then adjusting cell frequencies to conform first with one margin and then with another, iterating until convergence is obtained. The procedure is conceptually simple, but computationally tedious. Computer programs exist to perform this procedure (e.g., Fay and Goodman's ECTA).

We are searching for a model that does *not* give us significant G^2; that is, we are searching for nonsignificance. This means that we can do without terms that we drop from the fully saturated table. It is important to note that there is not just one G^2, but a different G^2 for each model. Now, here is where the statistics come in. Suppose we have two models, call them A and B. In the special case that B is a smaller model than A (i.e., it is A with some terms missing), as I have noted previously it is also the case that the difference in the two G^2's is asymptotically distributed as chi-square, with degrees of freedom equal to the difference in the sizes of A and B models (the difference in the number of parameters in the two models). This fact makes it useful to fit a hierarchical series of models to the data.

It is very important to reiterate that the goal in model fitting is to find a simple and interesting model that fits the data, that is, that produces a nonsignificant chi-square. The chi-square is not significant because the model provides a good approximation of the saturated table.

Perhaps the most commonly used technique for finding a model is the evaluation of a series of models that are arranged in a hierarchy so that each model is contained in a previous model. This is not the only set of models possible, but the hierarchical approach has some definite advantages.

It has become standard notation to write a model using brackets as follows. If we have three factors, A, B, and C, then a model that includes only A and B and their interaction would be written {AB}, and the model would be

$$\log (\hat{m}_{i,j,k}) = \hat{\mu} + (\hat{\lambda}_A)_i + (\hat{\lambda}_B)_j + (\hat{\lambda}_{A,B})_{i,j} \qquad (3)$$

The m_{ijk} are the cell frequencies and the λ's estimate the effects of each factor. Note that the presence of the interaction term implies the presence of the main effect terms. This is what makes the models hierarchical. In other words, the model in Equation (3) contains the following simple main effect model:

$$\log (\hat{m}_{ijk}) = \hat{\mu} + (\hat{\lambda}_A)_i + (\hat{\lambda}_B)_j \qquad (4)$$

Table 3 illustrates the 19 possible models for a three-way experimental design. Now, here is the beauty of the hierarchical arrangement: We can evaluate the effect of a term in the model by subtracting the G^2 for the models. For example, if the $LR\chi^2$ is 44.20 with 24 DF and the G^2 for model (4) is 200.70 with 39 DF, then the G^2 for the AB interaction term is $(200.70 - 44.20) = 156.50$ with $(39-24) = 15$ DF. (Recall this procedure uses IPF to compare [3] with the saturated table, i.e., the observed values.) This procedure shows that the term must probably be included in the model.

In this manner, each term in the full model can be evaluated. To summarize, each model yields its own likelihood-ratio G^2 term and DF. The difference between the G^2 and the DFs of two suitably selected models can produce an

TABLE 3. The 19 Possible Models for a Three-Way Table

Defining set of parameters	Parameters in the model							
	μ	A	B	C	AB	AC	BC	ABC
{ABC}	√	√	√	√	√	√	√	√
{AB} {AC} {BC}	√	√	√	√	√	√	√	
{AB} {AC}	√	√	√	√	√	√		
{AC} {BC}	√	√	√	√		√	√	
{BC} {AB}	√	√	√	√	√		√	
{A} {BC}	√	√	√	√			√	
{B} {AC}	√	√	√	√		√		
{C} {AB}	√	√	√	√	√			
{BC}	√		√	√			√	
{AB}	√	√	√		√			
{AC}	√	√		√		√		
{A} {B} {C}	√	√	√	√				
{A} {B}	√	√	√					
{A} {C}	√	√		√				
{B} {C}	√		√	√				
{A}	√	√						
{B}	√		√					
{C}	√			√				
{μ}	√							

assessment of the significance of a term in the full model. For example, in a two-dimensional table, if the {A} {B} model holds

$$\log \hat{m}_{i,j} = \hat{\mu} + (\hat{\lambda}_A)_i + (\hat{\lambda}_B)_j \tag{5}$$

yields $G^2 = 6.9$ with $1 = DF$ and the submodel {A} holds

$$\log \hat{m}_{i,j} = \hat{\mu} + (\hat{\lambda}_A)_i$$

yields $G^2 = 41.7$ with $2 = DF$, then the difference in the G^2s evaluates the (λ_B) term as $41.7 - 6.9 = 34.8$ with $DF = 2 - 1 = 1$. This result would suggest to us that we need to keep the (λ_B) term in the model.

Selecting a Model by Screening

Now, here's the rub. In contingency tables with more than two factors it is possible to find several pairs of models that will differ by the same simple parameter, and the difference in G^2 will not be the same. Why is this true? Because, in fact, the test of significance of a parameter is *conditional* on a specific set of parameters having been included.

Brown (1974) suggested a procedure called *screening* to decide whether to include each parameter in the final model. For each term, Brown suggested obtaining two estimates of significance. One estimate, called a *test of marginal association,* compares two simple models. For example, in a four-factor table, compare {AB} with {A} {B}. A second estimate, called a *test of partial association,* compares two complex models; for example, compare {AB} {AC} {AD} {BC} {BD} {CD} with {AC} {AD} {BC} {BD} {CD}. What's different in each comparison is the {AB} term, but the two comparisons will give different values for the significance of the {AB} term. The process of screening gives a range of significance values that can be used to decide whether to include a particular term in the final model.

Upton (1978) suggested using "forward selection" and "backward elimination." *Forward selection* means that, at each stage of the analysis, the most important term is included in the model. Backward elimination means that, at each stage, the least important term is excluded from the table. Hocking (1976) pointed out that neither procedure necessarily leads to a unique best model, if such a model even exists. The goal is to obtain a relatively simple *and interesting* model. Goodman (1971) wrote:

> By including additional λs in the model, the fit can be improved; and so the researcher must weigh in each particular case the advantages of the improved fit against the disadvantages of having introduced additional parameters in the model. Different researchers will weigh these advantages and disadvantages differently. (p. 41)

We now need some methods for assessing what specific sequences contribute to the effects that we decide are present after screening. I will review two sets of methods.

Contrasts

Plackett (1962) proposed that, because the estimated variance of the logarithm of a Poisson frequency is the reciprocal of the frequency, if λ is any weighted sum of the cell frequencies that is a linear contrast:

$$\hat{\lambda} = \sum_{i,j,k \ldots} a_{i,j,k} \ldots \log \hat{m}_{i,j,k} \ldots \tag{7}$$

Then an estimate of the variance of λ is

$$v(\lambda) = \sum_{i,j,k \ldots} \frac{(a_{i,j,k} \ldots)^2}{\hat{m}_{i,j,k} \ldots} \tag{8}$$

Furthermore, Goodman (1971) showed that the following ratio is asymptotically a unit normal distribution:

$$s(\hat{\lambda}) = \hat{\lambda} / \sqrt{v(\hat{\lambda})} \tag{9}$$

This method is a useful method for comparing cells in a table.

One option that we have once we have found an interesting model that nearly fits is to examine the table cell by cell and to look for cells that may be ruining the fit. To accomplish this analysis of residuals, we can use the Freeman–Tukey deviates or the components of chi-square (Bishop *et al.*, 1975). An alternative is to force cells to zero that we believe are "outliers," recompute G^2, and subtract our two G^2 terms; the difference in G^2 will have one degree of freedom.

Consider the data in Table 3. Let P = the prior or antecendent code; R = the result, or consequent code; S = satisfaction; and C = class. Then, Table 4 shows the results of a hierarchical log-linear analysis (I used the UCLA biomedical series program BMDP 4F). The model with all three-way interactions fits the data well (DF = 19, chi-square = 23.1) Freeman–Tukey deviates for this model show no significant cell. The model with the RPC term dropped is not bad; it is just marginally significant (chi-square = 55, DF = 38, P = .04). Even in this model, none of the Freeman–Tukey deviates are significant.

The RPS and RPC terms are of greatest interest theoretically. They suggest that the timetable varies with marital satisfaction and with social class, with satisfaction being a much larger effect than social class. Of greatest interest (see Gottman, 1979, on negative affect reciprocity) are sequences of extended conflict (negative affect). Table 5 illustrates the expected cell frequencies in the reduced model and proportions (divided by the frequency of the antecedent for that cell). Although the $S(\hat{\lambda})$ terms are quite large, the proportions would lead us to be cautious. We can suggest that (a) couples differ across class, independent of

TABLE 4. Hierarchical Log-Linear Analysis of the Data in Table 2

Effect	DF	Partial association		Marginal association	
		Chi-square	Probability	Chi-square	Probability
R	5	10223.8	.000		
P	5	10247.8	.000		
S	1	194.6	.000		
C	1	5.9	.015		
RP	19	1642.4	.000	1746.9	.000
RS	5	183.7	.000	204.4	.000
RC	5	136.3	.000	108.7	.000
RS	5	181.2	.000	203.1	.000
PC	5	137.5	.000	110.0	.000
SC	1	0.3	.585	3.6	.057
RPS	19	50.5	.000	44.1	.001
RPC	19	31.9	.032	27.3	.097
RSC	5	43.6	.000	31.1	.000
PSC	5	46.4	.000	31.4	.000

TABLE 5. Cell Frequencies and Conditional Probabilities in the Reduced Model (RPC Term Dropped)

Groups	Sequences			
	H− → W−	$S(\hat{\lambda})$	W− → H−	$S(\hat{\lambda})$
Blue collar	140.9 (.25)	4.26	143.5 (.28)	5.24
White collar	82.1 (.29)		87.5 (.17)	
Satisfied	71.0 (.19)	5.59	63.0 (.14)	7.08
Dissatisfied	152.0 (.31)		168.0 (.29)	

marital satisfaction, in that blue-collar husbands are more likely than white-collar husbands to reciprocate their wives' negative affect, and that (b) dissatisfied couples (husbands and wives), independent of class, are more likely than satisfied couples to reciprocate their partner's negative affect.

Another approach that is useful is Sackett's lag-sequence analysis. Here the Sackett z-score is examined for each target code at various logs from the criterion, regardless of what codes intervene. Each code plays the role of target and criterion code. The "probability profiles" are used to infer sequences of higher-than-chance expectation, compared to the full independence model. The method has advantages and disadvantages. It is a great savings in computation, and it makes it possible to do sequence analysis with many fewer data. Forming a two-step Markov contingency table with 40 codes gives $40 \times 40 \times 40$ cells = 64,000 cells, and most of us do not have enough data to be confident in our cell counts even for this two-step process. The disadvantage of the Sackett idea is that it is not logically identical to a full Markov analysis. To accomplish this analysis, the criterion has to become pairs of codes, triples, and so on. A procedure like this was used with great success by Revenstorf, (1980) for a small set of codes in studying affect in marital interaction. The Sackett approach is of great advantage in hypothesis generation, particularly if we are in the early stages of investigation or are using a coding system that hasn't yet been broken in.

There are issues of cells with "logical zeros" (e.g., some code combinations are logically impossible, such as a code following itself), sparse tables, and outlier cells that have state-of-the-art solutions (see Bishop et al., 1975). I will not review these issues in this chapter.

Figure 3 is a flowchart that summarizes this discussion. To form the indices of sequential connection, we need to create statistics that compare conditional with unconditional probabilities. A variety of indices are currently on the marketplace; they tend to be reasonably similar, so I will review only one of them, the one derived by Gottman (1980) and then subsequently by Allison and Liker (1982). A discussion of several other such statistics is given in Gottman and Roy (1986).

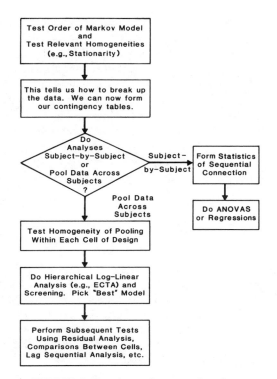

FIGURE 3. Flowchart of proposed analyses.

Indices of Sequential Connection

One index of sequential connection is based on the approximation to the binomial test by the normal distribution. Suppose one wishes to test whether a sequence, *AB*, is likely in the data at a lag, *k*. Form the statistic

$$z = \frac{p_k\,(B/A) - p(B)}{\sqrt{\dfrac{p(B)(1 - p(B))(1 - p(A))}{(n - k)\,p(A)}}}$$

This statistic is asymptotically normal, so that it can be compared to a normal distribution for sufficiently large *n* (e.g., it is significant at $p < .05$, if $Z > 1.96$). The $p_k\,(B|A)$ is the conditional probability of *B*, given that *A* has occurred *k* lags previously.

Several inappropriate analyses of sequential connection recur frequently in the literature. The most frequent incorrect index is the conditional probability itself. To establish sequential connection between an antecedent event, *A*, and the consequent event, B, the recommendation is to simply examine the conditional probability $p_k (B|A)$. The problem with this statistic is that it does not control for the *base-rate problem*. The base-rate problem is that it is meaningless to discuss the conditional probability without reference to the reduction over and above predicting the base rate of B, $p (B)$. Furthermore, the conditional probability alone is a poor statistic to use in comparing subjects (couples or families) because each subject will have a different base rate, $p (B)$. A conditional probability of 0.60 may be unimportant for one subject because the unconditional was .56, but it may be very important for another subject for which the unconditional was .40.

Also in use is the Freeman–Tukey deviate, FT, defined as

$$FT = \sqrt{O_i} + \sqrt{O_i + 1} - \sqrt{4E_i + 1}$$

where the E_i are usually the expected value under an independence model. The FT deviate is also asymptotically normal.

The suggestion in Figure 3 is that the indices of sequential connection be used as a measure and be subjected to the usual analyses of variance or regressions implied by the contextual design. The parametric analyses that do not pool data across subjects tend to be more powerful than the nonparametric analyses that do pool across subjects. For examples of both, see Gottman (1983). I urge the reader to examine examples that have used sequential analysis in order to understand the details of working with sequences.

SUMMARY

When we are interested in studying the temporal structure of behavior, two options are available. We can analyze the data subject-(dyad, family)-by-subject (dyad, family), using time-series statistics or indices of sequential connection. If we have enough data to have confidence in the stability of these statistics, this approach probably offers the most powerful set of alternatives. If we do not have enough data, or if we are interested in rare events, we will have to pool data across subjects. This chapter suggests that, for both options, techniques have been worked out that researchers who are interested in family interaction can learn. This chapter is intended primarily as an advertisement for the sequential analysis of observational data. For more useful and detailed information about the ins and outs of data analysis, as well as a discussion of available computer programs, readers are directed to Bakeman and Gottman (1986), Gottman (1981), and Williams and Gottman (1981).

REFERENCES

Allison, P. D., & Liker, J. K. (1982). Analyzing sequential categorical data on dyadic interaction: A comment on Gottman. *Psychological Bulletin, 91,* 303–403.

Anderson, T. W., & Goodman, L. A. (1957). Statistical inference about Markov chains. *Annals of Mathematical Statistics, 28,* 89–110.

Bakeman, R., & Gottman, J. (1986). *Observing behavior sequences.* New York: Cambridge University Press.

Bateson, G., Jackson, D. D., Haley, J., & Weakland, J. (1956). Toward a theory of schizophrenia. *Behavioral Science, 1,* 251–264.

Bishop, U. M. M., Fienberg, S., & Holland, P. W. (1975). *Discrete multivariate analysis.* Cambridge: MIT Press.

Brazelton, T. B., Koslowski, B., & Main, M. (1974). The origins of reciprocity: The early mother–infant interaction. In M. Lewis & L. A. Rosenblum (Eds.), *The effect of the infant on its caregiver.* New York: Wiley.

Brillinger, D. (1975). *Time series analysis.* New York: McGraw-Hill.

Brown, M. B. (1974). Identification of the sources of significance in two-way contingency tables. *Applied Statistics, 23,* 405–413.

Coulthard, M. (1977). *An introduction to discourse analysis.* London: Longman.

Cronbach, L. J., Gleser, G. C., Nanda, H., & Rajaratnam, N. (1972). *The dependability of behavioral measurements: Theory of generalizability for scores and profiles.* New York: Wiley.

Dindia, K. (1983). Reciprocity of self-disclosure: A sequential analysis. In M. Burgoon (Ed.), *Communication Yearbook* (Vol. 6). Beverly Hills, CA: Sage Publications.

Ekman, P., & Friesen, W. V. (1978). *The facial action coding system.* Palo Alto: Consulting Psychologists Press.

Fisher, R., & Ury, W. (1981). *Getting to yes.* New York: Houghton Mifflin.

Fleiss, J. L. (1971). Measuring nominal scale agreement among many raters. *Psychological Bulletin, 76,* 378–382.

Godel, K. (1932). *On formally undecideable propositions of Principia Mathematica and related systems.* London: Oliver & Boyd.

Gottman, J. M. (1979). *Marital interaction: Experimental investigations.* New York: Academic Press.

Gottman, J. M. (1980). Analyzing for sequential connection and assessing interobserver reliability for the sequential of observational data. *Behavioral Assessment, 2,* 361–368.

Gottman, J. M. (1982). *Time-series analysis: A comprehensive introduction for social scientists.* New York: Cambridge University Press.

Gottman, J. M. (1983). How children become friends. *Monographs of the Society for Research in Child Development, 48,* (201), 1–82.

Gottman, J. M., & Ginsberg, D. (1986). The conversations of college roomates. In J. M. Gottman (Ed.), *The conversations of friends.* New York: Cambridge University Press.

Gottman, J. M., & Mettetal, G. (1986). Friendships in middle childhood and adolescence. In J. M. Gottman (Ed.), *The conversations of friends.* New York: Cambridge University Press.

Gottman, J. M., & Ringland, J. (1981). The analysis of dominance and bidirectionality in social development. *Child Development, 52,* 393–412.

Gottman, J. M., & Roy, A. K. (1986). *Temporal form: Detecting sequences in social interaction.* New York: Cambridge University Press.

Gottman, J. M., & Roy, A. K. (1987). Untitled manuscript in preparation.

Gottman, J. M., Rose, F. T., & Mettetal, G. (1982). Time-series analysis of social interaction data. In T. Field & A. Fogel (Eds.), *Emotion and early interaction.* Hillsdale, NJ: Lawrence Erlbaum.

Goodman, L. A. (1971). Partitioning of chi-square analysis of marginal contingency tables and estimation of expected frequencies in multidimensional contingency tables. *Journal of American Statistical Association, 66,* 339–344.

Harper, R. G., Wiens, A. N., & Matarazzo, J. D. (1978). *Nonverbal communication: The state of the art.* New York: Wiley.

Hawes, L. C., & Foley, J. M. (1976). Group decisioning: Testing a finite stochastic model. In G. R. Miller (Ed.), *Explorations in interpersonal communication.* Beverly Hills, CA: Sage Publications.

Hocking, R. R. (1976). The analysis and selection of variables and linear aggression. *Biometrics, 32,* 1–49.

Koopmans, L. H. (1974). *The spectral analysis of time series.* New York: Academic Press.

Lederer, W. J., & Jackson, D. D. (1968). *The mirages of marriage.* New York: Norton.

Murstein, B. I., Cerreto, M., & McDonald, M. G. (1977). A theory and investigation of the effect of the exchange orientation on marriage and friendship. *Journal of Marriage and the Family, 39,* 543–548.

Parkhurst, J. T. (1986). Quantitative sociolinguistics in the requests of preschool children. In J. M. Gottman (Ed.), *The conversations of friends.* New York: Cambridge University Press.

Parkhurst, J., T. & Gottman, J. M. (1986). How children get what they want. In J. M. Gottman & J. Parker (Eds.), *Conversations of friends.* New York: Cambridge University Press.

Patterson, G. R., & Moore, D. (1979). Interactive patterns as units of behavior. In M. Lamb, S. Soumi, & G. Stephenson (Eds.), *Social interaction analysis: Methodological issues.* Madison: University of Wisconsin Press, 1979.

Plackett, R. L. (1962). A note on interactions and contingency tables. *Journal Royal Statistical Society, 24,* 162–166.

Porges, S. W., Bohrer, R. E., Cheung, M. N., Drasgow, F., McCabe, P. M., & Keren, G. (1980). New time-series statistic for detecting rhythmic co-occurrence in the frequency domain: The weighted coherence and its application to psychophysiological research. *Psychological Bulletin, 88,* 580–587.

Revenstorf, D., Vogel, B., Wegener, C., Halweg, K., & Schindler, L. (1980). Escalation phenomena in interaction sequences: An empirical comparison. *Behavior Analysis and Modification, 3,* 97–116.

Sackett, G. P. (1979). The lag sequential analysis of contingency and cyclicity in behavioral interaction research. In J. Osofsky (Ed.), *Handbook of infant development.* New York: Wiley.

Scherer, K. R., & Ekman, P. (Eds.). (1982). *Handbook of methods in non-verbal behavior research.* New York: Cambridge University Press.

Ting-Toomey, S. (1982, October). *An analysis of communication in differentially satisfied marital couples.* Paper presented at the annual convention of the International Communication Association, Boston.

Upton, G. (1978). *Analysis of cross-tabulated data.* New York: Wiley.

Williams, E. A., & Gottman, J. M. (1981). *A user's guide to the Gottman-Williams time-series analysis computer programs for social scientists.* New York: Cambridge University Press.

PART IV

FAMILY RESEARCH ON SPECIFIC PSYCHOPATHOLOGIES

CHAPTER 13

The Family and Schizophrenia

MICHAEL J. GOLDSTEIN AND ANGUS M. STRACHAN

The last 30 years have witnessed a steady growth of interest in family influences on the individual, in the operations of family systems, and in harnessing the power of the family in creating therapeutic change. Throughout this period, but particularly in the 1950s and 1960s, schizophrenia has been a major focus of family researchers and therapists and has received more attention from eminent scholars of the family than other forms of psychopathology.

One reason that the family of the schizophrenic has received such attention, other than the devastating effect of the disorder on the interpersonal functioning of the person and those around him or her, is related to the marked communicational problems of the person with schizophrenia. Many schizophrenics display such disorders in communication that their conversation is tangential or disjointed—at times, overly metaphorical and abstract, at other times, overly concrete and literal—and their affect contradictory or difficult to understand. Further, the major defining symptoms of schizophrenia—hallucinations and delusions (whether persecutory or grandiose)—can be conceptualized as difficulties in discriminating between the self and the outside world—a distortion in the boundary of the self. Because of these difficulties establishing clear boundaries and clear communication with the schizophrenic, scholars have focused on the family system because it is the primary arena in which children learn to communicate and to develop a sense of themselves as separate from but interdependent with others.

In the 1950s and 1960s, studies of the families of schizophrenics were seminal in the development of family systems theories and of family therapeutic approaches (e.g., Bateson, Jackson, Haley, & Weakland, 1956; Lidz, Cornelison, Fleck, & Terry, 1957; Wynne, Ryckoff, Day, & Hirsch, 1958). However, the

MICHAEL J. GOLDSTEIN AND ANGUS M. STRACHAN • Department of Psychology, University of California at Los Angeles, Los Angeles, CA 90024. Preparation of this chapter was supported, in part, by grants from the National Institute of Health, MH 08744 and MH 30911, and a grant from the MacArthur Foundation on Risk and Protective Factors in the Major Mental Disorders.

discovery that phenothiazine medication could significantly decrease the frequency and the intensity of schizophrenic phenomenology and symptomatology reduced interest in the search for causes of and solutions to schizophrenia in the family. Whatever the causes were, it appeared that medication could have dramatic effects on the most disabling symptoms of a schizophrenic disorder. The potent effects of neuroleptic drugs shifted interests from interpersonal to biological models of causation. This shift in emphasis was reinforced by the findings of twin and adoption studies (Rosenthal & Kety, 1968), which left the impression that schizophrenia was a disorder with a heavy genetic predisposition and with little room remaining for life experiences, particularly during early family life, to influence the likelihood of a schizophrenic disorder in late adolescence or early adulthood. Further, systematic family interaction studies were not providing convincing evidence of differences—other than in the area of communication clarity—between families of schizophrenics and families of normals and psychiatric comparison groups (e.g., Liem, 1980). It appeared that schizophrenia had been a siren that had lured boatloads of unsuspecting family researchers on to the rocks and into shipwreck.

After the disillusionment of the 1970s, however, there have been two important areas of development in research on the family and schizophrenia. Both areas have developed in the context of a stress-vulnerability model of schizophrenia (Lukoff, Snyder, Ventura, & Nuechterlein, 1984), which is now more generally accepted than the either/or models of naive genetic or naive family etiology that dominated the earlier studies. The first area of research grew out of the observations that the phenothiazines were not the cure-all they had appeared to be: psychotic symptoms were completely untouched by medication for 7% of patients, and 35% of patients relapsed within 2 years, even when they were maintained on medication (Leff & Wing, 1971).

This finding that phenothiazines were not a complete cure led to a resurgence of interest in the role of the family as a factor determining the course of the disorder once an episode had occurred. British researchers, in particular, sought to discriminate the kind of family environments that tended to protect the returning schizophrenic patients from relapse from those that tended to provoke relapse. They identified one measure of the family emotional environment termed *high expressed emotion* (high EE) as being particularly noxious (Brown, Birley, & Wing, 1972; Vaughn & Leff, 1976). The term *high expressed emotion* refers to attitudes of criticism and/or emotional overinvolvement expressed about a patient by a relative during an extensive interview. Patients who returned to high-EE homes were found to relapse at a significantly higher rate than those who returned to low-EE homes. The identification of these specific parameters of family life, which emphasize the impact of a negative affective climate within the family, has spawned several systematic outcome studies of the effectiveness of family intervention in aftercare (Anderson, Hogarty, & Reiss, 1980; Falloon, Boyd, McGill, Razani, Moss, & Gilderman, 1982; Goldstein, Rodnick, Evans, May, & Steinberg, 1978; Leff, Kuipers, Berkowitz, Eberlein-Fries, & Sturgeon, 1982, 1983) and has refocused interest in the role of family factors related to schizophrenia at a more general level.

In one sense, there is a sharp departure in emphasis between this newer research and the earlier studies. There is no presumption in the expressed-emotion studies that these family attitudes play an etiological role in the initial development of the disorder. The negative affective attitudes are presumed to be relevant only after schizophrenia has developed and do not necessarily possess continuity with the prepsychotic phase of family life. However, there is an important empirical question. We need to investigate whether there is such sharp discontinuity between affective attitudes expressed toward a relative from the pre- to the postpsychotic phases of their life. Perhaps the notable sensitivity of the schizophrenic person to intrafamilial criticism, for example, is based on a high level of exposure to such attitudes during the prepsychotic phase of his or her life.

The other area of development has been a move away from cross-sectional studies to more complex longitudinal research designs that explore the developmental course of schizophrenia. These so-called high-risk designs (Garmezy, 1974a,b) attempt to disentangle processes that precede from those that follow the onset of schizophrenia. Such a strategy is particularly important in the study of intrafamilial processes, as it is generally agreed that the presence of a psychotic relative has a major impact on family life. If we wish to draw reasonable conclusions regarding the contribution of intrafamilial processes to the development of schizophrenia, it is necessary to demonstrate with a prospective study that such processes do, in fact, antedate the onset of the disorder. These longitudinal, high-risk studies would be greatly enriched if we had behavioral or biological markers of the genetic vulnerability to schizophrenia, somewhat akin to the marker for the sickle-cell-anemia trait. The availability of such a marker would permit us to investigate how individuals predisposed to schizophrenia are affected by benign or pathological family relationships. At the present time, unfortunately, no valid markers of the diathesis for schizophrenia are available, although there are a number of possibilities on the horizon. Without such markers, it is extremely difficult for family researchers to indicate the degree to which disturbed family relationships play a contributory role in the development of schizophrenia.

One strategy that attacks this issue in a less direct way is the adoption study approach. This approach has been used primarily to establish that genetic factors influence the probability of schizophrenia. By establishing that the incidence of schizophrenia and of what have been termed *schizophrenia-spectrum disorders* was higher in the biological relatives of adopted schizophrenics than in adopted nonpsychiatric persons (Kety, Rosenthal, Wender, & Schulsinger, 1968), the evidence for genetic transmission was strengthened. However, this same strategy is currently being used by Tienari, Sorri, Lahti, Naarala, Wahlberg, Pohjola, and Moring (1985) to investigate possible gene–environment interactions. In this study, the Finnish Adoption Study, the psychiatric status of the adopted-away offspring of schizophrenic persons is contrasted with the status of adopted-away offspring of nonpsychiatric patients. However, unlike in the earlier Danish studies, a systematic attempt is being made to assess the psychiatric status of both the biological and the adoptive parents, as well as the family environment within the adoptive home. Although this study is still in progress, preliminary data are quite supportive of the stress–diathesis model, as the few cases of schizophrenia observed are seen only in the adopted-away offspring of schizophrenic patients, and such cases have appeared only in the most severely disturbed family environments. Further follow-up of this sample will clarify whether the level of family disturbance is a necessary condition for the emergence of schizophrenia or merely modifies the age of onset so that it is the early-onset cases that have appeared so far in these disturbed homes.

In the remainder of this chapter, after a historical overview of early family theories on schizophrenia, we shall discuss the family's role in schizophrenia in terms of a series of discrete but interrelated questions:

1. Is there any evidence that families of schizophrenics show patterns of intrafamilial communication and structure that are different from those of other families?
2. Is there any evidence that disturbed family relationships precede the onset of schizophrenia?
3. Is there any evidence that there are specific patterns of disturbed family relationships associated with schizophrenia as compared with other major psychiatric disorders?
4. Is there any evidence that family factors affect the course of schizophrenia?
5. Is there any connection between family factors that precede schizophrenia and those related to its course?
6. Is there any evidence that family relationships interact with a biological predisposition in the development of schizophrenia?

HISTORICAL OVERVIEW: THE DEVELOPMENT OF EARLY IDEAS ABOUT THE FAMILY AND SCHIZOPHRENIA

As in many other scientific fields, the history of theories about the family and schizophrenia parallels the history of epistemological developments in the philosophy of science. Early in this century, with the zeitgeist of Newtonian notions of energy conservation, ideas about schizophrenia were developed from Freud's theory of "intrapsychic energy," culminating in an object relations formulation of the development of schizophrenia (Guntrip, 1973). With the development of small-group theory and group therapy (Cartwright & Zander, 1968; Walton, 1971), the focus shifted to the interpersonal context of the schizophrenic, with a focus on family roles and norms. With the advent of the computer age came cybernetics (Wiener, 1965), with its focus on information, communication, feedback loops, and steady states, particularly in closed mechanical systems. Schizophrenia researchers began to investigate distorted communication patterns in the families of schizophrenics. Later, attention shifted to a consideration of open living systems as well (Miller, 1978), with their transactions across boundaries to other organic systems. These ideas had an impact on many fields: biology, economics, and ecology. However, although systems notions based on observations of families of schizophrenics have played a major role in the development of the new field of family therapy, they have had surprisingly little impact on research on families of schizophrenics. It appears that the operationalization of concepts derived from systems theory is not as simple as theorists originally implied.

In this section, these developments are outlined in detail.

Psychoanalytic Developments: Movement toward Interpersonal Theories

Freud explored the intrapsychic world of individuals, stressing the importance for personality formation of the conflict between innate instincts and drives, and societal expectations of appropriate behavior. To the extent that he also stressed the importance of early childhood events in the etiology of personality structure, particularly the shifting alliances at the time of the Oedipus–Electra stage, it could be said that he was a pioneer in emphasizing the importance of the family. It should be noted, however, that Freud focused exclusively on the internal conflicts generated within individuals and their fantasized representations of family figures and did not relate his theories to the observation of family transactions.

The cause of neurosis, according to Freud's theory, was unconscious intrapsychic conflict, which led to the repression of unacceptable unconscious impulses. This conflict model, however, was not useful in explaining psychosis. Therefore, psychoanalysts such as Federn (1952) advanced the idea that schizophrenia was due to a fragile ego with poorly developed defenses, so that, under stress, the defenses would break down and unconscious material would erupt into consciousness. The preferred treatment approach was to avoid transference interpretations and instead to focus on real relationships and support the patient's control and reality testing. Other American psychoanalysts, such as Eric Erikson, Karen Horney, Harry Stack Sullivan, and Nathan Ackerman, known as neo-Freudians, similarly expanded psychoanalytic theory to consider real interpersonal relationships. Another pioneer was Frieda Fromm-Reichman (1948), who described a "schizophrenogenic" mother as one who is overprotective but also cold, critical, and impervious to her child's needs, thus thwarting his or her ability to differentiate, to form a separate identity, and to develop close relationships.

Paralleling the development of neo-Freudian theory in America was the development of object-relations theory in Britain. This grew out of Melanie Klein's clinical work (Segal, 1973) with the fantasy life of emotionally disturbed 2- and 3-year-olds. Her work, which focused on the early mother–child relationship, emphasized the impact of a lack of "whole good internal objects" (fantasized representations of human relationships) in the development of severe forms of pathology, such as schizoid, borderline, narcissistic, and psychotic states, and led to the development of object-relations theory (Fairburn, 1954;

Guntrip, 1973; Kernberg, 1975). The theory suggested that damage to the early parent–child bond caused the formation of bad object-relations, which could lead to the defensive mechanisms of "splitting" and projection seen in schizophrenia and related disorders.

Thus, object-relations theory contributed to an interpersonal perspective on schizophrenia but focused on only one part of the family system, the mother–infant relationship.

The Family as a Small Group: Early Systems Thinking

It was in the aftermath of World War II that the notion of the family system was born. In the background was the "field theory" of Kurt Lewin (1951), a social psychologist who emphasized the importance of the context of the individual in determining behavior. During and after the war, veterans in Britain and the United States who needed counseling to deal with combat stress had to be seen in groups rather than individually because of the large numbers involved. Unexpectedly, it was found that the small groups were powerfully helpful. In addition to, but quite independent of, the development of group therapy for schizophrenics (Jones, 1953), the 1950s witnessed a rapidly developing interest in the systematic study of small groups—an area of interest that resulted in significant advances in role theory (Bales, 1950; Parsons & Bales, 1955) and small-group theory (e.g., Cartwright & Zander, 1968).

It was in this atmosphere that researchers began to think of the family as a special kind of small group, with values, norms, and interrelated roles. Extending psychoanalytic ideas, Lidz and his group of co-workers at Yale argued that, in families of schizophrenics, distortions in the role relationships between parents and between parent and child in terms of age and sex gave the child a distorted view of his or her own identity and unrealistic ideas about the outside world. This process was called the *transmission of irrationality*, and two major patterns of distorted parental roles were described (Lidz *et al.*, 1957): skewed and schismatic. In the former, the parents have markedly distorted sex-roles: the mother is dominant and cold in contrast with her husband, who is rather passive and ineffectual. The latter pattern, marital schism, is characterized by chronic hostility and criticism between the spouses and attempts to compete for the child's loyalty and affection.

At about the same time, Murray Bowen was hospitalizing schizophrenics with their families at the National Institute of Mental Health for observation and treatment. From this work, he developed the concept of *differentiation of self* and the *undifferentiated family ego mass*. Someone who is "differentiated" can be emotionally close to her or his own family members, or to anybody else, without "fusing into emotional oneness" (Bowen, 1978, p. 24). The undifferentiated family ego mass is the contagion of feeling within a family, so that, if one family member experiences an emotion, the emotion reverberates around the family. Bowen's theory of schizophrenia was multigenerational. Thus, whereas the grandparents may have been mature and differentiated, one offspring became immature and undifferentiated and, in turn, married an equally undifferentiated individual. The result of this pairing would be the creation of a very un-differentiated family ego mass, from which one or more of the children would be unable to escape and therefore would become schizophrenic.

Bowen (1978) later moved his theory to a more systemic level in his descriptions of the parts played by triangles in family interaction. Triangulation is a process in which two people form an alliance by focusing on a third. Bowen described the constantly shifting triangles in all families but argued that families of schizophrenics have much more rigid triadic patterns.

While Lidz was examining family roles, and Bowen was looking at family emotional contagion, another psychiatrist, Lyman Wynne (1963), was studying norms of communication in the families of schizophrenics. He noticed patterns of rapidly shifting alliances in which no two people ever got really close or really distant and angry. There was only what he called "pseudomutuality" or "pseudohostility" (Wynne, Ryckoff, Day, & Hirsch, 1958).

Wynne also observed another peculiar feature of the families of schizophrenics, which was that the boundary of the family appeared to be open to outsiders but, in fact, was impervious. He named this the "rubber fence." He explained that in these families there is a very strong norm against disagreement or difference. Children in these families have difficulty differentiating and thus may develop the distortions of reality testing seen in schizophrenics.

In summary, all three of these investigators moved from a purely psychodynamic approach to consider the family of the schizophrenic as a small group: Lidz examined roles; Bowen examined parental roles and emotional atmosphere; and Wynne examined family norms.

Parallel to advances in small-group theory that were occurring during the 1950s, there were also developments in information theory (e.g., Shannon, 1948), cybernetics (Wiener, 1965), and general systems theory (Bertalanffy, 1966). These contributed to new perspectives on psychopathology and the family, in terms of both communication in the family and systemic aspects of interaction. First, we will consider the communications perspective, in which psychopathology is redefined as a disorder in communication related to family functioning (Helmersen, 1983).

Distorted Family Communication: Toward a Theory of Transactions

Three groups of investigators focused directly on the transactions between schizophrenics and their families: Bateson's group, with their double-bind theory (Bateson et al., 1956); Laing's group, with their mystification theory (Laing & Esterson, 1964); and Wynne's group and communication deviance (Singer & Wynne, 1965a,b). At first, Singer and Wynne's theories focused on the impact of distorted parental communication on offspring who later became schizophrenic. Later, these investigators modified these linear formulations to incorporate recursive systems notions into a transactional perspective.

Gregory Bateson headed up a highly productive research group at the Palo Alto Veterans Administration Hospital including (among others) Don Jackson, Jay Haley, Paul Watzlawick, and John Weakland. This group initially attempted to understand communication in terms of multiple levels of meaning. They used Russell's theory of logical types (Whitehead & Russell, 1910), which proposed that all messages are accompanied by a statement about the message, or a meta-message at a higher level. The corollary of this proposition is that confusion of these levels can lead to contradiction and paradox.

In observing schizophrenic communication, the Bateson group noticed the frequent confusion between concrete and abstract thinking and suggested that the schizophrenic was confusing logical types. Speculating about the family environment in which this confused communication could have developed, Bateson and his colleagues developed the well-known theory of the double bind (Bateson *et al.*, 1956), in which a command at the overt meaning level is contradicted at the metalevel, perhaps by tone of voice or context. Further, comment on the contradiction is not allowed, and the receiver cannot withdraw. If these conditions were met, it was theorized, it would be impossible for the receiver to communicate logically, and the result would be the illogical communication known as schizophrenia.

In a theory similar to the theory of the double bind, Laing, Esterson, and Cooper developed the concept of *mystification* for explaining what they claimed were contradictory messages, denials, and vagueness in the communication of family members to their schizophrenic relative. These distorted transactions were illustrated in such books as *Sanity, Madness and the Family* (Laing & Esterson, 1964). Laing argued that schizophrenia was the only logical reaction to an illogical family situation.

Although this group did some conjoint family therapy in which the focus was on unraveling mystifying communication (Esterson, Cooper, & Laing, 1965), Laing and his colleagues are better known for their work at Kingsley Hall, in which individuals were allowed to regress in a group home with great respect for the meaning of their existential experience (see *Mary Barnes,* Edgar, 1979). Gradually, however, Laing began to see everyone as being mystified and himself disappeared into mysticism.

The other theory of transactions was that of Lyman Wynne and Margaret Singer. This is the only theory of the three to have received any scientific support. Singer and Wynne asserted that a necessary condition for communicating is a shared focus of attention that can then lead to shared meanings (Singer & Wynne, 1965a,b; Singer, Wynne, & Toohey, 1978). They formulated the concept of *communication deviance,* in which a "listener is unable to construct a consistent visual image or a consistent construct from the speaker's words" (Singer *et al.*, 1978, p. 500). They measured this construct from Rorschach protocols of parents by developing behavioral categories such as fragmented speech, amorphousness, lack of closure, and incorrect word usage. They have used these categories to reliably discriminate parents with schizophrenic offspring from parents with comparison offspring manifesting other forms of psychopathology, as well as from parents of normals. Parental communication deviance has also been found to be a successful predictor of the schizophrenia-spectrum disorders in a longitudinal high-risk design (Goldstein, 1985).

In summary, these three groups all followed the model that schizophrenia was a communication disorder and that this communication disorder was *caused* by distorted and confusing patterns of parental communication, whether described as double binds, mystification, or communication deviance.

Interestingly, these three groups developed their communicational theories with little direct observation of families (Hoffman, 1981). As the new systemic perspective emerged, they began actually to observe families. For example, Bateson and his colleagues had developed their double-bind theory solely from observations of the schizophrenic in psychiatric interviews. Only *after* their theory was published did they observe families through the one-way mirror. Such observations led to an outpouring of systemic theories about the family of the schizophrenic. For example, Jackson (1957) described these families as closed systems with homeostatic mechanisms that maintained the system through negative feedback. He also observed positive feedback in some families in which a small change led to exponentially larger changes, what he called a "runaway." Such observations led to clinical experiments with cognitive reframing and counterintuitive behavioral prescriptions. These clinical experiments attempted to counter homeostasis or to harness the power of family "resistance" and launched family therapy as a new form of therapy for all kinds of problems, not just schizophrenia (e.g., Jackson, 1968; Minuchin, 1974; Selvini-Palazzoli, Boscolo, Cecchin, & Prata, 1978).

As the implications of this new systemic perspective emerged, the linear causal communicational perspective on schizophrenia was modified. In a systemic perspective, it is assumed that any transaction (a two-person event) that is repeated depends on both parties' maintaining their side of the communication (one-person behaviors). Thus, Bateson *et al.* and Singer and Wynne changed their models to more sophisticated transactional models in which parental communication disorders and schizophrenia were seen as co-evolving over time (Bateson, Jackson, Haley, & Weakland, 1963; Singer & Wynne, 1965a,b). However, to date, little research has emerged that shows the contribution of pre-schizophrenic offspring's behavior to such repetitive transactions.

In conclusion, the search for family explanations of the etiology of schizophrenia has generated a range of intriguing observations and theories of family interaction and change. How productive these theories have been in terms of research data on the specificity of such processes is less clear, as will be discussed later.

In this brief historical overview, we have attempted to show that ideas about the family and schizophrenia have developed from an intrapsychic model to a more complex transactional, systemic model, and that these changes reflect broader paradigmatic shifts in scientific thinking in general. A careful analysis of the early family theories of schizophrenia can be found in Mishler and Waxler (1965), and the more recent advances in the systems perspective are presented at greater length in Hoffman's scholarly text on family therapy (1981). Theoretical perspectives on these developments are also provided in Helmersen's review (1983).

EMPIRICAL EVIDENCE ON THE FAMILY'S ROLE IN SCHIZOPHRENIA

We shall now turn to the empirical literature and examine the data relevant to the six questions outlined previously:

1. Is There Any Evidence That Families of Schizophrenics Show Patterns of Intrafamilial Communication and Structure That Are Different from Those of Other Families?

The new theories of Bateson, Wynne, and Lidz stimulated hundreds of family interaction studies. This activity reached a peak in the 1960s and has declined since. It is not our intention here to provide an exhaustive review of these studies. Rather, we will emphasize commonalities in the conclusions of previous reviewers and highlight areas of neglect.

We will focus on the more recent reviews of the quantifiable research on family interaction (Doane, 1978; Goldstein & Rodnick, 1975; Helmersen, 1983; Jacob, 1975; Liem, 1980; Riskin & Faunce, 1972).

Of all the reviewers, Riskin and Faunce (1972) and Jacob (1975) focused most attention on methodology and design. Both reviewers recommended, for example, having better standardization of diagnosis, better comparability of measures across studies, and more careful analysis, especially of comparisons between males and females. Jacob in particular pointed out that studies of schizophrenics were of poorer methodology than studies of other diagnostic groups.

Riskin and Faunce (1972) and Doane (1978) focused on the type of measures used. They suggested that "pure process" measures, such as interruptions, talking time, and frequency of laughter, are not powerful measures because of the ambiguity of interpretation; measures at the other extreme, such as ratings of "symbiotic" relationships, involve too much inference by coders, so that they are difficult to compare across studies. Thus, pleas were made for the use of qualitative process measures, which are at an intermediate level of abstraction, so that links can be made with theoretical constructs without too much inference.

In terms of substantive results, the reviews of Jacob (1975) and Goldstein and Rodnick (1975) were in substantial agreement. Both agreed that there were few consistent differences in the areas of dominance, conflict, or affective expression. However, both reviews also agreed that there were a fair number of consistent data that suggested that families of schizophrenics communicate with less clarity and accuracy than normal families.

The review of Liem (1980) 5 years later echoed these conclusions but emphasized that there are even more supporting data on communication deviance. In particular, findings are beginning to emerge of greater communication deviance in direct interaction with offspring, not only in individual parental Rorschach protocols.

Liem (1980) was also the first reviewer to describe the so-called artificial studies that have attempted to assess etiological versus responsive explanations of schizophrenic thought disorder. These innovative studies were initiated by Haley (1968) and have been followed by others, including Liem (1974, 1976). The designs involve mixing and matching schizophrenics and their parents with normals and their parents to see whether schizophrenic patients induce distorted communication in parents of normal offspring and, inversely, whether parents of schizophrenics show deviant communication when interacting with normal offspring from other families. The value of such studies lies in their ability to serve as preliminary investigations to select measures and procedures suitable for inclusion in (more expensive) longitudinal studies. Unfortunately, such studies have provided contradictory results. Furthermore, conclusions would be difficult to draw because the situation is artificial and communication may not reflect patterns that develop over years in actual family groups.

Doane's review (1978) has generated the most controversy. Doane took a different tack from other reviewers, refusing to accept the labels for constructs that investigators used. Instead, she grouped them according to her own understanding of their meaning. From this regrouping, she drew stronger conclusions than other reviewers. Not only did Doane note that families of schizophrenics show more communication deviance, but she also concluded that they were more likely to show weak parental-marital alliances and parent–child coalitions, unstable role-structures, and less flexibility in task performance. However, as Jacob and Grounds (1978) noted, these conclusions were based on a selective review of the findings.

Helmersen (1983) noted that there are now fewer programs of research but that they are more focused. Two programs at UCLA and Rochester are longitudinal studies and will be reviewed in another section. In general, Helmersen agreed that the strongest area of consistency is the area of communication deviance (CD). In particular, he emphasized the new study of Wynne, Singer, Bartko, and Toohey (1977) of 114 families with a variety of diagnoses. There is a steady increase in parental CD scores as the severity of the disorder increases from normal to schizophrenic.

Helmersen emphasized in particular the work of Blakar, who has led "the communication project" at Oslo, Norway, using a framework of social-cognitive psychology on language and communication as developed by Rommetveit and Blakar (1979) and the system-within-a-system model of Blakar and Nafstad (1981). The model used is similar to that of Wynne and Singer in that it is assumed that the central prerequisite of communication is a "shared social reality," which involves the ability to take the perspective of the other.

Blakar's task was designed so that both participants think they share the same reality, whereas, in fact, their realities are slightly different. In the task, each participant has a map in front of him or her that cannot be seen by the other. One person has to communicate two routes to the other: one is straightforward; the other passes through an area where, in fact, the maps are different. This task tests participants' abilities to "decenter."

In a series of studies, Blakar (1984) and his colleagues showed that families of schizophrenics are less able to decenter than other types of families. These studies are commendable for their attention to replication and their systematic efforts to examine background variables such as culture, sex, level of anxiety, and the variety of types of normal families.

The strength of this approach is that it is anchored firmly in theory: the European cognitive-social model of communication. A problem is the reliance on one method of assessment, the map problem, to the virtual exclusion of all other methods. This does reduce method variance in comparing studies but leaves questions about the generalizability of the findings. Nevertheless, it has been a clever way of studying communication, and the findings parallel and strengthen the findings on CD.

A final area is the research on the double bind. This research is reviewed most extensively in Sluzki and Ransom (1976). Other derivative research, on incongruence between nonverbal and verbal communication, has been reviewed thoroughly by Jacob and Lessin (1982). Helmersen (1983) observed that no conclusive evidence has been presented: the double bind is certainly not specific to schizophrenia, and there are no studies showing that double binds occur before the onset of schizophrenia.

Conclusions. In conclusion, the large number of cross-sectional family studies have produced one clear and consistent finding: Parents of schizophrenics show a deficit in their ability to share a focus of attention, to take the perspective of another, and to communicate meaning clearly and accurately.

Disappointingly, interactional studies of roles, affect, dominance, and so on have produced no clear and consistent finding. There may be a number of reasons, such as inadequate design, poor conceptualization, weak measures, bland tasks, or the coding of transcripts rather than tapes.

It may also be that such studies missed important group differences because they were searching for a single pattern that differentiated parents of schizophrenics from those of other groups. For example, Lewis, Rodnick, and Goldstein (1981) found that parents rated high in communication deviance tended to show several different patterns of interactional behavior, such as maternal dominance or dual parental focus ("dumping on the child"), all of which were distinctively different from groups low in CD. If Lewis *et al.* (1981) had been searching for only one pattern—say, maternal dominance—the results would have been negative because the various patterns would cancel each other out, producing a finding of no differences.

Alternatively, other designs may be required. Because brief family interactions may not pick up the subtlety of processes that occur over time, longitudinal designs may be more powerful. Our next question focuses on one longitudinal high-risk study.

2. Is There Any Evidence That Disturbed Family Relationships Precede the Onset of Schizophrenia?

The cross-sectional studies reviewed above suggest that deviant communication appears more commonly in families of schizophrenics.

However, such studies are incapable of discriminating between family behaviors that precede the onset of schizophrenia and the many accommodations that follow the onset of this severe disorder. A different approach is needed. The "high-risk" approach originally identified by Mednick (1960) was designed precisely to separate processes that antedate from those that follow the onset of a major psychiatric disorder. Families at high risk for developing schizophrenia in an offspring can be identified in a number of different ways, such as having a parent with schizophrenia (e.g., McNeil, Kaij, Malmquist, and Naslund, 1983).

Using a variant of that strategy, Goldstein and his colleagues (Goldstein, Judd, Rodnick, Alkire, & Gould, 1968) investigated a cohort of 65 families that were originally defined as being at risk for schizophrenia because they contained a mild to moderately disturbed teenager. Not all of the teenagers were considered at risk for schizophrenia, but those who showed patterns of behavioral disturbance that previous retrospective research (Nameche, Waring, & Ricks, 1964; Robins, 1966) had suggested was particularly notable in the premorbid phase of schizophrenia (social withdrawal or active family conflict) were initially hypothesized as being at highest risk, and the other disturbed teenagers were viewed as being a lower-risk comparison sample.

Extensive measures of family behavior were obtained at the time of the original contact, which included psychological tests as well as directly observed interactions among family members. The cohort of teenagers was then followed up into adulthood at two time periods: 5 and 15 years after the original contacts. The latter follow-up was recently completed, and the data have now been analyzed. At each follow-up, the young adults received psychiatric interviews and received diagnoses by clinicians blind as to any previous data on the families.

Two family measures received particular attention in this project as parental risk factors: communication deviance (CD) and what we have termed a *negative affective style* (AS). The former was based directly on the work of Singer and Wynne (1965a,b), who identified specific anomalies in communication in parents of families containing schizophrenic offspring. They found that CD was best measured from the transaction between the tester and the parent during the administration of the Rorschach projective test. Goldstein *et al.* (1968) followed this lead and used verbatim Thematic Apperception Test (TAT) protocols to score CD (Jones, 1977). AS, on the other hand, is based on codes applied to the verbal communications among family members during a series of family discussions stimulated by conflictual family problems. The negative AS codes represent interpersonal analogues of high-EE attitudes and reflect harsh criticism and/or intrusiveness expressed by one or more parents toward their teenager.

In a publication based on the 5-year follow-up data, Doane, West, Goldstein, Rodnick, and Jones (1981) grouped the young adults into two broad classes of psychiatric diagnoses: extended-schizophrenia-spectrum and nonspectrum groups. The use of a schizophrenia-spectrum category was used for two reasons: First, it paralleled the adoption studies of Kety *et al.* (1968), who found that this spectrum of disorder, rather than schizophrenia alone, was frequently noted in the biological relatives of adopted-away schizophrenic persons but rarely in the biological relatives of nonpsychiatric cases. Second, there were few schizophrenic cases in the sample (only two) at the time of this early follow-up, and the spectrum concept provided a more adequate basis for forming contrast groups. It should be recalled that, at the time of the 5-year follow-up, the sample was barely into the risk period for schizophrenia.

Doane *et al.* (1981) found that all of the families in which offspring were diagnosed within the extended schizophrenia spectrum had parents who had previously been rated as high in CD. In contrast, virtually all of the low-CD families had nonspectrum outcomes. However, there were a number of families defined as high CD whose offspring did not receive schizophrenia spectrum diagnoses at the 5-year follow-up. When those high-CD cases were contrasted on the AS factor, it was found that every one of the schizophrenia spectrum cases not only came from high-CD parents but were also recipients of negative AS behaviors when observed in direct interaction with their parents. The nonspectrum cases from high-CD homes had been spared such criticism and intrusive behavior and so had experienced something that the English investigators would term a *low-EE environment*.

Another study by Strachan (1982) looked at dyadic interactions between parents and adolescents. With regard to the 5-year follow-up data, it was found that, in benign-outcome families, parent–adolescent interaction was similar whether the adolescent was with the mother or the father. By contrast, in spectrum outcome families, there was a differential shift in the focus of the conversation: With the mother, the focus was shifted away from the mother's internal states and behavior and was shifted more toward the adolescent's experience, with the mother being critical, demanding, and questioning while disclosing little about herself. With the father, the opposite was the case, the father being deferent and avoiding confrontation. Interestingly, the adolescents, rather than being passive recipients of such communication, were actively involved: spectrum adolescents suppressed criticism of their mother and were more confronting with their father. Thus, this study sheds further light on the intrafamilial dynamics associated with global measures of affective interaction.

Since the time of these early reports, the cohort has been followed up again 15 years after the initial assessment. Data from parents and offspring have been obtained for 54 of the 65 original families. The most severe psychiatric disorder manifested by the target offspring during this period was used as an outcome criterion.

The diagnoses were divided into three groups: schizophrenia spectrum disorders, no mental illness, and other psychiatric disorders. The schizophrenia spectrum used here included schizophrenia as well as schizoid, schizotypal, paranoid, and borderline personality disorders. Three measure of the family environment were used as predictors: CD, categorized as high, intermediate, or low; AS, categorized as negative, intermediate, or benign; and a direct measure of EE, derived from the tape recordings of the interviews administered to the parents at the time of the initial contact. Because all of the cases came from intact homes, it was possible to classify the parents into two EE groups: dual high EE or dual low EE, in which both parents expressed a similar attitude, and a mixed group with one high-EE and one low-EE parent. Of this sample, 45 had all three parent measures available. As Goldstein (1985) reported, within that subsample, schizophrenia spectrum disorders were predominantly associated with the combined parental pattern of high CD, negative AS, and high EE. When follow-up data for siblings was included, the predictive value of CD was even greater.

Recently, Goldstein (in press) has reported an analysis of the predictive value of these three attributes. The three predictors were entered into a log-linear analysis to evaluate (a) how they related to the three outcome categories as independent factors and (b) how well they related when the variance in the other two predictors was partialed out. The distributions of outcomes are presented for each predictor at a time in Table 1.

As can be seen, all three variables significantly predicted outcome. However, when the log-linear procedure was used to test the contribution of each variable with the overlapping variance of the other variables removed, probabilities for the partial associations were .002 for CD and .001 for AS, but a clearly nonsignificant .789 for EE. Thus, when both affective measures were in the log-linear analysis, EE no longer added a significant contribution to the prediction of outcome.

If one examines these data on a case-by-case basis, it can be clearly seen that the overwhelming number of schizophrenia spectrum cases (8 out of 14) occurred when high CD and a negative AS profile were present at the time of the original family assessment. Three of the other spectrum cases occurred when a negative AS profile and an intermediate CD pattern coexisted at the original assessment. It is also important to note the protective role of low CD in parents, as the overwhelming majority of cases (8 out of 12) had no further mental disorder subsequent to their adolescent difficulties. Thus, the combination of a disordered communication style and a chronically critical attitude toward the teenager, which was also expressed directly to the already moderately disturbed teenager, was associated with a high risk for the subsequent development of a disorder in the extended schizophrenia spectrum.

During the follow-up interviews, siblings of the target offspring were interviewed and diagnosed if there was any indication that they might have a serious psychiatric disorder. These data were looked at in relation to CD, the only measure of the three that was not linked to a particular child in the family, so that it could be seen if any offspring of high-CD parents were at risk for schizo-

TABLE 1. Parental Communication as Predictors of Offspring Diagnosis

	CD[c]			AS[c]			EE[c]		
	NMI[a]	OPD	Spec	NMI	OPD	Spec	NMI	OPD	Spec
Low[b]	8	3	1	11	11	1	5	12	1
Intermediate	3	13	14	1	6	2	6	5	6
High	4	7	10	4	4	12	1	4	7

[a]NMI = No mental illness; OPD = Other psychiatric disorder; Spec = Extended schizophrenia spectrum, broad criterion which includes borderline personality disorder.
[b]For AS, comparable categories are benign, intermediate, and negative; for EE, dual low, mixed, and dual high EE.
[c]CD $p < .002$; AS $p < .0008$; EE $p < .04$.

phrenia spectrum disorders. The outcome variable was the "worst" case among the offspring in each family. The association with CD in this worst-case analysis was stronger than the association in the target offspring analysis. In fact, 14 out of 19 high-CD families had at least one spectrum case in the family, whereas only 10 spectrum diagnoses were found in the target offspring. Incidentally, no support was found for the hypothesis that the type of adolescent problem behavior was related to outcome.

In conclusion, these results suggest that the earlier research of Wynne and Singer, which emphasized deviant communication, is not a sufficient description of the preschizophrenic family. The affective component is also very important, as can be seen clearly in the results cited above.

It is interesting in light of these results to note that the seminal papers of Wynne and Singer in the mid-1960s emphasized affective as well as communicative difficulties in the families that these authors observed. However, possibly because the CD construct became operationalized first and became widely disseminated, the other parts of the model were obscured. In fact, Wynne (1984) recently reiterated and extended his model of family development to emphasize attachment and caregiving (affect), problem solving, and neutrality, as well as communication, as key processes in family development.

In summary, this important longitudinal study provides definitive answers to the question posed. Disturbed family relationships, indexed by the communication deviance measure, do, in fact, precede the onset of schizophrenia spectrum disorders. Other longitudinal studies, such as the one currently under way at Rochester, may help to confirm these results. This study overcomes some of the problems of the cross-sectional studies and definitely excludes the hypothesis that disturbed family communication is a result of relatives' reactions to psychotic behavior. However, it should be noted that it is still possible that relatives were reacting to some unmeasured aspect of the teenagers' behaviors that predicted schizophrenia spectrum outcomes. Nevertheless, the UCLA Family Project study has provided provocative evidence that disturbed communication and negative affect in families precede the development of schizophrenia spectrum disorders.

3. Is There Any Evidence That There Are Specific Patterns of Disturbed Family Relationships Associated with Schizophrenia as Compared with Other Major Psychiatric Disorders?

The review of cross-sectional studies under Question 1 suggested that there are differences between parents of schizophrenics and parents of normals and other psychopathological groups in the area of communication deviance. However, whereas Singer and Wynne's early study (1965) revealed clear separation between families of schizophrenics and normals, a replication in Britain by Hirsch and Leff (1971) found that, although parents of schizophrenics had significantly higher CD scores than parents of depressed offspring, there was considerable overlap between the groups. This finding challenged the notion of the specificity of CD to schizophrenia.

Subsequently, Wynne et al. (1977) conducted a larger study of 114 families of offspring with a variety of psychopathology, varying from normal to borderline to schizophrenic. They found that 32 of the 41 categories of CD each separately differentiated the parents of the schizophrenics from the other three groups. Further, there was no overlap between parents of normals and parents of schizophrenics in terms of total CD. This finding provides strong evidence of the specificity of CD to parents of schizophrenics. The discrepancy between the two earlier studies may have been due to differences in diagnostic procedures (Rutter, 1978).

Some evidence of specificity is also emerging from the UCLA project. Goldstein (in press) investigated whether CD and AS would segregate the non-mental-illness-outcome cases from all others, or whether they would actually identify those families with spectrum disorders, as distinctive from those containing offspring with some other form or psychiatric disorder. It was found that the most reliable separation of groups was between the spectrum cases and all others ($p < .003$); the segregation between the non-mentally-ill and other-psychiatric-disorder groups was only marginally significant ($p < .054$). This finding suggests that the combination of high CD and negative AS specifically identified a subset of families with a higher probability of spectrum disorders in particular, and not psychiatric cases in general.

Although there appears to be some specificity of prediction of a broad schizophrenia spectrum, predictions using the narrower spectrum of Kendler and Gruenberg (1984), derived from their reanalysis of the Danish Adoption Study Sample, were less successful (Goldstein, in press). One of two conclusions can be drawn. Either the high-CD–negative-AS family pattern is associated with very severe forms of psychopathology in adulthood but bears no specific link to schizophrenia *per se,* *or* the borderline and schizoid personality disorders (excluded from the narrow spectrum) share some common precursors with schizophrenia that have not been articulated in the prior adoption studies.

Another explanation of the apparent specificity of the high-CD–negative-AS pattern to schizophrenia spectrum disorders is that it may define the extremes of a very stressful family environment that could be associated with a high risk for psychosis but not necessarily schizophrenia. Unfortunately, the follow-ups in the Goldstein study have not yet revealed any cases of bipolar disorder, in either the manic or the depressive form, or any other disorders, such as unipolar psychotic depression. Thus, there may be a misleading illusion of a high degree of specificity in the aforementioned data. It is possible that the high-CD–negative-AS pattern defines a subset of families whose offspring are more likely to express one of this spectrum of disorders, but not those of another spectrum, such as that hypothesized for the mood disorders.

Two dissertation studies specifically address this possibility. Greene (1982) contrasted the parents of schizophrenics with the parents of depressed patients, both groups being diagnosed by research diagnostic criteria (RDC) (Spitzer, Endicott, & Robins, 1975). Greene did find highly significant differences in CD levels between the two groups of parents: the parents of schizophrenics scored much higher than the parents of depressives. Unfortunately, her sample included both unipolar and bipolar depressives, and no specific analyses were carried out for these two groups. Thus, it is ot possible to evaluate whethr the between-group differences were carried equally by the unipolar and the bipolar subsamples.

In the second study, Miklowitz (1985, in press) approached this issue by contrasting parents of young, recent-onset schizophrenics with those of young, recent-onset manic patients. Because both sets of cases had experienced clear-cut psychotic episodes of different forms, it was possible to establish whether CD was more likely to be associated with psychosis in general or with a particular type of psychotic disorder such as schizophrenia. The results showed that CD was equally high in both psychotic groups. However, families of schizophrenics showed significantly higher rates of criticism and intrusive behavior in direct interaction than families of manics. Further, in the manic sample, both EE and AS were moderately predictive of relapse separately; used as joint predictors, they predicted strongly. These results parallel the EE work on schizophrenia and relapse.

Thus, based on the very limited data available to date, we would have to conclude that there is only moderate evidence for the specificity of CD (or the CD–AS combination) to schizophrenia or even to schizophrenia spectrum disorders. There are suggestions from both the Goldstein 15-year follow-up study and the Greene report that CD is not prominent in the families with major depressive disorders. But the relationship of parental CD to other types of psychotic disorder in offspring has not been clarified.

Certain issues with regard to CD required additional critical data. We still do not know about the epidemiology of CD. How often are we likely to encounter high-CD parents in a survey of the general population? And what is the significance of such a pattern when no offspring are psychiatrically affected? This is not a simple issue to deal with, as offspring may not be affected at the time of measurement but could, as in the cases in the Goldstein study, manifest severe psychopathology at a later date. Despite this problem, it would still be valuable to include brief measures of CD (and EE as well) in such epidemiological surveys as those being currently carried out by the National Institute of Mental Health-Environmental Catchment Area (NIMH-ECA) program.

A second and related need is to establish the prevalence of CD within families with a schizophrenic index case. Many human genetic studies collect detailed histories of mental disorders in family lines in which there is at least one mentally ill relative. In the more elaborate of these studies, all first-degree relatives are interviewed by means of standardized diagnostic interviews. It would be very valuable if some method for indexing CD could be added to these assessments. It has frequently been suggested by genetically oriented investigators that CD relates to offspring schizophrenia because it represents a subclinical form of the genetic predisposition to the disorder. If that is the case, then family pedigree studies can be used to test this hypothesis by establishing the degree of association between the presence or absence of schizophrenia in parents' first-degree relatives and the presence of CD in parents and offspring.

4. Is There Any Evidence That Family Factors Affect the Course of Schizophrenia?

As highlighted in the introduction, a major reason for the renewal of enthusiasm in studying the family relationships of schizophrenics has been the research on the predictive value of expressed-emotion attitudes in the course of schizophrenia once it occurs.

A series of naturalistic studies at the Medical Research Council (MRC) Social Psychiatry Unit at the Institute of Psychiatry in London examined factors that protected patients from relapse once they had left the hospital (Brown, Birley, & Wing, 1972; Brown, Carstairs, & Topping, 1958; Brown, Monck, Carstairs, & Wing, 1962; Leff & Vaughn, 1981; Vaughn & Leff, 1976). These studies suggested that three important factors protect a patient from relapse. The most important is low EE in the relatives who live with them. As previously mentioned, EE is rated from attitudes spontaneously expressed to an interviewer by the relative during a semistructured interview about the patient, the Camberwell Family Interview. Patients who return to homes with one or more high-EE relatives have nine-month relapse rates of 51%; those who return to homes with low-EE relatives have a relapse rate of 13% (Vaughn & Leff, 1976).

The second protective factor is low contact with the high-EE relatives, defined as less than 35 hours per week of face-to-face contact.

The third protective factor is whether the patient is maintained on medication.

Of these three protective factors, low EE appeared to be the most important in that the nine-month relapse rates of patients with low-EE relatives were low, whether or not the patient was on drugs and irrespective of the amount of face-to-face contact. Nine-month relapse rates with high-EE relatives decreased with drug compliance and low contact, however, showing that they are important factors too.

One criticism of this work is that it is correlational, and the direction of effect could not be firmly established. It could be argued that the more deviant and disturbed the patient is, the more likely it is that relatives will react with anger, guilt, and overinvolvement, and that the patient will relapse. This alternative hypothesis was ruled out by Brown et al.'s analysis (1972), which partialed out the effect of behavioral disturbance and previous employment and showed that these had little effect on relapse compared with EE.

These data on EE have stimulated a number of replications in other countries. A study in California (Vaughn, Snyder, Jones, Freeman, & Falloon, 1984) basically replicated the findings in Britain. The California sample was a more chronic group and was more likely to be male. The relatives were more likely to be high-EE than in the British sample. Despite these differences, the relapse rate for patients returning to low-EE families was 17%, and that for patients returning to high-EE families was 56%, remarkably similar to the British relapse rates. Another study of Mexican-American schizophrenics (Jenkins et al., 1986) showed that, even though far fewer relatives were high-EE, the relapse rates were very similar for low- and high-EE relatives. Further cross-cultural studies are described in Leff and Vaughn (1985).

Although these findings are powerful, they are only correlational and thus cannot by themselves suggest that EE causes relapse. It could be, for example, that EE reflects parental frustration or worry in response to disturbing behavior that researchers have not yet identified. Thus, an experimental approach was required.

Leff et al. (1982, 1983) selected 24 schizophrenics who lived in high contact with high-EE relatives and randomly assigned them to a treatment condition or a treatment-as-usual condition. The relatives in the treatment group received psychoeducation about schizophrenia and then attended relatives' groups. After 9 months, 50% of the patients in the comparison group had relapsed, compared with only 8% in the treatment group, a significant difference. Further, these authors found that this treatment was associated with a significant decrease in critical comments, one component of EE.

Another study by Falloon and colleagues (Falloon, Boyd, & McGill, 1984) focused on in-home behavioral family therapy for improving communication and problem solving. This program significantly reduced relapse rates, too. It was found that these changes were significantly related to the style of direct affective expression as indexed by affective style (Doane, Falloon, Goldstein, & Mintz, 1985; Doane, Goldstein, Miklowitz, & Falloon, 1985).

Finally, a recently completed study by Hogarty, Anderson, Reiss, Kornblith, Greenwald, Javna, Madonia, and the EPICS Schizophrenia Research Group (1986) showed that a psychoeducational family treatment approach in conjunction with medication significantly decreased the likelihood of relapse. Further, these changes were significantly associated with changes in family EE from high to low levels.

Thus, all three programs provided evidence that altering negative affective family environments affects the course of schizophrenia and supported the hypothesis that family affective attitudes do, in fact, influence the short-term course of the disorder (see also Strachan, 1986).

5. Is There Any Correlation between Family Factors That Precede Schizophrenia and Those Related to Its Course?

Most of the EE studies were based on the notion that family attitudes such as criticism and/or emotional overinvolvement were relevant only after the family members had to contend with a mentally ill relative. The relationship of these attitudes to the development of the disorder was largely ignored.

The UCLA longitudinal study indicated that affective attitudes such as EE or analogous interactive behaviors were important contributors to the prediction of the course of psychiatric disorder from adolescence to young adulthood. This finding suggests that there is indeed some continuity between affective attitudes toward an offspring before and after a schizophrenic disorder appears. Of course, in both types of studies, parents were contending with a disturbed offspring (a disturbed teenager or a recently discharged schizophrenic patient), and the attitude may have reflected difficulties in coping with these stressful episodes rather than attitudes that preceded their development. We still do not know whether attitudes of criticism and/or emotional overinvolvement, expressed in the absence of notable psychiatric disturbance in an offspring, increase the likelihood of subsequent psychiatric disorder, including schizophrenia, in that offspring.

A more modest question has to do with whether high-EE attitudes expressed before the onset of schizophrenia reflect intrafamilial processes similar to those that transpire after a schizophrenic disorder has occurred. In one study, Miklowitz, Goldstein, Falloon, and Doane (1984) studied the interactional behavior of high- and low-EE parents of schizophrenics in a direct interaction task. The task was a modified version of the one used in the Goldstein *et al.* (1968) family assessment. Miklowitz *et al.* found that high-EE parents were significantly more likely than low-EE parents to express the negative AS behaviors of criticism and intrusiveness in this task. In a comparable study of families in Britain, Strachan, Leff, Goldstein, Doane, and Burtt (1986) studied the dyadic behavior of relative and patient. They found that EE attitudes paralleled direct interactional behavior, thus replicating the American study. Further, examining the families in the UCLA longitudinal study, Valone, Norton, Goldstein, and Doane (1983) also found a correspondence between EE attitudes and AS behavior toward the offspring.

These three studies indicate that affective attitudes expressed either before or after the onset of schizophrenia correspond to very similar patterns of intrafamilial behavior. Although it is very hazardous to combine, even at a conceptual level, data from different samples collected in the pre- and postpsychotic phases of that disorder, these data do suggest that high-EE attitudes may very well antedate the onset of schizophrenia. In fact, they may be augmented by the presence of a psychiatric disorder in an offspring.

The fact that high-EE attitudes are correlated with actual interactive behavior is important, but it still does not clarify the mechanism through which critical and/or overinvolved behavior heightens the probability of a schizophrenic episode or a relapse into a new episode once one has occurred. It may be, as first suggested by the original British investigators, that these behaviors raise the tension level within the home to a level exceeding the limited coping abilities of the recently remitted patient. However, it is also conceivable that these attitudes relate to some aspect of the patient's clinical picture that makes patients from high-EE homes more irritating or difficult to deal with.

One way to test this hypothesis of increased tension level in high-EE homes is to measure the psychophysiological reactivity of relatives to one another during a directly observed interaction task. This was the strategy used by Tarrier, Vaughn, Lader, and Leff (1979), who recorded skin conductance changes in the schizophrenic patient when interviewed in the presence of either a high- or a low-EE relative. These investigators found that the number of skin conductance responses remained high for patients interacting with a high-EE relative, whereas a progressive reduction (habituation) was noted for patients interacting with a low-EE relative. These results were replicated in a laboratory context by Sturgeon *et al.* (1981, 1984).

Recently, Valone, Goldstein, and Norton (1984) carried out a similar analysis of skin conductance changes before and during a directly observed interaction that was conducted during the initial phase of the Goldstein *et al.* (1968) longitudinal study of disturbed adolescents. These investigators went beyond the Tarrier and Sturgeon studies by recording parents' as well as offspring's skin conductance levels and reactivity during a series of interaction tasks. Valone *et al.* (1984) found that *both* parents and offspring from high-EE homes reacted more intensely to each other, as seen in the skin conductance measures, than did relatives from low-EE homes. Because none of these adolescents were schizophrenic at the time of this assessment, Valone's data show that the heightened reactivity of these high-EE parent–child dyads was not specific to a person who had already had an episode of psychosis.

The results of these three studies support the notion that the development and recurrence of schizophrenia are more likely in home environments characterized by a high level of negative affective exchanges and heightened psychophysiological arousal and reactivity level. When and how these heightened levels of negative arousal states arise within the history of high-EE families still remain unclear. Are they present from the earliest days of the offspring's life, or do they appear at a certain point, such as during adolescence, when pressures for achievement and autonomy are increased?

In summary, we conclude that the answer to our fifth question is also affirmative. There appears to be considerable continuity between those negative affective factors within the family that precede the onset of the disorder and those that are predictive of the course of the disorder once it occurs.

6. Is There Any Evidence That Family Relationships Interact with a Biological Predisposition in the Development of Schizophrenia?

This is, of course, the most challenging question of the six, touching most closely on the issue of the etiological model that best accounts for the development of the disorder. And yet, we have the least to say concerning this vital question. As indicated in the beginning of this chapter, research has been limited by the unavailability of a marker for the genetic predisposition to schizophrenia beyond that provided by knowledge of a family history of the disorder. Until such markers become available on either a biological or a behavioral level, it will be very difficult to tease apart the relative contributions of the family environment and the genetic predisposition.

The closest that we have come to a reasonable, yet indirect, approach is the adoption study design. Here, we will focus on two studies, one by Wynne, Singer, and Toohey (1976) and the other by Tienari *et al.* (1985).

Using data from the Wender, Rosenthal, and Kety (1968) study, Wynne, Singer, and Toohey (1976) reported a study of communication deviance in the adoptive parents of schizophrenics and parents who reared their biological schizophrenic offspring. There was a comparison sample of adoptive families of normal offspring. In the original study, mean psychopathology ratings for the biological parents of schizophrenics were significantly higher than those for the adoptive parents of schizophrenics (those for adoptive parents of normals were in between). If these ratings can be thought of as a genetic index of schizophrenia, the biological parents showed more of this index than the adoptive families, as would be expected.

However, when CD scores were examined, it was found that biological and adoptive parents of schizophrenics had equally high CD scores, which were significantly greater than the adoptive parents of normals. If CD is viewed as a rearing variable, this finding suggests an interaction between genetic and rearing variables.

Tiernari *et al.* (1985) have been studying a nationwide sample of all women in

Finland hospitalized for schizophrenia since 1960. They have focused on the 289 offspring who have been adopted and are now at risk for schizophrenia. These have been matched with adopted-away offspring without any biological risk. The adoptive families have been studied by means of the consensus Rorschach and the interpersonal perception method, among other measures. Global ratings of family functioning have been made, ranging from "healthy" families with clear communication, clear hierarchies, and an absence of conflict, to "severely disturbed" families with unclear boundaries, high anxiety, and conflict.

Of the 103 index cases rated so far, 7% have been diagnosed as psychotic, 17% as psychotic or borderline, and 30% as psychotic, borderline, or character disorders. However, of the offspring who have been reared in seriously disturbed adoptive families, these figures are doubled: 13% are psychotic; 38% psychotic or borderline; and 64% psychotic, borderline, or character disorders. In contrast, of the offspring who have been reared in healthy or mildly disturbed adoptive families, there are no psychotic, no borderline, and only two character disorders. This striking finding illustrates the interaction between a genetic vulnerability and the rearing environment.

Very young offspring are now part of the high-risk prospective-longitudinal study and will be followed up into the risk period of schizophrenia. In this phase of the research, it will be possible to determine whether family environment and offspring difficulties are present long before the onset of schizophrenia and also whether specific attributes of family life antedate the onset of schizophrenia in those offspring hypothesized to be at risk by virtue of mental disorder in their biological heritage. Undoubtedly, the results of this study will have a major impact on etiological theories concerning schizophrenia.

CONCLUSIONS

Design Considerations

Only in the area of communicational accuracy have cross-sectional comparison studies revealed consistent differences between families of schizophrenics and families of other types of offspring. It has not been possible to draw conclusions about measures of other constructs, such as role differentiation and affective communication because results from different studies are contradictory or difficult to interpret.

Goldstein and Rodnick (1975) concluded their review by making a plea for alternative designs, such as high-risk longitudinal designs. In this chapter, we have focused attention on one such study, the UCLA Family Project, because the results have been eagerly awaited from this prospective study.

It is important to note the preliminary data from other high-risk studies led by researchers such as Erlenmeyer-Kimling, Goodman, McNeil, Mednick, Mirsky, Sameroff, Weintraub, and Worland, recently reported at a meeting of the consortium of high-risk investigators. The report will appear as a special issue of the *Schizophrenia Bulletin* (Goldstein & Tuma, in press).

This is not to say that there is no value in cross-sectional studies. However, they could be improved, in a number of ways, first in terms of the task and, second, in terms of methods of analysis. In terms of design, the nature of the task is crucial. Thus, for example, the UCLA direct-interaction task may have been successful in producing predictive measures because topics were chosen with which the participants were currently struggling. The discussion may be more representative of interactional behavior around a fairly stressful topic than if a standard task is used. In terms of improvements in analysis, the use of summary frequency counts could be supplemented and extended by the use of sequential analyses of the flow of interaction. Such methods are still infrequently used.

Theoretical Considerations

More important than methodological issues' impeding progress has been the poverty of theoretical frameworks guiding research. Reiss, in particular, has called for greater attention to theory. For example, in his article subtitled "Fishing without a Net" (1975), Reiss pointed out that most research on family interaction and schizophrenia has been conducted using theories generated in the 1950s; little conceptual development has taken place since. Furthermore, data take on meaning only when they can fit into a "net" of propositions that form a theory. For example, a correlation between parental CD and offspring thought disorder makes sense only in the context of a theory of how forms of CD influence cognitive development. Reiss has followed his own advice and is thoughtfully collecting data linking family interaction with forms of individual thinking, as is shown by his chapter in this book. Wynne (1984) has proposed conceptual relationships between affective processes, communication, joint problem-solving, and mutuality that may also help guide future research. Finally, Dell's analysis (1980) of the family interaction research on schizophrenia focuses attention on the need for systemic theory. Perhaps with these recent moves toward a reconceptualization of family theories of schizophrenia, the widening gap between family researchers and family therapists may begin to narrow.

REFERENCES

Anderson, C. M., Hogarty, G. E., & Reiss, D. J. (1980). Family treatment of adult schizophrenic patients: A psychoeducational approach. *Schizophrenia Bulletin, 6*, 490–505.
Bales, R. F. (1950). *Interaction process analysis.* Reading, MA: Addison-Wesley.
Bateson, G. (1956). Toward a theory of schizophrenia. *Behavioral Science, 1*, 251–264.
Bateson, G., Jackson, D., Haley, J., & Weakland, J. (1956). Toward a theory of schizophrenia. *Behavioral Science, 1*, 252–264.
Bateson, G., Jackson, D., Haley, J., & Weakland, J. (1963). A note on the double bind. *Family Process, 2*, 154–161.
Bertalanffy, V. L. (1966). General systems theory and psychiatry. In S. Arieti (Ed.), *American handbook of psychiatry.* New York: Basic Books.
Blakar, R. M. (1984). *Communication: A social perspective on clinical issues.* Norway: Universitetsforlaget.

Blakar, R. M., and Nafstad, H. E. (1981, January 20–24). *The family as a unit in the study of psychopathology and deviant behavior: Conceptual and methodological issues.* Paper presented at a conference on Discovery Strategies in the Psychology of Action, Homburg, Federal Republic of Germany.

Bowen, M. (1978). *Family therapy in clinical practice.* New York: Jason Aronson.

Brown, G. W., Carstairs, G. M., & Topping, G. G. (1958). Post-hospital adjustment of chronic mental patients, *Lancet, 2,* 685–689.

Brown, G. W., Monck, E. M., Carstairs, G. M., & Wing, J. K. (1962). Influence of family life on the course of schizophrenic illness. *British Journal of Preventative and Social Medicine, 16,* 55–68.

Brown, G. W., Birley, J. L. T., & Wing, J. F. (1972). Influence of family life on the course of schizophrenic disorders: A replication. *British Journal of Psychiatry, 121,* 241–258.

Cartwright, D., & Zander, A. (Eds.). (1968). *Group dynamics: Research and theory* (3rd ed.). New York: Harper & Row.

Dell, P. (1980). Researching the family theories of schizophrenia: An exercise in epistemological confusion. *Family Process, 19,* 321–335.

Doane, J. A. (1978). Family interaction and communication deviance in disturbed and normal families: A review of research. *Family Process, 17,* 357–376.

Doane, J. A., West, K. L., Goldstein, M. J., Rodnick, E. H., & Jones, J. E. (1981). Parental communication and affective style: Predictors of subsequent schizophrenia-spectrum disorders in vulnerable adolescents. *Archives of General Psychiatry, 38,* 679–685.

Doane, J. A., Falloon, I. R. H., Goldstein, M. J., & Mintz, J. (1985). Parental affective style and the treatment of schizophrenia. *Archives of General Psychiatry, 42,* 34–42.

Doane, J. A., Goldstein, M. J., Miklowitz, D. M., & Falloon, I. R. H. (1986). The impact of individual and family treatment on the affective climate of families of schizophrenics. *British Journal of Psychiatry, 148,* 279–287.

Edgar, D. (1979). *Mary Barnes.* New York: Methuen.

Esterson, A., Cooper, D. G., & Laing, R. D. (1965). Results of family-oriented therapy with hospitalized schizophrenics. *British Medical Journal, 2,* 1462–1465.

Fairburn, W. R. D. (1954). *An object-relations theory of the personality.* New York: Basic Books.

Falloon, I. R. H., Boyd, J. L., McGill, C. W., Razani, J., Moss, H. B., & Gilderman, A. M. (1982). Family management in the prevention of exacerbations of schizophrenia. *New England Journal of Medicine, 306,* 1437–1440.

Falloon, I. R. H., Boyd, J. L., & McGill, C. W. (1984). *Family care of schizophrenia: A problem-solving approach to the treatment of mental illness.* New York: Guilford Press.

Federn, P. (1952). *Ego psychology and the psychoses.* New York: Basic Books.

Fromm-Reichmann, F. (1948). Notes on the development of treatment of schizophrenics by psychoanalytic psychotherapy. *Psychiatry, 11,* 263–273.

Garmezy, N. (1974a). Children at risk for the antecedents of schizophrenia: 1. Conceptual models and research methods. *Schizophrenia Bulletin, 8,* 14–90.

Garmezy, N. (1974b). Children at risk: The search for the antecedents of schizophrenia: 2. Ongoing research programs, issues and intervention. *Schizophrenia Bulletin, 9,* 55–125.

Goldstein, M. J. (1985). Family factors that antedate the onset of schizophrenia and related disorders: The results of a fifteen year prospective longitudinal study. *Acta Psychiatrica Scandinavica, 71,* 7–18.

Goldstein, M. J. (in press). Family interaction patterns that antedate the onset of schizophrenia and related disorders: A further analysis of data from a longitudinal study. In K. Hahlweg, & M. J. Goldstein (Eds.), *Understanding major mental disorder: The contribution of family interaction research.* New York: Family Process Press.

Goldstein, M. J., & Rodnick, E. H. (1975). The family's contribution to the etiology of schizophrenia: Current status. *Schizophrenia Bulletin, 14,* 48–63.

Goldstein, M. J., & Tuma, S. H. (Eds.). (in press). High-risk studies on schizophrenia. *Schizophrenia Bulletin.*

Goldstein, M. J., Judd, L. L., Rodnick, E. H., Alkire, A. A., & Gould, E. (1968). A method for studying social influence and coping patterns within families of disturbed adolescents. *Journal of Nervous and Mental Diseases, 147,* 233–251.

Goldstein, M. J., Rodnick, E. H., Evans, J. R., May, P. R. A., & Steinberg, M. R. (1978). Drug and family therapy in the aftercare of acute schizophrenics. *Archives of General Psychiatry, 35,* 1169–1177.

Greene, R. (1982). *The relationship of family communication deviance and attentional dysfunction in schizophrenia.* Unpublished doctoral dissertation, Florida Institute of Technology.

Guntrip, H. (1973). *Psychoanalytic theory, therapy and the self.* New York: Basic Books.

Haley, J. (1968). Testing parental instructions to schizophrenic and normal children: A pilot study. *Journal of Abnormal Psychology, 13,* 53–76.

Helmersen, P. (1983). *Family interaction and communication in psychopathology: An evaluation of recent perspectives.* London: Academic Press.

Hirsch, S. R., & Leff, J. P. (1971). Parental abnormalities of verbal communication in the transmission of schizophrenia. *Psychological Medicine, 1,* 118–127.

Hoffman, L. (1981). *Foundations of family therapy.* New York: Basic Books.

Hogarty, G. E., Anderson, C. M., Reiss, D. J., Kornblith, S. J., Greenwald, D. P., Javna, C. D., Madonia, M. J., & the EPICS Schizophrenia Research Group. (1986). Family psycho-education, social skills training and maintenance chemotherapy in the aftercare treatment of schizophrenia: 1. One year effects of a controlled study on relapse and expressed emotion. *Archives of General Psychiatry, 43,* 633–642.

Jackson, D. D. (1957). The question of family homeostasis. *Psychiatric Quarterly Supplement, 31,* 79–90.

Jackson, D. D. (Ed.). (1968). *Human Communication* (Vols. 1, 2). Palo Alto, CA: Science and Behavior Books.

Jacob, T. (1975). Family interaction in disturbed and normal families: A methodological and substantive review. *Psychological Review, 82,* 33–65.

Jacob, T., & Grounds, L. (1978). Confusions and conclusions: A response to Doane. *Family Process, 17,* 377–387.

Jacob, T., & Lessin, S. (1982). Inconsistent communication in family interaction. *Clinical Psychology Review, 2,* 295–309.

Jenkins, J. H., Karno, M., De La Selva, A., & Santana, F. (1986). Expressed emotion in cross-cultural context: Familial responses to schizophrenic illness among Mexican-Americans. In M. J. Goldstein, I. Hand, & K. Hahlweg (Eds.), *Treatment of schizophrenia: Family assessment and intervention.* Berlin, Heidelberg: Springer-Verlag.

Jones, J. E. (1977). Patterns of transactional style deviance in the TATs of parents of schizophrenics. *Family Process, 16,* 327–337.

Jones, M. (1953). *The therapeutic community.* New York: Basic Books.

Kendler, K. S., & Gruenberg, A. M. (1984). An independent analysis of the Danish Adoption Study of schizophrenia. *Archives of General Psychiatry, 41,* 555–565.

Kernberg, O. (1975). *Borderline conditions and pathological narcissism.* New York: Jason Aronson.

Kety, S. S., Rosenthal, D., Wender, P. H., & Schulsinger, F. (1968). The types and prevalence of mental illness in the biological and adoptive families of adopted schizophrenics. In D. Rosenthal & S. S. Kety (Eds.), *The transmission of schizophrenia.* Oxford: Pergamon Press.

Laing, R. D. (1965). Mystification, confusion, and conflict. In I. Boszormenyi-Nagy & J. L. Framo (Eds.), *Intensive family therapy.* New York: Harper.

Laing, R. D., & Esterson, A. (1964). *Sanity, madness and the family.* London: Tavistock.

Leff, J. P., & Vaughn, C. (1981). The role of maintenance therapy and relatives' expressed emotion in relapse of schizophrenia: A two-year follow-up. *British Journal of Psychiatry, 139,* 102–104.

Leff, J. P., & Vaughn, C. (1985). *Expressed emotion in families.* New York: Guilford Press.

Leff, J. P., & Wing, J. K. (1971). Trial of maintenance therapy in schizophrenia. *British Medical Journal, 3,* 599–604.

Leff, J., Kuipers, L., Berkowitz, R., Eberlein-Fries, R., & Sturgeon, D. (1982). A controlled trial of social intervention in the families of schizophrenic patients. *British Journal of Psychiatry, 141,* 121–134.

Leff, J., Kuipers, L., Berkowitz, R., Eberlein-Fries, R., & Sturgeon, D. (1983). Social intervention in the families of schizophrenics: Addendum. *British Journal of Psychiatry, 142,* 313.

Lewin, K. (1951). *Field theory in social science.* New York: Harper & Row.

Lewis, J. M., Rodnick, E. H., & Goldstein, M. J. (1981). Intrafamilial interactive behavior, parental communication deviance, and risk for schizophrenia. *Journal of Abnormal Psychology, 90,* 448–457.

Lidz, T., Cornelison, A., Fleck, S., & Terry, D. (1957). The intrafamilial environment of schizophrenic patients: 2. Marital schism and marital skew. *American Journal of Psychiatry, 114,* 241–248.

Liem, J. H. (1974). Effects of verbal communications of parents and children: A comparison of normal and schizophrenic families. *Journals of Clinical Consulting Psychology, 42,* 438–450.

Liem, J. H. (1976). Intrafamily communication and schizophrenic thought disorder: An etiologic or responsive relationship? *The Clinical Psychologist, 29,* 28–30.

Liem, J. H. (1980). Family studies in schizophrenia: An update and a commentary. *Schizophrenia Bulletin, 6,* 429–459.

Lukoff, D., Snyder, K., Ventura, J., & Nuechterlein, K. H. (1984). Life events, familial stress, and coping in the developmental course of schizophrenia. *Schizophrenia Bulletin, 10,* 258–292.

McNeil, T. F., Kaij, L., Malmquist-Larsson, A., et al. (1983). Offspring of women with nonorganic psychoses: development of a longitudinal study of children at high risk. *Acta Psychiatricia Scandinavica, 68,* 234–250.

Mednick, S. A. (1960). The early and advanced schizophrenic. In S. A. Mednick & J. Higgins (Eds.), *Current research in schizophrenia.* Ann Arbor, MI: Edwards.

Miklowitz, D. J. (1985). *Family interaction and illness outcome in bipolar and schizophrenic patients.* Unpublished doctoral dissertation, University of California, Los Angeles.

Miklowitz, D. J. (In press). The family and the course of recent-onset mania. In K. Hahlweg & M. J. Goldstein (Eds.), Understanding major mental disorders: The contribution of family interaction research. New York: Family Process Press.

Miklowitz, D. J., Goldstein, M. J., Falloon, I. R. H., & Doane, J. A. (1984). Interactional correlates of expressed emotion in the families of schizophrenics. *British Journal of Psychiatry, 144,* 482–487.

Miller, J. G. (1978). *Living systems.* New York: McGraw-Hill.

Minuchin, S. (1974). *Families and family therapy.* Cambridge: Harvard University Press.

Mishler, E. G., & Waxler, N. E. (1965). Family interaction processes and schizophrenia: A review of current theories. *Merrill-Palmer Quarterly of Behavior and Development, 11(4),* 269–315.

Nameche, G., Waring, M., & Ricks, D. (1964). Early indicators of outcome in schizophrenia. *Journal of Nervous and Mental Disease, 139,* 232–240.

Parsons, T., & Bales, R. F. (1955). *Family: Socialization and interaction process.* Glencoe, IL: Free Press.

Riess, D. (1975). Families and the etiology of schizophrenia: Fishing without a net. *Schizophrenia Bulletin, 14,* 8–11.

Riskin, J., & Faunce, E. (1972). An evaluative review of family interaction research. *Family Process, 11,* 365–456.

Robins, L. N. (1966). *Deviant children grow up.* New York: Williams & Wilkins.

Rommetveit, R., & Blakar, R. M. (Eds.). (1979). *Studies of language, thought and verbal communication.* London: Academic Press.

Rosenthal, D., & Kety, S. S. (Eds.). (1968). *The transmission of schizophrenia.* New York: Pergamon Press.

Rutter, M. L. (1978). Communication deviance and diagnostic differences. In L. C. Wynne, R. L. Cromwell, & S. Matthysse (Eds.), *The nature of schizophrenia.* New York: Wiley.

Segal, H. (1973). *Introduction to the work of Melanie Klein.* London: Heinemann.

Selvini-Palazzoli, M., Boscolo, L., Cecchin, G., & Prata, G. (1978). *Paradox and counterparadox.* New York: Jason Aronson.

Shannon, C. E. (1948). A mathematical theory of communication. *Bell System Technical Journal, 27,* 379–423, 623–656.

Singer, M. T., & Wynne, L. C. (1965a). Thought disorder and family reactions of schizophrenics: 3. Methodology using projective techniques. *Archives of General Psychiatry, 12,* 187–200.

Singer, M. T., & Wynne, L. C. (1965b). Thought disorder and family relations of schizophrenics: 4. Results and implications. *Archives of General Psychiatry, 12,* 201–212.

Singer, M., Wynne, L., & Toohey, M. (1978). Communication disorders and the families of schizophrenics. In L. C. Wynne, R. L. Cromwell, & S. Matthysse (Eds.), *The nature of schizophrenia.* New York: Wiley.

Sluzki, C., & Ransom, D. (Eds.). (1976). *Double bind: The foundation of communicational approach to the family.* New York: Grune & Stratton.

Spitzer, R. L., Endicott, J., & Robins, E. (1975). *Research Diagnostic Criteria (RDC) for a selected group of functional disorders* (2nd ed.). New York: Biometrics Research, New York State Psychiatric Institute.

Strachan, A. M. (1982). The focus, content, and style of dyadic communication in the families of adolescents at risk for schizophrenia spectrum disorders. Doctoral dissertation, University of California, Los Angeles, 1981. *Dissertation Abstracts International, 42*, 2087B. (University Microfilm No. 81–82, 858)

Strachan, A. M. (1986). Family intervention for the rehabilitation of schizophrenia: Toward protection and coping. *Schizophrenia Bulletin, 12*, 678–698.

Strachan, A. M., Leff, J. P., Goldstein, M. J., Doane, J. A., & Burtt, C. (1986). Emotional attitudes and direct communication in the families of schizophrenics: A cross-national replication. *British Journal of Psychiatry, 149*, 279–287.

Sturgeon, D., Kuipers, L., Berkowitz, R., Turpin, G., & Leff, J. (1981). Psychophysiological responses of schizophrenic patients to high and low expressed emotion relatives. *British Journal of Psychiatry, 138*, 40–45.

Sturgeon, D., Turpin, G., Kuipers, L., Berkowitz, R., & Leff, J. (1984). Psychophysiological responses of schizophrenic patients to high and low expressed emotion relatives: A follow-up study. *British Journal of Psychiatry, 145*, 62–69.

Tarrier, N., Vaughn, C., Lader, M. H., & Leff, J. P. (1979). Bodily reactions to people and events in schizophrenics. *Archives of General Psychiatry, 36*, 311–315.

Tienari, P., Sorri, A., Lahti, I., Naarala, M., Wahlberg, K-E, Pohjola, J., & Moring, J. (1985). Interaction of genetic and psychosocial factors in schizophrenia. *Acta Psychiatrica Scandinavica, 71*, 19–30.

Valone, K., Norton, J. P., Goldstein, M. J., & Doane, J. A. (1983). Parental expressed emotion and affective style in an adolescent sample at risk for schizophrenia spectrum disorders. *Journal of Abnormal Psychology, 92*, 399–407.

Valone, K., Goldstein, M. J., & Norton, J. P. (1984). Parental expressed emotion and psychophysiological reactivity in an adolescent sample at risk for schizophrenia spectrum disorders. *Journal of Abnormal Psychology, 93*, 448–457.

Vaughn, C., & Leff, J. P. (1976). The measurement of expressed emotion in the families of psychiatric patients. *British Journal of Clinical and Social Psychology, 15*, 157–165.

Vaughn, C. E., Snyder, K. S., Jones, S., Freeman, W. B., & Falloon, I. R. H. (1984). Family factors in schizophrenic relapse: A California replication of the British research on expressed emotion. *Archives of General Psychiatry, 41*, 1169–1177.

Walton, H. (Ed.). (1971). *Small group psychotherapy*. London: Penguin.

Wender, P. H., Rosenthal, D., & Kety, S. S. (1968). A psychiatric assessment of the adoptive parents of schizophrenics. In D. Rosenthal & S. S. Kety (Eds.), *The transmission of schizophrenia*. Oxford: Pergamon Press.

Whitehead, A. N., & Russell, B. (1910). *Principia mathematica*. Cambridge: Cambridge University Press.

Wiener, N. (1965). *Cybernetics*. Cambridge: MIT Press.

Wynne, L. C. (1984). The epigenesis of relational systems: A model for understanding family development. *Family Process, 23*, 297–318.

Wynne, L. C., Ryckoff, I. M., Day, J., & Hirsch, S. I. (1958). Pseudomutuality in the family relations of schizophrenics. *Psychiatry, 21*, 205–220.

Wynne, L. C., Singer, M. T., & Toohey, M. L. (1976). Communication of the adoptive parents of schizophrenics. In J. Jorstad & E. Vgelstad (Eds.), *Schizophrenia 75: Psychotherapy, family studies, research*. Oslo, Norway: Universitetsforlaget.

Wynne, L., Singer, M., Bartko, J., & Toohey, M. (1977). Schizophrenics and their families: Research on parental communication. In J. Tanner (Ed.), *Developments in psychiatric research*. London: Hodder & Stoughton.

CHAPTER 14

Depression

JAMES C. COYNE, JANA KAHN, AND IAN H. GOTLIB

The study of family interaction in depression is perhaps 20 years behind the study of such factors in schizophrenia, particularly if one judges from the lack of guiding concepts in depression research analogous to the double bind, pseudo-mutuality, schism, and skew. There have been efforts to describe depression as an interactional phenomenon (Coyne, 1976a; McPartland & Hornstra, 1964) and to identify the social role impairments (Weissman & Paykel, 1974) and social skills deficits (Libet & Lewinsohn, 1973; Youngren & Lewinsohn, 1980) of depressed persons. The association between marital disturbance and depression has been noted (Briscoe & Smith, 1973), and in general, there is a growing appreciation of the social environment as a factor in the etiology, maintenance, and treatment of depression (Brown & Harris, 1978). Yet, there is a puzzling lack of research involving actual observations of how depressed persons interact with the people who are significant in their lives. Of necessity, therefore, the present chapter focuses as much on building a case for the further study of marital and family interaction in depression and the issues that are likely to arise in this endeavor as on reviewing the meager interactional literature that has accumulated thus far.

If there is, as we shall argue, a compelling need to study marital and family interaction in depression, why has it been so seldom done? The reasons are complex, but worth considering. First, initial theory and research concerning the role of the family in psychopathology received its impetus from the work of Harry Stack Sullivan. Despite his insightful analysis of the communicational contexts associated with most forms of psychopathology, Sullivan had little to say about depression. He confessed that, in working with manic-depressives, "I did not get to first base in being able to deduce anything from the experience that

JAMES C. COYNE • Department of Family Practice, University of Michigan, School of Medicine, Ann Arbor, MI 48109-0010. JANA KAHN • Mental Research Institute, Palo Alto, CA 94301. IAN H. GOTLIB • Department of Psychology, University of Western Ontario, London, Ontario, Canada NGA 3K7.

was any good to me in terms of making a theoretical formulation" (Sullivan, 1956, p. 284).

Second, basic differences between depressed and schizophrenic persons in the configuration of significant relations probably discouraged any efforts to extend emerging concepts and methods in the study of schizophrenia to the study of depression. For example, whereas schizophrenics are likely to be brought to the hospital by their parents, depressives are more likely to be brought by their spouses (Vaughn & Leff, 1976). Furthermore, schizophrenia frequently has its onset in a protracted transition from adolescence to adulthood, and young schizophrenics are likely to live with their families of origin or to have left only recently. In contrast, clinical depression has a later onset and is more likely to afflict the married or the formerly married. It may arise for the first time in older adults who have previously functioned well and who have neither living parents nor a spouse. Depression theory and research must come to terms with the variety of interactional contexts in which depression can occur, and concepts and methods in the study of schizophrenic patients in interaction with their parents may not readily be applied to the study of depression.

A third, and perhaps the most important, reason for a lack of research examining marital and family interaction in depression is a long-standing bias in the field toward considering depressed persons and their complaints in isolation, out of any interactional context (Coyne, 1976a). Traditionally viewed as an affective disorder, depression has more recently been conceptualized with an emphasis on causal cognitions (Beck, 1974). The complaints of depressed persons are viewed as reflecting their biased or distorted thought processes, with little attention given to either the social context in which these complaints arise or the function that their verbalization may have in significant relationships. There has been a rapid accumulation of studies examining depressed persons' attributions and expectancies in questionnaire responses to laboratory tasks and in hypothetical and, occasionally, everyday life situations. Yet a recent review (Coyne & Gotlib, 1983) concluded that relatively little new is being learned. Overall, depressed persons present themselves negatively on a variety of questionnaire measures, but depressed–nondepressed differences have been smaller and less consistent than expected. There is little evidence that cognitive factors are causal, although tests of causal hypotheses have typically not employed adequate methodologies.

It may now be an appropriate time for a major redirection of research efforts. Despite the dominant biases in the current literature, an examination of questionnaire and interview studies strongly indicates that depression arises in a distressing social context, and further, that being depressed has a negative impact on social relationships. Although less satisfying than actual observations of interactions involving depressed persons, studies of their life circumstances can offer important indications of the need for interactional studies, the form they should take, and the issues and themes that are likely to arise. For our review of the literature, we begin with these interview and questionnaire studies. We next examine studies of interaction between depressed persons and strangers and then marital and family studies. Finally, we conclude the chapter with some suggestions for generating hypotheses about the interactions between depressed persons and their significant others.

QUESTIONNAIRE AND INTERVIEW STUDIES

Sex Differences in Depression

Consistent findings that women in the United States are 1.6 to 2 times as likely to be depressed as men in both community and clinical samples (Weissman & Klerman, 1977) have led many investigators to turn to marital and family roles for an explanation. Radloff (1980) reported that higher depression scores for women were limited to the married, divorced-separated, and never-married who were not heads of households (i.e., young people living with their parents). Men's scores were greater than women's for the widowed and never-married heads of households. Robertson (1974) and Porter (1970) found that there was a higher rate of neurotic depression among young married women than among comparable single women. Efforts to explain such findings have focused on sex differences in the demands and rewards that traditional marital and family roles provide.

Aneshensel, Frederichs, and Clark (1981) argued that the social roles of men and women are most similar in the absence of extensive family roles and in the presence of work roles, and that depression scores should reflect this similarity. Aneshensel *et al.* found that unmarried, employed men and women had comparable depression scores. Among married persons, gender differences in depression were limited to those with children. However, it appeared that overall sex differences were due to the exceptionally low scores of employed fathers rather than to the high scores of mothers. Similarly, the only significant effect for gender found by Gore and Mangione (1983) (i.e., a higher incidence of depression in women than in men) occurred in family situations in which the youngest child was between 6 and 12 years old. Paralleling the results of the Aneshensel *et al.* study, it was also in this group that fathers had their lowest scores. It seems, then, that both studies require a more complex explanation than simply that having children depresses women.

It has been argued that married men are less depressed than married women because they are more likely to be employed outside the home and thus to have access to the satisfactions of both this work and the family; housewives who are employed outside the home should therefore be less depressed than those who are not (the dual-role hyopthesis). Alternatively, it has been argued that being employed outside the home simply adds to the demands and responsibilities that women face as housewives and should therefore increase depression scores (the overworked-employed-housewife hypothesis). Existing studies are inconsistent in their results, and they do not allow a choice between these two possibilities (Roberts & O'Keefe, 1981; Rosenfield, 1980).

Stress and Depression

Findings from a large and growing literature relating stress processes to depression also highlight the need to consider marriage and the family. Depressed persons have an excess of recent life events, and this excess appears to be due to exits from the social field, rather than to entrances or other positive events, and to everyday experiences rather than to major catastrophes (Paykel, 1979). The most frequent event reported by depressed women is an increase in arguments with their spouses (Paykel, Myers, Dienelt, Klerman, Lindenthal, & Pepper, 1969). Schless, Schwartz, Goetz, and Mendels (1974) found that depressed patients reported feeling particularly vulnerable to marriage- and family-related stresses, a feeling that persisted after the patients had recovered. Corroborating this finding, Ilfeld (1977) found in a community survey that over 25% of the variance in depression scores was accounted for by the stresses of marriage and parenting.

It is unlikely that the relationship between marital disturbance and depression is a simple one (Arkowitz, Holliday, & Hutter, 1982; Bloom, Asher, & White, 1978; Coleman & Miller, 1975; Gotlib & Rusche, 1985; Kahn, Coyne, & Margolin, 1985). Briscoe and Smith (1973) interviewed 139 divorced individuals for the presence of primary affective disorders before, during, and after divorce. The interviewing psychiatrist judged that the symptoms of 17 of the 45 depressed individuals had contributed to the marital disruption rather than having been the result of divorce. People who had experienced a previous depressive episode were likely to have another one associated with the marital breakdown. Women tended to be more depressed during the marriage, whereas men tended to become depressed at the time of separation.

It is now generally recognized that life events such as marital disturbance provide only a partial explanation of the occurrence of depression. Recently, there have been attempts to develop more complex models of vulnerability and provoking agents (Brown & Harris, 1978) or, alternatively, stress and the buffering role of social support (Billings & Moos, 1982a). Brown and Harris (1978) identified four factors leaving women vulnerable to the provoking agents of life events and chronic difficulties: having three or more children under the age of 14, being unemployed, losing one's mother before the age of 11, and the lack of a confiding relationship with a spouse or boyfriend. The importance of not having an intimate confiding relationship as a risk factor for depression has also been replicated with other samples and for men (Brown & Prudo, 1981; Costello, 1982; Roy, 1978; Solomon & Bromet, 1982). Among the recently widowed, lacking a confiding relationship with children is virtually the only environmental difference between those who became depressed and those who did not (Clayton, Halikas, & Maurice, 1972).

The work of Brown and Harris (1978) is proving to be highly influential, but it has been subjected to intense criticism for its methodology, its conceptualization of variables, its mode of argument, and its statistical techniques (e.g., Cleary & Kessler, 1982; Everitt & Smith, 1979; Tennant & Bebbington, 1978). The most basic and recurring criticism has concerned the distinction between vulnerability and provoking agents as more theoretical than empirical. Re-analyses of the Brown and Harris data using alternative statistical techniques have shown that their "vulnerability factors" and "provoking agents" affect the risk of depression independently of each other (Cleary & Kessler, 1982; Tennant & Bebbington, 1978); thus, lacking a husband or boyfriend in whom to confide increases a woman's risk for depression independent of whether she has experienced a recent major life event.

Similar problems are being identified in efforts to conceptualize the benefits of social support as being primarily a buffer against the effects of life events. When an analysis-of-variance model is used, the interaction between level of stress and level of support is expected to predict depression. Although this interaction effect is sometimes found, it appears to be fragile across statistical methods and configurations of variables. The most robust finding in community surveys is that a lack of social support has a direct relationship to depression (Andrews, Tennant, Hewson, & Valliant, 1978; Aneshensel & Stone, 1982; Costello, 1982; Dooley, Catalano, & Brownell, 1980; Lin, Simeone, Ensel, & Kuo, 1979).

Depressed community-residing persons are more likely than nondepressed people to indicate that they seek social support in coping with everyday stressful incidents, but they perceive themselves as receiving less support (Coyne, Aldwin, & Lazarus, 1981; Schaefer, Coyne, & Lazarus, 1981).

Overall, the results of a number of studies suggest that depressed persons are lacking in positive involvement with others. Depressed outpatients report having half as many good friends and close relatives as do nondepressed individuals (Brugha, Conroy, Walsh, DeLaney, O'Hanlun, Donero, Hickey, & Bourke, 1982). They spend less time interacting with their friends and relatives (Brugha et al., 1982; Youngren & Lewinsohn, 1980) and report feeling uncomfortable when with them (Brugha et al., 1982; Weissman & Paykel, 1974). These findings, however, may not be unique to depression. Psychiatric controls also report more friction in interpersonal relationships than do nondepressed individuals (Lewinsohn, 1974; Youngren & Lewinsohn, 1980). Friends and relatives of depressed persons report that they spend less time discussing mutual interests with them than do friends and relatives of nondepressed persons. They indicate instead that their conversations tend to focus on the depressed person's problems, and that they have a tendency to be left feeling depressed themselves (Arkowitz, Buck, & Shanfield, 1979). Howes, Hokanson, and Lowenstein (1985) reported that roommates of depressed students themselves became progressively more depressed over the course of a semester.

There have been some attempts to examine the relationship between depression and particular dimensions of unsupportive family environments. Adults living in families low in cohesion and expressiveness and high in interpersonal conflict report more depressive symptoms (Billings & Moos, 1982b), as do adolescents in families low in cohesion and high in rigidity (Garrison, 1982). Wetzel (1978; Wetzel & Redmond, 1980) found that family support was the best discriminator between depressed and nondepressed women. From questionnaire and informal interview data, it was suggested that most of the depressed women were dependent but were in families insisting on autonomous behavior. However, depressed women scoring high on a measure of independence tended to perceive their family environments as not fostering autonomy. They perceived their husbands as supportive but unwilling to share responsibilities.

Questionnaire and interview studies clearly indicate relationships between depression and both disruptions in one's social relationships and a lack of social support. Increasingly, however, it appears that attempts to formulate simple causal models of these relationships will not be fruitful. Conventional methodologies and statistical techniques in this area of research have generally assumed that social support and life events are not related to each other, and specifically that assessment of one of these variables is not confounded by the other. However, few social ties or low social support may be the *result* of life events:

> Investigators who think that they are studying the effects of small social networks or low perceived support may actually be studying the effects of recent separation or bereavement—very profound sources of stress whose importance goes far beyond the mere loss of potential support. The psychological distress and dislocation in everyday living caused by bereavement or separation may differ in many respects from the long-term effects of being deprived of such relationships. (Schaefer *et al.*, 1981, p. 386)

It may be that life events prove depressing because they deprive a person of vital social resources (Thoits, 1982). Furthermore, rather than merely buffering the effects of life events once they have occurred, social support may decrease their likelihood of occurrence. Finally, efforts to model causally the relationship of stress and support to depression must generally invoke the simplifying assumption that changes in level of depression do not affect either the occurrence of stress or the perceived availability of support (e.g., Aneshensel & Stone, 1982), and this assumption may not be tenable. Being depressed may disrupt social relationships and reduce the availability of support (Briscoe & Smith, 1973; Coyne, 1976a,b).

In conclusion, studies of life events and social support may be seen as an important first step in understanding the relationship between social involvement and depression. Ultimately, however, these concepts and the relationships that theorists and researchers have constructed between them may prove to be oversimplifications of the complexities of social life and its role in depression. As Coyne and DeLongis (1986) noted in their review:

> If we attempt to describe what is going well or badly in [people's] lives . . . seemingly important distinctions between support and stress, coping, adaptational outcomes, and background characteristics become blurred. Ultimately, these distinctions may best be seen as a matter of theoretical and methodological convention, rather than anything that is reliably separable in the lives of our subjects. (p. 458)

Difficulties of Depressed Persons as Spouses

As we have already noted, depression is clearly associated with marital disturbance. The work of the Yale University Depression Research Unit has provided important data concerning the specific problems of depressed women both as wives and as mothers (Weissman & Paykel, 1974). Unfortunately, a comparable study of depressed men has yet to be done. Weissman and Paykel (1974) found in structured interviews that although the social difficulties of depressed women extended into all of their social roles, they were most impaired as wives and mothers. Their marriages were characterized by friction, poor communication, dependency, and diminished sexual satisfaction. They reported a lack of affection toward their husbands and considerable guilt and resentment. Hostility was frequently overt, and even when it was not, depressed women's unspoken misery was viewed by their spouses as an accusation (Bullock, Siegel, Weissman, & Paykel, 1972). These difficulties may persist well beyond the acute episode (Bothwell & Weissman, 1977) and may affect the outcome of treatment. Rousanville, Weissman, Prusoff, and Herceg-Baron (1979) reported that over half of their sample of depressed women presented with marital problems. Continued marital disturbance over the course of treatment was associated with less improvement and a greater tendency to relapse. On the other hand, women whose marital relationships improved showed greater recovery in their levels of depression and social functioning than those women who had not originally presented with marital problems.

Kahn *et al.* (1985) criticized the extent to which the Weissman group reduced the disturbed relationships between depressed women and their husbands to the role dysfunction of depressed women. Consistent with this criticism, Rush, Shaw, and Khatami (1980) noted that "the spouse of the depressed person cannot be considered neutral. He or she becomes frustrated, confused, overly solicitous, or angry, or withdrawn emotionally" (p. 105).

Leff, Roatch, and Bunney (1970) raised the question of whether spouses may be facing the same stressors as their depressed partners, and if so, why they are not depressed. These authors found that many of the depressed persons' stressors were initiated by their spouses (i.e., proposed moves); that the spouses used denial and projection more effectively; and that they responded with anger rather than depression when their sexual adequacy was threatened. Briscoe and Smith (1973) found that compared to nondepressed divorced persons, depressed divorced persons were more likely to have discovered adultery by the ex-spouse.

Coyne *et al.* (in press) found that 40% of the spouses of depressed persons currently in an episode were themselves distressed enough to meet a conventional criterion for a referral to psychotherapy. Furthermore, they felt burdened and upset by their depressed partners, and multiple-regression analyses indicated that the degree of the burden that they experienced accounted entirely for their greater distress than spouses of depressed patients who were not currently in an episode. In general, the sources of burden receiving the highest mean ratings by persons living with a patient who was currently in an episode were (in descending order of magnitude) the patient's lack of energy; the emotional strain on the respondent; the possibility that the patient would become depressed again; and the patient's feelings of worthlessness, lack of interest in doing things, and constant worrying.

It may indeed be difficult to live with a depressed person. Yet, if one takes these difficulties personally, or otherwise becomes emotionally overinvolved, the burden for both oneself and the patient can be aggravated (Coyne, Wortman, & Lehman, 1985). (Yet, questionnaire and interview studies have given relatively little attention to spouses of depressed persons and how they may be actively involved in the depressed persons' distress rather than passive victims of it.)

Depressives report difficulties communicating with their spouses (Freden, 1982; Wasli, 1977) and feel that their spouses' demands are too stringent (Freden, 1982). Spouses tend to respond to depressed persons with what they label as "constructive criticism," but what observers identify as simple hostility (McLean, Ogsten, & Grauer, 1973). Depressed persons are highly susceptible to characterological criticisms from their spouses. The number of critical comments made by a spouse bringing a depressed person for admission to a hospital have been found to be more predictive of outcome than is the patient's symptomatic status (Hooley, 1985; Vaughn & Leff, 1976). In general, depressed persons and their spouses report considerably more overt hostility toward each other than has generally been assumed (Arkowitz *et al.*, 1982; Kahn *et al.*, 1985; Kowalik & Gotlib, 1985; Weissman & Paykel, 1974). Kahn *et al.* (1985) found that depressed persons and their spouses did not differ from each other in their reports of how they typically handled disagreement, but that both were higher than normal controls in terms of aggressiveness and withdrawal and lower in constructive problem-solving.

Difficulties of Depressed Persons as Parents

McLean (1976) noted that depression may be incompatible with effective parenting. Weissman and Paykel (1974) concluded that "At the simplest level, the helplessness and hostility which are associated with acute depression interfere with the ability to be a warm and consistent mother" (p. 121). They found that, in comparisons with normal controls, the relationships between depressed women and their children were characterized by a lack of involvement and affection, impaired communication, friction, guilt, and resentment. The depressed women were even more hostile to their children than to their spouses. Other writers have also commented on the hostility of depressed mothers toward their children (Fabian & Donahue, 1956; Rutter, 1966). Although it is hardly a typical outcome of depression, Resnick (1969) found that almost three quarters of child-murdering mothers were depressed at the time of the murder, and that the victim was frequently the favored child of a loathed spouse.

Children of a depressed parent appear to be at risk for a full range of psychological symptoms, behavioral problems, and diagnosable disorders, and this has been found in assessments using parental reports, child self-reports, and teacher, peer, and clinician ratings (see Coyne & Gotlib, 1985, for a comprehensive review). As many as 40%–50% of the children of a depressed parent exhibit a diagnosable psychiatric disorder (Cytryn, McKnew, Bartko, Lamour, & Hamovit, 1982; Decina, Kestenbaum, Farber, Kron, Gargan, Sackeim, & Fieve, 1983; McKnew, Cytryn, Efron, Gershon, & Bunney, 1979; Welner, Welner, McCrary, & Leonard, 1977). Although some studies have reported increased rates of affective symptoms and diagnoses, others note attentional deficits and conduct disturbances. It has been found that the nature and severity of problems are similar to those found among the offspring of schizophrenics (Weintraub, Liebert, & Neale, 1978), although some studies have found more problems among the children of depressed parents (i.e., Rutter, 1966; Sameroff, Seifer, & Zax, 1982).

Children of neurotically depressed parents may be more symptomatic than are children of more severely depressed or psychotic parents (Fisher, Kokes, Harder, & Jones, 1980). Similarly, young children of unipolar depressed parents appear to be more dysfunctional than are offspring of bipolar parents (Cytryn *et al.*, 1982). Yet, children of bipolar parents show more diagnosable affective disturbances, but not more nonaffective disturbances, than do the adolescent offspring of psychiatric controls (Klein, Depue, & Slater, 1985). Such findings have been interpreted as suggesting a greater impact on the home environment of unipolar depression and a genetically determined later onset for bipolar disorder (Conners, Himmelhock, Goyette, Ulrich, & Neil, 1979).

Examining the mothers of children referred to a child guidance clinic, Fabian and Donahue (1956) found that one third were depressed. Griest, Wells, and Forehand (1979) found that mothers' ratings of the behavior problems of children referred to a clinic was more related to the mothers' levels of depression than to observers' ratings of the children's behavior. Walzer (1961) noted the frequency of mild depression in parents of children referred to a guidance clinic and suggested the usefulness of treatment for the parents to help the children. Patterson (1980) found that mothers of aggressive children showed elevated depression scores, which diminished after training in child management skills.

These studies suggest an association between maternal depression and child problems, but by themselves, they do not establish any simple causal model. It is likely, as various authors have suggested, that being depressed interferes with being an effective parent. However, having a child with behavior problems can be an important source of stress for a parent, and it can aggravate marital tensions. Alternatively, both maternal depression and child behavioral problems may be expressions of a more generally conflictful and unsupportive set of family circumstances.

The Contribution of Questionnaire and Interview Studies

Do the interview and questionnaire data that we have reviewed merely indicate the general tendency of people to evaluate themselves and their situations negatively when they are depressed? Some of the more global and highly inferential judgments that have been required of subjects may be particularly susceptible to such response biases. However, there are reasons for not dismissing out of hand the suggestions of these data.

When depressed and nondepressed subjects are presented with identical stimuli, the differences in their interpretation and recall are generally smaller than anticipated, and what differences do occur may not necessarily indicate depressed persons' biases (Coyne & Gotlib, 1983). Depressed persons' negative evaluations of their social relationships persist when they are no longer depressed (Lunghi, 1977), and interview measures of their social difficulties do not vary directly with recoveries and relapses in mood (Weissman & Paykel, 1974).

Depressed persons' reports of marital dissatisfaction and their own conflict behavior and that of their spouses are in general agreement with their spouses'
reports (Kahn *et al.*, 1985). The two major interview studies of depressed persons (Brown & Harris, 1978; Weissman & Paykel, 1974) have attempted to
control for the biasing effects of the depressed persons' distress and have produced validity data suggesting that they succeeded to a considerable degree.

Cautiously accepted as having the limitations of any self-report and interview data, the studies that we have reviewed can be used to shape the direction of
future research examining the marital and family interactions of depressed
persons. The studies suggesting a possible relationship between sex and marital
status and depression indicate the need to examine sex differences in the rewards, demands, and constraints of marital and family interaction, as well as the
need to examine the impact of women's employment on these factors. The stress
and coping literature indicates the need to examine disruption and support in
the significant relationships of depressed persons. Indeed, much of the ambiguity and confusion that has arisen in the literature may be resolved by going
beyond treating marital discord as a discrete "life event" and beyond global
assessments of support to examination of how conflict arises and support diminishes in the actual interactions of depressed persons. The difficulties that depressed persons have in spousal and parenting roles suggest contexts, tasks, and
target behaviors for studies that are more interactional in nature. It appears that
clinical folklore about the role of hostility in depression (i.e., that depression is
anger turned inward and that one should therefore not expect depressed persons to be overtly hostile) is misleading. The interpersonal dynamics of hostility
in the families of depressed persons need particular attention and may prove
critical in developing a family perspective on the disorder.

Turning to interactional studies of depression, we will now see that much of
the work that has been done has examined interactions between depressed persons and people who have not had long-term relationships with them. Many of
the studies involve fleeting encounters between strangers. Like the questionnaire
and interview studies, this work is not a substitute for research examining how
depressed persons actually interact with the people who are significant in their
lives, but it can prove important in suggesting hypotheses, methods, and general
foci for marital and family studies. Furthermore, studies of encounters with
strangers make studies of marital interaction more interpretable. Without such
data, we would have less of a basis for assuming that the negative marital interactions that have been observed are not merely the effects of mate selection or of
any preexisting conflict or negative attitudes that the depressed persons and
their spouses have toward each other (Coyne, 1985).

INTERACTIONAL STUDIES OF DEPRESSION

Interactions between Depressed Persons and Strangers

Behavioral-social-skills (Lewinsohn, 1974) and interactional-systems (Coyne,
1976a) conceptions of depression have stimulated the development of a growing
literature examining interactions between depressed persons and others. As we

will review, depressed persons have been studied in dyadic and group interactions, as they informally become acquainted with a stranger as well as while they participate in structured interviews, in the prisoners' dilemma game, and in Strodtbeck's revealed-differences task (1951).

Lewinsohn (1974) postulated that depression results when an individual receives a low rate of response-contingent positive reinforcement. This low rate occurs because the individual lacks the social skills necessary to elicit reinforcement from others. In a study of interaction in therapy groups (Libet & Lewinsohn, 1973), it was found that depressed persons were lower than nondepressed psychiatric patients and normal controls on measures of activity level, interpersonal range, rate of positive reaction emitted, and action latency. Other studies have found depressed patients to speak in a lower and more monotonous voice (Gotlib, 1982; Rehm, 1980); to make less eye contact and to have less pleasant facial expressions (Gotlib, 1982; Waxer, 1974); and to emit a greater proportion of adaptors and a smaller proportion of illustrators in their hand movements (Ekman & Friesen, 1974; Gotlib, 1982). Depressed students, too, have been found to have lower and more monotonous speech (Gotlib & Robinson, 1982) and to time their self-disclosures inappropriately (Jacobson & Anderson, 1982).

Anticipated differences between depressed persons and comparison-control groups are not always found. Coyne (1976b) found no differences between depressed outpatients, nondepressed outpatients, and normal controls in terms of activity level, approval responses, hopeful verbal content, genuineness, or ratio of time spent talking about one's partner in telephone conversations. Shrader, Craighead, and Schrader (1978) found no differences in the frequency or timing of reinforcement that depressed and nondepressed students indicated they would provide to a speaker whose speech had been taped. Rehm (1980) found no depressed–nondepressed differences in behavior during a structured interview for three categories of nonverbal behavior and six categories of paralinguistic behavior; the only difference found was that depressed persons smiled less and talked more softly. Both Gotlib (1982) and Youngren and Lewinsohn (1980) found that depressed persons differed from normal controls on a variety of verbal and nonverbal measures, but that they generally did not differ from nondepressed-patient controls.

The research we have reviewed has generally examined behaviors that can be reliably coded and that are likely to vary with mood. However, data demonstrating that these are socially significant behaviors have not yet been produced. It may be, for instance, that low-frequency but salient depressive verbalizations alienate others more than do the nonverbal and paraverbal behaviors that accompany them. Findings that depressed persons were negatively evaluated by partners and observers in the absence of differences on these behavioral measures suggest that critical behaviors were not being assessed (Coyne, 1976b; Youngren & Lewinsohn, 1980). Coyne (1976a,b) has been critical of the use of the term *social skills deficits* to describe the behavioral differences that have been found. He noted that, in the Libet and Lewinsohn (1973) data, there are correlations between behaviors that the subjects emit and the frequency with which they receive the same behaviors from others: "An alternative explanation for the apparent behavior deficits of depressed persons is that others are unwilling to interact with them and depressed persons lack the special skills necessary to overcome this" (Coyne, 1976b, p. 186).

The assumption that behaviors associated with depression may be interwoven and concatenated with a corresponding pattern in the response of others is central to an interactional conception of depression (Coyne, 1976a). As originally presented, the model posited that depressive symptoms are aversive and powerful in their ability to arouse guilt in others and to inhibit any direct expression of annoyance and hostility from them. Members of the social environment attempt to reduce the aversive behavior of depressed persons by manipulating them with nongenuine reassurance and support. At the same time, these same people reject and avoid the depressed persons. As the depressed persons become aware of the perception of others, they display more symptoms and distress, thereby further stimulating the depressive social process.

Although this model is an attempt to describe changes in the relationships of depressed persons over time, tests of it have generally focused on the emergence of such a system in fleeting contact between strangers. Coyne (1976b) found that subjects who talked with depressed outpatients on the telephone were more depressed, anxious, hostile, and rejecting than subjects who talked with nondepressed outpatients or normal controls. It was suggested that the negative mood that depressed persons induce in others may reduce the impact of any positive behaviors that depressed persons may emit. Strack and Coyne (1983) replicated these results in face-to-face interactions between depressed and nondepressed college students. Gotlib and Robinson (1982) failed to find differences in either self-reported mood or perception of their partners for subjects interacting with depressed or nondepressed college students. However, subjects interacting with depressed persons emitted more negative verbal and nonverbal behavior than those who interacted with nondepressed persons, and these differences were apparent after only three minutes of interaction.

Two studies have examined the relationship of the interpersonal behavior of mildly depressed persons to the response of others in a modified prisoners' dilemma game. In the first (Hokanson, Sacco, Blumberg, & Landrum, 1980), each player's relative power was manipulated, and opportunities for communication were provided during the game. In a high-power role, depressed persons tended to be exploitive and noncooperative, and they communicated more self-devaluation and helplessness. This behavior elicited noncooperativeness, extrapunitiveness, and expressions of helplessness from their nondepressed partners. Low-power depressed persons tended to blame their partners for their role, eliciting more friendliness and ingratiating behavior from them. The second study (Blumberg & Hokanson, 1983) varied the interpersonal roles played by confederates interacting with depressed and nondepressed college students. Confederates playing a critical-competitive role elicited more extrapunitiveness from depressed than from nondepressed subjects, and helpless-dependent confederates elicited more negative self-statements from the depressed than from the nondepressed subjects. Across confederate roles, depressed persons communicated high levels of self-devaluation, sadness, helplessness, and general negative content.

A number of other studies have supported hypotheses derived from an interaction-systems conception of depression, but they have tended to use transcripts describing the behavior of depressed persons, videotapes, or confederates, rather than examining the actual interaction between depressed persons and others. Hammen and Peters (1977), Winer, Bonner, Blaney, and Murray (1981), and Gotlib and Beatty (1985) all found that subjects responded more negatively to transcripts describing depressed persons than to ones describing nondepressed persons. Similarly, Boswell and Murray (1981) found that students reacted with more negative mood and rejection to audiotaped interviews with depressed psychiatric inpatients than to tapes of normals; schizophrenic inpatients elicited as much rejection, however.

Hammen and Peters (1977) found that subjects who conversed via an intercom with "depressed" confederates were themselves more depressed following the interaction than were subjects who had conversed with a confederate portraying a nondepressed role. "Depressed" confederates also elicited more personal rejection and less interest in further interactions than did "nondepressed" confederates. Howes and Hokanson (1979) examined the conversational responses of subjects interacting with confederates enacting a depressed, a physically ill, or a normal role, in the context of waiting for an experiment to begin. These investigators found that subjects who interacted with a "depressed" confederate, compared to subjects in the other two conditions, were more rejecting of their partners and responded with a higher rate of silences and directly negative comments and a lower rate of overall verbal responding. Finally, Yarkin, Harvey, and Bloxom (1981) showed subjects a videotape of a woman, either with or without the information that the woman was facing depressing circumstances and was worried about her mental health. When the subjects were given an opportunity to interact with the woman, those who were told that she was depressed sat further away, held less eye contact, engaged in more negatively valenced conversation, and spoke with her for a shorter period of time.

These studies suggest that depression manifests itself in even brief interactions with strangers, and that others react negatively. The Gotlib and Robinson (1982) study suggests that the negative reaction of others develops relatively quickly, and Yarkin *et al.* (1981) suggested that the mere anticipation that someone will be depressed is sufficient to produce withdrawal from her. Results thus far clearly indicate the usefulness of further study, but at present, we know little about what depressed people do that elicits a negative response from others or precisely how these others become involved in the perpetuation of depressed behavior. Questions remain about the specificity of negative responses to depression, as well as about the range of situations in which they occur. Depressed persons do not always elicit negative moods in others. There are likely to be situations in which one's depression has benefits for others; depressed persons are probably less likely to resist others who assume leadership in group tasks (Petzel, Johnson, Johnson, & Kowalski, 1981).

On the other hand, there are also situations in which the behavior of depressed persons may prove more aversive than in the casual acquaintance process. Ziomek and Coyne (1983) found that depressed persons' negative self-preoccupation interfered with their ability to be helpful listeners to others; despite, and perhaps because of their own support-seeking, they were unable or unwilling to be emotionally supportive. Thus, depressed persons may be ill-prepared to reciprocate the support they seek from others. Results from a study testing this hypothesis are currently being analyzed. Preliminary findings indicate that nondepressed helpers identified a high proportion of unhelpful behaviors in the responses of depressed persons.

Although it is a useful line of research, results of studies examining encounters between depressed persons and others may not generalize to interactions with intimate others. The social difficulties of depressed persons are more pronounced in close relationships (Weissman & Paykel, 1974), and in brief, casual exchanges, depressed persons may refrain from expressing their distress and dissatisfaction (Youngren & Lewinsohn, 1980). Existing studies of the marital interactions of depressed persons support these views, but they are few in number.

Marital Interaction in Depression

One of the first studies of depression and marital interaction was conducted by McLean *et al.* (1973), who examined the effects of a behavioral therapy on the valence of the marital communications of depressed patients. The 10 patients and their spouses in the behavior therapy group were given cue boxes to take home, with which they could provide their partner with immediate positive or negative feedback during their conversations. McLean *et al.* found a significant reduction in both the patients' and the spouses' use of negative feedback on the boxes following eight conjoint therapy sessions over 4 weeks. Each couple also participated in two half-hour interactions without the use of the cue boxes, one before and one following therapy. These interactions were rated with respect to negative interchanges, and the 10 couples in the behavior therapy group were compared to 10 couples who received either antidepressant medication combined with group or office psychotherapy, or no treatment at all. The analysis indicated that, although couples in both groups used significantly more negative remarks in responding to one another than in initiating conversation, couples in the behavior therapy group decreased their frequency of negative interchanges and increased their mood ratings significantly more than did couples in the other group.

In a series of studies, Hinchliffe and her colleagues (cf. Hinchliffe, Hooper, & Roberts, 1978) had 20 depressed inpatients interact with their spouses and with opposite-sex strangers while in the hospital, and again with their spouses after recovery. As controls, 20 nonpsychiatric surgical patients interacted with their spouses while in the hospital. Each dyad discussed a number of issues generated through Strodtbeck's Revealed Differences Technique Questionnaire (1951), and a 20-minute segment of each interaction was videotaped and coded on a number of dimensions of both verbal and nonverbal communication. It was found that the interactions of the depressed patients and their spouses were characterized by greater tension and negative expressiveness than were the interactions of the surgical patients and their spouses. Furthermore, whereas the depressed male patients after recovery resembled the surgical controls, the depressed women showed little change from hospitalization to recovery, continuing to exhibit an elevated degree of negative expressiveness. This finding is especially interesting in light of Weissman and Paykel's concordant observation (1974) that the relationship between the depressed women in their sample and their spouses continued to be characterized by interpersonal friction even when the women were no longer symptomatically depressed.

It was also found that the marital interactions of the depressed patients, in contrast to those of the surgical patients, were marked by high levels of disruption, negative emotional outbursts, and considerable incongruity between verbal statements and paralinguistic signals, such as voice tone. This latter finding supports Coyne's postulation (1976b) of a discrepancy between verbal and nonverbal responses to depressed individuals. Again, after recovery, the male depressives closely resembled the surgical patients, whereas the depressed female patients did not change on these measures between the hospitalized and the recovery sessions.

Perhaps the most important finding of Hinchliffe *et al.*'s study (1978) is their observation of the marked and consistent differences between the interactions of the depressed patients and their spouses and the depressed patients and strangers. On virtually every measure used in the study, the marital interactions of the depressed patients were more pathological, more "negative and uneven" than the interactions between these patients and strangers. As Hinchliffe *et al.* stated, the patterns of depressed behavior are

> created and sustained by the couple so that the internal world of the patient and the interpersonal world of the couple become fused together into a system governed by . . . the depressive rule (ambivalence of the depressive leading to distancing of the spouse). What we saw between spouse and stranger was interaction free of this system constraint. (p. 74)

Merikangas, Ranelli, and Kupfer (1979) examined interactions between depressed female inpatients and their spouses in six weekly sessions over the course of the patients' treatment. As in Hinchliffe *et al.*'s study, (1978), discussion between each couple was generated through the use of Strodtbeck's Revealed Differences Technique (RDT) Questionnaire, and a 15-minute segment of each session was audiotaped for subsequent coding. The interactions were scored on three measures: (a) the relative influence of the patient and the spouse over each other (i.e., the number of changes made by each person in their answers to the RDT Questionnaire in response to arguments made by their partner); (b) the frequency and duration of the speech of both patient and spouse and the total joint speech (i.e., interruptions); and (c) the motor activity of both patient and spouse, measured by a motion-sensing device worn on the wrist.

Merikangas *et al.* (1979) found that the spouses exerted significantly less influence over the patients at Session 6 than at Session 1. In the initial session, the patients changed 71% of their responses after joint discussion with their spouses. By Session 6, this amount was reduced to 50%, reflecting a more equal balance of power in the marital dyad following therapy. There was also a decrease over time of joint speech, or interruptions. Although it is not clear from the data whether the spouse or the patient was making the interruptions, the observed decrease in joint speech may be interpreted as another indication of the more equal roles of the two spouses. Finally, the motor activity of the patients increased over the course of therapy, perhaps indicating a greater use of illustrative hand movements (cf. Ekman & Friesen, 1974). Interestingly, spouses of the nonresponders—that is, of the patients who did not demonstrate clinical symptomatic improvement over therapy—showed a decrease in motor activity across therapy sessions. Citing this finding, Merikangas *et al.* (1979) suggested that

> ultimate treatment outcome for the patient may not only be determined by his own symptoms, but may also be predicted by the symptoms (or behavior) of his spouse. (p. 694)

Clearly, this position is compatible with the systems orientation outlined earlier by Coyne (1976a) and Hinchliffe *et al.* (1978).

Although the findings of Hinchliffe *et al.* (1978) and Merikangas *et al.* (1979) are important, there are a number of limitations on their interpretability and generalizability. The major difficulty concerns the absence of appropriate comparison-control groups. Merikangas *et al.* examined marital interaction with only a sample of nine depressed psychiatric patients. It is not clear whether their results are best generalized to couples with a depressed partner, to couples with a partner having any psychiatric condition, or to maritally distressed couples, and it is also unclear whether changes observed over time simply reflect practice effects or the effects of therapy on marital communication that are not specific to the treatment of depressed persons. Hinchliffe *et al.* (1978) included a comparison group of surgery patients and their spouses, but it is possible that the distress of surgical patients affects marital interaction in ways that are similar to, but smaller in degree than the effects of depression. Differences that were found may be fewer than those that would arise in comparison with a normal control group. Neither study included measures of marital adjustment or satisfaction, and it is possible that the deviant communication patterns observed in the depressed patients are more generally associated with marital difficulties.

In a study designed to address this issue, 26 married couples were selected from a larger group of 63 couples seeking marital therapy (Hautzinger, Linden, & Hoffman, 1982). Of these couples, 13 had one spouse with a severe, clinically significant unipolar depression, and in 13 couples, neither spouse exhibited depressive symptomatology. The two groups of subjects were matched with respect to severity of marital problems. For each couple, eight 40-minute conversations were recorded over a 3- to 4-week period. Each interaction was scored according to a 28-category system, reflecting 4 broad categories of behavior: nonverbal affect and mood expression, self-related verbalizations, partner-related verbalizations, and neutral conversation. Hautzinger *et al.* concluded that

> the interaction between couples without a depressed partner was positive, supportive, and reciprocal. In contrast, the couples with a depressed partner showed an uneven, negative, and asymmetrical communication. (p. 313)

Couples with a depressed spouse expressed more dysphoric and uncomfortable feelings, expressed more negative well-being, and in general talked more about well-being and asked questions about it. Hautzinger *et al.* noted some important asymmetries in the interactions between depressed persons and their spouses. The depressed persons spoke negatively of themselves and positively of their spouses, whereas their nondepressed spouses rarely spoke of their own well-being but evaluated their depressed partners negatively. The nondepressed spouses seldom agreed with their partners' statements, and although they offered their partners help, they did so with negative statements about them. Overall, the Hautzinger *et al.* data suggest that, even when level of marital distress is controlled, couples with and without a depressed partner differ in the quality of their interaction.

Three recent studies have found the interactions of depressed persons and their spouses to be characterized by hostility. All three studies involved couples with a depressed person discussing a topic that they had chosen from a list of possible areas of disagreement. Kahn *et al.* (1985) reported that partners in couples with a depressed spouse were more sad and angry following such marital interactions and experienced each other as more negative, hostile, mistrusting, and detached, as well as less agreeable, nurturant, and affiliative, than did nondepressed couples. The depressed persons and their spouses were remarkably similar in their reports of their own behavior. Further analyses of the congruence between depressed persons' self-reports and the reports by their spouses provided no evidence of the depressed persons' exhibiting any "depressive distortion": for some variables, the depressed persons presented themselves in a more positive light (Coyne & Kahn, 1984).

Arkowitz *et al.* (1982) found that, following interactions with their wives, husbands of depressed women reported feeling more hostile than did husbands of psychiatric and nonpsychiatric control subjects.

Finally, Kowalik and Gotlib (1985) examined the relative contributions of depression, global psychopathology, and marital distress to the quality of the interactions of depressed outpatients. Depressed and nondepressed psychiatric outpatients and nondepressed nonpsychiatric controls and their spouses participated in an interactional task, and as the partners interacted with each other, each spouse coded on a "talk table" (Gottman, Notarius, Markman, Berk, Yoppi, & Rubin, 1976) both the intended impact of their own behavior and their perception of their spouse's communications. The talk table is an apparatus that allows the speaker to register on a 5-point scale, from very negative to very positive, the intended impact of each message she or he sends and allows the spouse to simultaneously code the perceived impact of that message. Kowalik and Gotlib's results suggest that marital relationships of depressed psychiatric outpatients are characterized by negative interactions, and moreover, that this negative quality is specific to depression. The depressed patients emitted more negative intents and fewer positive intents than did the nondepressed patients and controls. Furthermore, although there were no differences in actual coding among the three groups of spouses, only the spouses of depressed patients recalled more negative intents than they actual coded, a finding suggesting that they felt hostile and anxious during interactions with their depressed spouses but tried to inhibit these negative feelings during the interactions.

The Marital Interaction Coding System (MICS; Weiss & Margolin, 1977) was used to code videotapes of the interactions. When the behavior codes were collapsed into positive and negative, verbal and nonverbal categories, no differences were found for verbal behavior; however, depressed women and their husbands had significantly lower rates of positive nonverbal behavior, and husbands of depressed and nondepressed patients had more negative nonverbal behavior. Taking behavioral coding and self-reports together, Arkowitz *et al.* suggested that the husbands of depressed women were feeling hostile and attempting to hide this feeling but leaking it nonverbally.

Studies of Depressed Persons in Family Interaction

Reports of observations of depressed persons interacting with more than one other family member present are rare. Lewinsohn and his colleagues (Lewinsohn & Atwood, 1969; Lewinsohn & Schaffer, 1971) collected some preliminary home observation data as part of an effort to gain baseline information with which to define treatment goals and to measure behavior change in psychotherapy. Observers used a coding system with 28 categories to score behavior. Summarizing observations of five families, four of them with children, Lewinsohn and Schaffer (1971) stated:

> Interpersonal patterns which have emerged as critical vary from the complete absence of any interaction between patient and spouse to very one-sided interactions. For instance, in one family, the patient rarely reinforced behavior directed toward him. In another family, a small proportion of time was devoted to topics of interest to the patient, and the patient's only topic was "depressive talk" (e.g., psychosocial and somatic complaints). (p. 89)

Lewinsohn and Schaffer suggested that their data are consistent with the hypothesis that a low rate of positive reinforcement is a critical antecedent of depressive behaviors, but they acknowledged having a small, unrepresentative sample with no comparison-control families. It should be further noted that these and other studies of "positive reinforcement" in the interactions of depressed persons have defined reinforcers in an *a priori* manner, rather than functionally (cf. Brokaw & McLemore, 1983). At the present time, we know very little about what is reinforcing for what behaviors in interactions involving depressed persons.

Finally, the Oregon Research Institute group has conducted the first study of the conditional responding of family members to depressed behavior in home interactions (Biglan, Hops, Sherman, Friedman, Arthur, & Osteen, 1985; Biglan, Hops, & Sherman, in press). Children of mothers who were depressed and maritally distressed emitted significantly more "irritated" affect (nonverbal behavior suggesting that they were angry) than did the children in normal or depressed-only families. In both depressed-only and depressed-maritally distressed groups, mothers' displays of dysphoric affect briefly reduced fathers' and children's irritated and sarcastic behavior; however, it also produced a suppression of caring behavior. In separate analyses of same data, Friedman (1984) found that both mothers' depressive behavior (both depressive content and dysphoric affect) suppressed children's aggressive and command-giving behavior. This research is important not only in providing the first systematic home observation of depressed persons and their families, but in its testing of hypotheses derived from an interactional model of depression (Coyne, 1976a,b) concerning the suppression of hostile behavior by displays of depressive behavior.

Evaluation of Marital and Family Interaction Studies

Only a small literature is available, but it is rather consistent in suggesting that marital interactions involving depressed persons are characterized by negative affect and tension. The negative attitudes of depressed persons and their spouses toward each other influence their interpretation of ongoing behavior, and there is evidence of both overt hostility and attempts to hide negative feelings when disagreements are being discussed. Interactions between depressed persons and their spouses are more negatively toned than interactions between depressed persons and strangers, and the negativity of the interactions of maritally distressed, depressed persons does not appear to be due merely to marital distress.

With the exception of the innovative studies being conducted at the Oregon Research Institute and some preliminary work conducted in the mid-1970s, there are no published home-observation studies of depressed persons in their families.

Only a narrow range of laboratory task situations has been sampled, and these are generally structured to elicit disagreement and conflict rather than supportive exchanges. Neither the task situations nor the behavioral coding systems that have been used have been validated against reports of frequent occurrences in the daily lives of depressed persons and their spouses, their perceptions of each other, or their presenting problems in psychotherapy. Data analysis has been limited primarily to comparisons of behavior frequencies, with little effort to look for the extended interactional patterns that Coyne (1976a) and others have suggested. Despite the strong suggestion of interview and questionnaire studies that examination of the marital and family interactions of depressed persons should prove theoretically and therapeutically useful, this line of research remains in its infancy.

SOME POSSIBLE FUTURE DIRECTIONS

Many of the conceptual, methodological, and statistical issues that depression researchers will face have been dealt with in more established literature examining marital distress and the role of marital and family factors in other forms of psychopathology. It would be unfortunate if depression researchers had to reinvent solutions that are available elsewhere, yet it would also be unfortunate if methods and measures were haphazardly borrowed without regard to theoretical relevance or the need to validate them with reference to the life situations of depressed persons and their families. It is likely that interactions between depressed persons and their families are negative in a variety of task situations and as assessed with a wide range of methods and measures. Hopefully, however, research will quickly move beyond demonstrating this to tests of more specific hypotheses with ecologically valid task situations and measures. Researchers need to establish that the differences they find are samples rather than mere signs of the difficulties of depressed persons.

At the present time, the theoretical background for marital and family studies of depression is underdeveloped. It is beyond the scope of the current chapter to tackle this problem (however, for some preliminary statements see Kahn, *et al.*, 1985; Coyne, in press), but the following suggestions may prove helpful:

1. Depression occurs in a variety of contexts, but a common element in them may be that depressed people are facing problems that are intractable to or are even maintained by their ways of coping. The marriages and families of depressed persons are likely to be implicated both as the locus of such problems and as inadequate sources of support. The apparent intractability of depressed persons' problems and the ineptness of their coping may be related to their family members' coping and the quality of the support they offer.

2. Interview and questionnaire studies, particularly the work of Myrna Weissman's group (Weissman & Paykel, 1974) suggest some specific difficulties of depressed persons in their intimate relationships. Rather than reifying these difficulties as "social role impairments," it would be useful to contextualize them in terms of hypotheses about what types of marital and family situations may perpetuate them and, in turn, what coping tasks they may pose for the intimate relations of depressed people. For instance, what home situations would perpetuate a communication style characterized by friction, inhibition, and indecisiveness, and, in turn, what is it like to live with someone who behaves in this way? That is, how do others cope, and what problems does this way of coping pose for the depressed persons?

3. Although it may ultimately be shown that living in certain circumstances may more dependably make someone depressed than being depressed produces distressing circumstances, it is important that researchers not prematurely commit themselves to linear causal hypotheses. Depressive patterns of interaction probably seldom occur only once, but persist, overlap, and recur with overwhelming complexity. As a provisional framework, a circular causal model is more appropriate than a linear one that artificially delimits sequences from the intricate patterns in which they occur (Coyne & Holroyd, 1982). It is likely that particular patterns of marital and family interaction may be seen as having formative, triggering, sustaining influences on the onset of depression, as well as being consequences of it.

4. Studies of marital and family interaction have given little attention to diagnostic issues and the heterogeneity of depressed persons, but this problem will undoubtedly be remedied as the field progresses. However, beyond traditional diagnostic considerations, it is likely that depressed persons may be usefully classified according to differences in interactional contexts. Many, but

not all, depressed persons face marital discord. Based on interview and question-naire studies, it may tentatively be suggested that conflict and discord, on one hand, and lack of support, on the other, may be independent contributors to depression, and these could prove to be useful provisional dimensions with which to characterize the close relationships of depressed persons.

REFERENCES

Andrews, G., Tennant, C., Hewson, D., & Valliant, G. (1978). Life stress, social support, coping style, and risk of psychological impairment. *Journal of Nervous and Mental Disease, 166,* 307–316.

Aneshensel, C. S., & Stone, J. D. (1982). Stress and depression: A test of the buffering model of social support. *Archives of General Psychiatry, 39,* 1392–1396.

Aneshensel, C. S., Frederichs, R. R., & Clark, V. A. (1981). Family roles and sex differences in depression. *Journal of Health and Social Behavior, 22,* 379–393.

Arkowitz, H., Buck, F., & Shanfield, F. (1979). *Interpersonal factors in depression: The reactions of family and friends to the depressed patient.* Paper presented at the Annual Meeting of the Western Psychological Association, San Diego.

Arkowitz, H., Holliday, S., & Hutter, M. (1982). *Depressed women and their husbands: A study of marital interaction and adjustment.* Paper presented at the Annual Meeting of the Association for the Advancement of Behavior Therapy, Los Angeles.

Beck, A. T. (1974). Cognition, affect, and psychopathology. In H. London & R. E. Nisbett (Eds.), *Thought and feeling.* Chicago: Aldine.

Biglan, A., Hops, H., Sherman, L., Friedman, L. S., Arthur, J., & Osteen, V. (1985). Problem-solving interactions of depressed women and their husbands. *Behavior Therapy, 16,* 431–451.

Biglan, A., Hops, H., & Sherman, L. (in press). Coercive family processes and maternal depression. In R. J. McMahon & R. DeV. Peter (Eds.), *Marriages and families: Behavioral treatments and processes.* New York: Bruner/Mazel.

Billings, A. G., & Moos, R. H. (1982a). Psychosocial theory and research on depression: An integrative framework and review. *Clinical Psychology Review, 2,* 213–237.

Billings, A. G., & Moos, R. H. (1982b). Social support and functioning among community and clinical groups: A panel model. *Journal of Behavioral Medicine, 5,* 295–311.

Bloom, B., Asher, S. J., & White, S. W. (1978). Marital disruption as a stressor: A review and analysis. *Psychological Bulletin, 85,* 867–894.

Blumberg, S. R., & Hokanson, J. E. (1983). The effect of another person's response style on interpersonal behavior in depression. *Journal of Abnormal Psychology, 92,* 196–209.

Boswell, P. C., & Murray, E. J. (1981). Depression, schizophrenia, and social attraction. *Journal of Consulting and Clinical Psychology, 49,* 641–647.

Bothwell, S., & Weissman, M. M. (1977). Social impairments four years after an acute depressive episode. *American Journal of Orthopsychiatry, 47*(2), 231–237.

Briscoe, C. W., & Smith, J. B. (1973). Depression and marital turmoil. *Archives of General Psychiatry, 29,* 811–817.

Brokaw, D. W., & McLemore, C. W. (1983). Toward a more rigorous definition of social reinforcement: Some interpersonal clarifications. *Journal of Personality and Social Psychology, 44,* 1014–1020.

Brown, G. W., & Harris, T. (1978). *Social origins of depression.* New York: Free Press.

Brown, G. W., & Prudo, R. (1981). Psychiatric disorder in a rural and an urban population: 1. Aetiology of depression. *Psychological Medicine, 11,* 581–599.

Brugha, T., Conroy, R., Walsh, N., DeLaney, W., O'Hanlun, J., Donero, E., Hickey, N., & Bourke, G. (1982). Social networks, attachments and support in minor affective disorders: A replication. *British Journal of Psychiatry, 114,* 249–255.

Bullock, R., Siegel, R., Weissman, M. M., & Paykel, E. S. (1972). The weeping wife: Marital relations of depressed women. *Journal of Marriage and the Family,* 488–492.

Clayton, P. J., Halikas, J. A., & Maurice, W. L. (1972). The depression of widowhood. *British Journal of Psychiatry, 120,* 71–78.

Cleary, P. D., & Kessler, R. C. (1982). The estimation and interpretation of modifier effects. *Journal of Health and Social Behavior, 23,* 159–168.

Coleman, R. E., & Miller, A. G. (1975). The relationship between depression and marital maladjustment in a clinic population: A multitrait–multimethod study. *Journal of Consulting and Clinical Psychology, 43,* 647–651.

Conners, C. K., Himmelhock, J., Goyette, C. H., Ulrich, M. S., & Neil, J. F. (1979). Children of parents with affective illness. *Journal of the American Academy of Child Psychiatry, 18,* 600–607.

Costello, C. G. (1982). Social factors associated with depression: A retrospective community study. *Psychological Medicine, 12,* 329–339.

Coyne, J. C. (1976a). Depression and the response of others. *Journal of Abnormal Psychology, 85,* 186–193.

Coyne, J. C. (1976b). Toward an interactional description of depression. *Psychiatry, 39,* 28–40.

Coyne, J. C. (1985). Studying depressed persons' interactions with strangers and spouses. *Journal of Abnormal Psychology, 94,* 231–232.

Coyne, J. C. (in press). Strategic therapy with couples having a depressed spouse. In G. Haas, I. Glick, & J. Clarkin (Eds.), *Family intervention in affective illness.* New York: Guilford Press.

Coyne, J. C., & DeLongis, A. M. (1986). Getting beyond social support: the role of social relationships in adaptational outcomes. *Journal of Consulting and Clinical Psychology, 54,* 454–460.

Coyne, J. C., & Gotlib, I. H. (1983). The role of cognition in depression: A critical appraisal. *Psychological Bulletin, 94,* 472–505.

Coyne, J. C., & Gotlib, I. H. (1985). *Depression and parenthood: An integrative review.* Unpublished manuscript.

Coyne, J. C., & Holroyd, K. (1982). Stress, coping, and illness: a transactional perspective. In T. Millon, C. Green, & R. Meager (Eds.), *Handbook of health care clinical psychology.* New York: Plenum Press.

Coyne, J. C., & Kahn, J. (1984). *Interpersonal perception in depression: The illusions of depressed persons, nondepressed persons—or depression researchers?* Paper presented at the Annual Convention of the American Psychological Association, Toronto.

Coyne, J. C., Aldwin, C., & Lazarus, R. S. (1981). Depression and coping in stressful episodes. *Journal of Abnormal Psychology, 90,* 439–447.

Coyne, J. C., Wortman, C., & Lehman, D. (1985). *The other side of support: Emotional overinvolvement and miscarried helping.* Paper presented at the Annual Convention of the American Psychological Association, Los Angeles.

Coyne, J. C., Kessler, R. C., Tal, M., Turnbull, J., Wortman, C., & Greden, J. (in press). Living with a depressed person. *Journal of Consulting and Clinical Psychology.*

Cytryn, L., McKnew, D. H., Bartko, J. J., Lamour, M., & Hamovit, J. (1982). Offspring of patients with affective disorders *Journal of the American Academy of Child Psychiatry, 21,* 389–391.

Decina, P., Kestenbaum, C. J., Farber, S., Kron, L., Gargan, M., Sackeim, H. A., & Fieve, R. R. (1983). Clinical and psychological assessment of children of bipolar probands. *American Journal of Psychiatry, 140,* 548–553.

Dooley, D., Catalano, D., & Brownell, A. (1980). *The relationship of social support and individual life change to depression.* Paper presented at the Annual Meeting of the Western Psychological Association, Honolulu.

Ekman, P., & Friesen, W. V. (1974). Nonverbal behavior and psychopathology. In R. J. Friedman & M. M. Katz (Eds.), *The psychology of depression: Contemporary theory and research.* Washington, DC: V. H. Winston & Sons.

Everitt, B. S., & Smith, A. M. R. (1979). Interactions in contingency tables: A brief discussion of alternative definition. *Psychological Medicine, 9,* 581–583.

Fabian, A. A., & Donohue, J. F. (1956). Maternal depression: A challenging child guidance problem. *American Journal of Ortho-psychiatry, 26,* 400–405.

Fisher, L., Kokes, R. F., Harder, D. W., & Jones, J. E. (1980). Child competence and psychiatric risk: 6. Summary and intergration of findings. *Journal of Nervous and Mental Disease, 168,* 353–355.

Freden, L. (1982). *Psychosocial aspects of depression: No way out?* New York: Wiley.

Friedman, L. S. (1984). *Family interaction among children of unipolar depressed mothers: A naturalistic observation study.* Unpublished doctoral dissertation, University of Oregon, Eugene.

Garrison, C. (1982). *Depression symptoms, family environment, and life change in early adolescents.* Unpublished doctoral dissertation, University of North Carolina.

Gore, S., & Mangione, T. W. (1983). Social roles, sex roles, and psychological distress: Additive and interactive models. *Journal of Health and Social Behavior, 24,* 300–313.

Gotlib, I. H. (1982). Self reinforcement and depression in interpersonal interaction: The role of performance level. *Journal of Abnormal Psychology, 91,* 5–13.

Gotlib, I. H., & Beatty, M. E. (1985). Negative responses to depression: The role of attributional style. *Cognitive Therapy and Research, 9,* 91–103.

Gotlib, I. H., & Robinson, L. A. (1982). Responses to depressed individuals: Discrepancies between self-report and observer-related behavior. *Journal of Abnormal Psychology, 91,* 231–240.

Gotlib, I. H., & Rusche, S. (1985). *Verbal and nonverbal communication patterns in couples with a depressed spouse.* Unpublished manuscript.

Gottman, J., Notarius, C., Markman, H., Berk, S., Yoppi, R., & Rubin, M. E. (1976). Behavior exchange theory and marital decision-making. *Journal of Personality and Social Psychology, 34,* 14–23.

Griest, D., Wells, K. C., & Forehand, R. (1979). An examination of predictions of maternal perceptions of maladjustment in clinic-referred children. *Journal of Abnormal Psychology, 88,* 277–281.

Hammen, C. L., & Peters, S. D. (1977). Differential responses to male and female depressive reactions. *Journal of Consulting and Clinical Psychology, 15,* 994–1001.

Hautzinger, M., Linden, M., & Hoffman, N. (1982). Distressed couples with and without a depressed partner: An analysis of their verbal interaction. *Journal of Behavior Therapy and Experimental Psychiatry, 13,* 307–314.

Hinchliffe, M., Hooper, D., & Roberts, F. J. (1978). *The melancholy marriage.* New York: Wiley.

Hokanson, J. E., Sacco, W. P., Blumberg, S. R., & Landrum, G. C. (1980). Interpersonal behavior of depressive individuals in a mixed-motive game. *Journal of Abnormal Psychology, 89,* 320–332.

Hooley, J. M. (1985). Expressed emotion: A review of the critical literature. *Clinical Psychology Review, 5,* 119–139.

Howes, M. J., & Hokanson, J. E. (1979). Conversational and social responses to depressive interpersonal behavior. *Journal of Abnormal Psychology, 88*(6), 625–634.

Howes, M. J., Hokanson, J. E., & Lowenstein, D. A. (1985). The induction of depressive affect after prolonged exposure to a mildly depressed individual. *Journal of Abnormal Personality and Social Psychology, 49,* 1110–1113.

Ilfeld, F. W. (1977). Current social stressors and symptoms of depression. *American Journal of Psychiatry, 134,* 161–166.

Jacobson, N. S., & Anderson, E. (1982). Interpersonal skills deficits and depression in college students: A sequential analysis of the timing of self-disclosure. *Behavior Therapy, 13,* 271–282.

Kahn, J., Coyne, J. C., & Margolin, G. (1985). Depression and marital conflict: The social construction of despair. *Journal of Social and Personal Relationships, 2,* 447–462.

Klein, D. N., Depue, R. A., & Slater, J. F. (1985). Cyclothymia in the adolescent offspring of parents with bipolar affective disorder. *Journal of Abnormal Psychology, 94,* 115–127.

Kowalik, D., & Gotlib, I. H. (1985). *Depression and marital interaction: Concordance between intent and perception of communications.* Unpublished manuscript, University of Western Ontario.

Leff, M., Roatch, J., & Bunney, L. E. (1970). Environmental factors preceding the onset of severe depression. *Psychiatry, 33,* 298–311.

Lewinsohn, P. M. (1974). A behavioral approach to depression. In R. J. Friedman & M. M. Katz (Eds.), *The psychology of depression: Contemporary theory and research.* New York: Halsted Press.

Lewinsohn, P. M., & Atwood, G. E. (1969). Depression: A clinical research approach. *Psychotherapy: Theory, Research and Practice, 6,* 166–171.

Lewinsohn, P. M., & Schaffer, M. (1971). The use of home observations as an integral part of the treatment of depression: Preliminary report of case studies. *Journal of Consulting and Clinical Psychology, 37,* 87–94.

Libet, J. M., & Lewinsohn, P. M. (1973). The concept of social skills with special reference to the behavior of depressed persons. *Journal of Consulting and Clinical Psychology, 40,* 304–312.

Lin, N., Simeone, R., Ensel, W. M., & Kuo, W. (1979). Social support, stressful life events, and illness: A model and an empirical test. *Journal of Health and Social Behavior, 20*, 108–119.

Lunghi, M. E. (1977). The stability of mood and social perception measures in a sample of depressed inpatients. *British Journal of Psychiatry, 130*, 598–604.

McKnew, D. H., Cytryn, L., Efron, A. M., Gershon, E. S., & Bunney, W. E. (1979). Offspring of patients with affective disorders. *British Journal of Psychiatry, 134*, 148–152.

McLean, P. D. (1976). Parental depression: Incompatible with effective parenting. In E. J. Marsh, C. Handy, & L. A. Hammerlynck (Eds.), *Behavior modification approaches to parenting.* New York: Brunner/Mazel.

McLean, P. D., Ogston, K., & Grauer, L. (1973). A behavioral approach to the treatment of depression. *Journal of Behavior Research and Experimental Psychiatry, 4*, 323–330.

McPartland, T. S., & Hornstra, R. K. (1964). The depressive datum. *Comprehensive Psychiatry, 5*, 253–261.

Merikangas, K. R., Ranelli, C. J., & Kupfer, D. J. (1979). Marital interaction in hospitalized depressed patients. *Journal of Nervous and Mental Disease, 167*, 689–695.

Patterson, G. R. (1980). Mothers: The unacknowledged victim. *Monographs of the Society for Research in Child Development, 45*(5, Serial No. 186).

Paykel, E. S., Myers, J. K., Dienelt, M. N., Klerman, G. L., Lindenthal, J. J., & Pepper, M. P. (1969). Life events and depression: A controlled study. *Archives of General Psychiatry, 21*, 753–760.

Petzel, T. P., Johnson, J. E., Johnson, H. H., & Kowalski, J. (1981). Behavior of depressed subjects in problem solving groups. *Journal of Research in Personality, 15*, 389–398.

Porter, A. M. W. (1970). Depressive illness in a general practice: A demographic study and controlled trial of Imipramine. *British Medical Journal, 1*, 773–778.

Radloff, L. S. (1980). Risk factors for depression: What do we learn from them? In M. Guttentag, S. Salasin, & D. Belle (Eds.), *The mental health of women.* New York: Academic Press.

Rehm, L. P. (1980). Detecting the dimensions of depression: Behavioral assessment in therapy outcome research. In K. Blankstein, P. Pliner, & J. Polivy (Eds.), *Assessment and modification of emotional behavior.* New York: Plenum Press.

Resnick, P. J. (1969). Child murder by parents: A psychiatric review of filicide. *American Journal of Psychiatry, 126*, 325–334.

Roberts, R. E., & O'Keefe, S. J. (1981). Sex differences in depression reexamined. *Journal of Health and Social Behavior, 22*, 394–400.

Robertson, N. C. (1974). The relationship between marital status and risk of psychiatric referral. *British Journal of Psychiatry, 124*, 191–202.

Rosenfield, S. (1980). Sex differences in depression: Do women always have higher rates? *Journal of Health and Social Behavior, 21*, 33–42.

Rousanville, B. J., Weissman, M. W., Prusoff, B. A., & Herceg-Baron, R. L. (1979). Marital disputes and treatment outcome in depressed women. *Comprehensive Psychiatry, 20*, 483–490.

Roy, A. (1978). Vulnerability factors and depression in women. *British Journal of Psychiatry, 133*, 106–110.

Rush, A. J., Shaw, B., & Khatami, M. (1980). Cognitive therapy of depression: Utilizing the couples system. *Cognitive Therapy and Research, 4*, 103–113.

Rutter, M. (1966). *Children of sick parents.* Oxford: Oxford University Press.

Sameroff, A. J., Seifer, R., & Zax, M. (1982). Early development of children at risk for emotional disorder. *Monographs of the Society for Research in Child Development, 47*(7, Serial No. 199).

Schaefer, C., Coyne, J. C., & Lazarus, R. S. (1981). The health-related functions of social support. *Journal of Behavioral Medicine, 4*, 381–406.

Schless, A. P., Schwartz, L., Goetz, C., & Mendels, J. (1974). How depressives view the significance of life events. *British Journal of Psychiatry, 125*, 406–410.

Shrader, S., Craighead, W. E., & Schrader, R. M. (1978). Reinforcement patterns in depression. *Behavior Therapy, 9*, 1–14.

Solomon, Z., & Bromet, E. (1982). The role of social factors in affective disorders: An assessment of the vulnerability model of Brown and his colleagues. *Psychological Medicine, 12*, 123–130.

Strack, S., & Coyne, J. C. (1983). Social confirmation of dysphoria: Shared and private reactions to depression. *Journal of Personality and Social Psychology, 44*, 806–814.

Strodtbeck, F. L. (1951). Husband—wife interaction over revealed differences. *American Sociological Review, 16,* 468–473.

Sullivan, H. S. (1956). *Clinical studies in psychiatry.* New York: W. W. Norton.

Tennant, L., & Bebbington, P. (1978). The social causation of depression: A critique of the work of Brown and his colleagues. *Psychological Medicine, 8,* 565–578.

Thoits, P. (1982). Conceptual, methodological, and theoretical problems in studying social support as a buffer against life stress. *Journal of Health and Social Behavior, 23,* 145–159.

Vaughn, C. E., & Leff, J. P. (1976). The influence of family and social factors on the course of psychiatric illness. *British Journal of Psychiatry, 129,* 125–137.

Walzer, H. (1961). Casework treatment of the depressed patient. *Social Casework, 42,* 505–512.

Wasli, E. L. (1977). Dysfunctional communication response patterns of depressed wives and their husbands in relation to activities of daily living. *Dissertation Abstracts International, 38*(1-B), 142.

Waxer, P. (1974). Nonverbal cues for depression. *Journal of Abnormal Psychology, 53,* 318–322.

Weintraub, S., Liebert, D., & Neale, J. M. (1978). Teacher ratings of children vulnerable to psychopathology. In E. J. Anthony (Ed.), *The child and his family: 4. Vulnerable children.* New York: Wiley.

Weiss, R. L., & Margolin, G. (1977). Assessment of marital conflict and accord. In A. R. Ciminero, K. S. Kalhoun, & H. E. Adams (Eds.), *Handbook of behavioral assessment.* New York: Wiley.

Weissman, M. M. & Klerman, G. L. (1977). Sex differences and the epidemiology of depression. *Archives of General Psychiatry, 34,* 98–111.

Weissman, M. M., & Paykel, E. S. (1974). *The depressed woman: A study of social relationships.* Chicago: University of Chicago Press.

Welner, Z., Welner, A., McCrary, M. D., & Leonard, M. A. (1977). Psychopathology in children of inpatients with depression: A controlled study. *Journal of Nervous and Mental Disease, 164,* 408–413.

Wetzel, J. W. (1978). The work environment and depression: Implications for intervention. In J. W. Hawks (Ed.), *Toward human dignity: Social work in practice.* New York: Bruner/Mazel.

Wetzel, J. W., & Redmond, F. C. (1980). A person—environment study of depression. *Social Service Review, 54,* 363–375.

Winer, D. L., Bonner, T. O., Blaney, P. H., & Murray, E. J. (1981). Depression and social attraction. *Motivation and Emotion, 5,* 153–166.

Yarkin, K., Harvey, J. L., & Bloxom, B. M. (1981). Cognitive sets, attribution, and social interaction. *Journal of Personality and Social Psychology, 41,* 243–252.

Youngren, M. A., & Lewinsohn, P. M. (1980). The functional relation between depression and problematic interpersonal behavior. *Journal of Abnormal Psychology, 1980, 89,* 333–341.

Ziomek, M. & Coyne, J. C. (1983). *Interactions involving depressed persons.* Paper presented at the Annual Convention of the American Psychological Association, Anaheim, CA.

CHAPTER 15

Alcoholism and Family Interaction

THEODORE JACOB AND RUTH ANN SEILHAMER

INTRODUCTION

A large portion of the literature relevant to family influences on alcoholism has focused on the status of individuals within the family complex, in particular, the personality, psychosocial, and psychiatric patterns characterizing the alcoholic's spouse and children. To a large extent, this literature has been individually focused and psychodynamically based, and investigators have endeavored to describe (a) personality patterns and traits of spouses that may predate the partner's alcoholism and/or result from extended periods of family life involving an alcoholic partner and (b) patterns of maladaption manifested by children raised within a family including an alcoholic parent.

In the first case, spouses of alcoholics came to attention when clinicians began to question wives' possible contribution to the emergence and perpetuation of their mates' alcoholism. In this context, wives were initially described as "disturbed personalities" who sought to satisfy their unconscious needs by dominating a male whose alcoholic drinking rendered him weak and dependent (Futterman, 1953; Kalashian, 1959; Lewis, 1937). With the advent of environmental perspectives, however, wives of alcoholics were recast as "victims" rather than "villains," and their psychological disturbance was considered a reaction to cumulative stress associated with living with an alcoholic spouse (Jackson, 1954; Jacob & Seilhamer, 1982). More recently, theoretical and empirical efforts have focused on individual–environmental associations in attempts to describe and categorize typical coping strategies as they relate to the husband's current drinking behavior (James & Goldman, 1971; Orford, Guthrie, Nicholls, Oppen-

THEODORE JACOB • Division of Family Studies, 210 Family and Consumer Resources Building, University of Arizona, Tucson, AZ 85721. **RUTH ANN SEILHAMER** • Department of Psychology, University of Pittsburgh, Pittsburgh, PA 15260.

heimer, Egert, & Hensman, 1975; Schaffer & Tyler, 1979; Wiseman, 1980b). Notwithstanding these interests, the data of most importance to exploring such relationships have been absent: the actual interactions between spouses that potentiate or maintain the abusive drinking. Regardless of emphasis, however, this literature has clearly implied that the alcoholic and his or her spouse exhibit unique relationship patterns, that these patterns are repetitive and identifiable, and that such interchanges are relevant to the emergence and perpetuation of abusive drinking.

Similarly, studies of the psychosocial and psychiatric status of alcoholics' offspring suggest that these children often exhibit a variety of interpersonal and cognitive difficulties as preadolescents and adolescents and that they are at high risk for alcoholism and general psychiatric disturbances as adults (Adler & Raphael, 1983; el-Guebaly & Offord, 1977; Jacob, Favorini, Meisel, & Anderson, 1978; Wilson, 1982). Although a lengthy list of maladjustments has been offered, empirical substantiation of child outcomes has been marked by a lack of consistent findings, sound research methods, and comprehensive conceptualizations. In addition to interest in the psychosocial impairments of alcoholics' offspring, observations that these children are at greater risk for developing alcoholism have spurred vigorous efforts to establish a genetic basis for transmission. Although findings in this area have been compelling, they are not completely explanatory. That is, the collective literature points to considerable variability among children of alcoholics—an observation that has led various researchers to hypothesize an interplay of multiple factors that influence child outcome. Again, the relevant literature implies that such outcomes are the result of the disturbed patterns of marital and parent–child interaction associated with family structures that include an alcoholic parent. Close examination of this literature, however, reveals few efforts that describe patterns of interaction that may mediate adverse child outcomes, or that document the temporal relationships between these processes and various child outcomes. What seems to be missing from much of the extant literature, then, is an effort to describe actual patterns of interchange between the alcoholic and members of his or her family that are related to the etiology, course, and perpetuation of alcoholism.

Similar to the literature on depression and drug abuse, and in contrast with studies of schizophrenia and childhood disorder, the study of family interaction in the alcoholism literature has been a relatively neglected area until the past decade. As noted, the reasons for this neglect can be related to various historical trends in the alcoholism domain, most important, the repeatedly emphasized view of alcoholism as an individual problem, notwithstanding the myriad interpersonal aspects that are associated with the disorder. Largely stimulated by the general interest in family interaction and psychopathology evident during the 1950s and 1960s, several preliminary reports on interactional views of alcoholics and on treatment of alcoholism within a family context began to appear in the late 1960s and early 1970s; soon thereafter, scattered observational studies of alcoholic–spouse interactions appeared in the literature, as well as the initiation of several programs of research on family influences on alcoholism. Notwithstanding the obvious interest in family interaction and alcoholism that has developed since the mid-1970s, the accumulated literature to date is still an extremely small one with only the beginning signs of a developing cumulative knowledge of this area through systematically designed, programmatic efforts. In fact, there have been less than 10 reported studies in this area since 1974, most of which can be considered preliminary and/or pilot efforts. Based on relatively small samples, and typically involving only alcoholics and their spouses in a laboratory game or discussion, these initial studies have described various outcomes and processes related to couples' problem-solving behavior and have introduced innovative methodologies and provocative conceptual frameworks.

In the following review, this small but developing literature is described and evaluated. Given the preliminary nature of this literature, it is not reasonable to expect major theoretical or substantive insights. Instead, the potentially important experimental designs and interactional hypotheses that have emerged from these efforts are discussed, as are the implications that such material has for subsequent work in this area. The studies of Steinglass and his colleagues represent the most programmatic contribution to date and are therefore given special attention. Finally, the ongoing research program of the current authors is presented in an attempt to highlight what we believe to be necessary research directions to be pursued in future studies.

Before beginning this review, it may be of interest to make explicit the potential importance of an interactional perspective to alcohol studies and the contributions that interaction research can make in untangling the admittedly complex association between alcohol abuse and the family matrix. Of first importance, empirically based *descriptions* of family interactions involving an alcoholic member can be viewed as *necessary building blocks* for theoretical, treatment, and prevention efforts to be forged in the years ahead. As noted previously, there are very few data of this sort in the extant literature, and for the most part, clinical theory and practice have been based on descriptions generated from self and spouse reports obtained within clinical contexts, involving samples of unknown reliability, validity, and representativeness. To what extent these "pictures" of alcoholic–family relationships correspond to observed patterns of interchange is unknown, although there is little reason to believe that reports of interchanges in which the reporter is a participant can be obtained in a scientifically sound manner. Beyond the many self-serving biases, memory distortions, and inattention to critical aspects of the field, self-report data, by their very nature, emphasize relatively global, imprecisely defined constructs rather than a set of discrete behaviors that are emitted and responded to over time. If one's interest is in developing theory and practice based on what family members actually do to one another over time and how such interchanges are, in turn, related to the development or perpetuation of such complex outcomes as "abusive drinking," it seems necessary to obtain comprehensive descriptions of interaction involving the alcoholic and his or her family.

Second, the identification of significant patterns of interaction characterizing (at least some types of) alcoholics and their families would provide a mechanism by which detailed interaction processes can be related to current or future states of the family or of individual members. Most important, the course of the alcoholic's abusive drinking and the psychosocial, psychiatric, and drinking status of the alcoholic's offspring should be related to (and precisely from) the nature of his or her interactions with family members. In addition, it would be important to relate these interaction patterns to broader levels of analysis. Interaction can be viewed as either a dependent or an independent variable, depending on one's research questions, time frame, and other identifiable sources of influence. In predicting offspring outcome or the course of the proband's alcoholism, for example, the interaction data would be viewed as an independent variable that, in conjunction with other effects (e.g., degree of alcohol dependence, family history of alcoholism, and child age and sex when parent drinking emerged), would be important to relate to future child and adult outcomes. On the other hand, the impact of external stress, alcohol ingestion, and situational variables (setting, interpersonal context, and so on) on emergent patterns of family interaction would cast the interaction level as the dependent measure, allowing for a variety of interesting and potentially important assessments to be conducted.

Third, the description and careful examination of interactions involving alcoholics and their families should provide data and insights that can be transformed into relevant programs of treatment and prevention more closely than with materials derived from indirect report procedures, clinical case studies, and personality assessments of individual members. In particular, the field of marital and family therapy has witnessed a vast expansion in theory and technique since the mid-1970s, involving a variety of approaches and models applied to a wide range of disordered behavior. Common to much of this literature is the emphasis on repetitive and maladaptive patterns of interchanges that can be observed and changed in order to allow for different modes of relating that do not support maladaptive behavior. In the alcoholism treatment arena, there seems to be increasing interest in applying and testing the limits of family therapy approaches to abusive drinking either as the major therapeutic intervention or as an adjunct to other concurrently instituted treatment modalities (O'Farrell, 1986). To the extent that interaction research can provide reliable and valid data regarding behaviors and sequences concerned with affective interchanges associated with alcohol and nonalcohol content areas, problem-solving style and effectiveness, dominance patterns and their variations, and parent–child socialization practices involving the triad of alcoholic parent, nonalcoholic parent, and child, it is increasingly likely that treatment (as well as prevention) programs will be founded on greater substance and less supposition than currently seems to be the case.

TRANSITIONAL STUDIES

Although based on self-report methodologies and generating relatively global and static trait descriptions, several investigations of alcoholic marriages have appeared during the past several decades that have attempted to move from individual assessments to descriptions of marital dyads involving an alcoholic spouse. Implied, although not directly studied, has been a focus on the relationship and on interchanges, and therefore, these efforts may be thought of as transitional studies that have acted as a bridge between the earlier individual assessments and subsequent investigations exploring actually observed and recorded processes characterizing alcoholic–spouse interchanges.

The earliest empirical attempt to study aspects of the alcoholic's *marital* relationship was reported by Mitchell (1959). Imbedded within a larger, multifocused study of the relationship between alcoholism and marital conflict (Mitchell & Mudd, 1957), the research strategy involved the application of interpersonal perception theory in order to probe the beliefs of alcoholics and their spouses regarding self and other appraisals. As noted by Mitchell (1959), "how a person perceives himself and others with whom he is interacting will largely determine how he carries out his role and the expectations he has of others in their role enactment" (p. 549). Perceptions regarding self and partner, then, are viewed as significantly closer to relationship issues than are individually defined trait descriptions, and as important bases on which studies of interaction *per se* can be developed.

The research strategy required each spouse to complete a "personality questionnaire" under two conditions: self-appraisal and appraisal of partner. Subjects were asked to rate 17 traits regarding their applicability to self and to spouse, a procedure that yielded measures of husband self-appraisal, wife self-appraisal, husband's appraisal of wife, and wife's appraisal of husband. The subjects included 28 couples in which the husband was an alcoholic and 28 matched controls characterized by significant marital conflict but without alcoholism. Although experimental and control couples were found to be quite similar on most measures, there did appear to be important group differences on dimensions concerned with control, dominance, and sensitivity; that is, the alcoholic was most likely to describe his wife as dominating, whereas she did not report herself in this manner, and the alcoholic was most likely to describe himself as easily hurt, whereas his wife did not share this perception of him.

Many aspects of this study can certainly be criticized, including the absence of formal statistical analyses of group differences and the absence of a nonpsychiatric control group. The major contribution of this study, however, was not a substantive one; instead, this early effort focused empirical attention on the marital relationship involving an alcoholic; introduced social-psychological methods and concepts to the study of such relationships; and provided a further stimulus for studies with a more direct focus on interaction *per se.*

Continuing this line of research, Drewery and Rae (1969) conducted analyses of perceptual-attributional differences between husbands and wives in alcoholic and control marriages. The authors' interpersonal perception technique involved completion of the Edwards Personal Preference Schedule (Edwards, 1959) from three perspectives: "myself as I am," "my spouse as I see him/her," and "myself as I think my spouse sees me." In this study, 22 alcoholics and their wives and 26 normal controls completed the procedure, allowing for a variety of rather sophisticated assessments of similarities and differences in the perception of the spouse. A variety of comparisons was conducted and described in great detail, although the most interesting findings related to differences between alcoholic and control groups regarding wives' descriptions of their husbands; that is, "the control wives describe their husbands in a way which accords well with the husband's self-description while the wives of patients do not" (p. 299). The authors' evaluation of this finding took them into a complicated series of secondary analyses that focused on explanatory possibilities involving the alcoholic's sociosexual role confusion and the attributions of each spouse regarding the partner's dependence–independence conflict. The logic and clarity of these analyses are certainly compelling, yet the researchers failed to move more fully onto the issues of *interaction* that can be implied or inferred from such descriptions—a criticism that has often been cited in reference to the earlier literature on personality characteristics of individual family members. Drewery and Rae's expressed interest, however, seems to have been quite different from that of earlier investigators, and for this reason, their shortcoming seems more disappointing. That is, if one is really interested in techniques "designed to measure how two people relate to each other," it would seem necessary to offer explanations and/or hypotheses that provide bridges between perceptions of self and others, on the one hand, and interaction between self and others, on the other. That such bridges have been difficult to design—let alone to build—provides further support for "entering" at the level of observed interactions.

Two additional studies, both of which must be considered pilot efforts, also involved perceptions of self and spouse in alcoholic couples. In these reports, however, the focus was on differences in perception of the alcoholic during sober and intoxicated states and spouse congruence regarding these differences. In a study conducted during the early 1970s (Tamerin, Toler, DeWolfe, Packer, & Neuman, 1973), 20 alcoholic inpatients and their spouses were asked to provide retrospective descriptions of moods and behaviors that characterized the alcoholic when he or she was sober and intoxicated. The two instruments used for this data collection were the NIMH Mood Scale (Lorr, McNair, Weinstein, Michaux, & Raskin, 1961) and the Katz Adjustment Scale (Katz & Lyerly, 1963). The major findings to emerge from this study were as follows: (a) both the alcoholic and the spouse described the alcoholic in generally positive terms when the alcoholic was sober; (b) both the alcoholic and the spouse reported significant changes from sober to intoxicated states characterized by an increase in negativism and depression; and (c) the increased negativity from sober to intoxicated states was reported significantly more often by the spouse than by the alcoholic. Subsequent (clinical) analyses of these data suggested several subgroups that appeared to differ importantly regarding the pattern of alcoholic–spouse agreement. In one group, for example, patient and spouse agreed that the alcoholic was hostile and negative when drinking but not when sober, whereas in another group, the patient and the spouse agreed about the alcoholic's negative behavior when drinking but disagreed about the patient's behavior during sober states. A considerable amount of time is spent describing these patterns of alcoholic–spouse agreement, noting the implications that these different couple styles hold for treatment interventions. The importance of this study resides in its effort to focus attention on the couple versus the individual and to argue that interpersonal perceptions are relevant to understanding interactions related to the expression and perpetuation of abusive drinking. Unfortunately, the results of this preliminary effort must be judged with extreme caution, because the work was seriously weakened by a small, unrepresentative sample; the absence of any comparison group; and the lack of psychometric data bearing on the instrument's reliability and validity. More important, there is no obvious and easy way to discern the relationship between interpersonal perceptions and actual interactions that must ultimately be identified in the pursuit of critical processes.

Based on the Tamerin *et al.* report, David (1976) conducted a second study of interpersonal perceptions associated with sober and intoxicated states. (In actuality, this paper is really a clinical case study that argues for a revised methodology and offers descriptive data on four couples in support of this procedure.) Specifically, the method included perception data obtained from both spouses while the alcoholic husband was sober and while he was intoxicated. In a third condition, spouses were sober but were asked to predict their responses if the alcoholic husband were intoxicated. The first and third conditions replicated the Tamerin procedure, whereas the second condition was novel. Furthermore, Davis had both spouses describe themselves and their partners in each of the three reporting conditions. In essence, these procedural modifications allowed the investigators to focus on discrepancies between the predicted and intoxicated reports, specifically, how the alcoholic believed he and his partner would act and feel while drinking versus how the alcoholic actually perceived himself and his spouse while drinking. That Davis noted a number of discrepancies between these two types of data should caution the investigator against relying too heavily on retrospective report data without corroboration based on observations actually made *within* the context of interest—in this case, perception during actual periods of drinking.

A final transition study, by Hanson, Sands, and Sheldon (1968), deserves brief mention because of its interest in communication patterns characterizing male alcoholics and their spouses. Drawing on Jourard's writings (1959) in the area of self-disclosure, Hanson's analysis of alcoholic marriages suggested that the male alcoholic communicates much less information about himself than the spouse does about herself; as a result, communication is more often unidirectional than bidirectional and therefore, the alcoholic knows more about the thoughts, feelings, and beliefs of the spouse than the spouse knows of her husband. To test this hypothesis, 19 alcoholic couples were assessed: each spouse completed a Personal Behavior Questionnaire on himself or herself and once again as he or she predicted his or her spouse would complete the form. Analyses clearly supported the primary hypothesis: Alcoholic husbands predicted their wives' responses more accurately than the spouses predicted their husbands' responses. Unfortunately, the study is characterized by various methodological weaknesses (Paolino & McGrady, 1977). Most important, previous findings have indicated that men in general do not disclose themselves as much as women, so that Hanson's failure to include any comparison group represents a particularly serious omission. That is, it is possible that the reported differences are not in any way unique to alcoholic marriages or even to generally distressed relationships; without some comparison groups, the reported findings can be viewed only as interesting hypotheses in need of verification.

INTERACTION STUDIES: OUTCOME MEASURES

As noted earlier, interaction studies of alcoholics and their families have emerged only since the mid-1970s, and, for the most part, represent preliminary efforts characterized by small samples, less than rigorous design features, a focus on marital versus family units, and single studies versus programs of research. Notwithstanding such limitations, these relatively few investigations have introduced important concepts and models relevant to interaction and have emphasized experimental designs involving the direct observation of couples and families in both laboratory and naturalistic contexts. Although having yielded only a small literature, this new direction of research has moved interest from individual descriptions to outcomes and processes associated with the ongoing interchanges of the alcoholic and her or his intimates.

As discussed elsewhere in this book, interaction research can emphasize and has emphasized process *per se* as well as specific outcomes that result from process over time. Three reported studies fall most comfortably into this latter grouping, in which couples have been engaged in laboratory games aimed at clarifying the nature of the role relationships, power structures, and communication styles characterizing alcoholic–spouse dyads.

The earliest and most important study in this group was conducted by Gorad (1971) and involved an analysis of the alcoholic's interaction style within a communication framework (Gorad, McCourt, & Cobb, 1971). Based on the communications-system framework emanating from the work of the Palo Alto group (Jackson, 1968a,b; Watzlawick, Beavin, & Jackson, 1967), the alcoholic's style of interaction is viewed as being characterized by a responsibility-avoiding feature. According to this view, communication is a multilevel process that includes two important components: the command aspect, which represents an overt, definable message, and a qualifying component, which provides a context within which the command aspect is to be interpreted. The latter, often referred to as a metacommunication (i.e., a message about a message), can be transmitted through various verbal, nonverbal, metaphorical, or contextual cues. In the case of the alcoholic, the key qualification that is made is "I am not responsible for what I say or do. I am under the control of the alcohol." The significance of such a communication, of course, is that the person can exert great control over relationships to the extent that actions can be taken for which one cannot be held responsible. As stated by Gorad, "drunkenness can be used as a maneuver whose function is to gain control of the setting of rules in a relationship. As such, it is a method of being 'one-up'" (p. 476). Through such indirect, responsibility-avoiding communications, the alcoholic can achieve an extremely influential status in relationship with those most likely to affect his or her day-to-day satisfaction.

To test this hypothesis, Gorad used a laboratory "game" that required spouses to send messages to one another within a relatively closed communication network. Twenty alcoholic men and their wives and twenty nonalcoholic control couples (matched on age, years married, family size, ethnic background, and religion) participated in the study. On each of 50 plays (rounds), each spouse sent one of three messages: "share," "win," or "secret win." Each combination of husband–wife messages resulted in a particular monetary payoff for the couple. Maximum personal gain was achieved by one spouse sending "win" or "secret win" and the other sending "share," whereas each spouse received a moderate and equal amount of money when both sent "share." When both selected "win" or "secret win," neither received any payoff. A particularly clever aspect of the design was Gorad's use of the "secret win" message; that is, couples were told that the experimenter could substitute "secret win" for a choice of "share" or "win" throughout the play. As a result, if a subject chose to use "secret win," his or her spouse would never know whether it was the subject's choice or that of the experimenter. In actuality, the experimenter never substituted any message for those selected by the subjects.

Within Gorad's theoretical framework, "win" and "secret win" choices were viewed as "one-up" messages, as use of these categories is an attempt to compete, dominate, or gain the "one-up" position. Alternately, the "share" choice represents a cooperative, compliant message, indicating that the subject desires an equal relationship. Finally, the "secret win" choice is viewed as a responsibility-avoiding message; that is, "to play this choice is to (a) send a message that attempts to place the sender in a 'one-up' position (just like win) and (b) attempt to shift responsibility for trying to be 'one-up' away from the sender and on to an external agent (the experimenter)" (p. 480).

The results provided strong support for Gorad's major hypotheses. The alcoholics used "secret win" significantly more often than did their spouses or normal husbands and normal wives, indicating more responsibility-avoiding behavior from the alcoholics than from the nonalcoholic subjects. In addition, couples with alcoholic husbands won less (total) money than normal couples; used the "share-share" pattern less often than the controls, and interacted with escalation of symmetry ("win-win," "win-secret win," or "secret win-secret win") more often than nondistressed couples. Further analyses indicated that both the alcoholic and his or her spouse used one-up messages more often than controls and "share" messages less often than controls, a finding indicating that both were "fighting hard to be one-up [in a] highly competitive battle" (p. 485).

The contributions of this study are several: the introduction of a general communication-systems framework to the study of communication styles, the involvement of couples with alcoholic husbands in an interaction paradigm, and the development of an objective, standardized observation procedure in which key constructs could be operationalized and measured in a highly reliable fashion. Gorad's emphasis was on measurement of the outcomes and consequences of hypothesized processes, and in this regard, his efforts represent an important contribution to the field. Design weaknesses, however, leave many unanswered questions for future investigations. Most important, the absence of a distressed, nonalcoholic comparison group makes it impossible to know how specific the results were to couples with alcoholic husbands. In this regard, it seems likely that some, if not most, of the features that differentiated alcoholic couples from normal controls reflected a general distress factor rather than patterns and properties specific to alcoholics and their spouses. Furthermore, the lack of detailed specifications regarding the selection and description of experimental and control couples limits our ability to generalize Gorad's findings to other alcoholic couples characterized by different alcohol abuse features, psychiatric difficulties, treatment histories, settings in which assessment was conducted, and variations in socioeconomic status (SES).

In an unpublished paper by Cobb and McCourt (1979), a variety of laboratory tasks was administered to alcoholic and normal couples in order to assess a range of problem-solving behavior. In part, this report represented an attempt to replicate the Gorad study, although Cobb and McCourt were generally more interested in exploring a range of problem-solving behaviors as reflected in the families of alcoholics. In brief, the argument advanced was that families of alcoholics—because of conflictual relationships and generally inadequate strategies for coping with difficulties during sober states—would be likely to exhibit problem-solving deficiencies across a variety of dimensions, including cooperation, flexibility, efficiency, openness, and evaluation. In this study, 36 families of alcoholics and 33 normal control families participated, with each family consisting of a husband, wife, and at least one child. The investigators indicated that groups were matched along a variety of SES variables. The laboratory task included Gorad's interaction game, a block-stacking game, a semantic differential task, and an unrevealed-difference task. The report of data analyses and results was often incomplete, so that definitive evaluations of this work are not possible. In general, however, the alcoholic and normal groups were found to be quite similar with a few exceptions. In particular, the alcoholic couples exhibited less cooperation and more competition and earned less total money than did the control couples in Gorad's laboratory procedure. Differences in responsibility-avoiding behavior, however, did not emerge.

The Cobb and McCourt work, although representing an attempt to extend the work of Gorad, is simply not presented with sufficient detail so that reasonable evaluations can be offered. Thus, there remains a range of explanations that may be relevant to their reported finding. In particular, the absence of group differences may simply reflect large error variance associated with generally unreliable experimental procedures, whereas the failure to replicate Gorad's avoidance-of-responsibility finding may be related to the procedural changes that were introduced. Specifically, Cobb and McCourt indicated that they used "an automated version of Gorad's (1971) interaction game" (p. 6), but they did not provide further specification regarding differences between this version and the original procedure. Furthermore, the nonsystematic inclusion of couple interactions and family interactions, as well as the unclear presentation of these various subsets and associated analyses, raises many unanswerable questions regarding the meaning of the presented findings.

In another study by Kennedy (1976), a "simulation" game was administered to couples in order to further evaluate the uniqueness of interaction styles in alcoholic couples. The "tax game" was originally used in social-psychological studies of conflict and was based on Kelly's theory of interpersonal relationships (Thiabut & Kelly, 1959). As revised by Kennedy, the task required spouses to negotiate the distribution of a fixed amount of money within a short period of time, and it involved multiple trials over which negotiations occurred. The dependent measures involved various game outcomes (e.g., profits, losses, and time scores), as well as several process and communication behaviors (e.g., first remarks, disclosures, and threats). Dyadic styles or patterns were defined *a priori* and focused on cooperative and competitive patterns. The design included three groups of couples: those in which the husband was alcoholic ($N = 11$), those in which both spouses were nondistressed ($N = 11$), and those in which the wife had received a diagnosis of neurotic or psychotic disorder and had been hospitalized within the past year ($N = 6$).

The initial assessments revealed a variety of significant effects, although subsequent analyses of covariance (controlling for length of marriage) resulted in significant group differences on only 2 of 14 contrasts. The investigator's secondary (qualitative) examination of obtained findings generated various interpretations relevant to alcoholic–spouse interactions, including the observation of great heterogeneity within the alcoholic group and potentially important subgroup differences related to the subjects' inpatient versus outpatient status. In general, however, the study provided little (statistical) support for the contention that alcoholic–spouse interactions can be differentiated from those of other couples; most important, the findings failed to replicate the earlier findings of Gorad to the effect that alcoholics can be distinguished from controls in terms of an emphasis on competitive versus cooperative patterns of interaction. Interpretation of Kennedy's data, as well as reconciling his findings with those of Gorad, however, is complicated because of deficiencies within the study itself, together with differences between the two sets of procedures. As discussed by Kennedy, several variables could have accounted for his failure to replicate Gorad's findings. Most important, the two samples of alcoholic couples were probably quite different regarding stage of addiction and socioeconomic status. In addition, the two experimental tasks (games) may have emphasized quite different behaviors and may have tapped "different dimensions of the relationship" (p 32). Regarding the limitations in Kennedy's design itself, the attempt to incorporate a psychiatric control group is certainly commendable, although the selection of distressed couples in which the wife was the index patient makes comparisons with other groups particularly difficult.

In overview, the work of Gorad, Cobb and McCourt, and Kennedy provided important contributions to the interaction literature involving alcoholics and their spouses. In particular, Gorad introduced provocative concepts from the communication-systems literature, suggesting that the alcoholic and his or her spouse are involved in repetitive interchanges concerned with issues of control and influence, and that the alcoholic exhibits a responsibility-avoiding style of communication. To assess these hypotheses, Gorad introduced precise methodologies borrowed from small-group research by which a carefully controlled series of interactions was created within a laboratory setting in order to assess alcoholic–spouse behavior along specific and relevant dimensions. In contrast with other research strategies, the use of a highly structured laboratory task guaranteed that each couple would interact in the same context and that emergent behaviors would be evaluated along common dimensions, thereby leaving less to clinical impression and subjective evaluation. Notwithstanding the highly objective and reliable nature of these assessments, as well as those of Kennedy and of Cobb and McCourt, this primary emphasis on structured laboratory tasks and game outcomes raises questions regarding the validity, the generalizability, and the completeness of the emergent characterizations of alcoholic–spouse relationships. In particular, one can question the correspondence between behavior exhibited in an atypical, highly structured laboratory setting and interaction between intimates in naturalistic settings. The potential influence of task structure, observation setting, and experimental demand characteristics can be significant indeed, resulting in findings that may be specific, distorted, and/or not particularly predictive of behavior evident in the day-to-day interactions of spouses. Furthermore, findings based on game outcomes do not clarify the nature of the ongoing processes and interactions associated with such outcomes. That is, the same outcome may arise from quite different processes, as the systems concept of equifinality reminds us, and depending on the particular process (set of interactions) involved, the interpretation of outcome and plans for intervention can be quite different.

Further discussion of types of measures—their strengths, limitations, and interrelationships—is presented elsewhere in this book and will not be pursued further at this time. The important points to be made, however, are that findings based on structured game procedures may be limited in their external validity, must be evaluated carefully regarding correspondence with alternative operations, and do not necessarily predict actual processes that result in particular outcomes.

INTERACTION STUDIES: PROCESS MEASURES

The earliest empirical study that focused on alcoholic–spouse interaction— the actual exchange of verbal and nonverbal behavior during an observed marital discussion—was reported in 1973 by Hersen, Miller, and Eisler. Using a behavioral perspective and motivated by a need to describe and identify marital behavior that may serve to maintain problem drinking, Hersen and his colleagues engaged four couples in a quasi-naturalistic interaction in which verbal and nonverbal behaviors were assessed. Specifically, alcoholics and their spouses were videotaped while they discussed topics that were related to or unrelated to their husband's abusive drinking, alternating drinking-related and drinking-unrelated topics every 6 minutes over a 24-minute period. Detailed coding of speech duration and looking were conducted. The results clearly indicated that the wives looked at their husbands more during discussion of drinking-related versus drinking-unrelated topics, a finding suggesting that the spouse's attention may support the pattern of abusive drinking.

In a follow-up to this preliminary report, Becker and Miller (1976) attempted to strengthen the initial design by including a larger sample of couples with alcoholic husbands ($n = 6$), a comparison group of nonalcoholic psychiatric patients and their spouses ($n = 6$), and a wider range of verbal and nonverbal dependent measures (duration of looks, duration of speech, number of negative statements, number of interruptions, touching, and requests for new behavior). In contrast with the visual inspection technique employed previously, Becker and Miller subjected the resultant data to analyses of variance in order to assess for group differences in a more rigorous manner. In general, very few significant effects were detected. Specifically, group classification was involved in only one significant main effect (and no significant interaction effects), indicating that alcoholic couples interrupted more frequently than did comparison couples regardless of the topic of conversation.

Several conclusions can be drawn from these two efforts. First, there is little reason to believe that the initially reported findings of differences in wives' looking behavior in alcohol-related versus alcohol-unrelated discussion are robust or replicable. Second, the similarity in interactions of alcoholic couples and nonalcoholic (but distressed) couples suggests that the relationship between psychopathology and marital interaction is of a general nature; that is, different types of individually defined disorders can exert similar effects on patterns of marital interaction. Third, more definitive statements regarding the interpretability of patterns found to characterize both groups of distressed couples require a design including a nonpsychiatric (normal) comparison group. Fourth, the generalizability of reported patterns may well be limited to certain subgroups of couples, with hospitalized husbands who are differentiated further according to the chronicity and severity of the husband's psychopathology.

As noted previously, family interaction research dealing with alcoholism is barely beyond its infancy, including less than a dozen studies that clearly fall within this literature. Moreover, the relatively few published studies are preliminary in nature; are characterized by small, unrepresentative samples, the absence of appropriate control groups and statistical analyses; and with few exceptions, are limited to marital subgroups with alcoholic husbands. Perhaps more important, identified studies have most often been scattered, "one-shot" efforts. Although innovative methodologies and interesting hypotheses have been introduced, programmatic features have been almost nonexistent. The work of Steinglass and his colleagues represents a major exception to this characterization and, as such, is presented in some detail.

If the alcoholism–family interaction field has a "father," Steinglass is certainly he. His interests in theory development and empirical study began nearly 14 years ago while he was associated with the intramural research branch at the National Institute on Alcohol Abuse and Alcoholism (NIAAA, Laboratory of Alcohol Research). During these early years, several related individuals (two brothers, a father, and a son) were taken into the inpatient unit and were involved in experimental drinking procedures over relatively long periods of time (Steinglass, Weiner, & Mendelson, 1971). From these clinical studies, together with related work probing the nature of "simulated" drinking gangs (Steinglass, 1975), Steinglass began to develop a conceptualization of abusive drinking based on concepts from general systems theory. Concepts of homeostasis, reciprocal causality, and circular feedback processes were proposed as key descriptive and explanatory principles, leading to an early formulation focused on "alcoholic" family systems. Subsequent observations of intact couples, also assessed in inpatient units where experimental drinking procedures were introduced, added further clarity and elaboration to the initial conceptualizations, leading to a more refined and sophisticated model linking the family process to the maintenance of abusive drinking. The third phase of Steinglass's efforts involved 31 families of alcoholics in a multifaceted, data-collection procedure involving laboratory observations around a structured problem-solving task, naturalistic home observations, and observations of small groups of alcoholic families in multiple-family group sessions (Steinglass & Robertson, 1983). The emphasis of Steinglass's conceptualizations now shifted to a more macroscopic view of alcoholism in which the family drinking phase (dry, wet, or transitional) was used as the basis for a typology aimed at clarifying the relationship between alcohol use and family development. Throughout these efforts, Steinglass has contributed both theory and methods that have shaped and guided this area of study since the mid-1970s. A detailed discussion of this work will now be presented.

During the late 1960s, Mendelson and Mello initiated a program of experimental drinking studies aimed at the direct examination of alcohol's impact on a variety of behavioral, cognitive, and physiological parameters (Mello, 1972). This program of research, based within the intramural laboratory of what was then NIMH, involved a paradigm consisting of a 28-day inpatient procedure: a 5-day period for the monitoring and collection of baseline data; a 14-day drinking period allowing for the consumption of up to 1 quart of 100-proof alcohol per day; and a 7-day withdrawal period involving the administration of needed medication and discharge procedures. The subjects were volunteers recruited from the surrounding area. For each 28-day "study," 6 subjects were admitted and observed, providing a unique opportunity to examine the acute effects of alcohol on group and interactional behavior. Earlier reports on these "simulated" drinking gangs suggested a variety of significant and unexpected effects of alcohol intoxication on the role relationships and communication patterns of group members. At least from a clinical perspective, these experiences strongly supported the view that much can be learned about the course, development, and maintenance of alcoholism if viewed and studied within the broader context of a system of interpersonal relationships.

As part of the experimental drinking studies, Steinglass and his colleagues had an opportunity to observe several pairs of related alcoholics who participated in the 28-day inpatient program (Steinglass & Robertson, 1983; Steinglass et al., 1971). In particular, an alcoholic father and his alcoholic son, as well as two pairs of alcoholic brothers (assessed in different study groups), represented the first instance in which family units (subgroups) were evaluated during periods of both intoxication and sobriety. As in experiences gleaned from observation of the drinking gangs, the investigators were struck by the significant and unexpected impact that alcohol had on the relationships of related individuals. Both affective and structural characteristics of the relationship changed dramatically during the experimental drinking period, involving significant role reversals and the intense and previously inhibited expression of positive affect. Beyond specific changes in the kind of behavior exhibited, the pattern of interaction was also seen to be markedly different during periods of intoxication, characterized as it was by greater patterning, organization, and structure than during sober states.

For Steinglass, these observations confirmed the significance of reciprocal effects involving alcohol and interpersonal interaction and led to a preliminary model of alcoholism based on family systems theory. Specifically, Steinglass *et al.* (1971) suggested that abusive drinking could serve two different functions. In one case, drinking is a signal or sign that individuals and relationships within the system are experiencing significant stress, a view that is not unlike the psychodynamic view that symptoms (individually defined) signal disturbance at other levels of functioning and act in part to relieve tension. For Steinglass *et al.* (1971), however, the "underlying" conflicts were not intrapsychic but interpersonal and part of the family system:

> In other words, in a malfunctioning system, the stress or strain created by conflicts within the system may be expressed through the drinking behavior of one member of the system. . . . In such instances, the drinking might be viewed as an attempt to relieve the strain within the system (an escape valve), or an attempt to alter some of the behavioral programs of the systems which are not functioning adequately. (p. 406)

In contrast with the "signal" function, which is most likely seen in families where abusive drinking has not been an ongoing process, drinking can also be seen as an integral part of a family system. In this case, Steinglass *et al.* (1971) talked about an "alcoholic system" to emphasize the key role that drinking plays in *maintaining* and *stabilizing* the family as an ongoing unit. In referring to observations of the several family pairs previously described, Steinglass *et al.* (1971) noted that alcohol appeared to effect very different behaviors in the different dyads; that is, alcohol was associated with the controlled release of aggression in one pair and with the clarification of dominance patterns in the other dyad: "Although the style was different, in each instance the end result was the stabilization of a dyadic system which might otherwise be expected to have been characterized by chaos" (p. 408).

The next phase of Steinglass's work involved the assessment of intact family units (marital pairs) within an experimental treatment program that included a 10-day inpatient period, the last 7 days involving experimental drinking procedures (Steinglass, Davis, & Berenson, 1977). The program began with a 2-week outpatient phase in which couples met in groups three times per week. Following this experience, two or three couples were admitted to the inpatient facilities, where they were encouraged to behave as normally as possible within the homelike atmosphere that had been created on the ward. The final phase of treatment involved a 3-week posthospitalization period during which the couples were involved in group meetings twice a week. Follow-up sessions were scheduled every 6 weeks during the 6-month period after the program had been completed.

The 10-day inpatient experience was the core component of the program, and it provided the opportunity to introduce couples to the experimental drinking procedures. Alcohol was made freely available throughout the last 7 days of this period, and videotaping of the therapy room and the living-dining area were conducted. The only structured and required activity for the participants was the daily 90-minute multiple-couple group-therapy session.

Ten couples participated in the program, the vast majority of whom volunteered out of desperation engendered by their current difficulties with alcoholism and their previous failures with other treatment programs. The couples were generally middle to upper-middle class and averaged 40 to 45 years of age, and most had been married for approximately 20 years. The sample included couples in which the husband, the wife, or both spouses were alcoholics.

The data on which the descriptions were based and the conclusions were drawn consisted of clinical observations made by the program staff and their attempt to organize these impressions and observations in the form of interaction summaries, that is, "a clinical assessment and formulation of drinking behavior in interaction terms" (Steinglass et al., 1977, p. 8). From the wealth of behavior available for staff observation and analysis, four foci become particularly salient: (a) the multiple-couple group-therapy meetings, with an emphasis on sober versus intoxicated interactional behavior: (b) the intoxication–sobriety cycle of behavior as played out within the apartmentlike environment on the ward; (c) patterns of drinking, social interactions with other couples, and housekeeping behavior in sober versus intoxicated states; and (d) feedback of videotaped interactions to couples as an aid in identifying and solidifying particularly critical processes related to abusive drinking.

As noted, earlier observations consisted of simulated drinking gangs and several family pairs, involving marginally adapting, chronic alcoholics with little, if any, contact of an intimate, ongoing nature. The study of relatively stable, intact family units, therefore, was an important and necessary extension, allowing for observation of family units, which at least theoretically should exhibit systematic and stable patterns of interaction—data assumed to be particularly relevant to theory development as well as to issues of treatment and prevention. Observations confirmed the earlier impressions and interpretations (Steinglass et al. 1971, 1977). Structurally and stylistically, intoxicated behaviors were more exaggerated (amplified) and more restricted in range than interactions seen in sober states. These characteristics, according to these researchers, enhanced the impression of regularity, pattern, and rigidity associated with periods of intoxication. Furthermore, striking differences in patterns of interaction were observed *between* sober and intoxicated periods, differences that appeared to serve important "adaptive" functions for the couple. That is, the behavior that emerged during intoxicated periods appeared to potentiate or inhibit certain aspects of the relationship that, in effect, reduced tensions through the temporary solution to a conflictual or stressful process. In one case, for example, a sexually inhibited couple became more expressive and affectionate during intoxicated states, whereas another couple became assertive and effective when sobriety gave way to intoxication. For a third couple, previously suppressed anger, frustration, and disappointment were more readily expressed during drinking than during nondrinking periods. The key feature of these observations was that intoxicated interaction seemed to provide a temporary solution to a problem for the spouses and for their relationship. Most important, the cycling between sober and intoxicated states and the emergence of intoxication-specific patterns appeared to be reinforced and perpetuated because these served an adaptive, problem-solving function.

Taken together, these observations suggested a second-generation theory: the "alcohol maintenance model." As conceptualized by Steingalss *et al.* (1977), problems (stress, tension, and so on) can arise from three sources: individual psychopathology as it impacts on the adjustment status of other family members; interactional conflicts that cannot be adequately explained by reference to individual member disturbances; and dislocations and stress emanating from the immediate social environment and its effect on family stability. Problems in any one of these areas can escalate until significant stress is experienced and substantial disruption to the family itself becomes likely. At this point, alcohol ingestion, intoxication, and associated interactions can function as a solution to the "problem." If intoxication is effective in reducing tension and/or temporarily solving a problem, short-term family stability can be achieved, and as a result, the change from sober to intoxicated interactional states can serve to stabilize an unstable system:

> In some families, equilibrium is restored by increasing interactional distance (the drinker goes off to drink in the basement), or diminishing physical contact (the nonalcoholic spouse refuses to have sex with someone who is drunk), or reducing tension in the family (family members' usual patterns of behavior are less tension provoking than unique patterns); whereas in other families alcohol might be associated with closer interactional distance (the nonalcoholic makes contact by fighting after the alcoholic spouse has been drinking), disinhibition (the use of alcohol permits ritualized sexual behavior), or maintaining distance from the social environment (the alcoholic fights with neighbors when drunk). (Steinglass, 1981, p. 300)

Regardless of the content of the interaction and the source of stress, then, alcohol serves to stabilize the family system by providing a solution to a problem. Given the repetitive and chronic nature of these problems, however, the solution offered by alcohol can be only a temporary one:

> Hence, a cycling would be established in which the long-term stability of the family system was dependent on the presence of both sober and intoxicated interactional behavior. . . . In other words, alcoholism maintains certain interactional patterns in families, which in turn maintain alcoholism. (Steinglass & Robertson, 1983, p. 269)

The third and current phase of Steinglass's work involves a more systematic and empirical effort that emphasizes a macroscopic, longitudinal review of drinking patterns over time. Embodied within a "life-history model of alcoholism" (Steinglass, 1980b), the theoretical emphasis is now focused on *alcohol phase,* suggesting that periods of sobriety and active drinking cycle over long time periods in the lives of most alcoholics. In contrast with the maintenance model, which referred to rapid changes from sober to intoxicated states and the associated change in patterns of interaction, the life history model draws heavily on family sociology in order to portray stage- or phase-related behavior in alcoholic families. Within each of five defined stages (premarriage, early marriage, mid-life plateau, mid-life crisis, and late resolution), alternative alcohol-involvement patterns are presented together with indications of the relative stability that characterizes a particular pattern of involvement. Three important phases are suggested: dry, wet, and transitional. Over a 20- to 30-year period, these phases can appear and reappear many times, characterized by differences in their apparent stability and time duration. For some families, there may be many occurrences of dry and wet periods and intervening transition phases, whereas for other families, there may be only one stable wet phase that is ultimately resolved into a stable dry phase or simply continues until death or divorce changes the structure of the family system.

The current life-history model incorporates the earlier maintenance model. That is, within the "wet" phase, there is the alternation between sober and intoxicated states, each associated with a distinct pattern of interaction and perpetuated because of the short-term solution provided by the intoxicated interactions, that is, because of the "adaptive" consequences that drinking has for stabilizing an unstable family system. A second, more macroscopic pattern of change operates over much longer time periods, in which phases of wetness, dryness, and transitions between the two extend over weeks, months, and years. A key implication of this broader framework is that the family fails to progress along a developmental course characterized by greater complexity and differentiation. That is,

> the family returns repeatedly to stages already experienced rather than moving ahead in stepwise fashion to deal with a progressive series of tasks and stages [suggested by a] family life cycle model. The cycling between stable wet and stable dry family life phases during the mid life period produces a plateauing effect that profoundly alters the customary slope of family development. . . . This is not to propose the total absence of customary patterns of family development in alcoholic families. Surely one is still able to perceive the effects of such developmental benchmarks as birth and death in such families. But the life history model proposes that the impact of such events on the developmental course of the alcoholic family would be blunted and very much colored by the family's current alcohol life phase and the behavioral patterns it tends to develop around this alcohol related issue. (Steinglass, 1980b, p. 225)

For Steinglass, it is this distortion and constriction of the family's natural growth and development that comes to be a major adverse outcome of alcoholism.

To explore the validity and implications of this life-history model and the associated typology, a large-scale observation study was undertaken. In total, 31 alcoholics and their families were conducted through the experimental pardigm, which consisted of three major components: naturalistic home observations in which observers recorded family behavior *in vivo* on nine separate occasions, each spanning a 4-hour block of time; a laboratory observation session involving the two parents and one of their children as they participated in a problem-solving task based on Reiss's pattern-recognition card-sort procedure (1981); and observation of multiple-family discussion groups involving six family groups that met on a weekly basis (held in the subject families' homes) over a 6-month period. The key independent variable was the family's alcohol phase while they were participants in the project.

The sample consisted of alcoholic families only, described as "white, middle-aged, well into their second decade of marriage, containing adolescent children, being middle-class and upper-middle class, highly educated, and representative of the general population regarding religious preference" (Steinglass, 1981, p. 290). The sample contained both male ($n = 23$) and female ($n = 8$) alcoholics, although these subgroups were quite similar in terms of sociodemographic characteristics. The diagnosis of alcoholism was carefully and rigorously conducted, although the alcoholic subjects, as well as their spouses, apparently could have manifested psychiatric disorders other than alcoholism. Families were recruited from a variety of community agencies and individual practitioners, and through newspaper advertisements.

The categorization of the families regarding drinking phase was based on weekly drinking records collected on the subjects during their 6-month participation in the study. By means of this material, the families were grouped into three "family drinking phases." Ten families were categorized as stable wet (SW), indicating that the identified alcoholic was drinking through the entire study period. Fourteen families, in which the index case remained abstinent during the 6-month study, were categorized as stable dry (SD). The seven remaining families were grouped into the transitional (TR) category, as the alcoholic "either started the study abstinent but resumed drinking by the end of data collection, or started the study drinking but became abstinent during the study and was still abstinent at the close of data collection" (Steinglass & Robertson, 1983, p. 274). According to Steinglass, the demographic characteristics of the three groups were the same.

Because the "life history model" describes between-phase variance as substantial, assessment of families in different phases should reveal reliable and meaningful differences in *family-level* (versus individual-only) functioning. The basic research strategy, therefore, was to group the families into SW, SD, and TR categories and then to assess for group differences in family interaction as exhibited in three contexts: the home setting, the interaction laboratory, and the multiple-family group meetings.

Home Interactions

To describe interaction patterns characteristic of family life in a familiar, naturalistic setting, Steinglass (1980a) conducted observations on sample families within the home setting. In total, nine four-hour periods of recording were performed, four during early evening hours of weekdays and three during weekend afternoons. The observation system that was used—the Home Observation Assessment Method (HOAM)—had been developed by Steinglass (1979b) and was heavily influenced by the methods of behavioral researchers assessing parent–child relationships (Patterson, 1982) and by systems theorists attempting to describe family interactive properties in terms of structural, noncontent measures of family behavior (Kantor & Lehr, 1975). Briefly, two trained observers remained in the family's home throughout the observation period. Each observer was "attached" to one of the spouses and, throughout the period, followed that target person during his or her movements in the house and recorded emergent behaviors. The coding system was structured in terms of two-minute recording blocks, and within each of these time periods, the following events or behaviors were recorded: (a) content codes, which included location within the house, persons in the field, interaction distance between target person and others, and to whom the target person was communicating; (b) behavioral characteristics, which described the activity occurring (e.g., meal, entertainment, telephone conversation, working, or physical contact); and (c) interaction codes, which detailed the type of interaction (problem-solving tasks, work tasks, or information exchange), affect (ranging from warmth to anger), and outcome (resolved or completed, unclear, unresolved or continued conflict). During each 2-minute block, the first verbal interchange between the target person and others in the field was called the "initial interaction sequence," and the observer coded this event in terms of all described categories. For all events occurring after the initial interaction sequence, the rater recorded, in sequence, the location, the persons in the field, the physical distance, and who-to-whom only. Only for the initial act, then, is there a complete description, including the coding of type, affective level, and outcome of interaction. Reliability assessments of the HOAM indicated adequate to excellent levels of interrater agreement as determined from percentage agreement and kappa indices (Steinglass, 1979b).

Guided by the investigator's interest in the structural characteristics of family systems, two major dimensions of interaction were thought to be most important: activity/engagement and variability. Based on this emphasis, 25 indices were calculated—measures that included scores relevant to physical location in the home, the people in the room with the subject, interaction distance, interaction ratios, the type of verbal exchange, the affective level of the verbal exchange, and the outcome of the verbal exchange. All scores were mean scores of husband-plus-wife behavior.

To further evaluate the relationship between the major dimensions of activity/engagement and variability and the 25 specific indices that were formed, a principal components analysis was performed on the sample of 31 families over the 25 constructed measures (Steinglass, 1980a). The results of this procedure suggested five orthogonal clusters that, in general, conformed reasonably well to the investigator's expectations. That is, measures of activity/engagement and variability generally loaded on different dimensions, although further differentiation was achieved beyond a simple two-factor solution. That is, a five-factor solution, accounting for 67% of the total variance, was found to be the most reasonable outcome:

1. *Intrafamily engagement.* The extent to which family members were in physical contact with each other and with coders, as well as the variability of the physical distances maintained while interacting with each other.
2. *Distance regulation.* The family's use of space in the house, including their proclivity for interacting with each other when in the same location, their

physical distance during these interactions, their rate of movement around the house, and the proportion of time they spent alone.

3. *Extrafamily engagement.* The extent to which nonfamily members were present during the coding session.

4. *Structural variability.* The family's variability of behavior during the coding session, including their verbal and physical interaction ratios, movement rate, and percentage of negative and positive outcomes of their verbal exchanges.

5. *Content variability.* The extent to which questions were raised during the coding sessions that required a decision to be made, as well as the affective level associated with the family interaction and the variability they displayed along these two dimensions.

With the use of these factor scores, analyses of differences across SW, SD, and TR groups were undertaken. Results from one-way ANOVAs indicated significant group effects for two of the five components, indicating an ordering of SW > SD > TR on distance regulation and an ordering of SD > SW > TR on content variability. Comparison among group means indicated significant differences between SW and TR on distance regulation and between SD and TR on content variability.

According to Steinglass's interpretation (1981a) of these two factor scores, the SW families were characterized by "a tendency of family members to disperse in the house, physically interacting only when they intend to talk with one another for some purposeful reason" (p. 581). That SW families fell midway between SD and TR families regarding content variability suggests a generally moderate degree of variability regarding content and affect of interactions. In contrast, SD families, by virtue of their high scores on content variability and their midrange scores on distance regulation, were viewed as exhibiting "relatively high rates of decision-making behavior and greater affective display, especially in the direction of allowing disagreements to be expressed" (pp. 581–582). TR families, manifesting extreme scores on both dimensions, were viewed as physically close "to a degree that gives them the appearance of huddling together for warmth and protection" (p. 582), and as manifesting a very narrow range of tasks, affect, and outcome.

Two additional analyses were performed in order to clarify the meaning of these obtained group differences. First, one-way ANOVAs were computed for each of the five factor scores in which selected developmental and demographic dimensions were related to variation on these composites. As expected, these analyses yielded significant effects, but on factors other than those that differentiated SD, SW, and TR groups. Specifically, years married was reliably related to intrafamily engagement (lower scores with greater years married), whereas family composition (childless, one child, or several children) was reliably related to structural variability (lower scores with larger families). For Steinglass, the importance of these findings was that family alcohol phase had a *selective* effect on family interactions rather than influencing all dimensions in a similar fashion.

Results from a discriminant function analysis further strengthened the contention that HOAM variables were importantly related to differences across the three groups. Specifically, application of this multivariate procedure to the previously described data yielded two significant factors. The first function, having heaviest loadings on structural variability, content variability, and distance regulation, produced a sharp differentiation between SW and SD groups, whereas the second function, with significant loadings on distance regulation and content variability, most clearly differentiated TR families from both SW and SD groups:

> The plot of the discriminant scores for the three groups strongly suggests that the distinction between interactional behavior in the home during SW versus SD phases is a polarity distinction; what is high during the SW phase is low during the SD phase and vice versa. . . . Transitional behavior on the other hand seems to follow a different pattern. (Steinglass, 1981a, p. 583)

Using the two discriminant functions to predict the group status of each family resulted in a correct clasification rate of 74.2%, indicating once again the importance of interaction patterns in differentiating the three groups and in predicting group status.

Laboratory Interaction

The second observation setting included in the Steinglass study was the interaction laboratory (Steinglass, 1979a). In this context, both parents and one of their children, 12 years of age or older, participated in Reiss's pattern-recognition card-sort procedures (1981)—a structured problem-solving task requiring family members to work individually and jointly on a novel problem presented by the experimenter. Briefly, the task involves a deck of 15 cards, each of which has printed on it a sequence of letters. The subject's task is to sort the cards into as many as seven piles, the basis on which such sorting is to be performed being completely up to the individual. In the first and third phase, each member independently and privately performs a sort. During the second phase (family sort), the family works on the task as a group within a semiclosed communication structure; that is, each member is in auditory (but not visual) contact with the other two members, so that verbal communication can occur as the three members simultaneously work on the sort task. Although it is not necessary for members to agree on the card placements on each successive trial or on the final sort, most families do work toward a common solution.

Two types of solutions are most common, one based on length and another based on pattern. In the former, cards are placed in different piles on the basis of number of letters, whereas in the latter, cards are grouped according to common patterns represented on the individual cards. Earlier work generated an "ideal length sort" and "ideal pattern sort" with which any obtained sort can be compared in quantitative form; in an analogous fashion, the individual and family sorts of the participating subjects can be compared and described in terms of degree of correspondence.

The card sort procedure yields two key measures. *Configuration* assesses the contribution made by the family on problem-solving effectiveness and includes two components: change in performance from initial sort to family sort and change in performance from initial sort to final sort. A positive score indicates that the family's interaction around the task resulted in a more sophisticated solution than the one the individual achieved working alone, and that the family's influence carried over to the individual's separate sort completed in private. In contrast, a negative configuration score can occur when the family involvement results in a deterioration in performance or change from a more to a less sophisticated and complex solution. *Coordination*, the second major variable, assesses the similarity among the sorts of individual family members and includes data from the family phase and from the final (individual) sort phase: "A positive coordination score implies that the family works as a coordinated group not only when they are directly communicating with each other (the family sort), but also when returning to the final individual sort" (Steinglass, 1979a, p. 431). (The conceptual and empirical details of this work are discussed in Reiss and Klein's chapter in this book—Chapter 6.)

The current assessment of laboratory problem-solving included only 17 of the original 31 families, as not all families had a child 12 years old or older living in the home (Steinglass, 1979a). Although detailed descriptions of this subset of families is not provided, subsequent analysis revealed that the configuration and coordination scores were not significantly related to the sex of the index case, the sex of the participating child, the number of previous marriages, or the birth order of the participating child. The major independent variable, however, did reveal a significant effect on one of the dependent variables: dry families ($n = 12$) scored significantly higher than wet families ($n = 5$) on coordination, whereas the groups were nonsignificantly different on the configuration variable. Additional analyses indicated another important relationship involving a drinking-related variable: families scoring highest on the Self-Administered Alcohol Screening Test (SAAST), a self-report inventory for assessment of alcoholism, had the highest Configuration scores. To the extent that high SAAST scores indicate more extreme or serious consequences associated with the alcoholic's drinking in the past and/or the present, family problem-solving was more effective in families with a more disturbed versus a less disturbed alcoholic member.

To help place these results in a broader empirical context, comparisons were conducted between the means and variances of scores obtained from this sample with other normal and disturbed samples previously studied by Reiss (1981). Although cross-study differences were not analyzed statistically, Steinglass's discussion of these various samples suggested that the alcoholics had a large variance on configuration scores comparable to the range seen in normal families, whereas the mean performance of alcoholic families was most similar to Reiss's sample of delinquent families. (The implication of these findings is discussed further in the chapter by Reiss and Klein.)

In discussing these findings, Steinglass (1979a) suggested that the coordination dimension can be seen to span two extreme positions: at one pole are families who strongly adhere to a strategy (rule) emphasizing uniformity of behavior, whereas at the other end of the continuum are families who adopted a laissez-faire attitude and an emphasis on individual performance. Viewed in this manner, members of wet families tended to behave in a relatively independent manner (low coordination), whereas individuals from dry families appeared to emphasize togetherness, agreement, and family solidarity (high coordination). Together with the tendency for wet families to obtain higher configuration scores than dry families, as well as the significant relationship between the SAAST scores and the configuration measure, Steinglass (1979a) suggested that the findings appeared consistent with earlier formulations of the alcoholic family's "biphasic" nature involving different patterns of interaction associated with intoxicated and sober states:

> The data suggested that during the wet phase, family members appeared isolated from one another and acted in a highly differentiated fashion, but appeared freed up in the process to behave more effectively in certain ways, whereas during the dry phase they emphasized family solidarity at the expense of problem solving. Either state . . . would appear to be relatively unstable as far as family life was concerned. Family behavior during the dry phase might be characterized as overly rigid, suggesting that family structure had an "eggshell" quality that might have made it relatively nonadaptive. During the wet phase the family, perhaps under the guise of its alcoholic member's drinking, was temporarily able to shelve the family line. (p. 435)

Without question, Steinglass's work since the mid-1970s has been the most influential force in this field of study, promoting, as it has, significant interest, theoretical development, and empirical investigation among an increasing number of investigators. His early observations of family dyads during intoxicated and sober periods represented the first report of experimental drinking procedures applied to family units. The interpretation of these novel data within a theoretical model emphasizing general systems concepts added a provocative framework to this work, which subsequently was used to develop more systematic studies of alcoholic family systems. Important theoretical papers (Steinglass, 1980; Steinglass *et al.*, 1977), attempting to elaborate on initial models and to integrate observations of alcoholic–family interaction with broader theoretical and empirical literatures, served as a guide to many workers in the field.

The most recent stage of Steinglass's (1979a, 1981a) work has involved an innovative experimental design in which intact families are observed in multiple settings, which allow the collection of behavior relevant to issues of family organization within the natural home environment and problem solving and adaptation in the more novel laboratory setting. This effort has yielded more contributions to the field, the most important of which have been (a) the development and initial testing of a new observational coding system of relevance to the general field of family studies; (b) the presentation of a major theoretical model that incorporates both macroscopic (drinking phase: dry, wet, and transitional) and microscopic (drinking state: intoxicated or sober) levels of analysis relevant to understanding the course and maintenance of alcoholism; and (c) the publication of empirical findings that discuss the viability of the proposed model and suggest necessary "next steps" in the examination of the model's validity and implications. Most assuredly, Steinglass's achievements have been significant.

The major limitation that has characterized Steinglass's efforts to date involves the experimental designs on which his models have been built and tested. As a result, substantive findings that have been reported must be viewed as extremely preliminary and tentative, notwithstanding the significant investment of time and expense that has been devoted to these efforts since 1972. Given the central position that Steinglass's work has assumed in the field, it is of particular importance to recognize those aspects of his investigation that place important limits on the internal and external validity of his reported findings. The result will be that theoretical speculation and empirical documentation can be more carefully differentiated so that the reported findings can be carefully evaluated and contrasted with work of other researchers in the field.

In general, Steinglass has not provided systematic and rigorous assessments of the assumptions and hypotheses that have emerged from his efforts of the early 1970s. Early reports were based on data obtained from several family dyads (Steinglass et al., 1977) and from a "sample of convenience," consisting of 10 couples conducted through the experimental inpatient observation–treatment protocol (Steinglass et al., 1977). Assessment of these family units relied heavily on clinical observation procedures rather than on the systematic collection and analysis of psychometrically reliable and valid measures. These samples were extremely small and highly selective, and it was not possible to conduct meaningful statistical analyses or to assess the generalizability of the findings. The data that Steinglass reported, interpreted, and used to develop conceptual models, then, were of a decidedly clinical nature, generated by sensitive and insightful clinical researchers who observed couples over extended periods of time; who sifted and distilled these observations in a search for pattern and purpose; and who interpreted and elaborated these characterizations by reference to impressions gleaned from various sources of data. Unfortunately, these clinical impressions slowly became transformed into empirical facts in the decade following their appearance in the literature. The reality of this program's development, however, was that no scientifically sound, empirical studies were ever conducted to test most of these clinical impressions.

The key infrastructure of Steinglass's theoretical developments is that interactional events are different in intoxicated versus sober states and that the intoxication-relevant patterns are sufficiently reinforcing to perpetuate or maintain cycles of abusive drinking. Inspection of Steinglass's work, however, indicates that these are assumptions drawn from his clinical observations of the early, small samples of family dyads and couples (1971, 1977), and that these observations were best viewed as hypotheses that had not yet been tested in a careful, scientifically rigorous design. Steinglass's next efforts, however, did not pursue these "tests" directly (1979a, 1981a). That is, his 31-subject data collection did not involve families in an experimental drinking procedure; instead, he observed the subject families in several observational settings (home, laboratory, and multiple-family group discussions). From this effort, Steinglass expanded his model to include the more macroscopic variable of family drinking phase ("dry" versus "wet"), yet still assumed that within the wet phase, the cycling of intoxicated and sober states is perpetuated because of the reinforcing ("adaptive") consequences that intoxication-relevant interactions have in family life. This assumption regarding the function of intoxication-related interaction remained a key component of the elaborated model; yet it was never subjected to adequate empirical tests. Notwithstanding the potential impact that such model building might exert on future empirical and theoretical developments, it is both unfortunate and notable that key tenets and assumptions have *never* been subjected to systematic empirical analysis.

Several conclusions can be drawn from this historical overview: (a) The basis on which Steinglass's early and most significant models were founded was one of clinical observation involving unsystematic observations of small, unrepresentative samples of family dyads and couples engaged in a highly unusual inpatient program containing both assessment and treatment components. (b) It is imperative that key aspects of his models be subjected to adequate empirical test. And (c) the related literatures must be carefully scrutinized with the aim of determining the nature and degree of support provided for Steinglass's conceptualizations.

As noted, Steinglass's recent work (1979a,b, 1981a) involves a more systematic, rigorous, and empirical approach to the study of alcoholic–family relationships than did his earlier studies. In particular, these efforts have included a reasonably large sample of alcoholics living within intact families ($n = 31$); have provided careful diagnoses of alcoholism status; have obtained objectively defined, reliably coded measures of interaction in home and laboratory settings; and have used conventional statistical analyses to assess for differences among the dry, wet, and transitional subgroups. Notwithstanding these advances, limitations in experimental design have characterized this work, which, in turn, raise questions about the strength and interpretability of the obtained findings. In describing such limitations, our intent is to offer qualifications regarding the findings that have emerged from this database; to direct attention to the research and theory development that must be undertaken to further advance this area of study; and to highlight issues of importance in our examination of other studies in this literature.

1. Although the subjects studied by Steinglass (1981a) represented the largest, most intensively assessed sample of alcoholic families that had been reported on up to that time, the issues of sample size and representativeness still remain a problem. In particular, the sample consisted of both male ($n = 23$) and female ($n = 8$) alcoholics who were classified into one of three drinking phases: stable dry ($n = 14$), stable wet ($n = 10$), and transitional ($n = 7$). Given these subgroupings, it is apparent that Steinglass was working with extremely small samples when key comparisons were conducted. Although Steinglass reported that the three subgroups were similar along various SES dimensions and that male and female alcoholic families were not significantly different regarding various outcomes, the very small samples would have required extremely large between-group differences in order for statistical significance to have been achieved. Even if borderline significant effects or trends were present, however, potential confounding of independent and demographic variables could have occurred, so that interpretation of the results would remain ambiguous. That sociodemographic variables are related to various dependent measures is clear; that is, "family composition" was significantly related to structural variability, whereas "years married" was reliably related to intrafamily engagement. In

considering these data, Steinglass concluded that family alcohol phase exerted "selective" effects on family life, as only the drinking phase, and not the SES variables, was related to interactional distance and content variability. Inspection of these data, however, raises some questions about this interpretation, as "family composition" tended to be related to variation in distance regulation ($F[2,28] = 2.46$, $p < .15$) and content variability ($F[2,28] = 2.51$ $p < .15$), and both demographics and drinking phase were *never* included in the same analyses. Thus, it is possible that an analysis of covariance (treating "family composition" as a covariate) might have yielded a nonsignificant effect for drinking phase, and/or that family composition and family alcohol phase interact in affecting patterns of family interaction. If either outcome had been obtained, Steinglass's reported findings could have been markedly different.

Relationships between family drinking phase and HOAM variables might also have been mediated through covariations with architectural variables. In particular, "average interactional distance" was significantly related to room size, whereas "location shifts per hour" were significantly related to house size. Both of these HOAM indices load on interactional variability, the key measure that differentiated the SW, SD, and TR groups. To the extent that large room size and large house size are related to family income or socioeconomic status, it is possible that some confounding could have occurred in Steinglass's study if the three groups differed along these dimensions.

Given the selection process involved in recruiting families and the type of data obtained on this sample, there are also uncertainties regarding the specific nature of the three groups and what population findings can be generalized. In particular, little information about the subjects' psychiatric status (other than alcoholism) was provided, nor do we know anything about psychiatric disorders among the spouses. Furthermore, the subjects in the "transitional" group exhibited a range of drinking patterns across their 6-month involvement in the study, so that this group was not only unstable but very heterogeneous as well. Finally, a majority of subjects were described as middle to upper-middle class whose primary motivation for participation in this experimental research and treatment program no doubt involved a mix of curiosity and help seeking. The major question that is raised by these sample characteristics and selection procedures concerns issues of replicability and generalizability. Of particular importance, to what extent are the reported findings unique to this unusual sample, and how would variations in the psychiatric, SES, and motivational status of the families serve to qualify the reported results?

It is unfair, of course, to expect one study to define and measure all possible sources of variance, and this is certainly not the demand we would place on the work of Steinglass. Given the less-than-complete—and, at times, uncertain—nature of his experimental procedures, however, our major conclusion seems clear: Steinglass's results are best viewed as preliminary findings in need of replication and extension; without verification of their dependability and unambiguous interpretation, they remain little more than interesting hypotheses.

2. Although acknowledged by Steinglass (1983) as a key need for future research, it is worth noting that his experimental design included neither a

psychiatric (nonalcoholic) nor normal (nondistressed) comparison group. Given the absence of these controls, the interpretation of the obtained group differences remains ambiguous. For example, it is possible that, once the stress of the alcoholic's disruptive drinking ceases, these families (SD) appear to be quite similar to any other nondistressed group—a conclusion that would be consistent with various recent findings comparing the adjustment patterns of "recovered" alcoholics and their spouses and children with groups containing active alcoholic and normal controls (Moos & Moos, 1984). In this case, we would assume an ordering of SW ≠ SD = NC (normal control). Alternatively, the SD families (or at least some subgroup among them) might continue to exhibit a nonnormal interaction style that perhaps "normalizes" over time. In this case, we would expect an SW = SD ≠ NC ordering. Similar uncertainty regarding the interpretability of current reports involves the relationships between family patterns characterizing alcoholic versus other psychiatrically disturbed (but nonalcoholic) subjects. The important question here is the extent to which observed patterns are at all unique to alcoholism rather than reflecting more general processes characterizing stressed and dysfunctional family units. To address this issue, which is certainly of great concern to the field, requires some type(s) of psychiatric comparison groups.

3. As noted, the development and the preliminary testing of the HOAM (Steinglass, 1979b) represent an important and general contribution to the field of family studies. That it is a new instrument, however, requires a more careful evaluation of its limitations, including discussion of information that it does and does not provide in its application. Other chapters in this book address a variety of issues involved in the development and validation of observational coding systems as well as problems regarding internal and external validity. In the present context, only several comments regarding the difficulties and limitations with the HOAM will be noted.

The first issue of concern with the HOAM is the absence of information regarding potential reactivity effects and resultant distortions in the collected data. Two observers enter the home for a 4-hour period, each becoming "attached" to one of the parents. Notwithstanding the long period of observation (4 hours) and the multiple observation periods ($n = 9$), the potential reactivity associated with this instrument could be significant. At this stage in the development of the HOAM, no information could be provided by Steinglass that would speak to this issue directly, and thus, it remains for future efforts to determine the extent and direction of these potential distortions.

A second issue concerns Steinglass's decision to use a "family mean" as the basic unit of analysis in which scores from the two parents were simply averaged (Steinglass, 1979b, 1981a). Although reducing the complexity involved in categorizing and describing intrafamilial events, the decision to use a family mean seems to limit the interpretability of the obtained findings. Specifically, this combining and averaging process tells us only about the total amount of behavior exhibited by two members, leaving unspecified the degree to which the two component scores (mother and father) are related. To the extent that there are significant level difference between the parents' scores (e.g., mothers shift locations frequently, whereas fathers rarely move) or low correlations between parents' scores (e.g., relatively frequent shifts by mothers are not related to relatively frequent shifts by fathers), interpretations of group differences become exceedingly difficult. For example, can the obtained differences between the SW and SD groups be explained by reference to the mothers' scores only or the fathers' scores only? Is this pattern the same across the various dependent measures, or is one parent's behavior more discriminating for some measures and the other parent's (or both parents') scores more discriminating for other measures? For measures that did not yield group differences, could the combining of the two parents' scores have "masked" group differences that might have emerged with scores from only one parent? These and other questions raise important issues regarding the interpretability of the group differences reported by Steinglass (1979b, 1981a) and, during subsequent study, should be addressed in a more systematic fashion. At present, there is no way to determine the validity of Steinglass's claim that family means describe family level characteristics. Whether or not these scores mask intramember inconsistencies, capitalize on extreme behaviors of one parent only, or reflect similarity of the two parents' behavior vis-à-vis one another and their children can be answered only through further research efforts.

INTERACTION STUDIES: ALCOHOL'S IMPACT ON INTERACTION

None of the interaction studies reported thus far assessed the acute effects of alcohol on family interaction—a particularly critical issue, given the importance that Steinglass (1980) ascribed to alcohol's role in stabilizing family structures. Given the limitations in Steinglass's own empirical assessments of the alcohol–interaction relationship, it appears critical, indeed, that empirical data be generated that can address the validity and explore the parameters of these proposed associations. Three studies that have included experimental drinking procedures with alcoholic families have been reported during the past several years.

In a laboratory interaction study conducted by Jacob, Richey, Cvitkovic, and Blane (1981), eight families containing an alcoholic father/husband and eight normal control families were assessed. Of particular importance, the assessments involved both parents and two of their children between 10 and 18 years old. On one evening, videotaped discussions included the serving of alcoholic beverages, and on a second evening of discussions, nonalcoholic beverages were served. For discussions involving mother–father, mother–children, and father–children, a relatively structured Revealed Difference Questionnaire (RDQ—Jacob, 1974) was used to generate interaction; in addition, the parents engaged in a second discussion involving more personally relevant items generated by the Areas of Change Questionnaire (ACQ—Weiss, 1980). For alcoholics, the mean number of ounces of absolute alcohol consumed was 1.56 (R = .40–2.40) whereas the mean postsession (BAC) was .08% (R = .01–.33). In contrast, five wives in the alcoholic group drank no alcohol, and each of the remaining wives drank approximately .70 ounces. Similarly, spouses in the control group drank only small amounts of alcohol; their mean BAC was .01% ($R = .01-.04$).

The primary analysis focused on affective and problem-solving communications as determined by application of the Marital Interaction Coding System (MICS—Weiss, 1976) to the various family interactions. Based on the ACQ discussion, the alcoholic couples were found to express more negative affect and less positive affect than the control couples. Of particular interest, the alcoholic couples were more influenced by the drinking condition than were the controls; that is, the alcoholic couples were more negative in the drink versus no drink condition, whereas the normals displayed similar levels of affect in the two conditions. Consistent with this "negativity-increasing" effect of alcohol in the experimental group, an agree-disagree measure yielded a three-way interaction (condition × group × spouse) in which the wives of alcoholics emitted more disagreement in the drink versus no drink condition, whereas the wives of normals exhibited less disagreement in drink versus no drink condition. Obviously, alcohol's impact is quite different in alcoholic versus control couples—in one case, increasing negativity and, in the other, increasing conviviality and positive mood.

In addition to group differences in affect expression, control husbands tended to engage in more problem-solving behavior than did their wives, whereas alcoholics and their wives were equally instrument in their behavior; that is, the sex-role stereotype of the husband's being the instrumental, problem-solving leader was evident in control couples but not in alcoholic couples.

Similar to the ACQ findings, the more structured RDQ discussion involving husband and wife also yielded a group × member interaction; that is, the husbands engaged in more problem-solving than the wives in the normal group and in less than the wives in the alcoholic group. Unlike the strong group differences in affect display on the ACQ, however, the RDQ yielded no significant differences between groups in positive affect, negative affect, or agree–disagree ratio.

For the two RDQ interactions involving children (father–children and mother–children), interesting and provocative effects were evident. In particular, the normal fathers were clearly more instrumental (that is, emitted more problem-solving behavior) than their children ($F > C$), whereas, the alcoholic and his children exhibited a relatively egalitarian structure ($F = C$). In contrast, the normal mothers and their children exhibited an egalitarian structure ($M = C$), whereas the mothers in the alcoholic group were more instrumental than their children ($M > C$). In brief, this pattern suggested an opposite influence structure in the experimental and the control families, the former characterized by a father who expressed or exhibited less leadership and problem-solving behavior than his normal counterpart and a mother who exhibited more of a directive influence on her family than her counterpart. Although the tetrad (father–mother–children) was not assessed, one could infer an $F > M = C$ influence structure in normal control families and an $M > F = C$ structure in alcoholic families. Such findings are not only consistent with clinical-theoretical accounts of the change in the alcoholic family structure (Jackson, 1954) but are compatible with other family interaction research suggesting that "fathers are more influential (especially vis-à-vis the child) in normal than disturbed family groups" (Jacob, 1975, p. 51). Although this study yielded a number of interesting findings, various limitations in design and analysis procedures were evident.

First, psychiatric interviews were not conducted with the parents, and it is possible that the alcoholics could have satisfied diagnostic criteria for alcoholism as well as other psychiatric disorders and/or that their spouses could have exhibited some type of psychiatric disturbance. If so, the observed differences may have been related more to psychopathology in general than to the specific impact of paternal alcoholism.

Second, this study included both parents and two of their children. In addition, analyses did not control for the sex of the participating children or for differences in age and sex combination across the experimental and control groups. Furthermore, there were no assessments of interactions including both parents and children. To the extent that these variables can effect emergent patterns of interaction, future research must examine and delimit these variables with greater care.

Third, and most important, the extremely small samples involved in this effort placed severe limitations on the types of analyses that could be considered and the confidence that can be placed in interpretations of the obtained findings. In particular, the (statistical) power associated with such small sample designs is extremely low, and it is not possible to perform cross-validations in order to determine the robustness of the identified relationships. Furthermore, homogeneous subgroups (types) can be identified and contrasted only when relatively large samples are available. Given the increasing attention directed toward alcoholism typologies and the clarity that such classifications can bring to psychosocial as well as biological investigations, considerable effort should be devoted to this issue in future research (Cloninger & Reich, 1982; Morey & Blashfield, 1981).

In a design similar to the one used in the Jacob *et al.* (1981) study, Billings, Kessler, Gomberg, and Weiner (1979) also conducted a laboratory interaction study involving couples with an alcoholic husband. Although only marital interactions were assessed, these investigators did include a distressed as well as a nondistressed (normal) control group in order to examine what, if any, unique effects alcoholism may exert on family life. Each of the three groups contained 12 couples, and the groups were matched on age of spouse, years married, family income, and employment status.

The laboratory procedures involved a standardized role-play procedure adapted from Raush's improvisational scenes (Raush, Barry, Hertel, & Swain, 1974), as well as the application of two relevant and reliable coding systems: the Interpersonal Behavior Rating System (IBRS) developed by Leary (1957) and the Coding Scheme for Interpersonal Conflict (CSIC) devised by Raush *et al.* (1974). All interactions were videotaped, and transcripts were made of the verbal interchanges that were associated with the taped discussions. Finally, alcoholic beverages were made available to the subjects during one evening's discussion, whereas only soft drinks were served during a second meeting.

The major finding to emerge from this study was that alcoholic and distressed couples exhibited remarkably similar patterns of interaction that were distinctly different from the behavior expressed by the normal controls. As noted by Billings *et al.* (1979), "both alcoholic and distressed couples communicated significantly fewer rational problem-solving statements and engaged in more negative and hostile acts than did nonalcoholic, maritally satisfied couples" (p. 193). In contrast with these marked differences related to diagnostic status, the experimental drinking condition exerted no significant impact on couple interaction with the exception that the alcoholic and distressed couples spoke more during the drinking versus the nondrinking sessions, whereas the normal controls were relatively unaffected.

Notwithstanding the noteworthy design and the analytic strategies characterizing this study, two major weaknesses must be noted, as they place important limits on the interpretability of the reported findings. First, like the weaknesses of the Jacob *et al.* (1981) study, subject selection procedures allowed for considerable heterogeneity in the obtained samples regarding the psychiatric status of both the male index case and his or her spouse. In particular, there is no clear description of the psychiatric status of the alcoholics (other than their drinking problem), nor is there a detailed description of the wives' psychiatric characteristics. For distressed couples, the major inclusion criterion was a score below 100 on the Marital Adjustment Test (MAT—Locke & Wallace, 1959), with no evidence of alcohol abuse, whereas the normal controls scored 100 or higher on the MAT and were defined as social drinkers. To what extent the distressed couples (husbands and/or wives) exhibited minor or major psychiatric disorders is unclear, and as a result, the interpretation of significant or nonsignificant effects becomes a problem.

Second, and more important, the experimental drinking procedure was an extremely weak manipulation, and thus, the absence of an alcohol effect has little meaning. Specifically, almost half the couples (in each of the three groups) chose not to drink at all during the drinking session. Furthermore, the vast majority of those who did drink consumed very little alcohol; that is, 80% of the drinking subjects consumed one or two drinks with BACs ranging from .019% to .026%. Notwithstanding the investigators' attempt to manipulate and assess alcohol ingestion as an independent variable, it seems clear that the actual implementation of this objective was unsuccessful. Thus, it would be unwarranted to draw *any* conclusions from the reported data regarding the impact of alcohol ingestion on marital interaction.

Notwithstanding these methodological weaknesses, the Billings *et al.* (1979) study did raise several important questions as well as introduce a potentially useful methodology to this area of study. The study's major finding suggests that different types of psychopathology can have a similar impact on family life; in particular, the stress and distress associated with various psychopathologies can increase marital strain and conflict, can limit effective and sustained problem-solving efforts, and can result in cycles of negativity that become increasingly difficult to untangle regarding the "affected" member's provocations and the spouse's responses. To the extent that a "general psychopathology" effect is manifested in the family interactions of individuals with different types of disorders, it may be valuable to develop typologies based on common patterns of interaction versus common diagnoses. At the very least, it would be imperative for investigators to include appropriate psychiatric controls in future research if the understanding of alcoholism's unique or specific effects on family life is to be advanced.

A final study, by Frankenstein, Hay, and Nathan (1985), also involved alcoholic couples in an experimental drinking procedure and assessed the emergent interactions with the Marital Interaction Coding System (MICS—Weiss, 1976). Again, a very small sample (8 couples) was studied, although the methods and findings of this preliminary effort highlight important design issues that should be addressed systematically in future research. Briefly, alcoholics and their spouses, recruited through newspaper advertisements, were involved in laboratory discussions of marital problems on two separate occasions, one involving alcohol ingestion and the other without an alcohol presentation. In contrast with the *ad lib* drinking procedures used by Billings *et al.* (1979) and Jacob *et al.* (1981), Frankenstein *et al.* administered a fixed dose of alcohol before the marital discussion—a dose that averaged 5.8 ounces of 80-proof beverage alcohol and yielded a mean BAC of .104%. Only alcoholics were administered alcohol, and the discussions involved topics assumed to vary in conflict intensity. All interactions were videotaped and rated via the MICS.

The dependent measures included the duration of talking as well as six summary scores based on various combinations of MICS codes: positive verbal, negative verbal, positive nonverbal, negative nonverbal, problem description, and problem solving. The major finding was that the couples exhibited greater verbal positivity in the alcohol versus the no-alcohol condition—a finding that was primarily a function of the spouse's significant change between sessions. That is, the alcoholic's affect expression was relatively constant across conditions, whereas the spouse became more positive when the alcoholic was intoxicated. In addition, the alcoholics were found to talk more, whereas their spouses talked less, in the alcohol condition as compared with their speech rates in the no-alcohol condition. Similarly, the alcoholics tended to make more problem description statements in the alcohol versus no-alcohol condition, whereas their spouses exhibited similar levels of behavior across sessions.

In discussing these findings, Frankenstein *et al.* (1985) suggested that the results provide general support for the reinforcing or adaptive effects that alcohol may exert on alcoholic family systems:

> Specifically, it has been hypothesized that certain benefits which accrue to an alcoholic's marriage over time result from and maintain drinking . . . [therefore, one important goal of treatment would be] to restore these benefits [e.g., decreased negativity or increased positivity accomplished through alcohol abuse] under conditions of sobriety. (p. 5)

The difference between the Frankenstein *et al.* findings and those of Jacob *et al.* (1981) deserves further comment, given what appears to be opposite results obtained by the two investigations. Specifically, Jacob *et al.* found that alcohol resulted in greater negativity and disagreement in alcoholic couples, whereas

Frankenstein *et al.* reported that alcoholic couples became more positive and agreeable during the experimental drinking session. How may this difference be explained? In considering this issue, Frankenstein *et al.* suggested that their subjects—because they were entering a treatment program as part of their participation in the study—could be viewed as "transitional" drinkers. In contrast, the subjects in the Jacob *et al.* (1981) investigation—who were active drinkers and were *not* seeking treatment—were best seen as "stable wet" drinkers. To the extent that transitional and stable wet drinkers have been shown to manifest different behaviors in laboratory and home observations (Steinglass, 1979b, 1981), the possibility is raised that this distinction may also account for the cross-study difference in alcohol's impact on marital interaction.

Although this explanation is an interesting possibility, the present authors do not find this argument compelling, given the great similarities in recruitment and sample characteristics in the two studies. Influences of seemingly greater importance would include the substantial differences between the two studies regarding the amount and administration of alcohol, the inclusion versus exclusion of spouses from the experimental drinking procedures, the presence versus absence of ongoing drinking during the discussion, and the specific measures used to assess interaction. Furthermore, an earlier, preliminary report by Frankenstein, Hay, and Nathan (1982), in which data from only 5 subjects were available for analysis, suggested that the positivity-increasing effects of alcohol did not characterize the behavior of most subjects; instead, this pattern was exhibited by only two of five couples. Notwithstanding the significant statistical relationships reported, it is nonetheless possible that only a subset of couples manifested and accounted for the reported relationships between drinking and positive affect—a suggestion that is consistent with the relatively large variance associated with spouse behavior in the alcohol condition.

Although an experimental drinking procedure was not included, a recent interaction study by O'Farrell and Birchler (1985) attempted to extend the findings of Billings *et al.* (1979) by increasing the sample size and using additional self-report and observational measures. Moreover, this study focused on a personally relevant, conflictual issue for videotaped interactions, rather than on the prescribed role-play procedure used in the Billings *et al.* study. Briefly, 26 couples in each of three groups were studied: (a) couples in which the husband was receiving VA treatment for alcoholism; (b) nonalcoholic, maritally conflicted couples evaluated for marital therapy at a VA facility; and (c) nonalcoholic, nonconflicted couples responding to a newspaper ad who were not currently in treatment. Measures included responses to the Areas of Change Questionnaire (Weiss, 1980) and the Marital Status Inventory (Weiss & Cerreto, 1980), as well as videotaped interactions coded with the MICS (Weiss, 1976).

The findings substantially supported the expectation that alcoholic and maritally conflicted couples would manifest more marital distress than nonconflicted couples—findings that were reflected in the self-reports and the behavioral observations. Moreover, there was little that differentiated the alcoholic and the maritally conflicted couples. The prediction that alcoholic couples would show unique patterns of wife dominance, perceptual inaccuracy, and greater responsibility-avoiding behavior by husbands was not supported.

Notwithstanding the noteworthy design features incorporated into this study (the larger sample, the multimethod assessment, and the personally relevant discussion topics), several methodological weaknesses are also evident. The most apparent are sampling issues: the use of treatment seeking subjects, an alcoholic group that had abstained for "at least a few weeks," and failure to assess other possible psychiatric influences. Finally, the lack of a drinking manipulation prohibits any conclusions about the generalizability of the interactions observed during nondrinking periods to patterns of interaction associated with drinking.

FUTURE DIRECTIONS

In overview, the literature on family interaction and alcoholism is still at a very early stage of development, characterized as it is by various methodological and conceptual immaturities. At the same time, there is a clear sense of excitement and potential reflected in these beginning efforts, as well as encouragement for the continued study of relationships between alcoholism and family interaction. To generate more reliable and valid data than those currently available, future investigations must address a range of issues through creative and rigorous research strategies. From our own perspective, the following research needs represent particularly important areas to be pursued:

1. The methodological foundations on which future studies are built must be broad and secure. The collection and report of small, unrepresentative samples must be replaced by large, clearly defined subject groups, involving careful descriptions of the psychiatric and alcohol abuse status of index cases, spouses, and offspring; the comparison of research samples with clinical samples to which experimental findings are to be generalized; and the inclusion of psychiatric and/or medical as well as nondisturbed control groups. Furthermore, large samples are necessary in order to cross-validate emergent findings and to justify the application of more powerful and clarifying multivariate techniques.

Equally important, experimental designs should endeavor to assess offspring status and parent–child interaction in addition to the spouse status and marital interaction. The role of children in the family system seems no less important than that of adult members insofar as it clarifies the family's role in perpetuating (maintaining) dysfunctional behavior. Furthermore, the child's future psychosocial and alcohol abuse status is theoretically and empirically linked to contemporary patterns of family life—a relationship of particular importance given the "high-risk" nature of alcohlics' offspring.

In light of the multidimensional nature of the alcoholism–family interaction complex, a comprehensive analysis of key issues must involve broad, multimethod assessment strategies. To this end, different levels of analysis should be considered, including small time frames (e.g., detailed interaction processes) as well as larger views (e.g., different stages of drinking and associated family patterns). Equally important, family influences should be related to other major determinants, most important, the impact of nonfamilial experiences on individual members and the interplay between genetic and environmental sources of influence.

2. Beyond the need for more adequate experimental designs, the generation and testing of theoretical models will be of major importance to the future credibility of the field. Since the mid-1970s, general principles drawn from systems and social learning theory have provided the major scaffolding on which preliminary formulations have been constructed. Although the hypotheses advanced thus far have been both provocative and heuristic, empirical studies of these propositions have only begun to emerge; as a result, the viability of these preliminary hypotheses has yet to be determined. The most important example of this "validity gap" involves the role that alcohol has been assumed to play in maintaining family structures and processes. As previously noted, Steinglass *et al.*'s hypothesis (1977) that alcohol use is reinforced because of some "adaptive" functions that are served within the alcoholic family system has been central to his theoretical model building yet has never been adequately tested. Beyond several clinical case studies and uncontrolled assessments of experimental drinking, only three empirical studies have attempted to assess the acute effects of alcohol on family interaction (Billings *et al.*, 1979; Frankenstein *et al.*, 1985; Jacob *et al.*, 1981), and as has been seen, all of these efforts have been characterized by significant methodological limitations.

In our view, future evaluations of alcohol's role in family interaction—its antecedents, concomitants, and consequences—will be greatly enhanced by the consideration and use of various research strategies. In addition, the identification and careful assessment of more homogeneous subgroups promise to add greater clarity to this research arena than studies that continue to assume that all alcoholics and/or all alcoholic families are alike. The relationship between alcohol abuse and family interaction is most certainly a multidimensional one that varies across different types of alcoholics and families; and no simple hypothesis nor single method is likely to provide an adequate explanation of such complex a phenomenon as the relationship between alcohol use and family stability. Recent efforts from the authors' ongoing studies of alcoholism and family interaction (Jacob, Rushe & Seilhamer, unpublished material) provide strong support for both of these recommendations.

Briefly, recent analyses of report data obtained from married alcoholics indicated that alcoholic husbands who had consumed relatively large versus small amounts of alcohol in the past month (a) tended to obtain low scores on various Minnesota Multiphasic Personality Inventory (MMPI) scales and to report high marital satisfaction and (b) had wives who (1) obtained relatively low scores on the MMPI and the Beck Depression Inventory and (2) reported relatively greater marital satisfaction on the Locke–Wallace Test and the Dyadic Adjustment Scale (Jacob, Dunn, & Leonard, 1983). Furthermore, the strength of these relationships was quite different in two subgroups of alcoholics, falling to nonsignificance for binge (B) drinkers and rising to highly significant and consistent effects for steady (S) drinkers.

Although various explanations of this outcome were considered, our interest in the interactional aspects of the family led to the following working hypothesis: marital and family relationships are more satisfying during high versus low consumption periods, and these consequences serve to maintain or perpetuate drinking to the extent that (a) the alcoholics husband's behavior is more predictable when he is consuming alcohol at a high rate than when he is not drinking; (b) the experience of stress in family life is minimized during periods of high consumption; and (c) the family has adapted to and incorporated high-rate drinking into its family life.

Given the limitations of these preliminary findings—in particular, the cross-sectional, retrospective nature of the data—our next effort attempted to assess drinking, psychiatric symptoms, and marital satisfaction on a day-to-day basis and to examine the actual covariation among these variables. For this assessment, a small group of eight married couples with alcoholic husbands who had previously participated in the core study were recruited (Dunn, 1985; Dunn, Jacob, Hummon, & Seilhamer, in press). The study was restricted to steady drinkers, as only this group had exhibited a significant association between alcohol consumption and marital stability in the original study. Because drinking location (in-home versus out-of-home) was correlated with the binge–steady categorization, our original findings could have resulted from differences on either or both dimensions. So that we could assess this issue more systematically, half of the selected subjects were in-home and half were out-of-home drinkers.

Procedurally, the eight couples were asked to provide daily records regarding alcohol consumption, psychiatric symptomatology, and marital satisfaction ratings over a 90-day period. Application of univariate and bivariate time series analyses was then undertaken with a particular interest in modeling the relationship between the husband's alcohol consumption and the wife's satisfaction ratings and daily consumption scores. The results of these analyses were quite striking and can be summarized rather succinctly: All four couples in the *out-of-home* group exhibited a negative relationship between the husbands' alcohol consumption and the wives' marital satisfaction (i.e., drinking resulted in a decrease in marital satisfaction), whereas two of the three clearly defined *in-home* drinkers exhibited a positive relationship betwen these two variables (i.e., the husbands' drinking resulted in an increase in marital satisfaction).

Based on these cross-sectional and time-series analyses, two conclusions seemed warranted: (a) the family's response to the alcoholic's drinking is quite different depending on the subgroups assessed, and (b) one's conclusions regarding the consumption–family-stability relationship becomes increasingly refined (and complex) as additional methodologies are brought to bear on this issue. Given the obtained relationship between drinking style and location, on the one hand, and variations in marital satisfaction, on the other, further examination of these dimensions and associated subgroups certainly seemed in order. From our perspective, an obvious testing ground for the emerging typology would be laboratory interactions that included an experimental drinking procedure—a paradigm that would allow for the assessment of alcohol's impact on family interaction in different drinking style and location subgroups. Just such data are now available from our research program, and although all analyses have not yet been completed, the available results clearly indicate the value of these subgroups in clarifying the relationship between alcohol and family stability.

Briefly, marital communications were generally negative and aversive among the binge (B) drinkers. Most of these negative communications came from the drinker himself rather than from his wife, and the interactions tended to become increasingly negative in the drinking session. In addition, these couples showed a decrease in problem-solving efforts during the drinking season, with a suggestion that the wife exhibited the more dramatic reduction in task focus. One implication that may be read into these data is that negativity (especially the husband's) during the drinking session leads to an increase in off-task talk, especially by the wife. That is, the alcohol's increasing anger and criticism result in the wife's "backing off" from direct attempts to deal with areas of conflict—a sequence that would suggest a coercive control mechanism at the center of this mode of relating. On the other hand, we could entertain the possibility of a negativity-accelerating process underlying the obtained findings in which cycles of negative reciprocity are of high strength and long duration. Obviously, other analytic procedures will be needed to determine which of these processes is operating.

For steady, in-home drinkers (SI), communication was generally less negative than with the B group. Although there was some increase in negativity in going from the no-drink to the drink condition, it was quite moderate in comparison with the negativity change we saw in the B group. Furthermore, problem solving actually improved a bit as a function of the drinking condition, whereas positivity increased noticeably during the drinking session. Given this pattern of outcomes, we can entertain the hypothesis that alcohol actually facilitates more problem-focused behavior, which is experienced as—or which is in the context of—a clearly positive mood.

Finally, the steady, out-of-home drinkers appeared to be the least stable type that we have examined so far, sometimes appearing more similar to the B drinkers and at other times operating more like the SI drinkers. Obviously, our small sample analyses must be followed by larger sample designs so that issues of stability and strength of findings can be determined more confidently than is now possible.

3. That children of alcoholics are at high risk for subsequent alcohol abuse has been extensively discussed and documented in the extant literature (Cotton, 1979; Jacob *et al.*, 1978; Wilson, 1982). Briefly, current knowledge suggests that genetic influences are probably crucial—and perhaps, even necessary—determinants for certain types of adult alcoholism. At the same time, there remains considerable uncertainty about the importance, of such influences across various forms, types, and degrees of alcohol abuse as well as about the nature of non-genetic influences (familial or nonfamilial) that serve to potentiate or minimize the emergence of alcoholism in genetically predisposed individuals. As concluded by Cloninger, Bohman, and Sigvardsson (1981),

> the susceptibility to alcoholism is neither entirely genetic nor entirely environmental, nor simply the sum of separate genetic and environmental contributions. Rather, specific combinations of predisposing genetic factors and environmental stress appear to interact before alcoholism develops in most persons. (p. 861)

Although the study of such gene–environment interaction involves various methodological and statistical difficulties, recent efforts of several investigative teams indicate the importance and potential of such work (see the review by Cloninger & Reich, 1982).[1]

In contrast with studies reporting on the familial nature of alcoholism, the literature concerned with the impact of parental alcoholism on the psychosocial and psychiatric status of offspring is numerically small and methodologically flawed. Most notably, this modest set of studies is characterized by the overrepresentation of subjects from nonintact, lower-SES, multiproblem families; the absence of appropriate comparison groups; and the dominance of indirect, self-report procedures in the assessment of child, parent–child, and family functioning. As a result of these design limitations, there remain considerable uncertainty and disagreement regarding the strength of these associations within more homogeneous, specifically defined subgroups; the relative influence of and interaction between family genetic and family environmental effects; the developmental patterns that characterize the emergence and expression of these outcomes; and the nature of the familial and nonfamilial variables that serve to protect a sizable proportion of these high-risk children from such adverse outcomes. In light of these considerations, it seems necessary for investigators to consider longitudinal studies of these high-risk offspring in order to provide further clarification of these issues.

4. Since the mid-1970s, an expanding literature on the drinking practices and problems of women has raised questions regarding the generalizability of

---

[1]Most attempts to elucidate environmental influences related to the transmission of alcoholism across generations have been relatively unelaborated and without empirical support, and therefore, Wolin and Bennet's work on family rituals is of special note (Wolin, Bennet, & Noonan, 1979; Wolin, Bennett, Noonan, & Teitelbaum, 1980). Rituals are the specific ways a family carries out everyday activities, the ways it marks transitional events, and the ways it celebrates special occasions. Specifically, these researchers have hypothesized that families that are able to maintain rituals despite a parent's alcohol problem are less likely to produce children with an alcohol problem. These families are labeled "distinctive" in contrast to "subsumptive" families, in which alcoholism has disrupted or altered family rituals. The results of an initial attempt to empirically substantiate these authors' model showed that, in addition to the subsumptive category (all rituals altered) and the distinctive category (no overall change in rituals), families also fall into an intermediate group in which approximately half their rituals are altered. Analyses showed that all transmitter families (those with a problem-drinker or alcoholic child) fell into the subsumptive or intermediate subsumptive categories. Also, almost all nontransmitter families (those with no children with alcoholic problems) fell into the distinctive or intermediate subsumptive categories. The intermediate transmitter families were fairly evenly dispersed across the three categories. Although these preliminary results are in need of replication with broader and larger samples, they underscore the viability of identifying distinct family behavioral patterns that lead to specific child outcomes.

findings based on male samples to issues of the etiology, course, expression, and treatment of alcoholism in females (Beckman, 1975; Blume, 1982; Gomberg, 1981; Greenblatt & Schuckit, 1976; Wilsnack & Beckman, 1983). A wide range of differences between male and female alcoholics has been reported, many of which strongly suggest that family processes related to the transmission and perpetuation of alcoholism, as well as the alcoholic's impact on family functioning, are likely to be markedly different for male and female alcoholics.

First, the alcoholic wife-mother versus the alcoholic husband-father is more likely to be "hidden," "ignored," or "protected" by family members, to drink at home, and to exhibit drinking patterns that are closely tied to family dynamics, crises, and developmental transitions (Beckman, 1975, 1976; Blume, 1982; Gomberg, 1981; Knupfer, 1982; Schuckit & Duby, 1983; Williams & Klerman, 1983). Taken together, such characteristics would predict that the determinants, concomitants, and consequences of maternal versus paternal alcoholism would be more closely tied to distinct family structures and processes and would be more amenable to change through family interventions.

Second, various reports indicate that the wife's versus the husband's drinking patterns are more influenced by the spouse's drinking behavior, and that the spouses of female versus male alcoholics are more likely to be abusers themselves (Schuckit & Morrissey, 1976; Wilsnack et al., 1982). Furthermore, Wiseman's insightful descriptions (1980a,b, 1981) of alcoholic–spouse relationships suggest that wives and husbands of alcoholic spouses respond very differently to the drinking of their mates. Given the importance that such characteristics can exert on theory development and clinical intervention—yet recognizing the speculative nature of these reports as well as the inconsistencies reflected in this literature (Corrigan, 1980; Wilsnack et al. 1982)—the need for rigorous, systematically designed investigations is of high priority.

Third, the impact of alcoholism on children is likely to be different with maternal versus paternal alcoholism. Mothers, for example, are usually the primary caretakers of the children, so that disruption of this function because of the debilitating effects of alcohol abuse can have serious consequences for the psychosocial development of children. To the extent that women alcoholics are more concerned about their parenting than male alcoholics (Gomberg, 1981) and experience depression and guilt during sober states (Corrigan, 1980), alcoholic mothers may be more likely than alcoholic fathers to overcompensate during sober periods. If so, inconsistent patterns of neglect and overindulgence may add to the adjustment problems of the offspring.

Fourth, results from the Swedish adoption studies have suggested two distinct forms of alcoholism differing in terms of family history and inheritance pattern (Cloninger et al., 1981). For one of these subgroups, the greatest risk to daughters occurs when the mother is alcoholic; when the mother's alcoholism does not involve an extensive treatment history (i.e., it is of a relatively mild form); and when the mother does not exhibit criminality requiring incarceration (Bohman, Sigvardsson, & Cloninger, 1981). The theoretical and clinical implications of these findings appear to be extremely important and certainly deserve continued study.

Overall, then, the available literature suggests many factors likely to distinguish families of alcoholic women from those containing male alcoholics. Clearly, such variables, if systematically related to the sex of the alcoholic spouse, can create significant differences in the marital and family patterns that are observed in families of male versus female alcoholics. Given the limited, indirect, and flawed nature of this literature, however, the tentative characterizations that have emerged from these preliminary efforts must be assessed more systematically and rigorously than has been accomplished thus far.

Finally, the field would benefit greatly from continued efforts to define homogeneous alcoholic subgroups that would provide a more differentiated and comprehensive understanding of the role of alcohol in family life. Examples of such efforts have been described in earlier sections of this chapter: Steinglass's typology based on stages of alcohol use, Wolin's efforts (1979, 1980) to understand cross-generational transmission in terms of the centrality of alcoholism in family life, and Jacob's recent finding on how drinking style and location impact on family relationships. Although provocative and informative, all of these efforts have used individually defined and/or static variables to distinguish groups. Only after classifications have been made (binge versus steady, wet versus dry, subsumptive versus distinctive) has the investigator attempted to describe the between-group differences in observed or inferred patterns of interaction.

An alternative strategy for developing a typology is to emphasize interaction (rather than common psychiatric diagnoses, personality structures, drinking phases, and so on) as the basis on which subjects are initially classified (Gottman, 1979; Miller & Olson, 1980; Raush *et al.*, 1974). This strategy is tenable not only on rationale grounds, but on the basis of two important developments: (a) a convergence around a limited number of dimensions thought to be relevant to descriptions of family interaction (Olson, Sprenkle, & Russell, 1979) and (b) a growing belief that different types of disturbances are associated with similar family patterns, suggesting a necessary (but probably not sufficient) set of family behaviors necessary for the development of some types of disturbances (Conger, 1980).

In our ongoing studies of alcoholic families, we are pursuing efforts to develop a typology based on interaction patterns. This investigation has involved 150 intact families in which the father is alcoholic ($n = 50$), depressed ($n = 50$), or normal ($n = 50$). Planned analyses will divide these 150 families into two replication samples, each sample containing 25 families from each of the three diagnostic groups. A broad range of report and observation procedures will be collected, but most central to this effort will be laboratory discussions in which an experimental drinking procedure is included (drink versus no-drink sessions). Discussions will involve four combinations of family members: mother–father, mother–child, father–child, and mother–father–child. Specifically, scores derived from an MICS coding of these videotaped sessions will generate a composite profile for each family. These profiles will serve as input for the clustering algorithm, which, in turn, will involve development of a preliminary grouping of types of family interaction.

Subsequent to the development of this basic typology, a series of validity studies are planned that will examine patterns of reciprocity, symmetry of predictability, and interactional variabilities. Also, generalization of the typology will be examined with respect to interactions that have been gathered in the home settings. Additionally, the impact of alcohol consumption on different family types will be examined with special interest in determining which family types are influenced in a positive versus a negative direction as a function of the drinking condition. Finally, the typology will be related to several indices of individual functioning in the personality, psychiatric, cognitive-academic, and drinking behavior domains.

It is anticipated that the assessment families of alcoholics in terms of their interactional patterns will aid in the clarification of subtle, ongoing phenomena that promote the emergence and maintenance of individual and systemic disturbances. Additionally, dysfunctional interactions that are unique to subgroups may be discerned, and such knowledge may then lead to the development of specific interventions and prevention strategies.

SUMMARY

In summary, the application of an interactional approach to understanding families of alcoholics has been extremely limited, and the confluence of these two domains is represented by a narrow stream of relevant empirical efforts. Moving from early, psychodynamically based reports that focused on individual characteristics of the alcoholic and his or her family members, the field advanced to inferring the quality of dyadic relationships from the retrospective self-reports of individual family members. Subsequently, direct observation became an increasingly preferred method for gathering data, although much of this research examined the interactive behavior of families in contrived laboratory situations. More recently, investigators have attempted to study families in less synthetic contexts by observing interactions during personally relevant, emotionally laden discussions and in naturalistic home settings.

Despite conceptual and methodological immaturity, these pioneering efforts have generated provocative hypotheses and have forged avenues for future pursuit. Suggested directions include the articulation and testing of more precise theoretical models, the implementation of more rigorous study methods, and the refinement and expansion of ancillary research areas that involve female alcohol abusers and the children of alcoholics. Currently, innovative designs that include experimental drinking, multimodal assessment, longitudinal data collection, and sophisticated analytical techniques have the potential for moving the field beyond its present embryonic state. Assuredly, such efforts will yield a broader and more thorough understanding of the complex association between familial processes and alcoholism.

REFERENCES

Adler, R., & Raphael, B. (1983). Children of alcoholics. *Australian and New Zealand Journal of Psychiatry, 17,* 3–8.

Becker, J. V., & Miller, P. M. (1976). Verbal and nonverbal marital interaction patterns of alcoholics and nonalcoholics. *Journal of Studies on Alcohol, 37,* 1616–1624.

Beckman, L. (1975). Women alcoholics: A review of social and psychological studies. *Journal of Studies on Alcohol, 36,* 797–824.

Beckman, L. J. (1976). Alcoholism problems and women: An overview. In M. Greenblatt & M. A. Schuckit (Eds.), *Alcohol problems in women and children.* New York: Grune & Stratton.

Billings, A., Kessler, M., Gomberg, C., & Weiner, S. (1979). Marital conflict-resolution of alcoholic and nonalcoholic couples during sobriety and experimental drinking. *Journal of Studies on Alcohol, 3,* 183–195.

Blume, S. B. (1982). Alcohol problems in women. *New York State Journal of Medicine, 82(8),* 1222–1224.

Bohman, M., Sigvardsson, S., & Cloninger, R. (1981). Maternal inheritance of alcohol abuse: Cross-fostering analysis of adopted women. *Archives of General Psychiatry, 38,* 965–969.

Cloninger, R., & Reich, T. (1982). Genetic heterogenity in alcoholism and sociopathy. In S. Kety, L. Rowland, R. Sidman, & S. Matthysse (Eds.), *Genetics of neurological and psychiatric disorders.* New York: Raven Press.

Cloninger, R., Bohman, M., & Sigvardsson, S. (1981). Inheritance of alcohol abuse: Cross-fostering analysis of adopted men. *Archives of General Psychiatry, 38,* 861–868.

Cobb, J. C., & McCourt, W. F. (1979, September). *Problem solving by alcoholics and their families: A laboratory study.* Paper presented at American Psychological Association Meeting, New York.

Conger, R. (1980). The assessment of dysfunctional family systems. In B. Lahey & A. Kazdin (Eds.), *Advances in child clinical psychology.* New York: Plenum Press.

Corrigan, E. M. (1980). *Alcoholic women in treatment.* New York: Oxford University Press.

Cotton, N. (1979). The familial incidence of alcoholism: A review. *Journal of Studies of Alcohol, 40,* 89–116.

Davis, D. I. (1976). Changing perception of self and spouse from sober to intoxicated state: Implications for research into family factors that maintain alcohol abuse. *Annuals of the New York Academy of Science, 273,* 497–506.

Drewery, J., & Rae, J. B. (1969). A group comparison of alcoholic and nonalcoholic marriages using the interpersonal perception technique. *British Journal of Psychiatry, 115,* 287–300.

Dunn, N. J. (1985). *Patterns of alcohol abuse and marital stability.* Unpublished doctoral dissertation, University of Pittsburgh.

Dunn, N. J., Jacob, T., Hummon, N., & Seilhamer, R. A. (in press). *Marital stability in alcoholic-spouse relationships as a function of drinking pattern and location. Journal of Abnormal Psychology.*

Edwards, A. (1959). *Edwards Personal Preference Schedule Manual.* New York: Psychological Corporation.

el-Guebaly, N., & Offord, D. R. (1977). The offspring of alcoholics: A critical review. *American Journal of Psychiatry, 134,* 357–365.

Frankenstein, W., Hay, W. M., & Nathan, P. E. (1982). *Alcohol's effects on alcoholics' marital interaction: Subjective and objective assessment of communication.* Paper presented at the American Psychological Association, Washington, D.C.

Frankenstein, W., Hay, W. M., & Nathan, P. E. (1985). Effects of intoxication on alocohlics' marital communication and problem solving. *Journal of Studies on Alcohol, 46,* 1–6.

Futterman, S. (1953). Personality trends in wives of alcoholics. *Journal of Psychiatric Social Work, 23,* 37–41.

Gomberg, E. S. (1981). Women, sex roles, and alcohol problems. *Professional Psychology, 12(1),* 146–155.

Gorad, S. (1971). Communicational styles and interaction of alcoholics and their wives. *Family Process, 10(4),* 475–489.

Gorad, S., McCourt, W., & Cobb, J. (1971). A communications approach to alcoholism. *Quarterly Journal of Studies on Alcohol, 32,* 651–668.

Gottman, J. (1979). *Marital interaction: Experimental investigations.* New York: Academic Press.

Greenblatt, M., & Schuckit, M. (Eds.). (1976). *Alcoholism: Problems in women and children.* New York: Grune & Stratton.

Hanson, P. G., Sands, P. M., & Sheldon, R. B. (1968). Patterns of communication in alcoholic married couples. *Psychiatric Quarterly, 42,* 538–547.

Hersen, M., Miller, P., & Eisler, R. (1973). Interaction between alcoholics and their wives: A descriptive analysis of verbal and nonverbal behavior. *Quarterly Journal of Studies on Alcohol, 34,* 516–520.

Jackson, D. (Ed.). (1968a). *Communication, family and marriage.* Palo Alto, CA: Science and Behavior Books.

Jackson, D. (1968b). *Therapy, communication and change.* Palo Alto, CA: Science and Behavior Books.

Jackson, K. (1954). The adjustment of the family to the crisis of alcoholism. *Quarterly Journal of Studies on Alcohol, 15,* 562–586.

Jacob, T. (1974). Patterns of family dominance and conflict as a function of child age and social class. *Developmental Psychology, 10,* 1–12.

Jacob, T. (1975). Family interaction in disturbed and normal families: A methodological and substantive review. *Psychological Bulletin, 82,* 33–65.

Jacob, T., & Seilhamer, R. A. (1982). The impact on spouses and how they cope. In J. Orford, & J. Harwin (Eds.), *Alcohol and the family.* London: Crown Helm.

Jacob, T., Favorini, A., Meisel, S., & Anderson, C. (1978). The spouse, children, and family interactions of the alcoholic: Substantive findings and methodological issues. *Journal of Studies on Alcohol, 39,* 1231–1251.

Jacob, T., Ritchey, D., Cvitkovic, J., & Blane, H. (1981). Communication styles of alcoholic and nonalcoholic families when drinking and not drinking. *Journal of Studies on Alcohol, 42,* 466–482.

Jacob, T., Dunn, N. J., & Leonard, K. (1983). Patterns of alcohol abuse and family stability. *Alcoholism: Clinical and experimental research, 7(4),* 382–385.

Jacob, T., Rushe, R., & Seilhamer, R. A. (n.d.). Alcoholism and family interaction: An experimental paradigm. Unpublished manuscript.

James, J. E., & Goldman, M. (1971). Behavior trends of wives of alcoholics. *Quarterly Journal of Studies on Alcohol, 32,* 373–381.

Jourard, S. M. (1959). Self-disclosure and other cathexis. *Journal of Abnormal and Social Psychology 59,* 428–431.

Kalashian, M. (1959). Working with wives of alcoholics in an outpatient clinic setting. *Marriage and Family, 21,* 130–133.

Kantor, D., & Lehr, W. (1975). *Inside the family.* San Francisco: Jossey-Bass.

Katz, M. M., & Lyerly, S. B. (1963). Methods for measuring adjustment and social behavior in the community: 1. Rationale, description, discriminative validity and scale development. *Psychological Reports, 13,* 503–535.

Kennedy, D. L. (1976). Behavior of alcoholics and spouses in a simulation game situation. *Journal of Nervous and Mental Disease, 162,* 23–34.

Knupfer, G. (1982). Problems associated with drunkenness in women: Some research issues. In NIAAA Alcohol and Health Monograph No. 4, *Special population issues.* U.S. Department of Health and Human Services (ADM) 82-1193, 3–39.

Leary, T. (1957). *Interpersonal diagnosis of personality.* New York: Ronald Press.

Lewis, M. (1937). Alcoholism and family casework. *Family, 18,* 39–44.

Locke, H., & Wallace, K. (1959). Short marital adjustment and prediction test: Their reliability and validity. *Marriage and Family Living, 21,* 251–255.

Lorr, M., McNair, D. M., Weinstein, G. J., Michaux, W. W., & Raskin, A. (1961). Meprobamate and chlorpromazine in psychotherapy. *Archives of General Psychiatry, 4,* 381–389.

Mello, N. K. (1972). Behavioral studies of alcoholism. In B. Kissin, & H. Begleiter (Eds.), *Biology of alcoholism* (Vol. 2). New York: Plenum Press.

Miller, B., & Olson, D. (1980). *Typology of marital interaction and contextual characteristics: Cluster analysis of the IMC.* Unpublished manuscript, University of Michigan.

Mitchell, H. E. (1959). The interrelatedness of alcoholism and marital conflict. *American Journal of Orthopsychiatry, 29,* 547–559.

Mitchell, H. E., & Mudd, E. H. (1957). The development of a research methodology for achieving the cooperation of alcoholics and their nonalcoholic wives. *Quarterly Journal of Studies on Alcohol, 18,* 649–657.

Moos, R. H., & Moos, B. S. (1984). The process of recovery from alcoholism: 3. Comparing functioning in families of alcoholics and matched control families. *Journal of Studies on Alcohol, 45,* 111–118.

Morey, L., & Blashfield, R. (1981, April). *The empirical classification of alcoholism: A review.* Paper presented at annual meeting of Classification Society, University of Florida, Gainesville.

O'Farrell, T. J. (1986). Marital therapy in the treatment of alcoholism. In N. S. Jacobson, & H. S. Gurman (Eds.), *Clinical handbook of marital therapy.* New York: Guilford Press.

O'Farrell, T. J., & Birchler, G. R. (1985). *Marital relationships of alcoholic, conflicted, and nonconflicted couples.* Paper presented at the American Psychological Association, Los Angeles.

Olson, D., Sprenkle, D., & Russell, C. (1979). Circumplex model of marital and family systems: I. Cohesion and adaptability dimensions, family types, and clinical applications. *Family Process, 18,* 3–28.

Orford, J., Guthrie, S., Nicholls, P. Oppenheimer, E., Egert, S., & Hensman, C. (1975). Self-reported coping behavior of wives of alcoholics and its association with drinking outcome. *Journal of Studies on Alcohol, 9,* 1254–1267.

Paolino, T. J., & McCrady, B. S. (1977). *The alcoholic marriage: Alternative perspectives.* New York: Grune & Stratton.

Patterson, G. (1982). *A social learning approach: Vol. 3. Coercive family processes.* Eugene, OR: Castalia Publishing.

Raush, H., Barry, W., Hertel, R., & Swain, M. (1974). *Communication, conflict and marriage.* San Francisco: Jossey-Bass.

Reiss, D. (1981). *The family's construction of reality.* Cambridge: Harvard University Press.

Schaffer, J. B., & Tyler, J. D. (1979). Degree of sobriety in male alcoholics and coping styles used by their wives. *British Journal of Psychiatry, 135,* 431–437.

Schuckit, M. A., & Duby, J. (1983). Alcoholism in women. In B. Kissin & H. Begleiter (Eds.), *The biology of alcoholism: The pathogenesis of alcoholism: Psychosocial factors* (Vol. 16). New York: Plenum Press.

Schuckit, M. A., & Morrissey, R. R. (1976). Alcoholism in women: Some clinical and social perspectives with an emphasis on possible subtypes. In M. Greenblatt & M. A. Schuckit (Eds.), *Alcoholism problems in women and children.* New York: Grune & Stratton.

Steinglass, P. (1975). The simulated drinking gang: An experimental model for the study of a systems approach to alcoholism: 1. Description of the Model; 2. Findings and implications. *Journal of Nervous and Mental Disease, 161,* 100–122.

Steinglass, P. (1979a). The alcoholic family in the interaction laboratory. *Journal of Nervous and Mental Disease, 167,* 428–436.

Steinglass, P. (1979b). The Home Observation Assessment Method (HOAM): Real-time observations of families in their homes. *Family Process, 18,* 337–354.

Steingalss, P. (1980). A life history model of the alcoholic family. *Family Process, 19,* 211–226.

Steinglass, P. (1981a). The alcoholic family at home: Patterns of interaction in dry, wet and transitional stages of alcoholism. *Archives of General Psychiatry, 8(4),* 441–470.

Steinglass, P. (1981b). The impact of alcoholism on the family. *Journal of Studies on Alcohol, 42,* 288–303.

Steinglass, P., & Robertson, A. (1983). The alcoholic family. In B. Kissin & H. Begleiter (Eds.), *The biology of alcoholism: Vol. 6. The pathogenesis of alcoholism: Psychosocial factors.* New York: Plenum Press.

Steinglass, P., Weiner, S., & Mendelson, J. H. (1971). A systems approach to alcoholism: A model and its clinical application. *Archives of General Psychiatry, 24,* 401–408.

Steinglass, P., Davis, D., & Berenson, D. (1977). Observations of conjointly hospitalized "alcoholic couples" during sobriety and intoxication: Implications for theory and therapy. *Family Process, 16,* 1–16.

Tamerin, J. S., Toler, A., DeWolfe, J., Packer, L., & Neuman, C. P. (1973, June). Spouses' perception of their alcoholic partners: A retrospective view of alcoholics by themselves and their spouses (pp. 33–49). In *Proceedings of the Third Annual Alcoholism Conference of the National Institute on Alcohol Abuse and Alcoholism*. Washington, DC: NIAAA.

Thiabut, J. W., & Kelly, H. H. (1959). *The social psychology of groups*. New York: Wiley.

Watzlawick, P., Beavin, H., & Jackson, D. (1967). *Pragmatics of human communication: A study of interaction patterns, pathologies and paradoxes*. New York: Norton.

Weiss, R. L. (1976). *Marital Interaction Coding System (MICS): Training and reference manual for coders*. Unpublished manuscript. University of Oregon, Marital Studies Program, Eugene.

Weiss, R. L. (1980). *The Areas of Change Questionnaire*. Eugene: Marital Studies Program, University of Oregon, Department of Psychology.

Weiss, R. L., & Cerreto, M. C. (1980). The Marital Status Inventory: Development of a measure of dissolution potential. *American Journal of Family Therapy, 8*, 80–85.

Williams, C. N., & Klerman, L. V. (1982). Female alcohol abuse: Its effects on the family. In S. Wilsnack, & L. J. Beckman (Eds.), *Alcohol problems in women*. New York: Guilford Press.

Wilsnack, S., & Beckman, L. (1983). *Alcohol problems in women*. New York: Guilford Press.

Wilsnack, R. W., Wilsnack, S. C., & Klassen, A. D., Jr. (1982, September). *Women's drinking and drinking problems: Patterns from a 1981 survey*. Paper presented at the Annual Meeting of the Society for the Study of Social Problems, San Francisco.

Wilson, C. (1982). The impact of children. In J. Orford & J. Harwin (Eds.), *Alcohol and the family*. London: Croom Helm.

Wiseman, J. (1980a). Discussion summary presented at NIAAA Workshop, Jekyll Island, Georgia, April 2–5, 1978. In NIAAA Research Monograph No. 1, *Alcohol and Women*. U.S. Department HEW, Publication No. (ADM) 80-835, 107–114.

Wiseman, J. (1980b). The "home treatment." The first steps in trying to cope with an alcoholic husband. *Family Relations, 29*, 541–549.

Wiseman, J. (1981). Sober comportment: Patterns and perspectives on alcohol addiction. *Journal of Studies on Alcohol, 42*, 106–126.

Wolin, S., Bennett, L., & Noonan, D. (1979). Family rituals and the recurrence of alcoholism over generations. *American Journal of Psychiatry, 136*, 589–593.

Wolin, S., Bennett, L., Noonan, D., & Teitalbaum, M. (1980). Disrupted family rituals: A factor in the intergenerational transmission of alcoholism. *Journal of Studies on Alcohol, 41*, 199–214.

CHAPTER 16

Family Factors in Childhood Psychology

Toward a Coercion–Neglect Model

ROBERT G. WAHLER AND JEAN E. DUMAS

The weaknesses of psychiatric diagnosis in terms of reliability, validity, and treatment implications have been spelled out in the behavioral literature (e.g., Kanfer & Saslow, 1969). Even recent refinements in the most widely used diagnostic system (DSM-III; American Psychiatric Association, 1980) have been found wanting, particularly in reference to childhood psychopathology (Cantwell, Russell, Mattison, & Will, 1979). Simply stated, there are serious concerns about the utility of this classification system as it is applied to troubled children. These concerns reflect not only the obvious problem of interrater agreement in classifying child problem behaviors but also questions of how to proceed in helping the child once a diagnosis has been made. That is, does the diagnostic classification have any implication for treatment? Suppose that reliable and valid diagnoses of child psychopathology were available to a therapist. Although these would then permit a designation of treatment targets, other important questions would still remain unanswered: (a) If a category encompasses multiple response excesses and deficits, are some of the components more crucial change targets than others? For example, a particular skill deficit in phobic children might prove to be a "keystone" component of its category—*keystone* in the sense that improvements in that particular deficit are reliably followed by improvements in the other components. (b) Do the categories differ as to the consequences in the environment that control them? This question addresses the stability of child problem behaviors, or the prognosis for change in these behaviors. For example, the same behavior categories for two children might differ in the likelihood that

ROBERT G. WAHLER • Child Behavior Institute, University of Tennessee, Knoxville, TN 37916. **JEAN E. DUMAS** • University of Western Ontario, London, Ontario, Canada NGA 3K7.

they can be changed, depending on the environmental contexts of maintaining contingencies. Thus, for two similarly aggressive children living in quite different environments, different treatment strategies may prove necessary.

The diagnostic issues of reliability, category breadth, and environmental context continue to spur interest in the empirical study of childhood psychopathology. If there is a trend in such study, we would say that the terms *inductive* and *empirical* provide the most appropriate descriptors of current guidelines. It is in this same methodological spirit that we offer a selective look at diagnostic issues as they pertain to children. Our examinations of the literature, along with our own research efforts, lead us to believe that much new information is available on childhood psychopathology as it develops in *family* contexts. Although that information might not be useful to therapeutic agents working in other child environments (e.g., schools and peer groups), we also suspect that these contexts may require selective study in their own right. The following material represents a review of the empirical data on troubled children as they develop in their family contexts. We hope to show that useful categories of psychopathology have been derived, and also that theoretical speculations on developmental processes can be derived from this approach. Although theory has not been a singularly important guideline in the more recent studies of childhood psychopathology, it is unlikely that continued progress in diagnostic classification can result from a purely inductive search strategy. As Barker (1965) pointed out in his summation of behavior ecology research, all investigators segment the "stream of behavior" into units that are derived, at least in part, from the investigator's conceptual bias. Even the most rigorous, "dust bowl" empiricist probably starts the search pattern with some theoretical notion about appropriate unit size. Thus, we think it importnat to spell out our own theoretical bias as an expanded version of the conceptual and methodological guidelines of applied behavior analysis (ABA).

A CONCEPTUAL EXPANSION OF APPLIED BEHAVIOR ANALYSIS (ABA): THE PERSPECTIVE FOR FAMILY CONTEXT IN CHILDHOOD PSYCHOPATHOLOGY

For an in-depth description of applied behavior analysis (ABA), we refer the reader to the classic position paper of Baer, Wolf, and Risley (1968). Our purpose in this section is to outline ABA guidelines as they apply to the study of childhood psychopathology, including some guideline expansions that we think will increase the productivity of such study.

If environmental factors must be included in a useful diagnostic classification of childhood problems, ABA offers appropriate guidance in the diagnostic process. From this viewpoint, the unit of choice includes child behavior *and* its stimulus contingencies. In the choice of this unit, ABA presents its most important conceptual directive: A behavior is significant to the extent that the investigator can demonstrate stimulus control over its occurrences and nonoccurrences. Such a directive will usually bias an observer in two ways: (a) If stimulus control must be demonstrated experimentally, the segment of behavior chosen for this analysis will probably be near the molecular end of the size continuum. A global or molar segment of child behavior (e.g., aggression) would be so widely spread over an environmental setting as to preclude a single experimental manipulation. (b) An unambiguous demonstration of stimulus control usually requires the identification of stimuli in close temporal proximity to the chosen behavioral segment. It stands to reason that causal explanations of behavior control become more difficult as the time lag between a behavior and its manipulated stimulus lengthens.

The choice of molecular behavior segments and their immediate stimulus contingencies is represented in the conceptual model of human development shared by many ABA proponents, namely, operant learning. At present, this model encompasses a three-term contingency that consists of a response and its antecedent and its consequent stimulus. Although response occurrences are determined ultimately by a consequent stimulus (or reinforcer), an antecedent stimulus adds to the response control if it predicts (is discriminative for) the consequent stimulus. That is, some stimuli serve to cue or signal the individual concerning likely outcomes if that person were to emit certain responses. A child's psychological development, then, should be governed by a process in which his or her various responses came into contingent relationships with various environmental stimuli. In this bidirectional process, a child's response repertoire becomes organized as a multitude of independent units, each operating on the basis of its stimulus contingencies. The operant assessor will be inclined to focus on molecular segments of behavior and to examine them in terms of stimulus–response combinations. When response–response associations are considered in assessment, the consideration is fairly selective; responses are considered in combination if they share a common stimulus contingency. If child behavior repertoires are built as operants, these units represent the influence of numerous molecular stimuli, each of which maintains a segment of that repertoire. Thus, the assessor would see little purpose in measuring contextual stimulus patterns; nor would the assessor monitor response interrelationships unless joint stimulus contingencies point to commonalities between or among responses.

A review of operant conceptualizations in applied work with children indicates that some ABA proponents prefer a broader definition of stimulus control than that defined in a three-term contingency. When Bijou and Baer (1961) published their highly influential *Child Development* texts, their conceptual guidelines were primarily Skinnerian. However, the authors also cited J. R. Kantor's *Interbehavioral Psychology* (1959) and attempted to integrate Skinnerian and Kantorian concepts. In reference to child assessment, the most important integration concerned Kantor's concept of the setting event (Bijou & Baer, 1961, p. 17). According to Kantor, setting events add a fourth term to operant contingencies—a term reflecting complex forms of control over other components in the contingency. Although deprivation and satiation operations were cited in Bijou and Baer as principal examples of setting events, it was also noted that social interactions can serve this function for later interactions by the same people.

Perhaps the most concise definition of a setting event is seen in Kantor's description (1959) of the phenomenon as those "immediate circumstances" that influence which of various stimulus–response relationships will occur. The crux of this definition is the stimulus control exercised by these "immediate circumstances." Given that a setting event materialized in the form of some quiet, peaceful interchange between child and parent, later interchanges involving these people might be predicted. For example, if father and child conclude a story-reading episode, it is likely that their next interchange will bear some similarity to the episode. More than likely, the pair will engage one another in passive style as opposed to assertive interchanges. This is tantamount to saying that the short-term stimulus control produced in the three-term operant contingency is partially governed by a setting event. Thus, an assessment geared to selective coverage of a child response and its immediate antecedent and its consequent stimuli could provide an incomplete picture of how that response is maintained.

Examples of setting-event control of operant contingencies are not yet commonplace in the ABA literature but are certainly available (see Wahler & Graves, 1983). Setting-event control even further removed in time from targeted parent–child interactions was depicted in correlational analyses by Wahler (1980). In this study, mothers' self-reported exchanges with friends were shown to predict reductions in their aversive child interactions occurring hours later. These examples certainly illustrate the possibility of stimulus control well beyond the "microstructure" so favored by traditional ABA proponents. By including setting events as a fourth term in the operant contingency, assessment guidelines in ABA must expand to include the environmental context in which these more molecular units are assessed.

More recent experimental analyses of setting-event control also create problems for traditional ABA explanations of stimulus control. Fowler and Baer (1981) and Simon, Ayllon, and Milan (1986) documented that changes in reinforcement schedules can function as setting events exerting stimulus control on child behavior in environments *not contingently related* to the reinforcement schedules. These rather puzzling effects illustrate the possibility that setting events may induce stable child–environment interactions that are only randomly connected with the setting events. These studies show that reinforcement control over a child's responses in one environment may also control that child's behavior in a second environment. Thus, preschool children in Fowler and Baer (1981) were shown to increase their sharing with peers in a free-play setting after a reinforcement schedule for sharing was made ambiguous in an earlier independent-play setting. Children in the Simon *et al.* (1986) study doubled their rate of schoolwork in one school classroom when reinforcement for schoolwork was eliminated in two other classrooms. If a child's various responses can covary dependably within and across environments *without* sharing some common stimulus contingency, then an assessor should not feel compelled to find such contingencies before examining response interrelationships. In other words, the setting-event conception requires a broadened view of response networks, just as it requires a broadened view of environmental networks. In our viewpoint, the *four*-term operant contingency provides some very useful guidelines in the study of childhood psychopathology.

Consider the implications of an expanded operant model with respect to family contexts and the psychological problems of children. The applied behavior analyst will seek to understand the child's problems as response classes marked by behavior excesses (e.g., fighting) and deficits (e.g., lack of sustained attention). In addition, because the behaviors are thought to be influenced by contiguous stimuli, the ABA diagnostician is likely to observe the reactions of parents and siblings when the child manifests his or her response style. In essence, dyadic interchanges between the target child and other family members would be considered the units of immediate diagnostic interest. However, in accepting a fourth term in the operant contingencies, these dyadic units are to be understood as figural parts of a larger, more fundamental unit in family operations. Each member in a dyadic exchange has also taken part in other exchanges within and outside the family. Because these "setting-event" experiences may well influence the functional quality of any dyadic exchange, it is reasonable to consider their influence in a triangular relationship with each member of a dyad. If such triads are to constitute the basic units of social exchange, one must recognize a quantum jump in complexity with regard to the unit paradigm. As we outlined earlier, the setting-event pole of a triad *does not* function as a simple discriminative stimulus by predicting reinforcement probabilities in the dyad. For example, a mother's abusive treatment of her noncompliant child may be worsened following arguments between her own mother and herself. But although the arguments are shown to predict her more abusive interchanges with her child, these setting events *do not* predict the child's contribution to the abuse exchanges (in contrast to the more complete predictive function of a discriminative stimulus). That is, the child's likelihood of provoking maternal abuse does not covary with the presence or absence of the mother's setting-event experiences. Although the mother acts *as if* her child's provocation is directly linked to the setting event, there is, in fact, no such link (see Wahler & Graves, 1983).

At present, there are no satisfactory explanations of setting-event functions based on the operating strategies of ABA. Unless one chooses to rely on hypothetical processes in understanding human behavior (see Chapter 4, by Robinson & Jacobson), ABA proponents must be content with a purely *descriptive* account of this phenomenon. Following the guidelines of this incomplete paradigm, the ABA diagnostician will be as interested in the contextual features of family interchanges as in the more figural dyad. Context, considered broadly as a third pole of any dyad, presents a formidable measurement task if one is to rely exclusively on the direct observation of molecular events—the favored methodology of ABA. Although there are certainly practical reasons to retain this measurement bias (i.e., the feasibility of the experimental manipulation of events), a shift to self-reports by the family participants does not violate ABA strategies as long as the reports can meet the usual reliability criteria of natural science. By then adopting self-report methods, as well as direct observation, the measurement of triads becomes feasible. Of course, once a dependable setting-event function is demonstrated through correlational analyses of the measures, the ABA diagnostician would wish to obtain a more molecular picture of the event in question.

Contextual stimuli in families have been assessed as demographic characteristics (e.g., income and parent education), parent self-reports about distress (e.g., depression), and parent self-reports about particular environmental experiences (e.g., conversations with friends) (see Griest & Wells, 1983). An often-favored view of such stimuli as they impinge on trouble families is seen in the term *life stressors,* those contextual events likely to influence pathological dyadic exchanges in a family. Some of these stressors, although reliably measured, are so global in content or stable in function as to preclude useful information for the ABA therapist (e.g., parent income and parent depression). But as assessment research has shown, the utility may lie in viewing these stressors as marker variables pointing the assessor to other, more manipulable events. For example, maternal self-reports of depression have been shown to function as setting events in the mother's judgments about her problem child (Griest, Wells, & Forehand, 1979). Then, Panaccopone and Wahler (1985) discovered that maternal depression was correlated with maternal reports about coercive interchanges with the spouse and/or with extended-family members. In addition, it was found that these interchanges served as setting events for the mother's child behavior judgments. Thus, maternal depression appears to be a marker variable for the diagnostician; its utility in assessment is to point the clinician to more molecular setting events in the family context.

In the course of assessment research based on a triadic unit of family functioning, some regularities have emerged with respect to troubled children and deviant families. We think that a case can be made for a developmental view of child problem behavior as emerging within two broadly construed processes of triadic function: coercion and neglect. Both processes refer to parent–child dyadic patterns of interchange that are marked either by aversive means of mutual control or by mutual indifference. At this point in our understanding of these processes, it would appear that the parent—the mother, in particular—is "triangulated" by a temperamentally difficult infant (too fussy or too passive) and a community of adults (e.g., her spouse and the extended family) who are likewise nonsupportive and/or aversive in their styles of response to her. Depending on how the mother reacts to these community stressors (irritable or passive responses) and what her infant's temperament amounts to (irritable or passive), we would predict the emergence of four classes of child problem behavior. These classes, overt and covert forms of conduct and dependency behaviors, seem to be associated with the unfortunate child-care styles of coercion and neglect. These maternal caretaking styles, in turn, seem to be influenced by the community context and the more figural infant behaviors just described. This chapter is geared to a description of the classes of childhood problems and our speculations on the processes leading to the development of these problems. We will begin with the descriptions.

MAJOR CLASSES OF CHILDHOOD DISORDERS: CONDUCT AND DEPENDENCY PROBLEMS

The majority of assessment findings in childhood psychopathology are based on adult summary reports of child behavior (see review by Quay, 1979). Although these judgments by parents and teachers do not therefore meet the molecular preferences of ABA, the measures do meet some fairly stringent psychometric criteria. Many checklist-type reports have been shown to be reliable (see Achenbach & Edelbrock, 1979), and their validity has been demonstrated in a number of ways. For example, when children are grouped into normal and deviant categories on the basis of parent and teacher reports, these groups also differ in intelligence test performance, academic achievement, and mental-health-center referrals (Eisenberg, Gersten, Langer, McCarthy, & Simcha-Fagan, 1976; Prior Boulton, Gayzago, & Perry, 1975). Thus, the summary-report measurement units that we are about to discuss are empirically well anchored. It is important to note, however, that few validity studies have focused on the molecular, direct observation covariates of these adult reports.

The studies that we found produced inconsistent relationships between the adult summary reports and the direct observational measures. Hendricks (1972) sampled mothers' summary reports of their children's conduct problem behaviors through a bipolar adjective checklist and then intercorrelated these ratings with home-based direct observations of the children. Maternal ratings were found to correlate significantly with the eight aggression codes of the Patterson, Ray, Shaw, and Cobb (1969) observation system (Pearson r's ranged from .46 to .54; $\bar{x} r = .49$). Using more specific parental ratings of children's daily conduct problems, Patterson (1974) found these ratings to correlate .69 ($p < .05$) with a composite index of the aggression codes in the Patterson *et al.* (1969) system. In support of these correlational findings, Durlak, Stein, and Mannarino (1980) examined relationships between teachers' ratings of their students' conduct problems and later direct observations of the students' in-class behaviors with the Wahler, House, and Stambaugh (1976) observation codes. When the children were grouped into high, medium, and low conduct problems based on the teachers' ratings, the aggression codes were five times more likely to appear in the high group than in the low group. Furthermore, a stepwise multiple-linear-regression analysis revealed that four of the direct observation codes accounted for approximately half of the variance in teacher ratings (multiple $R = .70$). The four codes, in order of predictive power, concerned the children's off-task behavior, approach to the teacher, and being out of sight of the observer, and the teacher's attention to the children.

Unfortunately, when Eyberg and Johnson (1974) compared parent daily ratings of child conduct problems with a revised version of the Patterson *et al.* (1969) observation system, these measures showed little convergence over the course of a home treatment program. Although the parent ratings revealed improvement in 94% of the children, the direct observations showed change in only 41% of the sample. Similarly, Forehand, Wells, and Griest (1980) found a lack of convergence in parent ratings and direct observations of child behavior using the Forehand coding system. In this study, the observational measures depicted behavior change over treatment, but the parent reports showed no change. Adding to these inconsistent findings, Forehand, Wells, and Griest (1980) compared pre- and posttreatment changes using Forehand's codes and two types of parent ratings systems. The results for 20 clinic-referred children showed consistent improvements in all three assessment measures. However, when the change scores from the three measures were later intercorrelated, there were no relationships across the different measurement systems. In other words, although the children as a group looked similar in terms of change on the ratings and observations, there was little day-to-day stability across these two sets of measures. Finally, in a school classroom study by Green, Beck, Forehand, and Vosk (1983), teacher ratings of children as conduct problems or normals were supported by direct observational differences in negative peer interactions between the groups. However, a second problem group composed of children said to be withdrawn on the basis of teacher ratings could not be differentiated from the normal group on the basis of the observational findings.

All in all, there is reason to believe that direct observational assessment of troubled children may yield a somewhat different picture from that produced by parent and teacher summary reports. Although both pictures can stand alone in terms of their respective psychometric qualities, one should not conclude that these assessment modes always tap the same aspects of child–environment interchanges. Thus, after we complete the following review and interpretation of parent summary report data, a different viewpoint, based on direct observational findings, will be presented.

Parent Ratings of Childhood Problems

A number of standardized checklists are available for research and clinical use, and a few of these have become popular choices for the systematic study of psychopathology. Of these latter devices, the Behavior Problem Checklist (BPC—Quay & Peterson, 1975), the Child Behavior Profile (CBP—Achenbach, 1979), and the Conners Parent Rating Scale (Goyette, Conners, & Ulrich, 1978) are frequently used in the research field.

When parental reports on standardized checklists are factor-analyzed, two global patterns typically emerge. One of these, which we choose to label *conduct problems,* summarizes a child's propensity to violate parent rules through assertive or passive behaviors. The second pattern, construed by us as *dependency problems,* summarizes a child's avoidance of general social contact by maintaining proximity to a parent or an apparent lack of interest in other people. These patterns have also been variously labeled as "undercontrolled" versus "overcontrolled" (Achenbach & Edelbrock, 1979) or "aggression" versus "inhibition" (Miller, 1967).

One also sees in our own summary descriptions of these patterns that two subcategories may be considered within each of the two global categories. Within the conduct problem pattern, the rule-violating children may commit their transgressions in overt or assertive ways, such as assaulting another person, or they may do so by covert or more passive means, such as stealing. Similarly, within the dependency problem pattern, nonsocial children may actively or overtly avoid social contact, such as by clinging to a parent and crying, or they may do so by covert or passive means, such as ignoring the approaches of other people. In effect, the overtly dependent child "demands" a selectively isolated relationship with certain adults, whereas the covertly dependent child may be equally isolated through social disinterest.

Although the subcategories show considerable overlap, their differences also stand out in factor-analytic studies. Thus, when Edelbrock and Achenbach (1980) administered the CBP to parents of clinic-referred children (ages 6–11; 1,050 boys and 500 girls), the parent reports fell into the expected conduct versus dependency groups, each of which could be broken into smaller groups. The boys who were grouped into conduct problems ("externalizing") appeared to be of two types, one reflecting on overt, active, disruptive pattern ("hyperactive") and the other reflecting the violation of family and community standards ("delinquent"). Although this latter type was said to sometimes commit their violations in assertive ways, many of the descriptions centered on covert behaviors such as stealing and running away. The dependency problem boys ("internalizing") were represented by four clusters reflecting both social withdrawal ("schizoid") and complaints ("somatic" and "depression"). The girls were not so clearly described as conduct or dependency problems, as about 10% had descriptors referring to both problem types. As was true of the conduct problem boys, "externalizing" girls presented behavior problems of an assertive, disruptive type ("hyperactive" and "aggressive-cruel") or a more covert type ("delinquent"). Similarly, the dependency problem girls were described as presenting combinations of withdrawal and complaining ("somatic" and "depression") behaviors.

Reviews of the parent rating literature have consistently supported the two general problem categories of child behavior just described (see Anthony, 1970). In addition, the overt-covert subcategories are rather consistently apparent, at least within the conduct problem category (see Quay, 1979). Our view of a similar dichotomy within the dependency problem category is less apparent. Although the obtained clusters encompassing this global factor do indeed include both overt (fears, complaints, and clinging) and covert (withdrawal, apathy, and social lack of interest) descriptors, they do not consistently fall into dichotomous groupings. Thus, in the Goyette, Conners, and Ulrich (1978) factor analysis of parent reports (Connors Rating Scale) on a normative (nonproblem) sample of children (mean age 9.9 years), the above descriptors of dependency problems were represented in two factors. However, one factor was comprised of somatic complaint descriptors ("psychosomatic"), and the other included fears, worries, and social withdrawal ("anxiety"). In comparison, Gersten, Langer, Eisenberg, Simcha-Fagan, and McCarthy (1976), using their own parent rating questionnaire with a normative sample (ages 6–18), found overt and covert groupings labeled, respectively, "regressive anxiety" and "isolation." Factor analyses also separated conduct problems into overt ("fighting" and "conflict with parents") and covert ("delinquency"—truancy, running away, and lying) descriptors. In addition, Gersten *et al.* (1976) provided longitudinal and cross-sectional analyses concerning the stability of the parent report categories. As expected from previous research (Robins, 1966), the conduct problems (conflict with parents, fighting, and delinquency) were likely to persist, particularly from ages 10 to 14. The least stable category concerned our overt dependency grouping (regressive anxiety), followed by its more covert associate (isolation). Interestingly enough, both of these dependency groupings showed increased stability within the adolescent years.

A further distinction between the adult rating-scale categories of conduct and dependency problems centers on some implicit "motivational" judgments about these children by labeling conduct problem children as impulsive, angry, and selfish, and dependency problem children as anxious, fearful, and schizoid. These labels do imply that two rather distinctively different motivational sources are assigned to these children by researchers. We found frequent references to conduct problem children as "unable to delay gratification," "acting out," or "psychopathic"—terms that imply a decidedly goal-oriented motivation. On the other hand, we found explanations of dependency problem children in terms such as "neurotic," "unable to separate from parent," and "guilt ridden"—all of which emphasize an avoidant class of motivation. The motivational biases concerning these children are most clearly seen in validity studies of parent ratings.

Borkovec (1970) suspected that dependency-problem children ought to demonstrate higher levels of autonomic-nervous-system arousal than would be true of conduct-problem children. In fact, clinic-referred children classified as dependent (Behavior Problem Checklist—Quay & Peterson, 1975) demonstrated significantly higher galvanic skin responses to tone stimuli than did conduct-problem children. In another study, Brown and Quay (1977) assessed the "impulsive" characteristics of conduct-problem children, assuming that they would respond faster and make more errors than normal children on a task requiring the matching of various stimuli. The results confirmed this expectation in that clinically referred conduct-problem children made significantly more errors on the task, although their response times were not shorter. Ellis (1982) argued that the impulsive, often antisocial actions of conduct-problem children are due to an absence of "empathy," a capacity to view or observe oneself in reference to others. The investigator then administered an empathy questionnaire to adjudicated delinquents (ages 12–18) and an age-matched group of normals. As predicted, the delinquents obtained significantly lower empathy scores, and within the delinquent sample, the overt problem types (e.g., assault) scored lower than did the covert types (e.g., theft). Finally, when Breit (1982) studied child referrals (ages 1–12) to an outpatient psychiatric clinic, she found a clear correspondence between mother ratings of the children (Louisville Behavior Checklist—Miller, 1973) and therapist motivational statements about the children's problems. Children rated by their mothers as dependent were also classified by therapists as "fearful" (in 86.1% of the cases). On the other hand, children rated by mothers as presenting conduct problems were likely to be judged *low* in fearful qualities by the therapists (in 76.9% of the cases).

In summary, there appears to be congruence among parents, teachers, and mental health agents in their summary ratings of disturbed children. These adults seem to agree in dividing most problem children into conduct and dependency categories and to have reasonable but more variable agreement on subdividing the two groupings into overt and covert types. With these categories as anchor points, there are further points of congruence. The conduct-problem children are also rated as less skillful in school-related tasks and in their social relationships with peers and adults than are the dependency-problem children. In addition, these latter children are judged to be motivated by avoidance processes, whereas their conduct-problem counterparts are seen as influenced by approach processes. We now turn to a review of these child problem categories from the perspective of direct observational assessment.

Direct Observation of Childhood Problems

In our review of the literature, we discovered that most direct observational assessments of troubled children have focused on conduct-problem children. In family settings, we could not find a single study that dealt with the naturalistic assessment of dependency-problem children. Fortunately, these children have received a fair amount of research attention in preschool and early-elementary-school settings. Thus, although the following comparisons are flawed by an absence of studies to contrast our two major problem categories in family settings, the two have been contrasted in school settings. Nevertheless, because of the importance we attach to the setting-specific nature of child psychopathology, we felt it necessary to conduct our own family-based comparison study. Although this single study is scarcely a drop in the empirical bucket of direct observational norms, we think the data add substance to the following speculations.

Naturalistic assessment of troubled children, like parent and teacher rating assessment, has been based on some popular measurement devices. These devices or coding systems enable the recording of several aspects of a child's behavior and of the behavior of his of her interaction partners (parents, teachers, siblings, and peers). The most commonly used system, called the Family Interaction Coding System (FICS—Patterson *et al.*, 1969; Reid, 1978), has an impressive documentation of its reliability and validity (see Patterson, 1977). Systems developed more recently by Forehand, King, Peed, and Yoder (1975), Wahler *et al.* (1976), and Burgess and Conger (1978) have also seen frequent use and have fared reasonably well in their respective psychometric evaluations. In school settings, the system described by Hartup, Glazer, and Charlesworth (1967) appears to be as popular as the Patterson *et al.* (1969) home system. In addition, the more recently derived codes reported by Greenwood, Walker, Todd, and Hops (1979) and by Strain, Shores, and Kerr (1976) are commonly used.

When clinic-referred children are described by their parents as troubled because of conduct-problem behaviors, one can be "reasonably" certain that an objective observer will see a predictable behavior pattern in the child's home. Comparisons of these children with matched controls indicate that the conduct-problem children are significantly more likely to tease, yell, noncomply, command in negative ways, disapprove, humiliate, and be physically negative (Patterson, & Cobb, 1971). Similar investigations by researchers using different coding systems lend support to this comparison (Delfini, Bernal, & Rosen, 1976; Horne, 1981; Lobitz & Johnson, 1975). In one study (Reid & Hendriks, 1973), the distinction between overt and covert forms of conduct problems was added to the normative comparisons. Clinic-referred children who stole, but who were nonaggressive, and who were classified solely as presenting problems in aggression, were compared with normal children. The results of these direct observations showed the overt-problem children to produce significantly higher rates of coercive behavior at home (Patterson *et al.*, 1969, observation coding system) than normals. The covert-problem children, however, could not be distinguished from the normals *or* the overt sample (stealers produced coercive rates midway between the other two samples). In Patterson's replication of this study (1982, p. 252), mean differences between these three groups did prove significant. Stealers behaved in a more coercive manner than normals, but in a less coercive manner than did the overtly aggressive children. These two studies also found that the problem children exhibited significantly fewer instances of prosocial behaviors such as cooperative play and work. Thus, the skill deficiency characteristics of conduct-problem children, described in the previous section of this paper, are also confirmed.

Perhaps the most fascinating aspect of the above comparisons concerns differences in how these children interact with their parents. Such differences bear on the "motivational" issue discussed earlier and the stimulus control issue presented still earlier within our applied-behavior-analysis model of assessment. Comparative studies indicate that mothers of conduct-problem children are significantly more aversive in their child-directed behaviors (Lobitz & Johnson, 1975; Patterson & Cobb, 1971) than are mothers of nonproblem children. More interesting still is the finding that conduct-problem children tend to respond to these maternal aversive stimuli by *increased* coercive behavior. In other words, the children act as if maternal yelling, disapproving, and hitting are positive reinforcers; their coercive behaviors, when following the maternal aversive stimuli, are likely to recur immediately. Patterson and Cobb (1971) and Kopfstein (1972) found this phenomenon in conduct-problem children, but not in normal children, and *only* in reference to these children's coercive actions. When the latter children's prosocial responses were followed by maternal aversive stimuli, a suppressive outcome was observed.

These findings led Patterson (1976) to formulate a "punishment acceleration" hypothesis to account for the high rates of coercive behaviors commonly seen in families of conduct-problem children. Accordingly, the rates may be due to "bursts" or sustained episdoes of child coercive responding, triggered by aversive social stimuli offered by family members. Presumably, these episodes of coercive interchange have some ultimate consequence that is predictable and reinforcing for any particular conduct-problem child (e.g., the mother's positive behavior or the mother's termination of her aversive responding). Although the process explanation of this burst phenomenon is debatable, the Patterson findings provide a reasonably solid descriptive answer to the stimulus control or motivational question: The coercive behavior of conduct-problem children appears to be closely tied to contiguous aversive stimuli offered by their mothers.

It was noted earlier that conduct-problem children have been shown to be deficient in prosocial behaviors, compared to normal children (e.g., Lobitz & Johnson, 1975). This finding is consistent with the parent rating data and does not constitute much of a surprising outcome. It is also evident from the observational studies that the organization of a child's prosocial behaviors with respect to his or her problem behaviors is sometimes predictable. These organizational properties refer to the previously outlined response interrelationship issue: the well-documented covariations among the responses comprising a child's behavior repertoire (see Kazdin's 1982 review). In the case of conduct-problem children, one broadly construed prosocial response, compliance with adult instructions, appears to stand as a "keystone" element in the organization of these repertoires. In virtually every observational study we surveyed, children who hit, teased, screamed, stole, or produced other components of the conduct-problem class were also children who were unlikely to comply with parental instructions. In fact, two intervention studies (Russo, Cataldo, & Cushing, 1981; Witman, Hurley, Johnson, & Christian, 1978) have demonstrated the functional properties of this inverse relationship between a deviant child's compliance and problem behaviors. When these investigators increased the likelihood of compliance in problem children, collateral reductions in the children's problem actions became evident. These findings are consistent with Patterson's hierarchical ranking (1982, pp. 250–251) of clinic-referred children who were noncompliant, told lies, stole, and set fires. Compared to the overall means across children who exhibit these conduct-problem behaviors, the probability of finding combinations of problem behaviors in children was revealing from a behavioral organization perspective. For example, although the base rate of fire setting in Patterson's sample was .23, its probability of occuring in those children who stole was .32. As expected, compliance appeared in this probability progression as a very obvious deficiency.

In closing this section on conduct-problem children, it is important to realize that observational evidence of behavioral deviance is not *always* found in these clinic-referred children. Even in the previously reviewed studies that reported different family interactions for conduct-problem and normal children, considerable overlap was generally obvious in the observational score distributions for the problem and normal groups (Delfini *et al.*, 1976; Griest *et al.*, 1979; Lobitz & Johnson, 1975). For instance, Forehand, Wells, and Griest (1980) were able to distinguish a group of mothers whose children behaved normally under home observation conditions, even though the mothers insisted on classifying the children as conduct problems. When Rikard *et al.* (1981) compared these mothers with another group whose clinic-referred children *did* demonstrate the expected deviance profile, the former mothers also described themselves as significantly more depressed on the Beck Depression Inventory. This lack of convergence between parent reports and observed child behavior was discussed in the previous section on parent ratings, and it constitutes a validity problem for both sets of measures. The fact that Forehand's research group was able to isolate some of these "false positives" (based on observation) in clinic referrals points to one of the major factors that contribute to the complexity of childhood assessment: the role of situational or setting factors in the occurrences of child and parent behavior and in the reports about such behavior. These factors will be discussed in the final section of this chapter.

Much of the observational research on dependency-problem children has been done in school settings, primarily within playground or other free-play subsettings. In most cases, the chosen child's problem description would fit our criteria for the covert dependency category. That is, the children have been viewed as needing help because of their withdrawn or isolated status with reference to their peers. For the most part, investigators appear to have been interested in evaluating the skill deficiencies of these children, instead of comparing them with conduct-problem children. Although some of these children might be labeled as anxious or phobic as well, their initial label has typically been limited to the global category *withdrawn*.

When teachers describe a child as withdrawn, objective observers do not find the same degree of behavioral consistency that is exhibited by conduct-problem referrals. One source of inconsistency concerns the problem child's rate of social interaction with peers. When Gottman (1977) used a modeling film to increase the social interaction rates of isolated preschool children, these increases were *not* accompanied by qualitative improvements (positive interchanges) or higher peer ratings in popularity. Greenwood *et al.* (1979) found that low-rated preschool interactors were judged by their teachers to be more deficient in verbal and social skills than their higher-rated counterparts. Likewise, Greenwood, Todd, Hopps, and Walker (1982) discovered that low-rated preschool interactors also demonstrated qualitatively different styles of social interaction: they initiated fewer interactions, received fewer peer approaches, were less verbal, and interacted more with adults. Actually, Gottman's findings appear to be more relevant to therapeutic issues than to natural covariations between the problem children's interaction rates and the quality of their interchanges. As Gottman, Gonso, and Schuler (1976) documented in another intervention study, treated children did not differ from controls in total interaction rate but did change interaction partners. From our assessment viewpoint, the Greenwood–Gottman findings appear compatible. Withdrawn children display certain interpersonal characteristics along with their low interaction rates. However, in looking further along the diagnostic track, appropriate intervention targets for these children (total rate vs. specific behaviors) are debatable.

Additional inspection of the naturalistic observational studies yields findings congruent with the adult ratings of dependency-problem children. Children labeled as withdrawn by their teachers are more likely to interact with adults (Strain & Shores, 1977) and, in contrast to conduct-problem children, are unlikely to engage others in a coercive manner (Gottman, 1977; Greenwood *et al.*, 1982). The "likability" of these children, compared to that of conduct-problem children, may also be inferred from observed peer responses in the above studies. Greenwood *et al.* (1982) found that aversive peer approaches to withdrawn children almost never occurred; rather, over 80% of the stimuli offered by peers were positive. Similarly, Green *et al.* (1983) discovered aversive peer interactions to be the *only* significant difference between teacher-nominated conduct- and dependency-problem (withdrawn) children. Once again, aversive techniques involving the latter children were very rare.

The motivational issue of social avoidance presented is difficult to address in these observational studies. Most of the coding systems did not include a "retreat" measure, and their child-aversive behavior measures could not be separated into aggressive (e.g., hit) versus distress (e.g., cry) measures. The most we can conclude from the above studies is that low-rate peer interactors are significantly less likely to reciprocate positive peer initiations than are higher-rate interactors. In essence, the motivational picture presented by the problem children seems to be one of lack of interest more than one of fear or avoidance. However, because the referrals centered on descriptors of withdrawal and isolation (covert dependency), these findings might be expected.

Kendall, Deardorff, Finch, and Graham (1976) reported one of the few observational studies in which avoidance measures were used in assessing referred problem children. In addition, the referral descriptors focused on overt dependency problems (anxiety neurosis and depressive neurosis) rather than on the more covert withdrawal descriptions. Two clinic-referred groups (overt conduct problems and overt dependency problems) and a group of normal controls were evaluated on an approach measure in terms of interpersonal distance from the peer confederate. In addition, all the children completed two self-report inventories measuring anxiety and locus of control. The results were surprising. The anxiety self-report measure and the child problem category proved to be unrelated to the children's observed approach distance. Both conduct-problem and dependency-problem children stayed a significantly greater distance from the peer than did normals. In addition, locus of control correlated with interpersonal distance in that children scoring high in external control kept a further distance than those scoring low on this measure. However, there were no differences between normal and problem children on the locus-of-control measure. Similar findings were reported by Weinstein (1965). Thus, from the standpoint of psychopathology, these observational studies shed little light on motivational differences in the two categories of overt-problem children.

Because we were unable to locate observational studies of how dependency-problem children behave in family settings, we decided to pursue the question by comparing previous clinic referrals to our research group (Child Behavior Institute, Knoxville, Tennessee). By examining intake interview records from 1979 through March 1983, it was possible to extract at least five children representing each of the four problem subcategories. These referral categories were relatively "pure" in terms of parent descriptors of child behavior. Because a number of other children in the referral list were said to demonstrate *both* overt and covert conduct problems, we decided to establish a fifth group called *mixed conduct problems* (after Loeber & Schmaling, 1986). The ages of the children in the five groups were comparable ($\bar{X} = 6.5$ years).

Table 1 summarizes the statistically significant group differences in 12 ob-

TABLE 1. Four Categories of Aversive Behavior Produced by 25 Clinic-Referred Children over 150 Baseline Observation Sessions (6 per Child) Conducted in the Children's Homes[a]

Referral group (5 per group)	Observation code level			
	Complaint	Opposition	Rule violation	Aversive opposition
Mixed conduct (MX)	16.05	9.31	4.06	4.37
Overt conduct (OC)	5.65	4.38	3.53	.86
Overt dependent (OD)	4.60	2.56	2.85	.48
Covert dependent (CD)	3.71	1.38	.30	.00
Covert conduct (CC)	1.13	.67	.03	.00
ANOVA, $df = 24,4$	$(F = 5.01c)$	$(F = 3.30b)$	$(F = 3.09b)$	$(F = 4.75c)$
Paired comparisons	MC > OC, OD, CD, CC; OC > CC	MC > OD, CD, CC; OC > CD, CC; OD > CC	MC > CD, CC; OC > CD, CC; OD > CC	MC > OC, OD, CD, DD; OC > CD, CC

[a]The children's baseline scores are presented as mean percentage occurrences for five child groupings. The groupings are based on referral descriptions. Although 12 behavior categories were examined, only the 4 shown above yielded significant differences between groups.
[b]$p < .05$
[c]$p < .01$

servational codes derived from the Wahler *et al.* (1976) coding system. Only the four coercive codes in Table 1 discriminated between groups. This finding indicates that the children did not differ in their overall social participation (three codes), independent activities (three codes), and autistic-like behaviors (two codes). This table suggests that most of the group differences resulted from the fact that the mixed and overt conduct-problem children acted more coercively than the other groups. The overt dependent group could not be distinguished from the overt conduct group, but the former proved to be more coercive than the covert conduct group. Perhaps the most consistent feature of the group rankings in Table 1 concerns the low incidence of coercive responding by both covert problem groups. These children were never observed to use physical force (aversive opposition) and rarely violated parental rules (rule violation). Only in their verbal complaints and noncompliance with parental instructions (opposition) did they show any semblence of coercive action. It is also evident that the two overt problem groups were similarly coercive on all four measures, and that the mixed conduct-problem group behaved quite differently in comparison with all other groups (see Loeber & Schmaling, 1986, for further discussion of this deviant group).

In summary, it seems obvious from our review of observational findings that little is known about the behaviors of dependency-problem children, particularly in family settings. In school settings, the covert subgroup appears withdrawn and uninterested in peer social contact, but the overt subgroup looks similar to the overt conduct-problem children. The other point of similarity in these overt-problem subgroupings concerns the motivational questions raised previously. There is little evidence to support a distinction between the groups in terms of social avoidance (anxiety). In contrast to the apparent social lack of interest of the covert dependent children, their overtly dependent counterparts appear to be motivated through social approach processes in much the same fashion as the overt conduct-problem children.

DEVELOPMENTAL SPECULATIONS I: PARENTAL ACCEPTANCE, CONTROL, AND CONSISTENCY

This section represents a speculative attempt to account for the role that the family plays in the development and maintenance of childhood conduct and dependency problems. This account focuses on both direct and indirect influences on child behavior and examines the role that children themselves may play in the development of their own psychopathologies. In other words, an attempt is made to discuss not only the family variables that presumably affect children directly (e.g., parental approval or disapproval), but also the contextual or setting variables that are believed to influence children indirectly, through their impact on caregivers (e.g., social isolation and marital conflict). Furthermore, the discussion assumes that children play an active role in the development of their own psychopathologies, and it examines the child variables generally associated with such development. We want to emphasize that the material that follows is speculative. It is presented here in an attempt to generate discussion and to stimulate research and not to summarize a set of well-established findings. We trust that it will be read in this spirit.

Coercion and Neglect

Our developmental speculations are set within the expanded ABA model presented earlier and are supported by data derived from parent ratings and direct observations. Specifically, we assume that two related developmental processes underlie the acquisition and maintenance of the pathological behavior patterns described in the previous section. One of these processes, called *coercion*, is defined as a person's attempt to modify the behavior of others in the course of day-to-day interactions in ways that are advantageous to that person but that are generally perceived as aversive by others. This commonly seen interchange pattern can, unfortunately, lead to *coercive entrapment*, in which two or more persons have learned to control each other's behavior by exchanging high rates of aversive responses. It is essential to note that the vast majority of these responses are not major events of crisis proportion. Rather, they are responses that, when considered in isolation, are rather innocuous (e.g., crying and yelling) but that can have disastrous cumulative effects when they are exchanged at a high rate by family members (Patterson, 1982).

In contrast to coercion, the process of *neglect* describes a chronic absence of interchange between two or more people who are members of a common group (a family). Whether these people report a dislike of one another of a lack of personal interest, their interpersonal style is the same: a low rate of social contact with each other. As in the case of coercion, the impact of *chronic neglect* on the people involved is cumulative and can be equally disastrous in terms of retarded skill development and motivation (Rothchild & Wolf, 1976). In addition, the affected group members are apt to look outside the group for approval, thus further diminishing the functional impact of the group on each individual.

Our definitions of coercive entrapment and chronic neglect put the emphasis not on the outward characteristic of conduct-problem and dependent children, but on the functional value of these behaviors to the children who display them. Although there are obvious differences in the topographies of these behaviors, they are assumed to share a dimension of functional versus neutral properties: some are aversive attempts to exercise *control* over the behavior of significant members of the environment, and others share a nonfunctional lack of control. In reference to the former response class, we view the regular crying episodes of an anxious or timid child as serving the same purpose and as being as aversive to other family members as the daily tantrums of a more aggressive or defiant counterpart. A less aversive class of responses—marked by withdrawl and apathy, on the one hand, and stealing and drug use, on the other—is thought to stem from an absence of control within the family. That is, a child's withdrawal is a likely product of parental neglect and permits the child's unchecked entry into other spheres of environmental influence (e.g., stealing).

Although the behavioral influences of coercion and neglect are quite different, the two processes often operate hand in hand. Coercive entrapment between people has been shown to be associated with a variety of interpersonal and intrapersonal phenomena. The participants are apt to report feelings of depression and low self-esteem (Feshbach, 1970; Patterson, 1980), and the quality of their social relationships may deteriorate as the entrapment continues (Parke, 1970). In terms of this latter outcome, a lower number of positive interchanges have been observed between coercively entrapped mothers and their children than between normals (Burgess & Conger, 1978). In addition, mothers who report personal entrapment with adults are likely to display an insensitive mode of infant care (Crockenberg, 1981). Thus, the relationship between coercive entrapment and neglect can extend beyond the boundaries of a dysfunctional parent–child relationship. If coercive entrapment leads the participants into dysphoric mood states, a generalized insensitivity to others may be expected. A depressed mother, regardless of how she developed this mood state, often proves to be an inattentive caretaker (Griest, Wells, & Forehand, 1979). As we will argue in the forthcoming material on family correlates of psychopathology, such insensitivity or inattentiveness may be equivalent to what has often been called *parental inconsistency*.

As we present our arguments for a coercion–neglect model, it will become apparent that we will use its hypotheses to account for differences between children's *overt* and *covert* problem behaviors. In our review of observational data on childhood psychopathology, we found reason to view overt conduct and dependency problems as functionally similar. Granted that the two categories consistute very different risk likelihoods in terms of future problem development, their more immediate functions as coercive behaviors set them together as a response class. We think that this commonality is important with respect to the treatment purposes of a diagnostic system—and it is with this purpose in mind that we dwell on the common functions of overt conduct and dependency behaviors. On the other side of this functional relationship, covert forms of the above behaviors are viewed as similar. We intend to present arguments for a developmental process in which parental neglect leads a child to lose interest in that parent and, in some cases, to look elsewhere for social involvement. Once again, there are many differences between the covert forms of conduct and dependency problems. But for treatment purposes, we think it important to assess their commonalities as behaviors linked to patterns of maladaptive parenting.

The database for the above conclusions is sparse and is limited to the few relevant findings reviewed earlier. However, if we also consider the developmental research on parental involvement in childhood aggression and dependency, further relevant information is made available. Although the information does not bear on the covert-overt distinctions, it does permit conclusions on relationships between conduct and dependency problems. Following this section, we will return to the covert-overt issue.

Family Correlates of Childhood Psychopathology

Any review of the literature on the relationship between family interaction and childhood psychopathology is necessarily affected by several methodological limitations. Although most of these limitations apply to the developmental literature in general and are well presented elsewhere (e.g., Achenbach, 1979; Hetherington & Martin, 1979), two of them are mentioned here because of their considerable impact on any conclusion we may draw from this review. The first and, we believe, the fundamental limitation of the literature is that it is essentially *noninteractive*. Although research on family interaction ultimately concerns the patterns of interaction among family members, most available studies fail to look at patterns. Rather, they report differences in *rates* of specific behaviors *within* individuals and use these differences to draw conclusions about the nature of the relationship *between* individuals. In other words, most studies of family interaction fail to directly study interactions by measuring how the behavior of one family member affects the behavior of another member over time, a point well made by Hetherington and Martin (1979) in their excellent review:

> Most of the studies of family interaction have yielded separate frequency measures of parent and child behavior that is recorded during the interaction. However, usually, investigators are interested in the etiology, the contingencies, and the sequencing of these observed behaviors and often generalize to such questions on the basis of inappropriate methodology. . . . *Such studies should look sequentially at interchanges involving chains of interpersonal exchanges and investigate shifts in probabilities of response in one family member as they are related to the specific behavior of others.* (p. 254; emphasis added)

A second, related limitation of the literature is that it focuses almost exclusively on dyadic relationships (e.g., mother–child and father–mother) and often ignores the influence that the *social setting* or *context* provided by other family members and by the larger community exercises on these relationships. Although many recent studies have attempted to assess the impact of contextual variables such as the influence of third parties (e.g., father, kin, or friend) on dyadic interactions (e.g., in the mother–child relationship), little is known about the processes responsible for such indirect influences (Caplan, 1976; Clarke-Stewart, 1973; Dumas & Wahler, 1983; Lynn, 1974). Thus, it would appear not only that the literature commonly fails to study parent–child interactions directly, but that it also tends not to measure or control the contextual variables known to influence these interactions. These and other methodological limitations, which will be mentioned in the course of the review, will be considered in our evaluation of the evidence.

Developmental Issues

Infants are born with a rich repertoire of behavioral capabilities that has been shown to influence their caretakers' behavior (discussed later). Given this repertoire and the fact that infants are capable of learning as defined by the principles of classical and operant conditioning (Lipsitt & Kaye, 1964), it would seem likely that the development of prosocial or deviant interpersonal characteristics becomes an observable process from the time of birth.

A tentative picture of such development can be found in the observational studies of infant–mother "attachment." These studies have examined both the quantity and the quality of mother–infant interchanges in a variety of common caretaking situations—some familiar to both parties and others involving unfamiliar or "strange" situations. The studies suggest that some mothers set contingencies that promote the development and maintenance of at least two common coercive behaviors in their infants: crying and noncompliance. As a signal promoting proximity, crying may be seen as an early form of attachment behavior (Bell & Ainsworth, 1972). In a study of 26 white, middle-class infant–mother pairs from intact families, Bell and Ainsworth recorded two measures of infant crying (the frequency of crying episodes per waking hour and the total duration of crying in minutes per waking hour) and two measures of maternal responsiveness (the number of crying episodes that a mother ignored and the duration of crying in minutes per waking hour without, or before, an intervention by the mother). These measures were taken on repeated occasions during the infants' first year and were grouped by quarters (i.e., 0–3 months, 4–6 months, and so on). The results indicated that the mothers were much more stable in their responsiveness to infant crying than the infants were in their tendency to cry. This was particularly true with respect to the length of time a baby cried without or before an intervention by the mother. Correlations between mother and infant measures showed that, from the beginning of the first year, maternal unresponsiveness in one quarter was significantly associated with a higher frequency of, and generally longer, crying episodes in subsequent quarters. In other words, although the young infants did not respond immediately to their mothers' ignoring (the within-first-quarter correlations were not significant) by crying more frequently, they tended to be more insistent in their crying from the beginning of the second quarter onward as a result of their past experience of maternal unresponsiveness. Conversely, it appeared that prompt maternal responsiveness fostered the development of more varied, less coercive means of communication in these infants. These results suggest that, by the end of the first year, individual differences in crying—a common form of coercive behavior in later life—reflect the history of maternal responsiveness to the child rather than constitutional differences in irritability.

Evidence gathered by the same research group indicates that maternal responsiveness is associated with the development of other aspects of social competence (Ainsworth & Bell, 1974; Stayton & Ainsworth, 1973; Stayton, Hogan, & Ainsworth, 1971). One such aspect is compliance. In a study conducted with 25 middle-class infants aged 9 to 12 months, Stayton et al. observed mother–child interaction in free-field home settings. They measured the probability of the infant's compliance with verbal commands and coded maternal behaviors directed to them into four classes: a global rating reflecting the mother's sensitivity to her child's behavior and the positive or aversive quality of her response style, the frequency of her verbal commands, the frequency of her discipline-oriented physical interventions, and the extent of floor freedom she gave the child. The results indicated that neither disciplinary practices (i.e., the two frequency measures) nor the extent of floor freedom was related to child compliance. However, the global rating of maternal sensitivity was positively and significantly correlated with compliance, account for 42% of the variance in this variable. The fact that this measure was not an index of selective attention to infant compliance but reflected maternal attention and responsiveness to a wide range of infant social

actions suggests that a prosocial interpersonal style is likely to emerge in a responsive social setting without extensive disciplinary intervention, and that a
more defiant, coercive style may be the result, at least in part, of repeated
interchanges with an insensitive and rejecting mother.

It would appear, on the basis of the evidence just reviewed, that most children, by the age of 1, display interpersonal behavior patterns that are distinguishable on a prosocial-coercive dimension. This is shown clearly in further
work by Ainsworth and colleagues (Ainsworth, 1979; Ainsworth, Blehar, Waters, & Wall, 1978; Stayton & Ainsworth, 1973) with the same children. Relying
on the use of the "strange situation" procedure, an assessment technique that
enables one to classify children according to the pattern of behavior they display
before, during, and after a brief period of separation from their mothers,
Ainsworth found that the quality of infant–mother attachment varied on a
security–anxiety dimension.

This procedure was used to classify infant–mother pairs into three groups:
Securely attached babies used their mothers as a base from which to explore
their environment. When separated from their mothers, their attachment behavior was intensified, as evidenced by a reduction in exploration and, commonly, crying. When reunited with their mothers, they sought close bodily contact or at least interaction before resuming exploration. Anxious-avoidant
infants, in sharp contrast, rarely cried when separated and generally avoided
their mothers when reunited, whereas their anxious-resistant counterparts
showed signs of anxiety even in the preseparation period and were greatly
distressed by the separation but were ambivalent when reunited with their mothers, seeking and resisting contact with them. Besides displaying higher rates of
crying and noncompliance than the securely attached babies, the two anxiously
attached groups were also found to be deficient in affectionate behaviors. On
reunion, they were unlikely to greet their mothers' approaches with smiling and
babbling and were similarly unlikely to respond positively to being held by them.
As would be expected from what was said earlier, the single most important
characteristic that distinguished the mothers of securely attached infants from
the mothers of anxiously attached infants was the extent to which they were "in
tune with" (i.e., sensitive to) their babies' behavioral cues. There seemed to be a
continuum of insensitivity among caretakers. Throughout the first year, the
mothers of the securely attached infants were more responsive to their needs,
more demonstrative in their display of affection, and more consistent in their
expectations than the mothers of the anxiously attached infants. Whereas the
latter were generally described as rigid and unresponsive, the mothers of the
avoidant babies were found to be particularly rejecting, emotionally code, and
hostile to any form of close bodily contact; the mothers of the resistant babies,
although not rejecting, were anxious and strongly interfering or were very inaccessible and exhibited serious depressive tendencies.

Although the direction of effects in the attachment studies is not unequivo-
cal, the greater stability of maternal behavior than of child behavior in the first
year and the fact that infant behavior in the first 3 months of life bore no
relationship to the mother's later social interchanges, but that the mothers' in-

fant-directed behaviors in the first few months did predict their infants' later social behavior, suggest that infant behavior in the first year of life is more a function of maternal responsiveness than vice versa (Ainsworth, 1979). If the maternal response hypothesis is correct, it would support the conclusion that a responsive (i.e., contingent and consistent) social environment in early life is inversely related to the later emergence of coercive behaviors such as crying and noncompliance, which are part of an overall behavior pattern characterized as insecure or anxious and as generally lacking in the display of positive emotions. In other words, it would appear that the contingent nature of a mother's responses to her infant is more important to the development of prosocial behaviors than the absolute amount of time she spends with the infant beyond some unknown threshold. The experience of a responsive social environment may enable the child to learn that his or her noncoercive behavior can reliably control the environment and ensure the availability of rewards and comfort in situations of distress.

This conclusion is supported by studies that have looked at other aspects of infant development besides the development of social behavior (Ainsworth & Bell, 1974; Beckwith, 1971; Bell, 1970; Clarke-Stewart, 1973; Lewis & Goldberg, 1969; Yarrow, Rubenstein, Petersen, & Jankowski, 1972). Empirical work by Arend, Gove, and Sroufe (1979), Matas, Arend, and Sroufe (1978), and Waters, Wippman, and Sroufe (1979) indicates that there is a continuity in social adaptation from infancy to early childhood. For instance, Arend *et al.* related individual differences in security of attachment at 1½ years to the dimensions of ego control and ego resiliency at age 4 to 5. This longitudinal project found some indication that children who had been described as anxious-avoidant as infants scored significantly lower on a composite measure of ego control than children who scored in between these two groups. If we make the admittedly tentative assumption that children in the first group were beginning to show evidence of undercontrolled, conduct-problem behaviors, and that children in the second group were showing evidence of overcontrolled, dependent behaviors, this study would indicate that these behavior patterns may have their origin in social interactions in early life.

We must conclude, on the basis of the evidence reviewed, that the infancy studies (except, possibly, for the last study just presented) tell us little about the family correlates of conduct problems and dependency in later childhood. Nevertheless, they clearly indicate that at least two maladaptive behavior patterns (which commonly accompany aggression and dependency in later childhood) have been reliably observed to develop in very young children and that these patterns are associated with maternal attributes such as noncontingency, coldness, rejection, and unavailability. It should therefore come as no surprise to find that these attributes have been implicated in the development of conduct problems and dependency in later life.

Because an almost unlimited number of parental variables has been reported to be associated with childhood psychopathology, the need for a reliable method of simplifying the description of relations among these variables has been recognized for some time. Following the theoretical impetus provided by

Schaefer (1959, 1961), several authors have relied on factor analysis to determine the smallest number of orthogonal dimensions of parental variables necessary to account for the major portion of the variance in child behavior (Baumrind & Black, 1967; Becker & Krug, 1964; Peterson & Migliorino, 1967). It would appear that these studies have all isolated at least two fairly independent dimensions of parental variables that, although they have often been labeled differently, clearly refer to comparable clusters of behavior. The first of these dimensions, which we will refer to as *parental acceptance*, is a bipolar dimension commonly labeled *acceptance* or *warmth*, on the one hand, and *rejection* or *hostility*, on the other. Typically, the accepting parent enjoys the child's presence, stresses the child's likable personality attributes and skills, uses much positive reinforcement, and is generally sensitive to the child's needs and ideas. The opposite obviously applies to the rejecting parent. The second dimension, which we will label *parental control*, is also bipolar; it is usually referred to as *permissiveness* versus *restrictiveness*. The permissive parent fails to state rules and consequences for violation clearly, is excessively lax and inconsistent in enforcing rules, and makes few demands for appropriate and mature behavior, whereas the restrictive parent expects more responsible behavior from a child and sets clear and consistent contingencies in the pursuit of this expectation. These dimensions are obviously difficult to isolate in natural settings and are themselves associated with other parental variables. As we have already seen, the most important of them are probably *consistency* and *contingency* (i.e., the extent to which one or both parents display their acceptance and control of the child in a reliable and predictable manner).

Parental Consistency as a Developmental Issue

We have already seen that consistent parental responsiveness appears to play a major role in the development of social competency in infancy. It should therefore come as no surprise that parental inconsistency and family disorganization, have often been related to child deviance in general, and to conduct problems in particular, in older populations (Bandura, 1962; Garmezy, 1974; Glueck & Glueck, 1950; Hetherington, Cox, & Cox, 1978; Langner, McCarthy, Gersten, Simcha-Fagan, & Eisenberg, 1979; McCord, McCord, & Zola, 1959; McCord, McCord, & Howard, 1961; Patterson, 1976, 1980). For instance, Langner *et al.* reported that the factor "mother excitable-rejecting" (a predictor partaking of aggressiveness and inconsistency) was highly and uniquely predictive of antisocial behavior both inside and outside the home for two samples of families. Similarly, in an earlier prospective study of delinquency, McCord *et al.* (1959) found that a low incidence of delinquency was so closely associated with consistency in parental discipline that the specific form of discipline (love-oriented or punitive) mattered less than the consistency with which it was applied. This study reported the lowest rates of delinquency in homes in which parents consistently disciplined their children in a love-oriented or punitive manner. In another study that looked at consistency in terms of family organization and supervision, Wilson (1974) found that, in severely disadvantaged families, strict and often intrusive and restrictive supervision was more effective in preventing delinquency than a warm, harmonious family atmosphere. She suggested that what is commonly considered "good" parenting may not be appropriate in certain situations. Rather, strict supervision may provide a form of consistency that is important for children living in conditions of severe deprivation, disorganization, and uncertainty.

This picture is confirmed and extended by observational and laboratory studies. It is useful, when considering this evidence, to distinguish between *intra-agent inconsistency,* or the extent to which the same person reacts differently to repetitions of the same behaviors, and *interagent inconsistency,* or the extent to which two or more persons react differently to the same behaviors. Let us consider intra-agent inconsistency first. Observations of parent–child interactions in normal and deviant families have repeatedly shown that parents tend to respond to aversive child behavior (in an aversive and inconsistent manner) more often than they respond to positive behavior. Johnson and his associates (Johnson, Wahl, Martin, & Johansson, 1973; Wahl *et al.*, 1973) found not only that the level of deviance of a sample of normal children was best predicted by the level of their parents' aversiveness, but also that the more deviant children got a higher level of parental attention (both positive and negative) than their better behaved counterparts. Support for this dual parental-response tendency can be found in Dumas and Wahler (1986) and in Herbert and Baer (1972), as well as in the studies of Patterson (1976) and Snyder (1977). A closely related form of intra-agent inconsistency is the discrepancy between the verbal and the nonverbal contents of a mother's message, as well as the lack of congruence between voice intonation and message content. Both forms of communicative inconsistency have been reported to be more common in distressed than in nondistressed families and to be associated with child aggression and withdrawal (Bugental & Love, 1975; Love & Kaswan, 1974).

Evidence regarding interagent inconsistency (excepting evidence on marital disharmony, to be discussed later) is less clear-cut. Nevertheless, Patterson (1980) presented data supporting the hypothesis (*post hoc*) that, whereas mothers and fathers share equally in the responsibility for child discipline in normal families, they do not in aggressive ones. Patterson's analysis of family interactions in the home showed that the fathers of clinic-referred boys aged 5 to 14 provided aversive consequences for their children's aversive behaviors at the same rate as did the fathers of normals. The mothers of the distressed sample, however, did not share their husbands' perceptions, as evidenced by the fact that they had almost twice as many aversive interactions with their sons than the mothers of normals. Moreover, their increased emphasis on aversive control was also reflected in the fact that they engaged in prosocial modes of interaction, such as approving, laughing, and talking at significantly lower rates. Another important aspect of interagent inconsistency pertains to parental roles. In this respect, Leighton, Stollack, and Ferguson (1971) and Love and Kaswan (1974) reported that their referred families were characterized by a lack of effective role-taking and role-relationships between parents. In these families, the cultur-ally appropriate role differentiations were blurred. Contrary to their nonre-ferred counterparts, the fathers failed to assume leadership in instrumental tasks and involved themselves instead in competing with their spouses or com-plying with the latters' demand that they accept the emotional management of the family. The mothers, for their part, took on the dominant role in the family and assumed several normally paternal responsibilities, an arrangement that led to repeated conflict among the parents as they attempted to control each other and their children.

Finally, the importance of consistency in child management has also been emphasized in laboratory studies of the effects of different schedules of rein-forcement and punishment on aggressive behavior. These studies indicate that inconsistent responding (i.e., approval and disapproval of the same aggressive responses), when compared to consistent punishment, leads to significantly more aggressive responses in young boys (Deur & Parke, 1970; Katz, 1971; Parke & Deur, 1972; Sawin & Parke, 1979). For instance, Sawin and Parke, besides being able to demonstrate the existence of a causal link between inconsis-tency and aggression, showed that inconsistent discipline led to more aggressive responses than either consistent reinforcement, punishment, or ignoring. Fur-thermore, it appears that inconsistency affects future prosocial learning. Cairns and Paris (1971) and Warren and Cairns (1972) showed that, compared to contingently reinforced children, children first exposed to rich schedules of noncontingent reinforcement had greater difficulty learning on later trials when reinforcement was made contingent on performance. Similarly, the experience of inconsistent punishment has been found to lead to increased resistance of the aggressive response to change under conditions of extinction and/or continuous, contingent punishment (Deur & Parke, 1970; Sawin & Parke, 1979). These findings closely parallel those of the studies described above in which infants first exposed to uncontrollability failed to learn control in later, controllable situations.

Parental Consistency in Childhood Dependency Problems

In comparison with the area of agression, relatively little evidence is avail-able on the family correlates of childhood dependency and withdrawal. This relative lack of data as well as the fact that the available evidence suffers from the same methodological limitations as the evidence just reviewed, makes any con-clusions in this area tentative at best. It would appear that the evidence can again be carefully reviewed under the headings of *acceptance, control,* and *consistency,* if we bear in mind that dependency and withdrawal, like conduct problems, are more likely to be associated with configurations of these parental dimensions than with these dimensions in isolation.

Measures of positive parental attitudes, such as warmth and acceptance, have generally been found to be unrelated to child dependency and withdrawal (Baumrind & Black, 1967; Kagan & Moss, 1962). However, measures of negative attitudes, such as hostility and rejection, appear to be moderately related to this syndrome (Langner *et al.*, 1974, 1977; McCord & Howard, 1961; Sears, Maccoby, & Levin, 1957; Smith, 1958; Winder & Rau, 1962). Although the evidence is difficult to compare because of major methodological differences between studies, it would seem that a cold and rejecting father may be more important than a cold and rejecting mother (Becker *et al.*, 1959, 1962; Jenkins, 1968; Rosenthal, Ni, Finkelstein, & Berwits, 1962), especially if he tends to be maladjusted (withdrawn or neurotic) himself. Relying on parental ratings and questionnaires, Becker *et al.* (1959) found fathers, but not mothers, of dependent children to be generally maladjusted and thwarting of their children's curiosity. These findings were later confirmed and extended (Becker *et al.*, 1962). An examination of the relationship separately for both sexes indicated that mothers who were hostile and punitive tended to have children, especially boys, who were rated as dominant rather than dependent, but that fathers who were hostile and punitive tended to have children, mostly girls, who were dependent, especially if their mothers themselves behaved in a submissive and dependent manner. Note that these sex differences appear to have been partly contradicted by Sears, Maccoby, & Levin (1957): Relying on teacher as well as parent ratings, these authors found that punitive and nonnurturant mothers tended to have dependent sons, but not daughters, in a preschool situation. Light was shed on this inconsistency by Martin and Hetherington (quoted in Martin, 1975), who found that mothers of withdrawn boys (9–12 years old) were as accepting of them as were mothers of normals and more accepting than mothers of aggressive boys; fathers of withdrawn boys, on the other hand, were less accepting than fathers of either normal or aggressive boys. Mothers of withdrawn girls showed less acceptance than mothers of normals, a difference not found in their fathers, however. As the authors indicated, these results suggest that a lack of acceptance by the same sex-parent, but average acceptance by the opposite-sex parent, may be related to child withdrawal and dependency. However, it should be noted that this has by no means been established and that further research is needed to clarify the nature of this relationship.

Withdrawn, dependent children are often described in terms that imply overcontrol on the part of their parents. Although several comparisons of child-rearing practices involving these children compared with those involving conduct-problem children indicate that the former parents are more restrictive than the latter (Bennett, 1960; Hewitt & Jenkins, 1946; Lewis, 1954; McCord *et al.*, 1961; Rosenthal *et al.*, 1962), this finding is difficult to interpret. First, it is contradicted by studies that did not obtain the same association (Bandura, 1962; Becker *et al.*, 1959, 1962; Martin, 1975). Second, even when the evidence shows that the parents of withdrawn children are more restrictive than the parents of conduct-problem children, it does not indicate, in the absence of control groups, whether the former differ in any way from the parents of normals. These studies, except that of McCord *et al.* (1961), had no control group. A well-designed and controlled study, which has already been quoted above in relation to conduct problems (Baumrind, 1967), throws light on the situation.

Baumrind's study is of considerable interest because of its methodological sophistication, in particular, its use of a control group and of direct observations in both structured and free-field settings. It will, therefore, be described in detail.

Relying on multiple assessment procedures, among which were 14 weeks of behavioral observations, three groups ($n = 32$) of children of both sexes were selected from a larger sample of 110 three- to four-year-olds attending nursery school. The children exhibited very different, stable patterns of interpersonal behaviors. Group 1 children ($n = 13$) were rated higher than the other two groups on self-control, self-reliance, approach to novel situations, cheerfulness, and positive peer interactions. Group 2 children ($n = 11$) ranked low on the approach, cheerfulness, and peer interaction dimensions and showed less self-control and self-reliance than Group 1 children, but more than Group 3. Group 3 children ($n = 8$) were rated low on self-control, self-reliance, and approach.

Given these three groups, parental behavior was assessed along four dimensions (nurturance, control, maturity demands, and communication clarity) and was compared across groups. If we make the assumption (not made by the author) that Group 2 children exhibited behaviors generally associated with dependency and withdrawal, and that Group 3 children showed behaviors associated with conduct problems, the study provides a comparison of child-rearing methods in the families of normal, dependent, and conduct-problem children. This comparison indicated that, in contrast with all other parents, the parents of Group 1 children scored high on the four child-rearing dimensions measured. Though not harsh or restrictive, they exercised much consistent control over their children and rarely yielded to their coercive demands. They were supportive and nurturant, however, as indicated by their greater reliance on positive reinforcement than on punishment and, thus, probably balanced the effect of their high level of control; in the same way, they balanced their high demands with clear communications about what they expected of their children, and with a willingness to be influenced by their requests. The parents of Group 2 children were less nurturant than the parents in the other two groups. Although they exercised less control than the Group 1 parents, they exercised more control than the Group 3 parents in a context in which they offered little support and affection for their children as indicated by their greater reliance on physical punishment, especially by fathers, and lack of concern about their children's needs and requests. The parents of Group 3 children exercised little control over them, were generally ineffective and inconsistent in disciplining them, and made few maturity demands on them. They were more nurturant than the Group 2 parents, however. Thus, the ratio of control to nurturance ran in opposite directions in Groups 2 and 3. The parents of Group 2 children were *controlling, but cold and unsupportive,* whereas the parents of Group 3 children lacked control over them but were comparatively warm. Although these differences are important, it should be noted that they are probably not as important as the differences between the parents of Group 1 and the parents of the children in the other two groups.

Regarding the issue of parental control, the results of the Baumrind study suggest that children who appear to exhibit behaviors associated with dependency and withdrawal have parents who are overcontrolling when compared to parents of more aggressive children, but who lack control and display little acceptance and warmth when compared to parents of normal children.

These results are indirectly supported in studies of social competence (Coopersmith, 1967; Shure & Spivack, 1979, 1980; Sigel, 1979; Wilton & Barbour, 1978) and parental dominance (Hetherington & Frankie, 1967) and overprotection (Jenkins, 1968; Kagan & Moss, 1962; McCord et al., 1961). Wilton and Barbour (1978), working with families of low socioeconomic status, reported that mothers of high-risk (low-competence) 2- to 4-year-old children, when compared to a low-risk contrast group, engaged less often in direct didactic teaching, showed less encouragement of their children's activities, and more often failed in their attempts to control them. Coopersmith (1967) conducted a study of maternal variables associated with self-esteem in boys. Relying on interview and questionnaire measures, the study found that high-self-esteem boys had mothers who themselves had a positive self-concept and who generally enjoyed a harmonious relationship with their spouse and child. Their child-rearing practices were characterized by the use of positive reinforcement, reasoning, and discussion, rather than punishment, in a context in which they had high expectations for their children and enforced rules and discipline in a firm and consistent manner. As both low competency and low self-esteem are common correlates of withdrawal and dependency, we may assume that dependent children probably have parents who generally fail to exhibit such high levels of control *and* nurturance.

Hetherington & Frankie (1967) measured interpersonal dominance and conflict in families with a delinquent son or daughter. They found that the families of neurotic delinquents were generally characterized by maternal dominance, and the families of social delinquents, by paternal dominance. Maternal dominance in the former families appeared to be accepted by the children, but not by the fathers, as evidence by repeated conflict between them and their spouses. Similarly, Martin and Hetherington (Martin, 1975) found the homes of withdrawn preadolescent boys to be dominated by mothers more often than the homes of aggressive or normal boys, and to be characterized by low restrictiveness by both parents, especially fathers, and low father acceptance. Because we know that children are most likely to imitate parents who are of high reinforcement value and who are able to exercise immediate control, whether through reinforcement or punishment (Hetherington & Frankie, 1967; Wahler & Nordquist, 1973), these results suggest that dependent children, especially boys, may acquire some of their maladaptive behaviors through a process of imitation of some of their mothers' feminine characteristics. It would appear that this imitation may be most likely to take place in the context of a fairly positive mother–child relationship and a lack of closeness with a more passive, nonnurturant, or distant father.

Finally, some studies have described as overprotective the type of parental control exercised in families of dependent children. For example, Jenkins (1968), relying on psychiatric case-note data, reported that the mothers of overly anxious children tended to be described as anxious, overprotective, and infantilizing, whereas their fathers tended to be passive and to have neurotic problems themselves. Comparable results can be found in Kagan and Moss (1962); Mc-

Cord *et al.* (1961); Rosenthal *et al.* (1962); and Sears (1961). However, the fact that other studies failed to find the same association (Becker *et al.*, 1959) or found it only in a subgroup of dependent children, namely school phobics, raises questions about the importance of overprotection as a correlate of child dependency. One of the first studies in this area (Levy, 1943), as well as more recent findings gathered from school phobics (Eisenberg, 1958; Hersov, 1976), suggests that, more than the degree of control as such, overprotection may reflect a situation in which an anxious parent, usually the mother, makes few maturity demands on the child, provides little emotional support, and generally restricts the child's social autonomy, whereas the other parent adopts a rather passive role and may personally suffer from emotional maladjustment. If this suggestion is correct, *overprotection* would be a summary term describing a social context similar to the one described in the studies of parenting and social competency presented earlier in this section.

Although direct measures of parental consistency in families of withdrawn, dependent children are almost nonexistent, the limited evidence available suggests that the parents of such children may be inconsistent. However, it should be noted that this evidence does not indicate whether there are differences in the level of inconsistency between parents of dependent children, on the one hand, and parents of conduct-problem or normal children, on the other. Sears *et al.* (1957) found that their young subjects were most likely to be dependent if their mothers were both highly rewarding and highly punishing of dependency. This finding, which parallels the finding that highly aggressive children are most likely to have parents—or at least mothers—who reward and punish their behavior at high rates, can be understood if one assumes that inconsistency training teaches the child to persist in the display of dependent behaviors, even in the face of parental ignoring or punishment, in the knowledge that such behaviors will eventually be reinforced.

There is also limited evidence of interagent inconsistency in families of dependent children. In a study that was part of Project Re-Ed (a residential treatment program for disturbed children), Weinstein (1965) compared three groups of children (normal, aggressive, and withdrawn) on a series of measures. One comparison indicated that the withdrawn children saw themselves as being pulled apart by their parents, whom they perceived as having very different expectations of them. Such a perception is in keeping with the finding, reported in the previous two sections, that parents of dependent children appear to relate to them in a discrepant manner. Whether their child-rearing practices are measured in terms of acceptance (Martin, 1975), dominance (Hetherington *et al.*, 1971), or overprotection (Levy, 1943), it has repeatedly been found that, in such families, mothers tend to exercise a more assertive, dominant role and fathers a more passive one, and that this situation is commonly associated with high levels of marital conflict. Although discrepancy and conflict were not directly measured in these studies, it would seem reasonable to expect such discrepancy and conflict between parents to be reflected in inconsistent handling of their children. This conclusion is supported by findings of greater interparental inconsistency in communication studies that compared normal and clinical samples (Love & Kaswan, 1974; Murrell & Stachowiak, 1967), even though the clinical samples were not limited to families with withdrawn, dependent children.

Conclusions: The Need for Interactive Research

Based on the evidence just reviewed, we can tentatively conclude that the family correlates of childhood conduct problems and dependency overlap considerably and that no single family variable has been found to distinguish reliably between them. Consider this conclusion in light of our developmental speculation that a dual process underlies the development and maintenance of these two dimensions of psychopathology.

First, this conclusion may reflect the essentially noninteractive nature of the literature. The parents of both conduct-problem and dependent children may share broad behavioral characteristics such as a lack of acceptance, control, and consistency, but they may differ in the manner in which they express them in their interactions with their children. In other words, the study of broad dimensions of parental behavior may tell us little about specific parent–child interactions.

Second, the conclusion may also reflect the fact that most studies have focused on isolated dimensions of parental behavior and have failed to measure interdependencies in these dimensions. Studies that have measured interdependencies in parental acceptance, control, and consistency (e.g., Baumrind, 1967) suggest that important response covariations may exist. If this is true, parents of conduct-problem and dependent children may share comparable behavioral characteristics but may differ in the way in which these covary as the parents interact with the children.

Third, the considerable overlap in the family correlates of childhood psychopathology may reflect the fact the children may react differently to the same parental behaviors. This possibility is suggested by studies of temperamental differences (discussed later), which indicate that some children may respond to adverse parental behavior by withdrawing and others may react by becoming aggressive (Rutter, 1979), a fact that points to the importance of studying response covariations in children also. Finally, our conclusion is likely to reflect the fact that the large majority of family interaction studies ignore the wider social context in which children learn to behave aggressively or dependently. In other words, these studies ignore the setting in which parents and children interact, as well as its impact on their behavior.

These considerations, which are obviously not mutually exclusive, underline the need for research that will consider not only parent–child interactions but also the response covariations within parents and children. Although little is known about such covariations in disturbed children and their parents, there is increasing evidence about the importance of the social setting in the development and maintenance of the adverse parental behaviors generally associated with childhood aggression and dependency. We will discuss this evidence, which provides the background of our coercion–neglect model. In other words, we turn to the fourth term of the expanded operant model described at the beginning of the chapter.

DEVELOPMENTAL SPECULATIONS II: SETTING EVENTS IN COERCION AND NEGLECT

The evidence just reviewed indicates that parental aversive and inconsistent behavior is associated with the presence of maladaptive behavior patterns in children at all stages of development. Thus far, in our speculations, we have made a case for the presence of these parent–child associations in the emergence of both conduct and dependency problems. At this point, we think it appropriate to carry these arguments a step further into a look at the overt and covert forms of both childhood problem categories. One might recall our earlier stated contention that the overt-covert distinction in these problem categories is both reasonable and useful in terms of treatment planning. We also noted that the developmental process of coercion and neglect may have a formative impact on the overt and covert manifestations of conduct and dependency problems. A more complete description of the process requires an understanding of why a parent would interact with his or her developing child in an aversive and inconsistent manner. Following this speculative explanation, we will attempt to provide a fit between the coercion–neglect processes and the covert and overt forms of childhood conduct and dependency problems.

Setting Events

A parent obviously experiences several sources of social input besides the immediate discriminative stimuli provided by the child in the course of interaction. Although the importance of such input is commonly acknowledged, little effort has been made to study parent–child relationships in a truly social context. The limited evidence available—most of it gathered from mothers—indicates that child rearing, at best a challenging task, is made easier or more difficult depending on the setting functions served by the child and the adults that are part of the mother's social system (e.g., Caplan, 1976; Cochran & Brassard, 1970; Lynn, 1974). Specifically, it would appear that mothers who fail in their child-rearing task receive more aversive and fewer positive social inputs than mothers who succeed, and that this unsupportive environment sets the occasion for the development and maintenance of inconsistent and aversive responding. The circumstances that make social input differences likely can generally be found if (a) the child is temperamentally irritable or "difficult" to manage or (b) other persons in the mother's social network are constant sources of aversive interchanges. Both of these aversive stimulus sources have been shown to function as "setting events" for the mother, in the sense that their presence predicts which of a number of specific interchanges between mother and child is most likely to follow. If we recall the arguments in the first section of this chapter, the

Kantorian (Kantor, 1959) setting-event concept implies that two behaviorally similar mother–child dyads can develop quite different interaction patterns depending on environmental context factors such as (a) and (b) previously mentioned. Research findings relevant to this conclusion are now presented.

It has been recognized for some time that from birth, the infant influences his or her environment (e.g., Bell, 1968). Although crying is the neonate's major means of influencing caretakers, the infant soon acquires another means of social control: smiling. There are considerable individual differences among infants in the likelihood of these responses—differences commonly referred to as *temperamental differences* (Brazelton, 1973; Carey, 1970). Consider the effect of crying on a mother. Frodi, Lamb, Leavitt, and Donovan (1978) reported both self-report and psychophysiological data that support the commonsense notion that a crying infant acts as an arousing and aversive stimulus. Although this type of stimulus commonly increases the likelihood that an aggressive response will follow, in most cases the arousal remains limited and the aversive situation is terminated by relieving the cause of the infant's discomfort.

However, the situation is more complicated when one is dealing with a "difficult" infant. As reviews of temperamental differences indicate (Bates, 1980; Thomas, Chess, & Birch, 1970), these infants cry for longer periods and often seem inconsolable despite their caretakers' repeated efforts. As a result and through a process of conditioning, the child may become an aversive stimulus whether he or she is crying or not (Lamb, 1978), leading the mother to become less responsive and consistent in her caretaking behavior (Donovan, Leavitt, & Balling, 1978; Milliones, 1978). The infant's aversive actions may indeed elicit avoidance responses in the mother and may increase the likelihood that she will exhibit a variety of aversion-reducing behaviors (e.g., picking the infant up or scolding the infant). Given a number of similar mother–child interchanges, the infant's entire range of social actions may come to function as a class of conditioned aversive stimuli eliciting maternal avoidance and/or setting the occasion for her performance of those aversion-reducing responses that in the past have been successful in "turning off" the infant's aversive actions. If this avoidance hypothesis is correct, we would expect "difficult" infants to set the stage for maternal inconsistency and aversiveness by conditioning their mothers to generally disregard their signals and/or to respond to them aversively. Under such circumstances, a mother may develop a negative perception or a summary report of her child's behavior and may generally evaluate and respond to most of her child's social actions in light of this report.

The literature indicates that these undesirable maternal responses can also be under the control of temporally distant stimuli that may have no direct, contingent relationship with the responses in question. For example, a mother's confrontation with her husband or with her own mother in the morning may be shown to increase the likelihood that she will interact aversively with her child in the afternoon, even though the two events are not contingently related (Wahler & Graves, 1983). Similarly, a mother's history of depression or her ability to tolerate her child's aversive behavior may lead her to describe her child as behaviorally "deviant," even though the child's behavior does not differ from that of normal children on objective behavioral measures (Delfini *et al.*, 1976; Griest *et al.*, 1979; Lobitz & Johnson, 1975).

. A study by Egeland and Sroufe (1981) illustrates this process of indirect influence. The authors compared a group of 31 mother–infant dyads with a known history of abuse and neglect with a group of 33 dyads in which maternal care was judged to be excellent. Home observations of mother–infant interactions were conducted when the children were 12 and 18 months old. As expected from the research reviewed above, the first comparison indicated that the maltreated children were more likely than their counterparts to interact with their mothers in coercive and avoidant ways. However, 6 months later, the two groups no longer differed. This was so because, although the control infants had not changed, some of the maltreated infants had become significantly more prosocial. Life stress interviews independently obtained from the mothers when the infants were 12 and 18 months old showed that infants who had become significantly more prosocial over this 6-month period had mothers who reported significant reductions in stressful life events over the same period. Specifically, this change seemed to be associated with maternal reports of greater support from social agents outside the family.

The impact of a mother's social contacts on her child's behavior has also been reported in epidemiological (Kellam, Ensminger, & Turner, 1977; Kolvin, Garside, Nicol, Macmillan, Wolstenholme, & Leitch, 1977; Lagerkvist, Laruitze, Olin, & Tengvald, 1975) and clinical (Wahler, 1980; Wahler, Hughey, & Gordon, 1981; Wahler, Leske, & Rogers, 1979) studies of older populations. Wahler's work is of particular interest here. This work relies on the concept of *insularity*. *Insularity* may be defined as a specific pattern of social contacts within the community that is characterized by a high level of negatively perceived coercive interchanges with relatives and/or helping-agency representatives and a low level of positively perceived supportive interchanges with friends. As mentioned above, differences in maternal patterns of social contacts are associated with differences in deviant child behavior, at least among aggressive, noncompliant children. Specifically, Wahler and his colleagues found not only that insular children exhibited higher rates of aversive behavior than their noninsular counterparts, but also that insular mothers were more aversive and inconsistent (Dumas & Wahler, 1985), more negative in their perception of their children (Wahler & Afton, 1980), and less likely to benefit from a parent training program aimed at teaching them to relate in more prosocial ways to their children (Dumas & Wahler, 1983) than noninsular mothers. Furthermore, Wahler (1980) provided evidence that these differences reflect the existence of a covarying relationship between maternal community contacts and mother–child interactions at home, rather than the effect of a third, undetermined factor on both variables.

Although the specific operational characteristics of setting events are far from being understood, the limited evidence just presented indicates that a parent's—or at least a mother's—aversiveness and inconsistency directed at a child are not only a function of the immediate stimulus events presented by the child. They are also under the influence of setting events that may bear little or no temporal or contingent relationship to these child-provided stimuli. Setting events play a major role in the coercion–neglect model that follows.

Setting-Event Influences on Coercion and Neglect

If a mother lives within an environmental context marked by the previously described setting events, we would assume that she is apt to provide a similar context for her child. An aversive and inconsistent parental caretaking style, as we have noted repeatedly, is implicated in the development of childhood psychopathology. The next question of interest centers on the fourfold forms of these developmental problems. How could troubled children develop behaviorally and functionally different forms of psychopathology from this common ground? We suspect that the temperamental characteristics of the child and the mother's response style are key elements in the different developments that result from this pathological baseline. In our view, individual response differences promote different likelihoods of coercion and neglect as major or minor facets of the growth process.

Previously reviewed research indicates that infants display temperamental differences early in the first year of life (e.g., Thomas *et al.*, 1970). We also reviewed research showing response-style differences across mothers, particularly in self-reports of depression (e.g., Griest *et al.*, 1979). Both sets of findings reflect the fact that infants and mothers display somewhat generalized response characteristics. Although we have argued a setting-event cause of these temperament and mood styles, it is equally reasonable (highly probable in the infant's case) to infer genetic influences. Whatever the causes, it is clear that infants differ greatly in their generalized tendencies to be irritable, unresponsive, and affectionate. Similarly, mothers differ greatly along these same dimensions. Consider, for example, Patterson's analyses (1982, p. 277) of maternal "irritability" as a reaction to groups of normal children and those classified as overt and covert conduct-problem children. Given that the children acted in an aversive manner (e.g., nagging and yelling), there were significant differences between groups in the mothers' likelihood of counterattack. The mothers of the overt conduct-problem children were more likely to respond in kind than were the mothers in the other two groups. These mothers (of normals and covert conduct-problem children) did not differ in their counterattack probabilities. However, once a child–mother coercive episode had started, the mothers of both conduct-problem groups were twice as likely to continue responding aversively, *regardless of how their children responded.* The latter finding adds confirmation to the indiscriminate or inconsistent aversive response styles of mothers of deviant children. The former finding is of greater interest at this point because it suggests that mothers of overt conduct-problem children are of more irritable temperament than those of covert conduct-problem and normal children.

Figure 1 provides a schematic view of our coercion–neglect model. The model presumes that various combinations of parent mood and infant temperament will lead to parent–child entrapment marked by either coercion or neglect. Although they are not illustrated in the Figure 1, we presume broad differences in the response styles of "irritability" and "unresponsiveness." Thus, an irritable–irritable matchup between parent and infant could involve the coercive responses of crying and clinging or the equally demanding forms of pushing and hitting. The latter, more aggressive types of coercion ought to establish the child

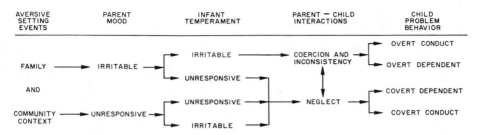

FIGURE 1. Developmental sequences leading to child problem behaviors of overt and covert types. According to the progressions described, the pathology-inducing parent lives in an environment marked by aversive setting events. Depending on that parent's mood and that infant's temperament, the two individuals will develop interpersonal relationships characterized by coercion and inconsistency or chronic neglect. Finally, coercive entrapment is seen to produce two functionally similar child problem behaviors: overt-conduct and dependency-response classes. Chronic neglect, on the other hand, ought to produce the covert forms of these problem behaviors.

problem class *overt conduct disorder,* and the former would lay the foundation for an *overt dependency disorder.* In the three other combinations of parent–infant mood and temperament matchups, a lack of social influence would be expected. In two of these, marked by an unresponsive infant, we would expect the child's development of isolated behavior (covert dependency). The third matchup of irritable infant and unresponsive mother ought to foster the child's development of alternative social relationships. Given the availability of antisocial peers, siblings, or adults, these alternative relationships (covert conduct problem) could develop without hindrance by the uninterested parent.

It is also important to notice the two-pronged arrow joining the coercion and neglect terms of Figure 1. We argued earlier that these interpersonal processes are often linked together in the sense that coercion can lead to neglect. Our major assumption about psychopathology centers on the notion that people act in ways that are *averisve* to one another. It is reasonable to expect some parent–child entrapments in which coercion and neglect are equally apparent, as well as those in which one of the two processes is dominant. As we showed in Table 1, clinic-referred children who manifest both overt and covert conduct problems may also be expected to display greater deviance within the family. In fact, Loeber and Schmaling (1986) found that these "mixed" conduct-problem children were at greater risk of becoming delinquent than either overt or covert conduct-problem children. In reference to another overt-covert "mixture," Ledingham (1981) studied the developmental course of children who manifested both overt conduct and covert dependency behaviors. When this group was compared to problem children representing "pure" forms of overt conduct and covert dependency, the former was rated by teachers, mothers, and peers as more deviant and less likable.

Conceivably, the comparatively poorer adjustment of the mixed-problem children is due to the combined effects of coercion and neglect. From the standpoint of our conceptual model, these processes produce cumulative adjustment problems. In essence, neglect leads to the child's withdrawal from the uninterested parent and thus deprives the child of the potential benefits of that parent's teaching. Coercion, on the other hand, is viewed as an active teaching process in which the child learns a very narrow, aversive interpersonal style. Consider the probabilities that children in the four subgroups will behave in a manner that will alienate adults and peers. According to our model, the overt conduct and overt dependent children are most likely to display coercive interpersonal styles. However, although the adult and peer audience is likely to judge the styles as aversive, we have also seen in the summary-report-rating literature that the overt conduct-problem children are more likely to be assigned motivational causes of selfish and harmful intent (e.g., "psychopathic"). On the other hand, the topographically different coercive actions of overt dependent children will usually lead an audience to assign less antisocial intent to these behaviors (e.g., "neurotic"). Thus, in all probability, these latter children are apt to elicit sympathy and concern, whereas their overt counterparts are apt to elicit dislike and anger. On a dimension of likability or popularity, the overt conduct-problem child would be expected to repel adults and peers—an expectation born out in the previously reviewed literature.

The skill deficiencies of troubled children constitute another risk factor in psychological development. In reference to this factor, neglect would be expected to contribute to the process as much as, or more than, coercion. In our Figure 1 model, neglect will be most pervasive when the child is of an unresponsive temperament. Whether the parent be irritable or unresponsive, we would expect a chronic absence of interchange between parent and child under these conditions—given, of course, that the parent is entrapped in the setting-event contect depicted in Figure 1. Neglect conditions of this sort ought to lead to the child's development of covert dependency problems, those characterized by social withdrawal and apathy. From our previous literature review of direct observational studies in school settings, these children are clearly marked by social skill deficiencies. However, because we have yet to see a skill deficiency comparison between covert dependent and overt conduct-problem children, the differential extent of this deficiency is unknown. It is evident, however, that the covert dependent children are better liked than are the overt conduct-problem children. Despite the skill deficiencies of the former children, it seems probable that their noncoercive reputations stand them in good stead in terms of a potential entry into adaptive peer relationships.

Another facet of the neglect process is highlighted in the interpersonal styles of covert conduct-problem children. Following our temperament assumptions of Figure 1, these children are viewed as interested in social contact but are apt to engage others coercively during infancy. However, because their troubled parents are of an unresponsive temperament, the children must look elsewhere for social stimulation. Because the children have not been shaped to behave coercively, one would not expect them to approach other adults and peers with the same level of coercion as their overt conduct counterparts. However, at the same time, these unsupervised and socially active children are not hindered in their progressive experimentation with commonly seen rule violations, such as stealing, truancy, and vandalism. Thus, we would assume that the children's newly formed social relationships would include the continued practice of these covert conduct-problem behaviors. One would expect the children to be fairly skilled in social relationships, reasonably popular because of their nonconfrontive nature, and quite stable in their output of moral, ethical, and legal transgressions. Because the transgressions are often sanctioned by the children's peers (who tend to be of similar problem status), there is good reason to expect maintenance of the pathology (see Robins & Ratcliff, 1980).

A final risk consideration in the coercion–neglect process concerns parental contributions to the process. As outlined in Figure 1, the impact of parent and child temperament in coercion and neglect depends on the influence of setting events on the parent's caretaking behavior. The parents who are entrapped within other family and community interchanges are those most likely to adopt an indiscriminate and aversive caretaking style. We have argued elsewhere (Dumas & Wahler, 1985) that this caretaking style is a keystone of childhood psychopathology. There are several lines of evidence to support this contention. First, there are suggestions that the degree of inconsistency in the parent's caretaking style is correlated with the severity of the parent–child entrapment. Patterson (1976) and Snyder (1977) both discovered that the mothers of overt conduct-problem children were significantly more indiscriminate in their aversive responses to the children than were samples of mothers in normal mother–child dyads. Second, Dumas and Wahler (1985) found similar differences in two samples of clinic-referred families that differed in the mothers' self-reports of personal entrapment. The mothers who reported more coercive encounters with adults in their family and community contexts were shown to be significantly more indiscriminate in their caretaking style than the mothers who reported a smaller number of such encounters. Because Dumas and Wahler (1983) also discovered that the former mothers fared more poorly in a parent–child treatment program, the pathology-inducing power of these setting-event influences is given further credence.

A summary of this section will highlight several assessment findings on differing forms of child problem behaviors and their possible maintenance sources. Conduct and dependency problems appear to share some important commonalities in their overt and covert forms. The overt forms of child conduct and dependency behaviors may both be considered demands for parental compliance. If so, the interventions of choice would be similar in a functional sense. In both cases, the coercive exchanges between child and parent would be targeted for interruption, and the two individuals would be helped to develop more cooperative interchanges. On the other hand, a family treatment strategy for the covert forms of these child problems would be quite different if neglect is indeed the functional social property. In both covert problems, a means of promoting reciprocal interest between parent and child would follow. But regardless of the specific treatment targets within the parent–child relationship, it is also evident that these relationship problems have contextual determinants as well. Both members of the dyad may be influenced, to varying degrees, by the setting-event context of other adults and peers. These indirect social influences must be regarded as assessment targets of the same priority as those more obvious sources of control lying within the family.

These brief suggestions regarding treatment strategies bring us back full circle to our use of an expanded operant model with its emphasis on a triadic conception of family psychopathology. As we have outlined the model, a mother represents the pivotal factor in a triangle formed by her children, on the one hand, and her community of adult interaction associates, on the other. Her *style* of child care has been implicated in the child's development of dependency and conduct problems, including the more subtle overt and covert forms of these behaviors. When that style fits the process criteria of coercion and/or neglect, one ought to be seriously concerned about the child's future development. In translating that concern into diagnostic assessment, we have outlined a fairly complicated picture of the process. Not only is the complexity marked by our imperfect understanding of setting-event operations, but we are also unsure about how to explain the stimulus influence of maternal inconsistency as it impinges on the child's developing problems. In some respects, the assessment picture bears little relationship to the familiar operant perspective that has guided applied behavior analysis for so many years. Consider an example from our clinical experience: An unwed mother is confronted by the caretaking demands of a temperamentally irritable infant, lack of money and education, and a protective but critical extended family. The coercive triangles formed by these problems are highlighted by one in particular: her own mother is a constant companion, offering advice, solace, and warnings with respect to the care of her infant and how she ought to conduct herself with men. Her baby cries frequently and squirms when she holds him, and his sleep cycle is sporadic. Whenever this young mother has prolonged contact with either her mother or her infant, she becomes "preoccupied" with thoughts of her prior contacts with them, thoughts of how unfair her predicament is, and thoughts about her happier past. An observer would be struck by her seemingly insensitive, routine response to her infant; her actions toward the baby, although sometime elicited by the child's aversive behavior, are for the most part irrelevant to what the infant says and does. The same observer would be equally impressed by the mother's childlike stance toward her mother, marked by impetuous outbursts of anger at the older woman or periods of clinging obedience.

As the baby grows, his irritability shifts in quality from crying and squirming to more focused "attacks" on his mother. He whines, nags, and yells at her, particularly on those days on which she is preoccupied and therefore indiscriminate with respect to the boy's approaches to her. His coercive actions, however, are always successful in generating predictable matching responses from her; she *threatens* him, screams at him, and, on occasion, slaps him. These episodes of escalating coercive exchanges are especially noticeable following visits between the mother and her own mother. After one of these setting-event experiences, not only is the mother preoccupied, but her threshold for aversive response to the youngster's demands seems lower.

The triangular entrapment just described is difficult to comprehend on the basis of simple reinforcement probabilities. As we argued at the beginning of this chapter, setting events are not discriminative stimuli. Although this mother's coercive child-care style is most likely to materalize following a setting-event experience with her own mother, the experience does not predict or signal the child's probability of taking part in the coercive matchup. That is, he is just as likely to respond coercively to her behavior on days on which the setting events have not been in operation; if she is indiscriminate and/or aversive, he will respond coercively, regardless of what her antecedent experiences have been. The sequence of interdependent steps appears to be as follows: The mother has a temper outburst with her mother when the older woman critiques her choice in men; the mother leaves her mother's home crying and obsessively reviewing the previous discussion and temper flareup; her child comes home from school in a hurry to have a snack and then watch television; the mother, still reviewing her prior experience, responds aimlessly to the child's chatter and occasional demands; the child responds to her indiscriminate attention by "boring in" with the unreasonable demand, "Bake me a pie"; the mother shouts at her child, "You two are just alike!"; the child cries and throws his glass of milk on the floor; the mother slaps the child.

As further research on triadic entrapment proceeds, we suspect that new principles of stimulus–response functions will be demonstrated, ultimately leading to our better understanding of the stimulus control process. In our opinion, two functions are likely to be documented: (a) An "uncertainty" principle may account for some aspects of the child's coercive interpersonal style (see Wahler & Hann, 1984, 1986). According to our view of the principle, children react to indiscriminate parental attention as aversive stimuli. When faced with this sort of social context, a child will resort to those behaviors that generate predictability. Of course, coercive responses such as nagging and yelling are highly effective means of capturing predictable forms of parental attention, typically of an "in-kind" nature. (b) If we remove *time* as a dimension of triadic operations, it may prove useful to conceptualize setting-event functions as instances in which maternal response is governed by the *relational* properties of two simultaneously presented stimuli. In the case of our clinical example, the mother's indiscriminate attention to her child may be shown to be a dependable response to a stimulus best described as a commonality between the grandmother's critique and the child's chatter (e.g., "Both expect me to comply"). Thus, a diagnostic assessment of this mother's child-care behavior would have to include her specific stimulus experiences *and* some index of their functional similarity.

We realize that much of our clinical anecdote and our conceptual argument is liberally sprinkled with "cognitive" terms such as *thoughts, preoccupations,* and *obsessions.* Our use of these terms is geared only to a poetic license to communicate some important behavioristic concepts. We think that applied behavior analysis is a viable operating strategy in the conceptualization of family psychopathology. Even though terms such as *uncertainty* and the *relational properties of stimuli* are abstractions, they do not require hypothetical constructs to be understood.

REFERENCES

Achenbach, T. M. (1979). Psychopathology of childhood: Research problems and issues. *Journal of Consulting and Clinical Psychology, 46,* 759–776.

Achenbach, T. M., & Edelbrock, C. S. (1979). The classification of child psychopathology: A review and analysis of empirical efforts. *Psychological Bulletin, 85,* 1275–1301.

Ainsworth, M. D. S. (1979). Attachment as related to mother–infant interaction. In J. S. Roxenblatt, R. A. Hinde, C. Beer, & M. Busnel (Eds.), *Advances in the study of behavior* (Vol. 9). New York: Academic Press.

Ainsworth, M. D. S., & Bell, S. M. V. (1974). Mother–infant interaction and the development of competence. In K. Connolly & J. Bruner (Eds.), *The growth of competence.* New York: Academic Press.

Ainsworth, M. D. S., Blehar, M. C., Waters, E., & Wall, S. (1978). *Patterns of attachment: A psychological study of the strange situation.* Hillsdale, NJ: Lawrence Erlbaum.

American Psychiatric Association. (1980). *Diagnostic and statistical manual of mental disorders* (3rd ed.). Washington, DC: American Psychiatric Association.

Anthony, E. J. (1970). The behavior disorders of childhood. In P. H. Mussen (Ed.), *Carmichael's Manual of Child Psychology.* New York: Wiley.

Arend, R., Gove, F., & Sroufe, L. A. (1979). Continuity of individual adaptation from infancy to kindergarten: A predictive study of ego-resiliency and curiosity in preschoolers. *Child Development, 50,* 950–959.

Baer, D. M., Wolf, M. M., & Risley, T. R. (1968). Some current dimensions of applied behavior analysis. *Journal of Applied Behavior Analysis, 1,* 91–97.

Bandura, A. (1962). Social learning through imitation. In M. R. Jones (Ed.), *Nebraska symposium on motivation.* Lincoln: University of Nebraska Press.

Barker, R. G. (1965). Explorations in ecological psychology. *American Psychologist, 20,* 1–14.

Bates, J. E. (1980). The concept of difficult temperament. *Merrill-Palmer Quarterly, 26,* 299–319.

Baumrind, D. (1967). Child care practices anteceding three patterns of pre-school behavior. *Genetic Psychology Monographs, 75,* 43–8.

Baumrind, D. (1971). Current patterns of parental authority. *Developmental Psychology Monographs, 41 (1),* Part 2.

Baumrind, D., & Black, A. E. (1967). Socialization practices associated with dimensions of competence in preschool boys and girls. *Child Development, 38,* 291–327.

Becker, W. C., & Krug, R. S. (1964). A circumplex model for social behavior in children. *Child Development, 35,* 371–396.

Becker, W. C., Peterson, D. R., Hellmer, L. A., Shoemaker, D. J., & Quay, H. C. (1959). Factors in parental behavior and personality as related to problem behavior in children. *Journal of Consulting and Clinical Psychology, 23,* 107–118.

Becker, W. C., Peterson, D. R., Luria, Z., Shoemaker, D. J., & Hellmer, L. A. (1962). Relations of factors derived from parent-interview ratings to behavior problems of five-year-olds. *Child Development, 33,* 509–535.

Beckwith, L. (1971). Relationships between attributes of mothers and their infants' IQ scores. *Child Development, 42,* 1083–1097.

Bell, R. Q. (1968). A reinterpretation of the direction of effects in studies of socialization. *Psychological Review, 75,* 31–95.

Bell, S. M. (1970). The development of the concept of object as related to infant–mother attachment. *Child Development, 41,* 291–311.

Bell, S. M., & Ainsworth, M. D. S. (1972). Infant crying and maternal responsiveness. *Child Development, 43,* 1171–1190.

Bennett, I. (1960). *Delinquent and neurotic children: A comparative study.* New York: Basic Books.

Bijou, S. W., & Baer, D. M. (1961). *Child development: Vol. 1. A systematic and empirical theory.* New York: Appleton.

Borkovec, T. D. (1970). Autonomic reactivity to sensory stimulation in psychopathic, neurotic and normal juvenile delinquents. *Journal of Consulting and Clinical Psychology, 35,* 219–222.

Brazelton, T. B. (1973). *The neonatal behavioral assessment scale.* Philadelphia: Lippincott.

Breit, M. (1982). Separation anxiety in mothers of latency-age fearful children. *Journal of Abnormal Child Psychology, 10,* 135–144.

Brown, R. T., & Quay, L. C. (1977). Reflection-impulsivity in normal and behavioral disordered children. *Journal of Abnormal Child Psychology, 5,* 457–462.

Bugental, D. B., & Love, L. (1975). Nonassertive expression of parental approval and disapproval and its relationship to child disturbance. *Child Development, 46,* 747–752.

Burgess, R. L., & Conger, R. D. (1978). Family interaction in abusive, neglectful and normal families. *Child Development, 49,* 1163–1173.

Cairns, R. B., & Paris, S. G. (1971). Informational determinants of social reinforcement effectiveness among retarded children. *American Journal of Mental Deficiency, 76(3),* 362–369.

Cantwell, D. P., Russell, T., Mattison, R., & Will, L. (1979). A comparison of DSM-II and DSM-III in the diagnosis of childhood psychiatric disorders: 1. Agreement with expected diagnosis. *Archives of General Psychiatry, 36,* 1208–1213.

Caplan, G. (1976). *Support systems and community mental health.* New York: Behavioral Publications.

Carey, W. B. (1970). A simplified method of measuring infant temperament. *Journal of Pediatrics, 77,* 188–194.

Clarke-Stewart, K. A. (1973). Interactions between mothers and their young children: Characteristics and consequences. *Monographs of the Society for Research in Child Development, 38,* 6–7.

Cochran, M. M., & Brassard, J. A. (1970). Child development and personal social network. *Child Development, 50,* 601–616.

Coopersmith, S. (1967). *The antecedents of self-esteem.* San Francisco: Freeman.

Crockenberg, S. (1981). Infant irritability, mother responsiveness and social support influences in the security of infant–mother attachment. *Child Development, 52,* 857–865.

Delfini, L. F., Bernal, M. E., & Rosen, P. M. (1976). Comparison of deviant and normal boys in home settings. In E. J. Mash, L. A. Hamerlynck, & L. C. Handy (Eds.), *Behavior modification and families.* New York: Brunner/Mazel.

Deur, J. L., & Parke, R. D. (1970). Effects of inconsistent punishment on aggression in children. *Developmental Psychology, 2(3),* 403–411.

Donovan, W. L., Leavitt, L. A., & Balling, J. D. (1978). Maternal physiological response to infant signals. *Psychophysiology, 15,* 68–74.

Dumas, J. E., & Wahler, R. G. (1983). Predictors of treatment outcome in parent training: Mother insularity and socioeconomic disadvantage. *Behavioral Assessment, 5,* 303–313.

Dumas, J. E., & Wahler, R. G. (1985). Indiscriminate mothering as a contextual factor in aggressive-oppositional child behavior: "Damned if you do and damned if you don't." *Journal of Abnormal Child Psycholgoy, 13,* 1–17.

Durlak, J. A., Stein, M. A., & Mannarino, A. P. (1980). Behavioral validity of a brief reacher rating scale (the AML) in identifying high-risk acting-out schoolchildren. *American Journal of Community Psychology, 8,* 101–114.

Edelbrock, C. S., & Achenbach, T. M. (1980). A typology of child behavior profile patterns: Distribution and correlates for disturbed children aged 6–16. *Journal of Abnormal Child Psychology, 8,* 441–470.

Egeland, B., & Sroufe, L. A. (1981). Attachment and early maltreatment. *Child Development, 52,* 44–52.

Eisenberg, J. G., Gersten, J. C., Langer, T. S., McCarthy, E. D., & Simcha-Fagan, O. (1976). A behavioral classification of welfare children from survey data. *American Journal of Orthopsychiatry, 46,* 447–463.

Eisenberg, L. (1958). School phobia: A study in the communication of anxiety. *American Journal of Psychiatry, 114,* 712–718.

Ellis, P. L. (1982). Empathy: A factor in antisocial behavior. *Journal of Abnormal Child Psychology, 10,* 123–134.

Eyberg, S. M., & Johnson, S. M. (1974). Multiple assessment of behavior modification with families: Effects of contingency contracting and order of treated problems. *Journal of Consulting and Clinical Psychology, 42,* 594–606.

Feshbach, S. (1970). Aggression. In P. H. Mussen (Ed.), *Carmichael's Manual of Child Psychology* (Vol. 2). New York: Wiley.

Forehand, R., King, H. Peed, S., & Yoder, P. (1975). Mother–child interactions: Comparison of a noncompliant clinic group and a nonclinic group. *Behavior Research and Therapy, 13,* 79–84.

Forehand, R., Wells, K. C., & Griest, D. L. (1980). An examination of the social validity of a parent training program. *Behavior Therapy, 11,* 488–502.

Fowler, S. A., & Baer, D. M. (1981). "Do I have to be good all day?": The timing of delayed reinforcement as a factor in generalization. *Journal of Applied Behavior Analysis, 14,* 13–24.

Frodi, A. M., Lamb, M. E., Leavitt, L. A., & Donovan, W. L. (1978). Fathers' and mothers' responses to infant smiles and cries. *Infant Behavior and Development, 1,* 187–198.

Garmezy, N. (1974). The study of competence in children at risk for severe psychopathology. In E. J. Anthony & C. Koupernik (Eds.), *The child and its family: Children at psychiatric risk.* New York: Wiley.

Gersten, J. C., Langner, T. S., Eisenberg, J. G., Simcha-Fagen, O., & McCarthy, E. D. (1976). Stability and change in types of behavioral disturbances of children and adolescents. *Journal of Abnormal Child Psychology, 4,* 111–128.

Glueck, S., & Glueck, E. T. (1950). *Unraveling juvenile delinquency.* New York: Commonwealth Fund.

Gottman, J. M. (1977). Toward a definition of social isolation in children. *Child Development, 48,* 513–517.

Gottman, J. M., Gonso, J., & Schuler, P. (1976). Teaching social skills to isolated children. *Journal of Abnormal Child Psychology, 4,* 179–197.

Goyette, C. H., Conners, C. K., & Ulrich, R. F. (1978). Normative data on revised Conners Parent & Teacher Rating Scales. *Journal of Abnormal Child Psychology, 6,* 221–236.

Green, K. D., Beck, S. J., Forehand, R., & Vosk, B. (1983). Validity of teacher nominations of child behavior problems. *Journal of Abnormal Child Psychology, 11,* 221–232.

Greenwood, C. R., Walker, H. M., Todd, N. M., & Hops, H. (1979). Selecting a cost-effective screening device for the assessment of preschool social withdrawal. *Journal of Applied Behavior Analysis, 12,* 639–652.

Greenwood, C. R., Todd, N. M., Hops, H., & Walker, H. M. (1982). Behavior change targets in the assessment and treatment of socially withdrawn preschool children. *Behavioral Assessment, 4,* 273–297.

Griest, D. L., & Wells, K. C. (1983). Behavioral family therapy with conduct disorders in children. *Behavior Therapy, 14,* 37–53.

Griest, D. L., Wells, K. C., & Forehand, R. (1979). An examination of predictors of maternal perceptions of maladjustments in clinic-referred children. *Journal of Abnormal Psychology, 88,* 277–281.

Hartup, W., Glazer, J., & Charlesworth, R. (1967). Peer reinforcement and sociometric status. *Child Development, 38,* 1017–1024.

Hendricks, A. F. C. J. (1972). *Reported versus observed deviance.* Unpublished manuscript, University of Nijmegen, Netherlands.

Herbert, E. W., & Baer, D. M. (1972). Training parents as behavior modifiers: Self-recording of contingent attention. *Journal of Applied Behavior Analysis, 5,* 139–149.

Hersov, L. School refusal. (1976). In M. Rutter & L. Hersov (Eds.), *Child psychiatry: Modern approaches.* Oxford: Blackwell.

Hetherington, E. M., & Frankie, G. (1967). Effects of parental dominance, warmth, and conflict on initiation in children. *Journal of Personality and Social Psychology, 6(2),* 119–125.

Hetherington, E. M., & Martin, B. (1979). Family interaction. In H. C. Quay & J. S. Werry (Eds.), *Psychopathological disorders of childhood* (2nd ed.). New York: Wiley.

Hetherington, E. M., Cox, M., & Cox, R. (1978). The aftermath of divorce. In J. H. Stevens & M. Matthews (Eds.), *Mother–child, father–child relations.* Washington, DC: National Association for the Education of Young Children.

Hewitt, L. E., & Jenkins, R. L. (1946). *Fundamental patterns of maladjustment: The dynamics of their origin.* Chicago: State of Illinois.

Jenkins, R. L. (1968). The varieties of children's behavioral problems and family dynamics. *American Journal of Psychiatry, 124,* 1440–1445.

Johnson, S. M., Wahl, G., Martin, S., & Johansson, S. (1973). How deviant is the normal child?: A behavioral analysis of the preschool child and his family. In R. D. Rubin, J. P. Brady, & J. D. Henderson (Eds.), *Advances in behavior therapy* (Vol. 4). New York: Academic Press.

Kagan, J., & Moss, H. A. (1962). *Birth to maturity.* New York: Wiley.

Kantor, J. R. (1959). *Interbehavioral psychology.* Granville, OH: Principia Press.

Katz, R. (1971). Interactions between the facilitative and inhibitory effects of a punishing stimulus in the control of children's hitting behavior. *Child Development, 42,* 1433–1446.

Kazdin, A. E. (1982). Symptom substitution, generalization and response covariation: Implications for psychotherapy outcome. *Psychological Bulletin, 91,* 349–365.

Kellam, S. G., Ensminger, M. E., & Turner, R. J. (1977). Family structure and the mental health of children. *Archives of General Psychiatry, 34,* 1011–1022.

Kendall, P. C., Deardorff, P. A., Finch, A. J., Jr., & Graham, L. (1976). Proxemics, locus of control, anxiety and type of movement in emotionally disturbed and normal boys. *Journal of Abnormal Child Psychology, 4,* 9–16.

Kolvin, I., Garside, R. F., Nicol, A. R., MacMillan, A., Wolstenholme, F., & Leitch, I. M. (1977). Familial and sociological correlates of behavioral and sociometric deviance in 8-year-old children. In P. J. Graham (Ed.), *Epidemiological approaches in child psychiatry.* London: Academic Press.

Kopfstein, D. (1972). The effects of accelerating and decelerating consequences on the social behavior of trainable retarded children. *Child Development, 43,* 800–809.

Lagerkvist, B., Laruitze, S., Olin, P., & Tengvald, K. (1975). Four-year-olds in a new suburb: The need for medical and social care. *Acta Paediatrica Scandinavia, 64,* 413–420.

Lamb, M. E. (1978). Social interaction in infancy and the development of personality. In M. E. Lamb (Ed.), *Social and personality development.* New York: Holt, Rinehart & Winston.

Langner, T. S., Gerston, J. C., Greene, E. L., Eisenberg, J. G., Herson, J. H., & McCarthy, E. D. (1974). Treatment of psychological disorders among urban children. *Journal of Consulting and Clinical Psychology, 42,* 170–179.

Langner, T. S., McCarthy, E. D., Gersten, J. C., Simcha-Fagan, O., & Eisenberg, J. G. (1979). Factors in children's behavior and mental health over time: The Family Research Project. *Research in Community and Mental Health, 1,* 127–181.

Ledingham, J. E. (1981). Developmental patterns of aggressive and withdrawn behavior in childhood: A possible method for identifying preschizophrenics. *Journal of Abnormal Child Psychology, 9,* 1–22.

Leighton, L. A., Stollack, G. E., & Ferguson, L. (1971). Patterns of communication in normal and clinic families. *Journal of Consulting and Clinical Psychology, 36,* 252–256.

Levy, D. M. (1943). *Maternal overprotection.* New York: Columbia University Press.

Lewis, H. (1954). *Deprived children.* London: Oxford University Press.

Lewis, M. L., & Goldberg, S. (1969). Perceptual-cognitive development in infancy: A generalized expectancy model as a function of mother–infant interaction. *Merrill-Palmer Quarterly, 15,* 81–100.

Lipsitt, L. P., & Kaye, H. (1964). Conditioned sucking in human newborn. *Psychonomic Science, 1,* 29–30.

Lobitz, W. C., & Johnson, S. M. (1975). Parental manipulation of the behavior of normal and deviant children. *Child Development, 46,* 719–726.

Loeber, R., & Schmaling, K. B. (1986). *Empirical evidence for overt and covert patterns of antisocial conduct problems.* Unpublished paper, Oregon Social Learning Center, Eugene, Oregon.

Love, L. R., & Kaswan, J. W. (1974). *Troubled children: Their families, schools, and treatments.* New York: Wiley.

Lynn, D. B. (1974). *The father: His role in child development.* Monterey, CA: Brooks/Cole.

Martin, B. (1975). Parent–child relations. In F. D. Horowitz, E. M. Hetherington, S. Scarr-Salapatek, & G. M. Siegel (Eds.), *Review of child development research* (Vol. 4). Chicago: University of Chicago Press.

Matas, L., Arend, R. A., & Sroufe, L. A. (1978). Continuity of adaptation in the second year: The relationship between quality of attachment and later competence. *Child Development, 49,* 547–556.

McCord, W., McCord, J., & Zola, I. K. (1959). *Origins of crime.* New York: Columbia University Press.

McCord, W., McCord, J., & Howard, A. (1961). Familial correlates of aggression in nondelinquent male children. *Journal of Abnormal and Social Psychology, 62,* 79–93.

Miller, L. C. (1967). Louisville Behavior Checklist for males, 6–12 years of age. *Psychological Reports, 21,* 897–903.

Miller, L. C. (1973). *Louisville Behavior Checklist manual.* Los Angeles: Western Psychological Services.

Milliones, J. (1978). Relationship between perceived child temperament and maternal behavior. *Child Development, 49,* 1255–1257.

Murrell, S. A., & Stachowiak, J. G. (1967). Consistency, rigidity, and power in the interaction patterns of clinic and nonclinic families. *Journal of Abnormal and Social Psychology, 72,* 265–272.

Panaccione, V. F., & Wahler, R. G. (1986). Child behavior, maternal depression and social coercion as factors in the quality of child care. *Journal of Abnormal Child Psychology, 14,* 263–278.

Parke, R. D. (1970). The role of punishment in the socialization process. In Ronald A. Hoppe (Ed.), *Early experiences and the process of socialization.* New York: Academic Press.

Parke, R. D., & Deur, J. L. (1972). Schedule of punishment and inhibition of aggression in children. *Developmental Psychology, 7,* 266–269.

Patterson, G. R. (1976). The aggressive child: Victim and architect of a coercive system. In E. J. Nash, L. A. Hamerlynck, & L. C. Handy (Eds.), *Behavior modification and families: 1. Theory and research.* New York: Brunner/Mazel.

Patterson, G. R. (1977). Accelerating stimuli for two classes of coercive behaviors. *Journal of Abnormal Child Psychology, 5,* 335–350.

Patterson, G. R. (1980). Mothers: The unacknowledged victims. *Monographs of the Society for Research in Child Development, 45,* 5.

Patterson, G. R. (1982). *A social learning approach: Vol. 3. Coercive family process.* Eugene, OR: Castalia Publishing.

Patterson, G. R., & Cobb, J. A. (1971). A dyadic analysis of "aggressive" behaviors. In J. P. Hill (Ed.), *Minnesota Symposia on Child Psychology* (Vol. 5). Minneapolis: University of Minnesota Press.

Patterson, G. R., Ray, R. S., Shaw, D., & Cobb, J. A. (1969). *A manual for coding of family interactions, 1969 revision.* Available as document 01234 from ASIS/NAPS, 440 Park Avenue South, New York, NY 10016.

Peterson, D. R., & Migliorino, G. (1967). Pancultural factors of parental behavior in Sicily and the United States. *Child Development, 38,* 967–991.

Prior, M., Boulton, D., Gayzago, C., & Perry, D. (1975). The classification of childhood psychosis by numerical taxonomy. *Journal of Child Psychology and Psychiatry, 16,* 321–330.

Quay, H. C. (1979). Classification, In H. C. Quay & J. S. Werry (Eds.), *Psychopathological disorders of childhood* (2nd ed.). New York: Wiley.

Quay, H. C., & Peterson, D. R. (1975). *Manual for the behavior problem checklist.* Unpublished manuscript.

Reid, J. B. (1978). *A social learning approach to family interaction: Vol. 2. A manual for coding family interactions.* Eugene, OR: Castalia Publishing.

Reid, J. B., & Hendricks, A. F. (1973). A preliminary analysis of the effectiveness of direct home interventions for treatment of predelinquent boys who steal. In L. Hamerlynck, L. Handy, & E. Mash (Eds.), *Behavior therapy: Methodology, concepts and practice.* Champaign, IL: Research Press.

Robins, L. (1966). *Deviant children grown up.* Baltimore: Williams & Wilkins.

Robins, L. N., & Ratcliff, K. S. (1980). Childhood conduct disorders and later arrest. In L. N. Robins, P. Clayton, & J. Wing (Eds.), *Social consequences of psychiatric illness.* New York: Brunner/Mazel.

Rosenthal, M. J., Ni, E., Finkelstein, M., & Berwits, G. K. (1962). Father–child relationships and children's problems. *Archives of General Psychiatry, 7,* 360–373.

Rothchild, J., & Wolf, S. (1976). *The children of the counter culture.* New York: Doubleday.

Rovee-Collier, C. K., & Lipsitt, L. P. (1981). Learning, adaptation, and memory. In P. M. Stratton (Ed.), *Psychobiology of the human newborn.* New York: Wiley.

Russo, D. C., Cataldo, M. F., & Cushing, P. J. (1981). Compliance training and behavioral covariation in the treatment of multiple behavior problems. *Journal of Applied Behavior Analysis, 14,* 209–222.

Rutter, M. (1979). Protective factors in children's responses to stress and disadvantage. In M. W. Kent & J. E. Rolf (Eds.), *Primary prevention of psychopathology: Vol. 3. Social competence in children.* Hanover, NH: University Press of New England.

Sawin, D. B., & Parke, R. D. (1979). Inconsistent discipline of aggression in young boys. *Journal of Experimental Child Psychology, 28,* 525–538.

Schaefer, E. S. (1959). A circumplex model for maternal behavior. *Journal of Abnormal and Social Psychology, 59,* 226–235.

Schaefer, E. S. (1961). Converging conceptual models for maternal behavior and for child behavior. In J. C. Glidewell (Ed.), *Parental attitudes and child behavior.* Springfield, IL: Charles C Thomas.

Sears, R. R., Maccoby, E. E., & Levin, H. (1957). *Patterns of child rearing.* Evanston, IL: Row & Peterson.

Shure, M. B., & Spivack, G. (1979). Interpersonal cognitive problem solving and primary prevention: Programming for preschool and kindergarten children. *Journal of Clinical Child Psychology, 2,* 89–94.

Shure, M. B., & Spivack, G. (1980). Interpersonal problem solving as a mediator of behavioral adjustment in preschool and kindergarten children. *Journal of Applied Developmental Psychology, 1,* 29–44.

Sigel, I. E. (1979). Consciousness-raising of individual competence in problem solving. In M. W. Kent & J. E. Rolf (Eds.), *Primary prevention of psychopathology: Vol. 3. Social competence in children.* Hanover, NH: University Press of New England.

Simon, S. J., Ayllon, T., & Milan, M. A. (1986). Behavioral compensation: Contrastlike effects in the classroom. *Behavior Modification, 13,* 101–110.

Smith, H. T. (1958). A comparison of interview and observation measures of mother behavior. *Journal of Abnormal and Social Psychology, 57,* 278–282.

Snyder, J. J. (1977). A reinforcement analysis of intervention in problem and nonproblem children. *Journal of Abnormal Psychology, 86*(5), 528–535.

Stayton, D. J., & Ainsworth, M. D. S. (1973). Individual differences in infant responses to brief, everyday separations as related to other infant and maternal behaviors. *Developmental Psychology, 9,* 226–235.

Stayton, D. J., Hogan, R., & Ainsworth, M. D. S. (1971). Infant obedience and maternal behavior: The origin of socialization reconsidered. *Child Development, 42,* 1057–1069.

Strain, P. S., & Shores, R. E. (1977). Social reciprocity: Review of research and educational implications. *Exceptional Children, 43,* 526–531.

Strain, P. S., Shores, R. E., & Kerr, M. M. (1976). An experimental analysis of "spillover" effects on the social interaction of behaviorally handicapped preschool children. *Journal of Applied Behavior Analysis, 9,* 31–40.

Thomas, A., Chess, S., & Birch, H. G. (1970). The origin of personality. *Scientific American, 223,* 2, 102–109.

Wahler, R. G. (1980). The insular mother: Her problems in parent–child treatment. *Journal of Applied Behavior Analysis, 13,* 207–219.

Wahler, R. G., & Afton, A. D. (1980). Attentional processes in insular and noninsular mothers. *Child Behavior Therapy, 2,* 25–41.

Wahler, R. G., & Dumas, J. E. (1986). "A chip off the old block": Some interpersonal characteristics of coercive children across generations. In P. Strain (Ed.), *Children's social behavior: Development, assessment, and modification.* New York: Academic Press.

Wahler, R. G., & Fox, J. J., III. (1980). Solitary toy play and time-out: A family treatment package for children with aggressive and oppositional behavior. *Journal of Applied Behavior Analysis, 13,* 23–39.

Wahler, R. G., & Graves, M. G. (1983). Setting events in social networks: Ally or enemy in child behavior therapy? *Behavior Therapy, 14,* 19–36.

Wahler, R. G., & Hann, D. M. (1986). A behavioral systems perspective in childhood psychopathology: Expanding the three-term operant contingency. In N. Krasnegar, M. Catado, & E. Rastah (Eds.), *Child Health Behavior, 1,* 146–167.

Wahler, R. G., & Nordquist, V. M. (1973). Adult discipline as a factor in childhood imitation. *Journal of Abnormal Child Psychology, 1,* 40–56.

Wahler, R. G., House, A. E., & Stambaugh, E. E. (1976). *Ecological assessment of child problem behavior.* New York: Pergamon Press.

Wahler, R. G., Leske, G., & Rogers, E. S. (1979). The insular family: A deviance support system for oppositional children. In L. A. Hamerlynck (Ed.), *Behavioral systems for the developmentally disabled: Vol. 1. School and family environments.* New York: Brunner/Mazel.

Wahler, R. G., Hughey, J. B., & Gordon, J. S. (1981). Chronic patterns of mother–child coercion: Some differences between insular and noninsular families. *Analysis and Intervention in Developmental Disabilities, 1*(2), 145–156.

Warren, V. L., & Cairns, R. B. (1972). Social reinforcement satiation: An outcome of frequency or ambiguity? *Journal of Experimental Child Psychology, 13,* 249–260.

Waters, E., Wippman, J., & Sroufe, L. A. (1979). Attachment, positive affect, and competence in the peer group: Two studies in construct valuation. *Child Development, 50,* 821–829.

Weinstein, L. (1965). Social schemata of emotional disturbed boys. *Journal of Abnormal Psychology, 70,* 457–461.

Wilson, H. (1974). Parenting in poverty. *British Journal of Social Work, 4,* 241–254.

Wilton, K., & Barbour, A. (1978). Mother–child interaction in high-risk and contrast preschoolers of low socioeconomic status. *Child Development, 49,* 1136–1145.

Winder, C. L., & Rau, L. (1962). Parental abilities associated with social deviance in preadolescent boys. *Journal of Abnormal and Social Psychology, 64,* 418–424.

Yarrow, L. J., Rubenstein, J. L., Peterson, F. A., & Jankowski, J. J. (1972). Dimensions of early stimulation and their different effects on infant development. *Merrill-Palmer Quarterly, 18,* 205–218.

CHAPTER 17

Psychopathology

A Behavior Genetic Perspective

Michael F. Pogue-Geile and Richard J. Rose

The central task in family studies of psychopathology is the identification of the causes of individual variation and familial resemblance. Why and how do behavior disorders exhibit familial aggregation? How and why do siblings who are reared together exhibit differences in behavioral outcome?

We recognize that environmental factors, including those shared with family members and those specific to an individual, can contribute importantly to the onset and course of behavior disorders. We recognize also that genetic differences can influence the development of lifestyles and can modulate the effect of environmental events. Accordingly, there is widespread recognition that twin-family studies offer incisive tools in our efforts to identify genetic predispositions to psychopathology and the genetic modulation of environmental stress.

In this chapter, we describe in a nontechnical fashion these behavior genetic methods for the investigation of psychopathology, discussing first the analysis of genetic variation and then the evaluation of environmental influences. The applications of these methods are illustrated with substantive examples from a range of psychopathologies.

FAMILIAL AGGREGATION OF PSYCHOPATHOLOGY

Psychopathologies, like most other biological and behavioral characteristics, exhibit significant familial aggregation. In the case of schizophrenia, Gottesman

MICHAEL F. POGUE-GEILE • Department of Psychology and Department of Psychiatry, University of Pittsburgh, Pittsburgh, PA 15260. RICHARD J. ROSE • Department of Psychology and Department of Medical Genetics, Indiana University, Bloomington, IN 47405. Completion of this chapter was supported in part by Biomedical Research Support Grant RR07084-20 from the National Institute of Health awarded to the first author, and grant NIAAA-6232 and Senior Fellowship (TW1019) from the John E. Fogarty Foundation awarded to the second author.

and Shields (1982) estimated the lifetime risk for schizophrenia as 12.8% in offspring of one schizophrenic parent, and as 10.1% in siblings of schizophrenic probands, compared to a risk of 1% in the general population—an approximately 10-fold increase in risk for close family members of a schizophrenic proband. A similar situation obtains for unipolar depression, in which a morbid risk in first-degree relatives of unipolar probands has been reported as 18.4%, compared to 5.9% in relatives of normal controls—an approximately three-fold increase (Weissman *et al.*, 1984). First-degree relatives of alcoholic probands have similarly been estimated as having at least a five-fold increase in their risk for alcoholism compared to the general population (Goodwin, 1979).

Such demonstrations of familiality are not surprising and are only the first step in the study of the etiology of any characteristic that shows variation in a population. The basic question concerns the determinants of these observed familial correlations: Why does psychopathology run in families?

THE ANALYSIS OF GENETIC INFLUENCES

The Classic Twin Study

In the nuclear family studies cited above, the origins of familiality are difficult to specify because both genes and experiences are shared among family members. Because nuclear family studies alone are usually not sufficient to disentangle the relative roles of genetic and environmental influences, twin and adoption strategies have been developed to detect genetic influences.

The classic twin study has been the most common strategy used for the analysis of genetic influences on psychopathology. Its rationale lies in the comparison of phenotypic resemblance between two sibling relationships that differ in genetic similarity, but that are assumed to be equivalent in relevant environmental similarity. Monozygotic (MZ) twins share 100% of their genes, whereas dizygotic (DZ) twins, like other siblings, share only, on average, 50% of their genes. If MZ co-twins share no more environmental experiences relevant to the development of psychopathology than do DZ co-twins, any increased similarity, or concordance, of MZ co-twins compared to that shown by DZ co-twins must be attributed to their greater genetic similarity.

The validity of this inference depends on several assumptions. First, twins are assumed to be representative of the general population for the trait under study—an assumption that must be tested because twins differ from nontwins in several potentially significant ways. Specifically, factors associated with the twinning process may be associated with the risk for psychopathology. DZ twinning is related to maternal age and parity. Furthermore, the placentation of most MZ twins differs from that of DZ twins and singletons, and placental differences may be related to variables of importance. The birth weight and size of twins systematically differ from those of singletons, and early in development, these factors predict motor and mental growth. Tests of these potential biases must be made by evaluating the prevalence of the disorder in twins relative to singletons, and by testing the generalizability of inferences drawn from twin data to results obtained from other data sets. Additionally, experiences unique to being a twin may influence the development of some behavioral traits or psychopathologies. Thus, it was suggested that experience unique to MZ twins impairs the development of their personal identity and creates elevated risk for schizophrenia (Jackson, 1960). Again, the obvious test is a comparison of the prevalence of a particular disorder (e.g., schizophrenia) among twins in general and among monozygotic twins in particular with its prevalence among singletons. For schizophrenia, the risks appear to be equivalent (Rosenthal, 1960). Twins do differ from singletons in some aspects of early behavior development, including language fluency, but such differences dissipate with age, and by puberty, few consistent differences remain. On standardized personality, interest, and aptitude scales, twins obtain scores that are indistinguishable from those of nontwins, and in the face of such evidence, it appears unlikely that experiences peculiar to twins have systematic effects on personality development and psychopathology.

Beyond the assumptions necessary for valid generalizations from twins to nontwins, a second set of assumptions is necessary for valid comparisons of the two twin types. The first assumption is that the prevalence of the disorder under study is not associated with twin type—a premise that can be evaluated by a test of the difference in relative frequencies of affected individuals in representative samples of MZ and DZ twins.

The second assumption necessary to the classic twin method is equality of environmental covariance in MZ and DZ twin pairs. No aspect of the twin method has been challenged more frequently than this assumption of "equal environments," and in recent years, no assumption has been tested more rigorously. MZ twins do have more similar experiences than do DZs. They are more likely to sleep in the same room during childhood, are more likely to play together, are more likely to share a similar circle of adolescent friends, and so on. The important question, of course, is whether such shared experiences systematically influence the development of psychopathology and personality. Consider the question: Are within-pair differences in experience correlated with intrapair differences in dimensions of personality? For example, some identical twins dress alike, but others do not. Given a large set of identical twins, we can test whether the tendency to dress alike is associated with similarity in personality. Extensive tests (e.g., Loehlin & Nichols, 1976) suggest a negative answer for this aspect of experience and for all others so tested.

Other tests of the equal-environments assumption have led to the same conclusion. For example, an approach introduced by Scarr (1968) and later replicated by Matheny (1979) studied twin pairs misclassified for zygosity. Many twin children are misidentified by themselves and their parents, usually on the basis of erroneous placental information at the time of delivery. An evaluation of such misclassified twin pairs reveals that behavioral differences in twins relate to their true zygosity.

In short, equality of relevant environmental covariance appears to be a tenable assumption, and there is no consistent evidence of important differences in attitude or experience of MZ and DZ twins. In their large sample of adolescent twins, Loehlin and Nichols (1976) found that only 5 of 1,600 discrete variables reliably distinguished the two twin types, and only one item consistently differed in both sexes. What item? Pretending to be one's twin!

Twin designs have been extensively used in the study of psychopathology. For example, 11 major twin studies of schizophrenia have been completed, and although differing in methodological rigor and diagnostic criteria, these studies have been unanimous in finding concordance rates for schizophrenia that are three to five times higher among MZ twins than among DZ twins. In a compilation of the five recent twin studies, Gottesman and Shields (1982) estimated the overall concordance rates weighted by sample size for MZ twins to be 46% and that for DZ twins to be 14%. Such robust findings, replicated across investigators, countries, and time periods, provide extremely persuasive evidence for a role of genetic influences in the etiology of schizophrenia. Similarly, average concordance rates across the seven twin studies of affective disorders have been estimated as 65% for MZ and 14% for DZ twins (Nurnberger & Gershon, 1982). The case for alcoholism appears to be somewhat more complex, with two studies reporting MZ concordances greater than DZ concordances, one reporting no difference, and one being equivocal (Goodwin, 1985; cf. Murray, Clifford, & Gurling, 1983). Although comparison of such concordance rates between MZ and DZ twins serves to detect the presence of genetic influences, much more information is available if the prevalence of the psychopathology in the general population is also known (Gottesman & Carey, 1983).

MZ Twins Reared Apart

The study of MZ twins reared apart (MZA) represents a hybrid twin-adoption design that provides a direct estimate of the importance of genetic influences in the absence of shared experience because only the influence of shared genotype contributes to the similarity between MZAs, assuming independent placement. Obviously, the representativeness of such rare MZAs must be scrutinized carefully, and only systematically ascertained MZAs should be studied. The concordance rates for schizophrenia among the 12 MZA pairs in the literature have been calculated as 58% (Gottesman & Shields, 1982) and as 67% for affective disorders in 12 published pairs (Price, 1968).

Adoption Studies

In addition to the twin designs, adoption strategies have also been developed to estimate the importance of genetic influences. The rationale for adoption studies is in some sense complementary to that for twin studies. Whereas the twin study compares two groups of siblings who differ in genetic resemblance although both share a family rearing environment, the basic adoption study of genetic influences investigates the association between genetically related individuals who are reared in uncorrelated environments, such as biological parents and their adopted-away offspring. Because biological parents and their adopted-away offspring share half their genes but no family environmental experiences, any significant association between the two may be attributed to their shared genotype. Biological siblings who are reared apart provide a similar comparison.

As in the twin designs, this inference depends on several important assumptions. First, adoptees are assumed to be representative of the general population of nonadoptees for the trait under study. However, children who are adopted tend to be born to young, unmarried women, and maternal age as well as circumstances of prenatal care, pregnancy, and delivery could be causally relevant to major psychopathology. Furthermore, adoptive parents may be selectively screened by adoption agencies so that their personal and familial characteristics distinguish them from the larger population of nonadopting parents.

A second major assumption is that genetic background and rearing environment are uncorrelated for factors relevant to the development of the specific psychopathology under study. For selective placement to invalidate the inference of genetic influence, adoption agencies would have to selectively place offspring of affected biological parents in adoptive homes that demonstrated psychopathology-inducing characteristics. In this case, any correlation between psychopathology in the biological parents and the adoptees would be spurious and would be secondary to selective placement. Given our current inability to identify psychopathology-inducing environments, the likelihood of selective placement by adoption agencies on such putative characteristics would seem minimal.

For relatively rare disorders, two different proband ascertainment strategies have been developed to investigate the association between the biological parents' phenotype and the phenotype of their adopted-away offspring, whereas for more common disorders, an unselected sample of adoptees can be efficient. The cohort, or adoptees, method begins with the affected biological parents with adopted-away offspring as probands. The rate of psychopathology in their adopted-away offspring is then compared to that found in the adopted-away offspring of control parents who exhibit no psychopathology. The second ascertainment strategy has been termed the *adoptees' families design* because affected adoptees serve as the probands and the rate of psychopathology among their biological relatives is compared to that among the biological relatives of normal control adoptees. This approach may be considered a variation on case-control sampling (Pogue-Geile & Harrow, 1984). The adoptees' families design depends on the screening of affected adopting biological parents being minimal. Such screening might occur if affected parents wishing to adopt away as a resolution to an unwanted pregnancy were recommended an abortion instead of adoption. An additional screen may occur because parents in general appear to be screened for mental health compared to nonparents. For example, rates of psychopathology in parents of probands often are lower than those for siblings. Thus, the adoptees' families design may be expected to have a relatively low yield of psychopathology in biological parents, given the possibility of these two screenings for health in adopting parents. To ensure against this problem, other biological relatives, such as siblings and half-siblings, who are less likely to be screened, are also generally assessed in adoptees' families designs.

To date, one ongoing and two complete studies with normal control groups have investigated genetic influences on schizophrenia using the adoptees design.

The first study, completed by Heston in Oregon and reported in 1966, found a morbid risk for schizophrenia of 16.6% among the adopted-away offspring of chronic schizophrenic biological mothers. This risk was significantly higher than the 0% found among adopted-away offspring of normal control biological parents. Rosenthal and colleagues, in a similar study in Denmark, reported rates of borderline or definite schizophrenia in index adoptees of 18.8% versus 10.1% for control adoptees ($p \leq .06$) (Rosenthal, Wender, Kety, Schulsinger, Welner, & Rieder, 1968; Rosenthal, Wender, Kety, Welner, & Schulsinger, 1971; Wender, Rosenthal, Kety, Schulsinger, & Welner, 1974). The third major adoptee study of schizophrenia is currently in progress, directed by Tienari in Finland. A recent preliminary report also shows increased rates of psychosis or borderline disorder in index adoptees with schizophrenic biological parents (16.5%) compared to control adoptees with normal biological parents (7.7%) (Tienari, Sorri, Lahti, Naarala, Wahlberg, Pohjola, & Moring, 1985).

Kety and colleagues in Denmark have completed the largest series of adoptees' families studies of schizophrenia. In their first study, the biological and adoptive relatives of schizophrenic and normal adoptees from the Greater Copenhagen area were diagnosed based on institutional records (Kety, Rosenthal, Wender, & Schulsinger, 1968). After that report, the investigators personally interviewed the relatives, and in this Greater Copenhagen Interview Study (Kety, Rosenthal, Wender, Schulsinger, & Jacobsen, 1975), rates were found for their "hard" schizophrenia spectrum of 12.1% in the biological parents of schizophrenic adoptees, compared to 6.2% in the biological parents of normal control adoptees. Similarly, elevated rates of schizophrenia-spectrum disorders were found among biological half-siblings of schizophrenic adoptees (19.2%) compared to half-siblings of normal adoptees (2.9%). This project was then extended to include all schizophrenic adoptees in Denmark, and a preliminary report was published (Kety, Rosenthal, Wender, Schulsinger, & Jacobsen, 1978). This Danish National Case Record Study has also found increased rates of schizophrenia-spectrum disorders among all biological relatives of index adoptees (5.9%) compared to controls (1.0%).

There have been three adoption studies of affective disorders to date. A small adoptees study by Cadoret (1978) in Iowa reported that 3 of 8 adoptees of biological mothers with affective disorder also showed depression at follow-up, compared to 4 depressed adoptees of 43 normal control biological parents ($p \leq .07$). A much larger adoptees' families study by Mendlewicz and Rainer (1977) in Belgium used adoptees with bipolar mania-depression as probands. Affective disorder was concentrated in the biological parents of bipolar adoptees compared to the biological parents of normal control adoptees. Contradictory findings have been reported in a second adoptees' families study using the Stockholm adoption register and institutional records (von Knorring, Cloninger, Bohman, & Sigvardsson, 1983). The rate of affective disorder in the biological parents of depressed adoptees was not significantly greater than that found in the biological parents of control adoptees. This contradiction between the Swedish adoption-study results and other twin and adoption data on affective disorders is difficult to resolve and requires further study.

Potential genetic influences on susceptibility to alcoholism have also been investigated in four studies using adoption methods. Adoptee studies have been carried out in the United States (Roe, 1944), in Denmark (e.g., Goodwin, Schulsinger, Knop, Mednick, & Guze, 1977), and in Iowa (e.g., Cadoret, Cain, & Grove, 1980), and an unselected, total sample of adoptees has been studied in Sweden (e.g., Bohman, Sigvardsson, & Cloninger, 1981; Cloninger, Bohman, & Sigvardsson, 1981). Three studies have reported a significant association between biological parent and adoptee alcoholism; one found no association (Roe, 1944). These studies have also provided evidence for the heterogeneity of alcoholism, with some forms possibly being primarily genetically influenced, and others being less so.

Models of Genetic Transmission

Because the focus of this chapter is on a behavior genetic perspective of family–environment research, we will not discuss in detail the methods and findings of studies that have attempted to describe the specific nature of these genetic influences on the various psychopathologies. Clearly, demonstrating the presence of genetic influences is merely the first step, and the identification of the mode of genetic transmission, the localization of genetic loci, and the characterization of gene products are the primary goals of study. Although this progression has been completed for many disorders, research has yet to unequivocally identify the mode of genetic transmission for any of the major psychopathologies. A number of studies have attempted to model the genetic mode of transmission of schizophrenia, with generally equivocal results (Faraone & Tsuang, 1985), although fully penetrant single-major-locus (SML) genetic models can be rejected. However, most studies have found it difficult to choose among various SML models with reduced penetrance, multiple loci models, mixed models, and multifactorial models, although often the multifactorial model shows some advantages. The multifactorial model (Falconer, 1965) will be briefly described because of its potential relevance to the disorders discussed in this volume.

The multifactorial model hypothesizes the existence of a continuous and normally distributed dimension of liability to a certain psychopathology. Although this liability is present in some degree in all persons, only those beyond a certain threshold would be clinically diagnosed. The degree of liability is hypothesized to be determined by *both* multiple genetic and multiple environmental influences. The effects of these putative influences are often hypothesized to be equal and additive, so that a value for an individual on the dimension of liability is the sum of the relevant genetic and environmental influences. Thus, for example, clinical schizophrenia (i.e., a suprathreshold value on the liability dimension) may arise because of either the presence of a number of "schizogenes" with few environmental insults, a moderate dose of both morbid genes and environmental influences, or a large number of "schizophrenogenic" environmental insults with little genetic contribution. As can be seen, this is quite a general model, and few of its characteristics are specified. Nevertheless, it is a useful conceptual model for continuously distributed characteristics and common disorders.

Estimates of the heritability of liability to psychopathology may be calculated from the multifactorial model. *Heritability* refers to the proportion of variation in liability in the population that may be attributed to genetic variation. Heritability estimates are thus time- and population-specific and will change if relevant environmental or genetic variation is altered. Thus, such estimates imply nothing concerning the malleability of a behavior disorder or its responsiveness to therapeutic treatments, but they do provide an overall estimate of the importance of genetic factors assuming polygenic transmission. First calculated for schizophrenia by Gottesman and Shields (1967), estimates of the heritability of schizophrenia generally range between 60% and 70% (e.g., Fulker, 1973; McGue, Gottesman, & Rao, 1983). Such figures suggest that genetic variation accounts for the majority of variation in the liability to schizophrenia, with only approximately 30% to 40% being due to environmental influences of some type. In the balance of the chapter, we review methods relevant to understanding such environmental influences.

THE ANALYSIS OF UNSPECIFIED ENVIRONMENTAL INFLUENCES

As the twin and adoption studies cited above make clear, genetic influences play a role in the etiology of a variety of different psychopathologies. However, in no psychopathology have genetic factors alone been found to be sufficient. In all psychopathologies, the behavior genetic evidence suggests some role for environmental variation. The issue, of course, is the characterization of these influences.

We should make clear that we will be discussing evidence for environmental influences on the etiology of psychopathologies, not on their course. Although etiology and course are not entirely distinct, the demonstration of environmental effects on the course of a disorder (e.g., treatment) does not imply that similar environmental experiences are relevant to its etiology. In addition, it should be clear that *environmental* does not necessarily mean "psychological." Exposure to viruses and perinatal insult are also environmental experiences that may be as relevant as—or more relevant than—poor mothering to the etiology of some psychopathologies.

Shared Family Environmental Experience

We will first present methods for investigating unspecified environmental influences using the behavior genetic distinction between shared family experiences and nonshared experiences (Jinks & Fulker, 1970). Like genetic influences, environmental influences may contribute both to family resemblance and to differences within a family. Data on this broad distinction may make the search for specific environmental experiences relevant to psychopathologies more informed.

Although, specific estimates of shared family experiences made from a number of different designs are discussed below, let us first examine a rough upper-bound estimate of this influence based on sibling–sibling or DZ twin concordances or correlations. Such data provide an upper-bound estimate because we know from the data cited above that at least some of this familiality among siblings is due to shared genetic influences. In the case of schizophrenia, the risk in the siblings and the DZ co-twins of schizophrenic probands is approximately 10% to 14% (Gottesman & Shields, 1982). DZ concordance for affective disorders is in a similar range (14%—Nurnberger & Gershon, 1982), as is that for hospitalized alcoholics (11%—Hrubec & Omenn, 1981). These figures indicate that the overall familiality for these psychopathologies is rather low, and given that at least some of it is due to shared genetic influences, the potential portion to be attributed to *shared* environmental influences may not be large.

Adoptive Siblings Reared Together. One of the most direct estimates of the importance of shared rearing experiences is provided by the correlation between biologically unrelated siblings who are reared together. This method involves the comparison of genetically unrelated adoptive siblings of affected adoptees (who share their rearing environment, but no genes) to adoptive siblings of normal adoptees (who share neither genes or environment with an affected proband). Although valuable, unexpectedly few data relevant to this strategy have been reported in the study of psychopathology. For schizophrenia, data from Kety's Greater Copenhagen Interview Study showed no significant increase in risk among adoptive siblings of schizophrenic adoptees, although the sample sizes were small (Kety *et al.*, 1975). Publication of appropriate data from the larger Danish National sample based on either institutional records (Kety *et al.*, 1978) or interviews (Kety, 1983) would address this issue more precisely with larger sample sizes. Karlsson's Icelandic study (1966) also assessed the adoptive siblings of schizophrenic adoptees. No schizophrenic patients were identified from 28 adoptive siblings of schizophrenic adoptees. Similarly, in a larger study, Kallman (1946) found only one schizophrenic among adoptive siblings of schizophrenic probands.

Mendlewicz (1981) reported similar data from his adoption study of bipolar affective disorder. Only 1 unipolar depressive was identified from 12 adoptive siblings of bipolar probands. However, a comparable figure for adoptive siblings of normal adoptees was not reported. To date, only data on the parents and not on adoptive siblings of adoptees have been reported from the Stockholm adoption study of depression (von Knorring *et al.*, 1983).

As regards alcoholism, the Danish adoptees' study by Goodwin has not reported data on adoptive siblings of adoptees. Cadoret and colleagues in Iowa found no correlation for alcoholism among adoptive siblings in their first two adoptees studies (Cadoret & Gath, 1978; Cadoret *et al.*, 1980), but in a more recent study, they reported a nonsignificant trend for increased alcohol problems in the adoptive siblings of alcoholic adoptees (Cadoret, O'Gorman, Troughton, & Heywood, 1985). Unfortunately, these adoptive siblings were not interviewed directly, and instead, information was gathered via nonblind interviews with adoptive parents and adoptees. To date, no data have been reported for adoptive siblings of adoptees from the Stockholm adoption study. Although preliminary, these data do not provide evidence of major main effects for rearing environment in the absence of shared genotype for these psychopathologies. However, the limited sample sizes make such conclusions tentative. This can be a quite informative method that should be exploited more fully in the study of psychopathology.

   Biological Siblings: Reared Together and Reared Apart. Other methods are also informative regarding the effects of shared rearing environment, although within the context of shared genotypes. These designs compare the risk of psychopathology in relationships in which genotypes are shared, along with rearing environment, to those in which only genotypes are shared. Such strategies assess whether a shared rearing environment has any *additional* effect over that provided by shared genotypes.

   The first example of this general strategy is the comparison of concordance rates between MZ twins reared together (MZT) versus the rare MZA twins. Whereas similarity among MZA twins is due only to their shared genotype, concordance for MZT twins may be a function of both shared genotype and shared experience. The extent to which concordance rates are higher among MZTs than among MZAs provides an estimate of the additional importance of shared environment in the context of shared genotype.

   For schizophrenia, Gottesman and Shields's estimate (1982) of a 58% concordance rate for MZA twins is *not* lower than that generally found for MZT twins (46%). Similarly, concordance among MZAs for affective disorder has been estimated at 67% (Price, 1968), compared to an average across studies of 65% for MZTs (Nurnberger & Gershon, 1982). Data on systematically ascertained MZA twins with alcoholism are not available. Such comparisons obviously rest importantly on the comparability of the diagnostic criteria and on an unbiased ascertainment of MZA and MZT twins. Nevertheless, with these caveats in mind, these data provide no positive evidence for a major role of shared environment in schizophrenia or affective disorders.

   A second methodological variation on this theme is the comparison of risks for psychopathology between biological siblings (or half-siblings) of affected probands who are reared together and those biological siblings (or half-siblings) reared apart from affected probands. Data relevant to this issue for schizophrenia have been collected in Kety and colleagues' adoptees' families study in Denmark, where a matched sample of nonadoptees was also studied. Unfortunately, the data have been reported only in summary form, and not specifically for siblings or half-siblings. However, based on institutional records, these authors reported no difference in rates of schizophrenia-spectrum disorders between all biological relatives of schizophrenic adoptees and all biological relatives of nonadopted schizophrenic probands (Kety *et al.,* 1978). In a small Icelandic study, Karlsson (1966) similarly reported a rate of schizophrenia in biological siblings reared with schizophrenic probands that was no higher than that found in reared-apart biological siblings of probands.

Mendlewicz and Rainer's adoption study of bipolar affective disorder also presents some data relevant to this method. They reported that 5 of 9 biological siblings who were reared apart from their bipolar siblings showed affective disorders. Unfortunately, the rates in matched siblings reared together were not available. Similar data have not been reported from the Stockholm adoption study of depression, and this comparison has also not been reported from the adoption studies of alcoholism. However, in a study of half-siblings of alcoholics, Schuckit, Goodwin, and Winokur (1972) presented evidence that half-siblings reared with an alcoholic proband are not at increased risk for alcoholism compared to those reared apart from alcoholic probands.

Nonshared Environmental Experience

In contrast to shared experiences, which serve to increase family resemblance, nonshared experiences are those that do not happen to all family members and thus serve to decrease family resemblance. For many dimensions of behavior and personality characteristics, such nonshared experiences, along with genetic influences, appear to be much more important than experiences shared within a family (Rowe & Plomin, 1981). A primary method of estimating the importance of such nonshared experience in the etiology of psychopathology is the degree of dissimilarity among MZ twins reared together. This method provides a direct estimate of the importance of nonshared environment because only experiences that are not shared by MZ co-twins contribute to differences between them. As was mentioned above, twin studies of schizophrenia, affective disorders, and alcoholism generally have found approximately half of MZT twins to be discordant, thus indicating some role for the influence of nonshared experience in these psychopathologies.

What does the distinction between shared and nonshared experiences actually imply for the investigation of environmental risk factors for psychopathology? First, it is clear that no specific environmental experience is necessarily shared within a family. For instance, exposure to the virus responsible for measles tends to cluster within families (shared experience), although exposure is also possible from outside the family (nonshared). In contrast, the death of a parent is always an experience shared among offspring. Thus, it is likely that different specific environmental experiences vary in their probability of being shared or not shared within families. As important as this issue appears to be, little research has investigated it.

Are there any other strategies that may help to characterize even further the nature of these nonshared experiences? Perhaps the method most frequently used for this purpose involves the study of MZ twins discordant for psychopathology. Here, we are searching for those experiences that are not shared by approximately half of MZ twins. What kinds of experiences, or their combination, would be so infrequent that they would not be shared by half of MZ twins reared together in the same family? When the question is framed this way, we have considerably narrowed the range of potential candidates from the universe of all possible environmental events. This strategy has been most used in research on schizophrenia, and the findings have been that affected members of discordant pairs appear to have experienced increased rates of obstetrical complications (McNeil & Kaij, 1978). Investigations of other psychopathologies have exploited this method less often.

Other methods of further characterizing relevant nonshared experiences include the comparison of concordance rates for psychopathology between same-sex DZ twins and same-sex nontwin siblings. Both groups share an average 50% of their genotype, so that differences in concordance between the two groups can be ascribed to some difference in environmental experiences. A higher concordance rate for DZ twins may be due to increased shared experiences that are specific to being twins, or to the greater age displacement of siblings compared to age-matched DZ twins. Such a situation may imply that relevant environmental experiences are age-dependent, and that their impact depends on the "critical period" in which they are experienced. The effects of such environmental experiences, dependent on the age of those exposed, would serve to increase DZ twin resemblance, relative to age-displaced siblings. In general, differences between DZ-twin and sibling concordances tend to be slight for most psychopathologies, although such comparisons depend critically on the similarity of diagnostic criteria between the two groups.

THE ANALYSIS OF SPECIFIED FAMILY EXPERIENCES

The methods discussed above estimate the importance of *unspecified* environmental influences, by analyzing differences in correlations among groups of siblings that vary in their environmental and genetic relatedness. Specific environmental experiences are not actually measured, but their importance is deduced from the amount of residual variation that is not due to genetic influences. As an initial strategy, this traditional behavior genetic approach has many advantages. For example, we do not need to have accurate hypotheses about specific environmental influences in order to study their general importance. Although efficient and informative, this approach also has obvious limits; until environmental characteristics are actually measured, we cannot know which *specific* experiences may be important. In contrast, most traditional family–environment research has started with this more difficult problem and has emphasized the measurement of specifically hypothesized rearing characteristics. Thus, whereas most traditional behavior genetic research has studied the simple correlation of the same characteristic, such as schizophrenia, in different relatives, family–environment research has focused on the cross-correlation of some hypothesized rearing characteristic, such as parental communication deviance, and a second characteristic, such as schizophrenia in the offspring.

Most family–environment research on psychopathology has investigated such cross-correlations between parental rearing characteristics and disorder in offspring within the context of nuclear families (reviewed by Hirsch & Leff, 1975; Jacob, 1975; Liem, 1980). However, as was discussed earlier, when an association is observed in such a study, its interpretation is causally ambiguous. It might have arisen because of the genes shared by parents and offspring, the offspring's influence on the parents, or the parents' influence on the offspring. Nuclear family studies, even prospective longitudinal ones, cannot rule out the genetic alternative explanation. In fact, Plomin, Loehlin, and DeFries (1985) demonstrated that much of the influence of rearing characteristics on normal children is genetically mediated. Therefore, however useful they may be for hypothesis generation and as preliminary screening research, such studies do not provide evidence concerning the importance of specific environmental experiences in the etiology of psychopathology. Accordingly, our discussion emphasizes the more powerful adoption studies.

Main Effects of Family Environment

Adoption studies in which adoptive parents provide the rearing environment but not the genes for the adoptees represent a major advance over the nuclear family study. Where the correlation discussed above between biological parent and adoptee provided information on genetic influences, the correlation between features of the adoptive rearing environment and adoptee psychopathology sheds light on potential "main effects" of family–environment, when studied without regard to the adoptees' genetic background. In the absence of selective placement, an association between a hypothesized rearing characteristic in the adoptive parents and psychopathology in adoptees cannot be attributed to shared genotypes. Of course, the possibility that the parental characteristic is a reaction to offspring psychopathology still cannot be ruled out.

Inferences regarding environmental influences drawn from adoption designs depend on several assumptions. First, there should be no selective placement for relevant aspects of the adoptive environment. Just as selective placement may invalidate genetic inferences, it may also complicate environmental conclusions. Selective placement produces a correlation between the characteristics of the biological parents and aspects of the adoptive home that may produce a spurious association between adoptive environment and adoptee psychopathology if genetic influences are important. For example, adoption agencies often selectively place adoptees in adoptive homes based on similarity of hair color in the biological and the adoptive parents. In this case, a correlation for hair color will be found between adoptees and adoptive parents. However, this correlation reflects not the possible rearing effects on hair color, but the effect of selective placement. An estimate of the importance of selective placement may be provided by the correlation between the relevant characteristics of the biological parents and the adoptive home environments. A second methodological aspect of adoption studies concerns how representative adoptive home environments are of nonadoptive homes. Adoptive parents are generally screened by adoption agencies for health and stability. Therefore, it may be that adoptive homes do not represent the range of relevant nonadoptive rearing environments. To the extent that screening on trait-relevant characteristics occurs, adoption studies may underestimate the importance of normal family–environment variation. For example, suppose extremely low social class were an environmental risk factor for delinquency. Then, if adoptive parents were screened to be middle and upper class, the correlation between adoptee delinquency and adoptive-parent social class would be attentuated because of the reduced variation in adoptive homes. Another important methodological point concerns "blindness" between evaluation of the adoptive home and assessment of adoptees. Independence of assessment of adoptees and adoptive environment is particularly difficult to maintain if the adoptees still reside in the adoptive home.

For relatively common disorders, the identification of an unselected sample of adoptees is optimal. In this case, the adoptive parents studied are obviously representative of adoptive parents in general. For rarer disorders, however, such a strategy can be quite wasteful, particularly when the assessments are time-consuming. If genetic influences are important, one common approach in this situation involves the adoptee design described earlier, in which the probands are groups of affected and normal biological parents who have adopted away their offspring. In the absence of selective placement, the adoptive parents identified by this approach should be representative of adoptive parents in general. Additionally, as in the adoptees' families design, ascertainment may be through affected and control adoptees, with their adoptive homes being compared.

When the potential influence of a family–environment characteristic that is relatively rare among adoptive parents is to be studied, another strategy should be considered. In this case, adoptive homes with the hypothesized characteristic and matched control homes are selected, and the rates of disorder in the two groups of adoptees are compared. Because adoptive homes were specifically selected for the characteristic of interest, this strategy is robust to potential screening of adoptive parents and can potentially evaluate the effect of relatively rare family environments.

Of the various family–environment influences, rearing by an affected parent has been the most investigated. Obviously, the presence of parental psychopathology does not encompass all of the potentially psychopathology-inducing environments, but it is certainly a likely candidate, given the importance often ascribed to social modeling.

The Stockholm adoption study of alcoholism is one of the few examples of approaches to this issue that have used an unselected sample of adoptees (Bohman *et al.*, 1981; Cloninger *et al.*, 1981). The investigators reported no significant association, based on public records, between alcohol abuse in adoptive parents and in adoptees. This result has also been found in studies using subjects ascertained via the biological parents' alcohol status (e.g., Cadoret & Gath, 1978; Cadoret *et al.*, 1980; cf. Cadoret *et al.*, 1985).

Adoptees' families approaches have also been used to investigate the issue of the effect of parental psychopathology. For example, Kety and colleagues' Danish adoption study of schizophrenia found no difference in schizophrenia-spectrum disorders between adoptive parents of schizophrenic and normal adoptees. (Kety *et al.*, 1975). In their NIMH adoption study, Wender and colleagues (Wender, Rosenthal, & Kety, 1968; Wender, Rosenthal, Zahn, & Kety, 1971) reported similar results using this strategy. In contrast, for depression, there is an indication from the Stockholm adoption study that rates of affective disorders are increased in adoptive fathers of depressed adoptees, compared to adoptive fathers of normal adoptees (von Knorring et al., 1983). However, this does not seem to be the case for bipolar disorder, as Mendlewicz and Rainer (1977) reported similar rates of affective disorder in adoptive parents of bipolar adoptees and controls. However, as noted earlier, the sensitivity of these designs to the screening of adoptive parents weakens somewhat the impact of the negative findings. For example, if almost all prospective adoptive parents with psychopathology were not allowed to adopt, then studies using unselected samples would require very large sample sizes to ascertain those few disturbed adoptive parents.

Other approaches to the issue of rearing by an affected parent have ascertained groups on the basis of the rearing parents' psychopathology in order to reduce the problem of screening the adoptive parents. One strategy addresses the potential effect of the rearing parents' psychopathology on adoptee psychopathology in the absence of any genes shared with an affected relative. In this design, the biological parents are normal, and the rates of psychopathology in the adoptees are compared between those reared by normal adoptive parents and those reared by affected adoptive parents. This strategy has been used in schizophrenia by Wender and colleagues (1974) in their adoption study in Denmark. Those rare adoptees of normal biological parentage who were reared by schizophrenic adoptive parents were found to be no more often schizophrenic than were adoptees reared by normal adoptive parents.

A complementary approach also controls biological parentage and varies rearing-parent psychopathology, but in this case, all biological parents are affected. The comparison of interest is that between the rates of psychopathology in adoptees with affected biological parents who are reared by normal adoptive parents and offspring who are reared by their affected biological parents. Offspring reared by their affected biological parents are used because of the rarity of adoptees with affected biological parents who are reared by affected adoptive parents. This design thus addresses the question of to what extent rearing by an affected parent increases the risk for psychopathology in offspring over that conferred by an affected biological parent. If the environmental experience requires a genetic predisposition to show an effect, then this design should detect it.

The Danish adoption study of alcoholism by Goodwin and colleagues (1974, 1977) provides an example of this approach. Similar to the findings reported earlier, these investigators found no difference in rates of alcoholism between offspring of alcoholic biological parents who were reared by normal adoptive parents, and those reared by their own alcoholic parents. The same approach has also been used to investigate the effect of rearing by a schizophrenic parent (Higgins, 1966, 1976; Rosenthal, Wender, Kety, Schulsinger, Welner, & Rieder, 1975), with similar results. An ingenious variation on this design was used by

Fischer (1971) in her twin study of schizophrenia in Denmark. In this report, she compared the rate of schizophrenia among offspring of a schizophrenic MZ twin with the rate of schizophrenia among offspring of an unaffected, discordant MZ co-twin. Thus, both groups of offspring shared genes with a schizophrenic parent, but only one group was reared by an affected parent. Fischer found no difference in rates of schizophrenia between the two groups of offspring.

Adoption studies have also been used to investigate a variety of environmental influences beyond rearing by an affected parent. However, because most adoption studies have been genetically oriented, more attention has been paid to assessing biological relatives than to evaluating the adoptive environment. Therefore, the range of family–environment measures of adoptive families has not been as rich as it might be, considering that the strength of the adoption study is in the investigation of environmental influences. We briefly survey examples of these studies below.

The association between adoptive family social class and adoptee psychopathology has been studied in several disorders. In schizophrenia, adoptees studies (Heston & Denney, 1968; Wender, Rosenthal, Kety, Schulsinger, & Welner, 1973) and adoptees' families studies (Wender *et al.*, 1973) have found no relationship between adoptive social class and schizophrenia in adoptees. In contrast, lower social class of adoptive parents was found to be associated with increased risk for alcoholism in adoptees in the Stockholm adoption study (Bohman *et al.*, 1981; Cloninger *et al.*, 1981).

Several adoption studies, particularly those on schizophrenia, have also evaluated characteristics that are more along the lines that traditional family–environment researchers often assess. For example, associations have been reported between family disturbance or poor parent–child relationships in the adoptive family and psychosis or psychopathology in adoptees (Rosenthal *et al.*, 1975; Tienari *et al.*, 1985), although these findings are based on nonblind assessments of adoptive families and adoptee psychopathology. Wender and associates' pilot adoption study at the NIMH (1971) also reported an increased rate of mild psychopathology, but not psychosis, among the adoptive parents of schizophrenic adoptees, compared to the adoptive parents of normal offspring. Although no differences were found on parental responses to the Thematic Apperception Test, the Object Sorting Test, or the Proverbs Interpretation Test, Singer and colleagues analyzed these same adoptive parents' Rorschach protocols for evidence of communication deviance, which they hypothesized to be a schizophrenogenic rearing factor (Wynne, Singer, & Toohey, 1976). In this analysis, the adoptive parents of schizophrenic adoptees showed significantly greater communication deviance than the adoptive parents of normal controls. However, these findings were not replicated in a later study (Wender, Rosenthal, Rainer, Greenhill, & Sarlin, 1977). In any case, as was mentioned above, the demonstration of an association between adoptee psychopathology and adoptive environmental characteristics may rule out genetic mediation, but it does not resolve the issue of whether parents primarily influence offspring or vice versa. Prospective, longitudinal adoption studies are best suited to the study of such issues.

Gene–Environment Interaction

In addition to investigations such as those above of the "main effect" of family-environment on psychopathology without regard to genetic background, full adoption designs in which both adoptive and biological relatives are assessed are uniquely suited to an exploration of the possibility of gene–environment interaction (Jinks & Fulker, 1970; Plomin, DeFries, & Loehlin, 1977). In general, gene–environment interactions imply that the effects of experience are modulated by genetic influences, and vice versa. This notion has great intuitive appeal to researchers in psychopathology and development, with a disorder such as favism providing a classic example. In this case, the predisposition to favism, an anemia, depends on an X-linked gene that is expressed only when an individual's diet includes the fava bean, which is a common staple in the Mediterranean region (Gottesman & Shields, 1982). If fava beans are absent from the diet, no anemia is produced, and in normal individuals without the rare mutant gene, the fava bean produces no ill effects. Thus, the effects of relevant genes and experience are not additive; rather, they interact statistically. The popular diathesis–stress model of the etiology of psychopathology is also an instance of a hypothesized gene–environment interaction in which environmental stressors have a particularly deleterious effect on only those individuals with a genetic diathesis, or predisposition, to a particular psychopathology.

Family–environment researchers have been especially interested in a particular type of gene–environment interaction in which genes differing within a family interact with environments that are shared by a family. As has been mentioned above, a major difficulty of theories of family–environment influence is how to account for differences in outcome within the family. A gene × family–environment interaction in which the "pathogenic" effect of some family environments would be expressed in only those offspring who were genetically vulnerable might represent one possible mechanism to explain differences among siblings in the presence of an influential family environment.

Despite the theoretical importance of these interactions, the analysis and detection of gene–environment interactions in human behavior and psychopathology are in an early state of development. Most gene–environment models assume additivity of effects and no interactions. Aside from the early proposal by Jinks and Fulker (1970), which relied on the correlation between score sums and differences for MZA twins, most analytic methods have required the measurement of specific environmental experiences. Eaves (1984) suggested some preliminary analytic strategies for use with nuclear family pedigrees, but most work to date has emphasized the full adoption-study design in which both biological and adoptive parents are assessed (Erlenmeyer-Kimling, 1972; Plomin *et al.*, 1977; Rosenthal, 1971). In analysis-of-variance (or multiple-regression) terms, the characteristics of the biological parents (e.g., affected or normal control) represent the genetic "factor," and the presence of some hypothesized rearing characteristic in the adoptive parents represents the environmental factor. The frequency or severity of psychopathology in the adoptees would thus be considered the "dependent" measure, and the statistical interaction term estimates the extent to which genetic and family environmental effects depend on one another. Such studies investigate the interaction between genes shared by families and environments shared by families, but they should also be relevant to those interactions involving the genes differing within families and the environments shared by families that are most theoretically important to family–environment researchers. Although generally not used in this manner, these designs could also elucidate interactions between genes and those experiences that are not shared by families. A further consideration is that adoption strategies have generally assumed that the genes predisposing to a disorder are also those responsible for modulating sensitivity to the environment. As suggested by Eaves (1984; Eaves & Eysenck, 1976), this is not necessarily the case. Therefore, exclusive emphasis on the diagnostic status of the biological parents as an index of the genotype predisposing to a disorder may not detect all important gene–environment interactions. Therefore, exploration of interactions between environmental indices measured in the adoptive homes and nondiagnostic characteristics of the biological parents may also prove informative on such questions.

Of the adoption studies relevant to such issues, surprisingly few have performed analyses to specifically investigate gene × family–environment interactions. The Finnish adoption study of schizophrenia by Tienari and colleagues (1985) is one of the few to focus on detecting such interactions. Although this project is still ongoing, preliminary reports suggest an interaction between adoptive family disturbance and schizophrenia in the biological parents on quantitative ratings of psychopathology in the adoptees. Adoptive family disturbance was more associated with adoptee psychopathology in the index group with schizophrenic biological mothers than in the control adoptees with normal biological parents. However, complete data were not provided in this preliminary report for diagnoses of psychosis in the adoptees, and tests of significance were not presented. The forthcoming reports from this ambitious project will be important in more fully evaluating the importance of gene × family–environment interactions in the etiology of schizophrenia. The Stockholm adoption study of alcoholism also provides a sophisticated example of the analysis of gene × family–environment interactions (Bohman *et al.*, 1981; Cloninger *et al.*, 1981). In this study, the adoptive parents' low social class was associated with increased alcohol abuse only among those male adoptees whose biological parents showed mild or severe alcohol abuse.

Gene–Environment Correlation

Gene–environment correlation is another instance of joint gene–environment action. Plomin and colleagues (1977) distinguished among three kinds of gene–environment correlation. "Passive" gene–environment correlation is that which may occur between genes and family environments that are transmitted to offspring in nuclear families. Thus, disordered parents may pass to their offspring not only genes, but also stressful environmental experiences that contribute to psychopathology in the offspring. Such a situation would tend to increase the differences between nuclear families but would not contribute to within-family differences. Adoption serves to eliminate this source of gene–environment correlation. In contrast, "reactive" gene–environment correlation may act to increase differences within families. In this case, genetically determined attributes of individuals influence environmental reactions to these individuals. For example, children who may be temperamentally difficult for genetic reasons may elicit few affectionate responses from parents, siblings, and nonfamily members, thus potentially exaggerating genetically influenced differences within families in a positive-feedback manner. The related "active" gene–environment correlation may also serve to increase differences among offspring. This would occur when genetically influenced attributes lead individuals to actively expose themselves to selected environmental experiences. For instance, children with potentially genetically mediated antisocial tendencies may become involved in criminal activities that, by virtue of peer and societal influences, also contribute to the likelihood of further criminal behavior. Although potentially important for theory, relatively few analytic methods have been developed to detect such gene–environment correlations (cf. Kendler & Eaves, 1986; Plomin *et al.*, 1977), and none have yet been applied in empirical studies of psychopathology.

CONCLUSIONS

We hope that this survey of methods and empirical examples has been informative concerning environmental influences both on psychopathology and on general ways of investigating genetic and environmental influences. Despite some recent pioneering attempts in both normal behavior (e.g., Plomin & DeFries, 1985; Plomin *et al.*, 1977, 1985; Rowe & Plomin, 1981; Scarr & McCartney, 1983) and psychopathology (Cloninger *et al.*, 1981; Gottesman & Shields, 1982), behavior genetic and family–environment traditions have generally run on parallel tracks, with collisions being their only interactions. It should now be clear that both traditions are studying the same phenomena and that each can enrich the other. That enrichment can take place both conceptually and methodologically. For example, the conceptual distinction between shared and nonshared experiences used by biometricians (Jinks & Fulker, 1970) is an important one, with far-reaching theoretical consequences that are only beginning to be assimilated by the general psychological community (Rowe & Plomin, 1981). Similarly, the behavior genetic tradition can be enhanced by an emphasis on measuring specific aspects of the environment (Plomin *et al.*, 1985).

The growing challenge posed by behavior genetic findings in psychopathology to family–environment researchers is in developing and evaluating theories that will account for differences within families. Simple conceptions of general rearing influences do not fit the data on schizophrenia or many other phenotypes. We require more sophisticated environmental models that will depend increasingly on adoption and other behavior genetic designs (Plomin, DeFries, & McClearn, 1981) for their evaluation. And the emerging dialogue between behavior genetic and family–environment investigations will serve us all.

REFERENCES

Bohman, M., Sigvardsson, S., & Cloninger, C. R. (1981). Maternal inheritance of alcohol abuse. *Archives of General Psychiatry, 38*, 965–969.

Cadoret, R. J. (1978). Evidence for genetic inheritance of primary affective disorder in adoptees. *American Journal of Psychiatry, 135*, 463–466.

Cadoret, R. J., & Gath, A. (1978). Inheritance of alcoholism in adoptees. *British Journal of Psychiatry, 132*, 252–258.

Cadoret, R. J., Cain, C. A., & Grove, W. M. (1980). Development of alcoholism in adoptees raised apart from alcoholic biologic relatives. *Archives of General Psychiatry, 37*, 561–563.

Cadoret, R. J., O'Gorman, T. W., Troughton, E., & Heywood, E. (1985). Alcoholism and antisocial personality: Interrelationships, genetic, and environmental factors. *Archives of General Psychiatry, 42*, 161–167.

Cloninger, C. R., Bohman, M., & Sigvardsson, S. (1981). Inheritance of alcohol abuse. *Archives of General Psychiatry, 38*, 861–868.

Eaves, L. J. (1984). The resolution of genotype × environment interaction in segregation analysis of nuclear families. *Genetic Epidemiology, 1*, 215–228.

Eaves, L. J., & Eysenck, H. J. (1976). Genotype × age interaction for neuroticism. *Behavior Genetics, 6*, 359–362.

Erlenmeyer-Kimling, L. (1972). Gene–environment interactions and the variability of behavior. In L. Ehrman, G. Omenn, & E. Caspari (Eds.), *Genetics, environment, and behavior: Implications for educational policy*. New York: Academic Press.

Falconer, D. S. (1965). The inheritance of liability to certain diseases, estimated from the incidence among relatives. *Annals of Human Genetics, 29*, 51–71.

Faraone, S. V., & Tsuang, M. T. (1985). Quantitative models of the genetic transmission of schizophrenia. *Psychological Bulletin, 98*, 41–66.

Fischer, M. (1971). Psychoses in the offspring of schizophrenic monozygotic twins and their normal co-twins. *British Journal of Psychiatry, 118*, 43–52.

Fulker, D. W. (1973). A biometrical genetic approach to intelligence and schizophrenia. *Social Biology, 20*, 266–275.

Goodwin, D. W. (1979). Alcoholism and heredity. *Archives of General Psychiatry, 36*, 57–61.

Goodwin, D. W. (1985). Alcoholism and genetics. *Archives of General Psychiatry, 42*, 171–174.

Goodwin, D. W., Schulsinger, F., Moller, N., Hermansen, L., Winokur, G., & Guze, S. B. (1974). Drinking problems in adopted and nonadopted sons of alcoholics. *Archives of General Psychiatry, 31*, 164–169.

Goodwin, D. W., Schulsinger, F., Knop, J., Mednick, S., & Guze, S. B. (1977). Psychopathology in adopted and nonadopted daughters of alcoholics. *Archives of General Psychiatry, 34*, 1005–1009.

Gottesman, I. I., & Carey, G. (1983). Extracting meaning and direction from twin data. *Psychiatric Developments, 1*, 35–50.

Gottesman, I. I., & Shields, J. (1967). A polygenic theory of schizophrenia. *Proceedings of the National Academy of Sciences, 58*, 199–205.

Gottesman, I. I., & Shields, J. (1982). *Schizophrenia: The epigenetic puzzle*. New York: Cambridge University Press.

Heston, L. (1966). Psychiatric disorders in foster home reared children of schizophrenic mothers. *British Journal of Psychiatry, 112*, 819–825.

Heston, L., & Denney, D. (1968). Interactions between early life experience and biological factors in schizophrenia. In D. Rosenthal & S. S. Kety (Eds.), *The transmission of schizophrenia*. New York: Pergamon Press.

Higgins, J. (1966). Effects of child rearing by schizophrenic mothers. *Journal of Psychiatric Research, 4*, 153–167.

Higgins, J. (1976). Effects of child rearing by schizophrenic mothers: A follow-up. *Journal of Psychiatric Research, 13*, 1–9.

Hirsch, S. R., & Leff, J. P. (1975). *Abnormalities in parents of schizophrenics*. New York: Oxford University Press.

Hrubec, Z., & Omenn, G. S. (1981). Evidence of genetic predisposition to alcoholic cirrhosis and psychosis: Twin concordances for alcoholism and its biological endpoints by zygosity among male veterans. *Alcoholism: Clinical and Experimental Research, 5,* 207–214.

Jackson, D. D. (1960). A critique of the literature on the genetics of schizophrenia. In D. D. Jackson (Ed.), *The etiology of schizophrenia.* New York: Basic Books.

Jacob, T. (1975). Family interaction in disturbed and normal families: A methodological and substantive review. *Psychological Bulletin, 82,* 33–65.

Jinks, J. L., & Fulker, D. W. (1970). Comparison of the biometrical genetical, MAVA, and classical approaches to the analysis of human behavior. *Psychological Bulletin, 73,* 311–349.

Kallman, F. J. (1946). The genetic theory of schizophrenia: An analysis of 691 schizophrenic twin index families. *American Journal of Psychiatry, 103,* 309–322.

Karlsson, J. L. (1966). *The biologic basis of schizophrenia.* Springfield, IL: Charles C Thomas.

Kendler, K. S., & Eaves, L. J. (1986). Models for the joint effect of genotype and environment on liability to psychiatric illness. *American Journal of Psychiatry, 143,* 279–289.

Kety, S. S. (1983). Mental illness in the biological and adoptive relatives of schizophrenic adoptees: Findings relevant to genetic and environmental factors in etiology. *American Journal of Psychiatry, 140,* 720–727.

Kety, S. S., Rosenthal, D., Wender, P. H., & Schulsinger, F. (1968). The types and prevalence of mental illness in the biological and adoptive families of adopted schizophrenics. In D. Rosenthal & S. S. Kety (Eds.), *The transmission of schizophrenia.* New York: Pergamon Press.

Kety, S. S., Rosenthal, D., Wender, P. H., Schulsinger, F., & Jacobsen, B. (1975). Mental illness in the biological and adoptive families of adopted individuals who have become schizophrenic: A preliminary report based on psychiatric interviews. In R. R. Fieve, D. Rosenthal, & H. Brill (Eds.), *Genetic research in psychiatry.* Baltimore: Johns Hopkins University Press.

Kety, S. S., Rosenthal, D., Wender, P. H., Schulsinger, F., & Jacobsen, B. (1978). The biologic and adoptive families of adopted individuals who become schizophrenic: Prevalence of mental illness and other characteristics. In L. C. Wynne, R. L. Cromwell, & S. Matthysse (Eds.), *The nature of schizophrenia: New approaches to research and treatment.* New York: Wiley.

Liem, J. H. (1980). Family studies in schizophrenia: An update and a commentary. *Schizophrenia Bulletin, 6,* 429–459.

Loehlin, J. C., & Nichols, R. C. (1976). *Heredity, environment, and personality.* Austin: University of Texas Press.

Matheny, A. P. (1979). Appraisal of parental bias in twin studies: Ascribed zygosity and IQ differences in twins. *Acta Geneticae Medicae et Gemellologiae, 28,* 155–160.

McGue, M., Gottesman, I. I., & Rao, D. C. (1983). The transmission of schizophrenia under a multifactorial threshold model. *American Journal of Human Genetics, 35,* 1161–1178.

McNeil, T. F., & Kaij, L. (1978). Obstetric factors in the development of schizophrenia. In L. C. Wynne, R. L. Cromwell, & S. Matthysse, (Eds.), *The nature of schizophrenia: New approaches to research and treatment.* New York: Wiley.

Mendlewicz, J. (1981). Adoption study in affective illness. In C. Perris, G. Struwe, & B. Jansson (Eds.), *Biological Psychiatry 1981.* New York: Elsevier/North-Holland Biomedical Press.

Mendlewicz, J., & Rainer, J. D. (1977). Adoption study supporting genetic transmission in manic-depressive illness. *Nature, 268,* 327–329.

Murray, R. M., Clifford, C., & Gurling, H. M. (1983). Twin and alcoholism studies. In M. Galanter (Ed.), *Recent developments in alcoholism.* New York: Gardner Press.

Nurnberger, J. I., & Gershon, E. S. (1982). Genetics. In E. S. Paykel (Ed.), *Handbook of affective disorders.* New York: Guilford Press.

Plomin, R., & DeFries, J. C. (1985). *Origins of individual differences in infancy.* New York: Academic Press.

Plomin, R., DeFries, J. C., & Loehlin, J. (1977). Genotype-environment interaction and correlation in the analysis of human behavior. *Psychological Bulletin, 84,* 309–322.

Plomin, R., DeFries, J. C., & McClearn, G. E. (1981). *Behavioral genetics: A primer.* San Francisco: W. H. Freeman.

Plomin, R., Loehlin, J. C., & DeFries, J. C. (1985). Genetic and environmental components of "environmental" influences. *Developmental Psychology, 21,* 391–402.

Pogue-Geile, M. F., & Harrow, M. (1984). Strategies for psychopathology research. In A. S. Bellack & M. Hersen (Eds.), *Research methods in clinical psychology.* New York: Pergamon Press.

Price, J. (1968). The genetics of depressive behavior. *British Journal of Psychiatry Special Publication* (2), pp. 37–54.

Roe, A. (1944). The adult adjustment of children of alcoholic parents raised in foster homes. *Quarterly Journal of Studies on Alcohol, 5,* 378–393.

Rosenthal, D. (1960). Confusion of identity and the frequency of schizophrenia in twins. *Archives of General Psychiatry, 3,* 297–304.

Rosenthal, D. (1971). A program of research on heredity in schizophrenia. *Behavioral Science, 16,* 191–201.

Rosenthal, D., Wender, P. H., Kety, S. S., Schulsinger, F., Welner, J., & Ostergaard, L. (1968). Schizophrenics' offspring reared in adoptive homes. In D. Rosenthal & S. S. Kety (Eds.), *The transmission of schizophrenia.* New York: Pergamon Press.

Rosenthal, D., Wender, P. H., Kety, S. S., Welner, J., & Schulsinger, F. (1971). The adopted-away offspring of schizophrenics. *American Journal of Psychiatry, 128,* 307–311.

Rosenthal, D., Wender, P. H., Kety, S. S., Schulsinger, F., Welner, J., & Rieder, R. O. (1975). Parent–child relationships and psychopathological disorder in the child. *Archives of General Psychiatry, 32,* 466–476.

Rowe, D. C., & Plomin, R. (1981). The importance of nonshared (E_1) environmental influences in behavioral development. *Developmental Psychology, 17,* 517–531.

Scarr, S. (1968). Environmental bias in twin studies. *Eugenics Quarterly, 15,* 34–40.

Scarr, S., & McCartney, K. (1983). How people make their own environments: A theory of genotype–environment effects. *Child Development, 54,* 424–435.

Schuckit, M. A., Goodwin, D. W., & Winokur, G. (1972). A study of alcoholism in half siblings. *American Journal of Psychiatry, 128,* 1132–1135.

Tienari, P., Sorri, A., Lahti, I., Naarala, M., Wahlberg, K-E., Pohjola, J., & Moring, J. (1985). Interaction of genetic and psychosocial factors in schizophrenia. *Acta Psychiatrica Scandinavica Supplementum, 71(319),* 19–30.

von Knorring, A.-L., Cloninger, R., Bohman, M., & Sigvardsson, S. (1983). An adoption study of depressive disorders and subtance abuse. *Archives of General Psychiatry, 40,* 943–950.

Weissman, M. M., Gershon, E. S., Kidd, K., Prusoff, B. A., Leckman, J. F., Dibble, E., Hamovit, J., Thompson, D., Pauls, D. L., & Guroff, J. J. (1984). Psychiatric disorders in the relatives of probands with affective disorders. *Archives of General Psychiatry, 41,* 13–21.

Wender, P. H., Rosenthal, D., & Kety, S. S. (1968). A psychiatric assessment of the adoptive parents of schizophrenics. In D. Rosenthal & S. S. Kety (Eds.), *The transmission of schizophrenia.* New York: Pergamon Press.

Wender, P. H., Rosenthal, D., Zahn, T. P., & Kety, S. S. (1971). The psychiatric adjustment of the adopting parents of schizophrenics. *American Journal of Psychiatry, 127,* 53–58.

Wender, P. H., Rosenthal, D., Kety, S. S., Schulsinger, F., & Welner, J. (1973). Social class and psychopathology in adoptees. *Archives of General Psychiatry, 28,* 318–325.

Wender, P. H., Rosenthal, D., Kety, S. S., Schulsinger, F., & Welner, J. (1974). Cross-fostering: A research strategy for clarifying the role of genetic and experiential factors in the etiology of schizophrenia. *Archives of General Psychiatry, 30,* 121–128.

Wender, P. H., Rosenthal, D., Rainer, J. D., Greenhill, L., & Sarlin, B. (1977). Schizophrenics' adopting parents. *Archives of General Psychiatry, 34,* 777–784.

Wynne, L. C., Singer, M. T., & Toohey, M. L. (1976). Communication of the adoptive parents of schizophrenics. In J. Jorstad & E. Ugelstad (Eds.), *Schizophrenia 75: Psychotherapy, family studies, research.* Oslo: Universitetsforlaget.

Index